Dioscorides, De materia medica, translated by Lily Y. Beck

Altertumswissenschaftliche
Texte und Studien

Band 38

# Pedanius Dioscorides of Anazarbus

# De materia medica

Translated by
Lily Y. Beck

Olms - Weidmann
Hildesheim · Zürich · New York
2020

# Pedanius Dioscorides of Anazarbus

## De materia medica

Translated by
Lily Y. Beck

Fourth, enlarged edition

Olms - Weidmann
Hildesheim · Zürich · New York
2020

Die Deutsche Nationalbibliothek verzeichnet diese Publikation in der Deutschen Nationalbibliografie; detaillierte bibliografische Daten sind im Internet über *http://dnb.d-nb.de* abrufbar.


www.olms.de

Printed in Germany
Gedruckt auf säurefreiem und alterungsbeständigem Papier
Umschlaggestaltung: Inga Günther, Hildesheim
Herstellung: KN Digital Printforce GmbH, Ferdinand-Jühlke-Straße 7, 99095 Erfurt
ISSN 0175-8411
ISBN 978-3-487-31194-4

In memory of
Curt W. Beck

# CONTENTS

# ABBREVIATIONS AND SIGNS

For full bibliographical information see Bibliography

## A. General

A. = André, Jacques, *Les noms des plantes dans la Rome antique*
*ANRW* = *Aufstieg und Niedergang der römischen Welt*
Bk. = book
*Bull. Soc. Bot. Fr.* = *Bulletin de la Société Botanique de France*
Cels. = Celsus, *De medicina*
ch. = chapter
Dsc. = Dioscorides, *De materia medica*
*H. P.* = Theophrastus, *Historia Plantarum* = *Inquiry Into Plants*
*JHS* = *Journal of Hellenic Studies*
LSJ = Liddell, Scott, *A Greek-English Lexicon*. Rev. by Jones
Mabberley = Mabberley, D. J., *The Plant-Book*
n. = note
*N. H.* = Pliny, *Natural History*
p., pp. = page(s)
P.W. = Pauly-Wissowa-Kroll
s. = see
sp. = species
s.v. = *sub verbo,* under the word
~ = perhaps
< > = added by Max Wellmann
[ ] = bracketed by Max Wellmann

## B. Botanical

Adans. = Adanson, Michael
Aiton = Aiton, William
All. = Allioni, Carlo
Andrz. = Andrzejowski, Antoni Lukianowicz
Baker = Baker, John Gilbert
Benth. = Bentham, George
Berg = Berg, Ernst von
Bernh. = Bernhardi, Johann Jakob
Bertol. = Bertoloni, Antonio
Birdw. = Birdwood, George Christopher Molesworth

Boiss. = Boissier, Pierre Edmond
Bory = Bory de Saint-Vincent, Jean Baptiste Georges Geneviève Marcellin
Buhse = Buhse, Fedor Aléksandrovich
Cass. = Cassini, Alexandre Henri Gabriel de
C. C. Gmel. = Gmelin, Carl (Karl) Christian
Chiov. = Chiovenda, Emilio
Crantz = Crantz, Heinrich Johann Nepomuk von
Curtis = Curtis, William
DC. = Candolle, Augustin Pyramus de
Desr. = Desrousseaux, Louis Auguste Joseph
Dryand. = Dryander, Jonas Carlsson
Dunal = Dunal, Michel Félix
Ehrh. = Ehrhart, Jacob Friedrich
Engl. = Engler, Viktor
Fisch. = Fischer, Friedrich Ernst Ludwig von (Fedor Bogdanovic)
Forssk. = Forsskaol, Pehr (Peter)
Gaertn. = Gaertner, Joseph
Gawler = Ker Gawler, John Bellenden
Gilib. = Gilibert, Jean-Emmanuel
Griseb. = Grisebach, Augustus Heinrich Rudolph
Heldr. = Heldreich, Theodor Heinrich Hermann von
Hoffm. = Hoffmann, Georg Franz
Horn. = Hornemann, Jens Wilken
Huds. = Hudson, William
Jacq. = Jacquin, Nicolaus (Nicolaas) Joseph von
Juss. = Jussieu, Antoine Laurent de
Koch = Koch, Wilhelm Daniel Joseph
L. = Linné, Carl von
Labill. = Labillardière, Jacques Julien Houtou de
Lag. = Lagasca y Segura, Mariano
Lam. = Lamarck, Jean-Baptiste Antoine Pierre de Monet de
Link = Link, Johann Heinrich Friedrich
Mig. = Miguel, J. R.
Miller = Miller, Philip
Moench = Moench, Conrad
Moris = Moris, Giuseppe Giacinto (Joseph Hyacinthe)
P. B. = Palisot de Beauvois, Ambroise Marie François Joseph

Pall. = Pallas, Peter (Pyotr) Simon von
Pell. = Pellegrini, Gaetano
Pers. = Persoon, Christiaan Hendrik
Rafin. = Rafinesque-Schmaltz, Constantine Samuel
Retz. = Retzius, Anders Jahan
Rich. = Richard, Louis Claude Marie
Rchb. = Reichenbach, Heinrich Gottlieb Ludwig
R. Br. = Brown, Robert
Roscoe = Roscoe, William
Roxb. = Roxburgh, William
Russ = Russ, Georg Philip
Sart. = Sartorelli, Giovanni Battista
Savi = Savi, Gaëtano
Schipcz. = Schipczinski, Nicolaj Valerianovich
Schott = Schott, Heinrich Wilhelm
Schrader = Schrader, Heinrich Adolph
Schreb. = Schreber, Johann Christian Daniel von
Scop. = Scopoli, Giovanni Antonio
Ser. = Seringe, Nicolas Charles
Sibth. = Sibthorp, John
Sm. = Smith, James Edward
Stokes = Stokes, Jonathan S.
Spach = Spach, Édouard
Spreng. = Sprengel, Curt (Kurt, Curtius) Polycarp Joachim
Targ.-Tozz. = Targioni Tozzetti, Giovanni
Vill. = Villars, Dominique
Willd. = Willdenow, Carl Ludwig von

## Weights and Measures (after J. Berendes)

| Name | Greek name | Weight/Volume |
|---|---|---|
| Ceration | κεράτιον | 0.189 g |
| Thermos | θέρμος | 0.378 g |
| Obol | ὄβολος | 0.568 g |
| Dichalcon = 2/3 obol | δίχαλκον | 0.379 g |
| Cyamos Aigyptios | κύαμος Αἰγύπτιος | 0.852 g |
| Gramma | γράμμα | 1.137 g |
| Triobolon | τριώβολον | 1.794 g |
| Drachme | δραχμή | 3.411 g |
| Holce | ὁλκή | 3.411 g |
| Caryon Ponticon | κάρυον Ποντικόν | 3.40 g |
| Caryon basilikon | κάρυον βασιλικόν | 13.644 g |
| Oungia | οὐγχία | 27.288 g |
| Xestes | ξέστης | 54.58 g |
| Tetarton | τέταρτον | 81.86 g |
| Litra | λίτρα | 327.45 g |
| Mna, Minai (pl.) | μνᾶ/μίναι | 436.6 g |
| Cheme | χήμη | 0.0114 l |
| Cochlarion | κοχλιάριον | 0.012 l |
| Cyathos | κύαθος | 0.0456 l |
| Mystron | μύστρον | 0.068 l |
| Oxybaphon | ὀξύβαφον | 0.0684 l |
| Tetarton | τέταρτον | 0.137 l |
| Cotyle | κοτύλη | 0.274 l |
| Xestes | ξέστης | 0.547 l |
| Choinix | χοῖνιξ | 1.094 l |
| Chous | χοῦς | 3.282 l |
| Ourna | οὔρνα | 13.130 l |
| Amphoreus | ἀμφορεύς | 26.260 l |
| Ceramion | κεράμιον | 26.260 l |
| Metretes | μετρήτης | 39.360 l |

Tryblion = Oxybaphon

# INTRODUCTION

Professor Lily Beck has accomplished something most important in both classical studies and the History of Medicine and Pharmacy: with her accurate and contemporary English translation of Dioscorides' fundamental *Materia medica*, she has made accessible to the wider world of physicians, pharmacists, historians of the botanical sciences, and to classical scholars at large, the most influential work in the history of the medical sciences to emerge from the early days of the Roman Empire. One can argue that Dioscorides is more an authority in medicine and pharmacology than even Galen of Pergamon (A.D. 129 – after 210) in the centuries after the demise of Rome and the long eras of Byzantine, classical Islamic, and Renaissance and Enlightenment European medicine, and it is surprising that Dioscorides has received so little attention in modern scholarship.

To be sure, the *Materia medica* remained a "living text" until the early nineteenth century, and continual augmentations altered details through the centuries, so that the original non-alphabetical Greek version first set down by the master pharmacologist from Anazarbus became festooned with accretions of an always "local" herbal and drug lore; scholars have thus recognized the difficulties in establishing a reliable Greek text from the welter of known manuscripts, some of which have descended in Latin and Arabic translation (these are important since the earliest of these were rendered from Greek originals of late Roman and early Byzantine times, and the Arabic versions produced in the so-called Golden Age of Translations in ninth- and tenth-century Baghdad were founded on Byzantine Greek copies procured from Constantinople, and which, in turn, became ancestral to the Arabic Dioscorides still in circulation today). Yet even with the general rejection by later medical writers of Dioscorides' prescient "drug affinity system" (as described by John Riddle in his remarkable 1985 *Dioscorides on Pharmacy and Medicine*) in favor of a more traditional listing of drugs by letters of the Greek alphabet, the amazing collection of details by Dioscorides on all aspects of pharmacology survived almost intact through the millennia.

The earliest Greek text we have is an alphabetical version, the magnificent Juliana Anicia Codex (dated A.D. 512), currently the major treasure in Vienna's Nationalbibliothek, and it has numerous illuminations of medicinal plants, some painted from nature, others not. From time to time, the sixth-century artists allow us to solve species identifications, so accurate are the depictions in various instances, and it is this combination of written text with field botany that makes the *Materia medica* quite unusual in antiquity: Dioscorides insists that a physician has to be not merely a master of the sources of medical botany extant in written form, but he also must also become an expert on herbal lore as derived from personal experience of plants in all of their variations of growth, from seedling to maturity, not to mention the stages in between, as well as how and why given plants grow where they do (an early form of botanical geography) to explain different properties of the drugs manufactured from them. And by dismissing then-current philosophical theories to explain drug actions, Dioscorides establishes a pharmacology firmly resting on empirical data, but suggesting that such facts could change as the practitioner added his own experiences in the field and with patients. "Hearsay" and folk traditions were also important to him, but he normally makes sure the reader understands when he has not "tested" the remedies for himself, or that he has simply "heard" about them, recording such matters when the details seem to warrant further investigation.

Unlike much of the ornate Greek used in learned works in the Roman Empire, Dioscorides' syntax and style are marked by almost studied simplicity, a directness attempting precise description of drugs and their effects so that one could use his book as a sure guide to therapeutics in the first century. The obvious exception to his habit of clarity in his writing is the elaborate and difficult Preface to the *Materia medica,* addressed and dedicated to a teacher and colleague from Tarsus, and through him to a high-ranking Roman official. Once finished with the flowery verbiage then deemed necessary in such dedicatory tracts, Dioscorides' Greek displays a limpid and crystalline quality. Of course in summarizing the thousands of details on all aspects of pharmacology (botany accompanied by mineralogy, medical entomology, the technologies of mining and metallurgy, drugs manufactured from aquatic creatures, the basics of anatomy, acknowledgement of local traditions, a precise comprehension of topography, etc.) he assumes a vocabulary rather removed from the usual literature in Greek characteristic of the first century, and this "technical language" has disquieted most classicists, who do not come to the text equipped with a control of botany, medicine, and the kindred technologies. So it takes a special kind of classical scholar to do what Lily Beck has done. Botany is the key. And her translation shows a mastery of modern botany, from that sense of getting one's fingers muddy as the first seeds are set into place, to the arcane lore of scientific (viz. Linnaean) nomenclature so essential in classification of plants, indicating their consequent chemical constituents grouped into what we call the "active principles" in pharmacy.

If the *Materia medica* (Grk. Περὶ ὕλης ἰατρικῆς) is a well-known work throughout Roman, Byzantine, Classical Arabic, and early modern European times, its apparently energetic and gifted author is almost a complete blank, in terms of biographical details. The testimonia in Galen's writings secure his birthplace as the city of Anazarbus, a sometime rival to the more prosperous Tarsus, about eighty miles due southwest along a major highway in the Roman province of Cilicia. Dating Dioscorides is reasonably certain by comparing parallel passages in Pliny the Elder's *Natural History* with similar extracts in the *Materia medica*, and since both quote from the works of Sextius Niger — and do so independently — it is probable that Dioscorides was born sometime in the reign of Tiberius or Caligula, and wrote up his observations on pharmacology in the same decade as Pliny composed his encyclopedia. From the spare references in the Preface to the *Materia medica*, one teases out that Dioscorides studied pharmacology at Tarsus, and that here was a gathering of teachers who taught herbal pharmacology and medical botany; one of these early and respected instructors was named Arius, and it is to him that Dioscorides dedicates his own work. Other texts, including Galen, note that Arius was a famous teacher in Tarsus in the right decade, and the *Materia medica* probably indicates teaching centers in the eastern half of the Roman Empire, cities that had reputations for given subjects available for instruction (Alexandria in Egypt long remained such a center for the teaching of medicine, and there were other municipalities that boasted their own collection of medical instructors; Roman Asia Minor had several of these urban clusters of medical learning, including Laodicea, Ephesus, and probably Smyrna).

The *Materia medica* shows that Dioscorides had traveled widely throughout the Greek-speaking eastern half of the Roman Empire, and it is likely that he visited Greek communities in Sicily, southern Italy, and perhaps southern Gaul. There is no indication that he was part of the circles of the rich and famous of his own day, although Arius' connections with the consular Bassus could suggest intermittent contacts. And the six words in Preface, 4, οἶσθα γὰρ ἡμῖν στρατιωτικὸν τὸν βίον, do not mean that Dioscorides was a military physician, but perhaps had served in an eastern legion for short periods as a civilian doctor, a fairly common practice among the legions of the western Empire. In fact, the more we learn about military medicine in the Roman Empire, the less it seems there is any uniform or standard organizational guidelines for medical care of the soldiers, even though there were hospital facilities constructed in the larger military encampments. "My soldier's life" probably suggests that Dioscorides lived like a soldier as he traveled from region to region, listening to the natives of each, and surviving with the minimum of food, drink, and clothing; perhaps he made his living as an itinerant physician, in the mold of the famous medical travelers recorded in the works under the name of Hippocrates.

Dioscorides arranges his material into five books, stating in the Preface that his manner of organization is far better than any previous compilation of drugstuffs, but he never explicitly explains this new method. The clues are in the inclusion of "similars" in each book, or as he writes in Preface, 3, "…[not] using the alphabetical arrangement which splits materia medica and their properties from those which they are closely related," or to put it positively, drugs will be classed according to the δυνάμεις almost always "properties" to Dioscorides) they display as pharmaceuticals, especially as they "act" in or on the body of a patient. Crucial are the senses:[1] olfactory sensations allied

[1] Dioscorides may reflect the long-term influence of concepts derived from Theophrastus' *De causis plantarum*, VI, 4. 1 and following, where the philosopher-botanist attempts definitions of tastes (αἱ δὲ ἰδέαι τῶν χυλῶν ἑπτὰ δοκοῦσιν εἶναι [καθάπερ καὶ τῶν ὀσμῶν καὶ τῶν χρωμάτων]). Occasionally χυλοί is rendered as "flavors," attempting in English to preserve the subtle shadings suggested by Theophrastus. Much of Theophrastus' *On Odors* (mostly about the technologies of ointment- and perfume-production) assumes similar definitions, and fourth-century

with tastes identify the particulars in Book I, which include aromatic oils, salves, trees, and shrubs, and the strongly fragrant liquids, gums, and fruits produced by them; Book II takes up animals and parts of animals, drugs made from various creatures and larger denizens, both wild and domestic, and then Dioscorides incorporates cereals, pot herbs, and other herbs which have "sharper" characteristics, and in Book II there seems to be a shading of olfactory sensations into the less prominent perceptions of taste in turn shading into herbal acidity, perhaps in contrast to the bland matter of poultices made from barley and the like; Book III continues with further roots, juices, and seeds, and Book IV gives the qualities of roots and herbs not discussed in the previous books; finally in Book V, Dioscorides provides details about wines and mineralogy, suggesting that he knew the technical specifics that went with the skills of a vintner, since much of ancient wine production was in the struggle to produce a beverage that did not become "sour" (viz. turn into vinegar), and the "additives" in Book V incorporate a priceless list of ingredients Greeks and Romans used to flavor their wines, or were substances employed in hopes to regulate what we call 'fermentation,' (not until the nineteenth century would vintners speak of the must [freshly pressed juice] as containing sugars, organic acids, tannin, proteins, mineral salts, pectin, mucilage, yeasts, bacteria, and fungi). It is in Book V that Dioscorides ranges far beyond what moderns would expect in a work on pharmacology: here are the technologies of quicklime, the salient properties of minerals as they are manufactured into pharmaceuticals and other products, and why one has to know the best sites of the mining and smelting of fine ores in order to

---

B.C. philosophy wrestled frequently with the meanings of "odors" and "tastes," or "flavors," as specific sensations. *Vide* Plato, *Timaeus*, 65 B-66C; Aristotle, *On Sense*, 442a12-28 and 443b7-11, and *On the Soul*, 422b10-14. A millennium later, Aetius of Amida (a physician active in the reign of Justinian [A.D. 527-565]), suggests why tastes and odors remained essential in drug classification, and Aetius sets down the long-lived "drugs by degrees," which was how pharmacists 'knew' drugs until the early 19th century. *Vide* John Scarborough, "Early Byzantine Pharmacology," *Dumbarton Oaks Papers*, 38 (1984), 213-232, esp. 224-225, with translation of Aetius of Amida, Sixteen Books, I *prooemium*; although Dioscorides had rejected theoretical notions of "particles" to explain drug-action, Roman and Byzantine pharmacologists and physicians reincorporated this philosophical concept, and Aetius' summation mirrors a long tradition that includes Theophrastus, Dioscorides, and Galen.

procure good mineral drugs, and how knowledge of these metallurgical particulars enables the pharmacologist to discern the best remedies (as contrasted to some common poisons, also derived from minerals); and there is no better account of "pure water" than in *Materia medica*, V, 10, "if it is clean and sweet, free of any quality whatsoever" (trans. Beck). Here too are the multitudinous details about the production of dozens of wines and their medicinal values, and why the evergreen tang of good wine can mean the long aging of the finest (our turpentine is a strong version of the flavors and tastes of Roman wines, since pine resin both flavored and preserved wines).

The complete *Materia medica* is a huge compaction of well over 600 items fused into about 2000 recipes and formulas, and its bulk guaranteed that it would be modified and augmented according to local requirements. It is unlikely that the *Materia medica* carried illustrations in its original form, but once papyrus rolls had been replaced by codices (basically our "book"), scribes and artists soon produced handsome versions of the work, with the Codex Juliana Anicia of A.D. 512 our earliest exemplar. First to mention Dioscorides in an alphabetical format was Oribasius, physician and friend of Julian the Apostate (reigned A.D. 361-363), and it may be that Oribasius is the author of that first alphabetical version in Greek. Papyri of an earlier date, however, indicate that recensions of Dioscorides had begun to vary as early as the second century.

Extremely complex is the history of the transmission of the *Materia medica* through the centuries until the *editio princeps* appeared in an Aldine text (1499), and various versions had appeared in Latin translation by the sixth century. Unlike the sumptuous Greek copies produced in Constantinople — also alphabetical — the Latin translations were not illuminated, except for some crude representations, and those pictures have no relation to the textual transmission of illuminations in the Greek manuscripts.[2] Complicating the text were many "scholia" and "synonyms" added by scribes and

---

[2] Essential for these aspects is John M. Riddle, "Dioscorides," in F. Edward Krantz and Paul Oskar Kristeller, eds., *Catalogus Translationum et Commentariorum: Mediaeval and Renaissance Latin Translations and Commentaries*, Vol. IV (Washington, D.C.: Catholic University Press of America, 1980), pp. 1-143.

practicing physicians, and as the centuries passed, the marginal commentaries (the "scholia") wandered into the text itself. In themselves, some of these scholia and synonymn-lists (called *notha* or "glosses" by specialists) are valuable documents attesting to an ongoing practice of medicine, and the *notha* frequently became grouped at the heads of sections as "synonyms" in various languages, while some scholia remained within the text. The best editions of the Greek text have carefully delineated both the *notha* and the scholiastic commentaries, and the occasionally lengthy if anonymous commentaries in Wellmann's apparatus criticus are fascinating glimpses into how physicians through the centuries valued and challenged the tract in front of them.[3] Several other tracts on drugs came to be part of the manuscript tradition, and much debate continues about the "genuine" corpus of Dioscorides' writings. One on toxicology, or perhaps two separate works on the topic, the Περὶ δηλητηρίων φαρμάκων ("Poisons"), and Περὶ ἰοβόλων ("Poisonous Animals"), are certainly Pseudo-Dioscorides, since the earliest manuscript linking the poison-lore with the full *Materia medica* is from the eleventh century,[4] and may bear close relationship to a toxicological handbook produced in Constantinople during the reign of Constantine VII Porphyrogenitus (913-959).[5] Needless to say, much work remains to be done on the vast number of recensions and redactions of Dioscorides that descended into the printed versions of the Renaissance.

Latin translations of Dioscorides were common in the Renaissance, and there are numerous editions known from the first printing in 1478,[6] through a publication of a Latin translation in Madrid

---

[3] That the scholia on Dioscorides can be very useful in assessing Byzantine employment of the *Materia medica*, is neatly demonstrated by John M. Riddle, "Byzantine Commentaries on Dioscorides," *Dumbarton Oaks Papers*, 38 (1984), 95-102.

[4] Escorialensis [Madrid] III R 3.

[5] Sibylle Ihm, *Der Traktat* περὶ ἰ βόλων θηρίων καὶ δηλητηρίων φαρμάκων *des sog. Aelius Promotus* (Wiesbaden: Ludwig Reichert Verlag, 1995), and Alain Towaide, "Les deux traités de toxicologie attribuès à Dioscoride. Tradition manuscrite, établissement du texte et critique d'authenticité," in Antonio Garzya, ed., *Tradizione e ecdotica dei testi medici tardoantichi e bizantini* (Naples: D'Auria Editore, 1992), pp. 291-335.

[6] Riddle, "Dioscorides," p. 8.

in 1733. Translations into vernacular languages soon followed, with Castlilan Spanish (1555), Dutch (1520), French (1553), Italian (by Mattioli in 1544 and later editions to 1597), and German (1546), but not into English. Sometime between 1652 and 1655, John Goodyer made a translation into English from an uncertain circulating printed text (probably a Latin translation),[7] but it was not published until 1934 (Hafner: London and New York), in a lightly edited version by Robert T. Gunther. And until Lily Beck's translation into English, the Goodyer-Gunther has served the English-speaking world as the only rather wobbly version of Dioscorides, a version that may have a kind of Elizabethan charm, but which does not do justice to the precise medical botany and pharmacology so characteristic of the *Materia medica* in Greek. A recent "updating" of the Goodyer-Gunther by Tess Anne Osbaldeston,[8] 'fancifies' the book with out-of-copyright lithographs, and loses the Elizabethan charm without improving the translation.

Establishing a good Greek text defied classical scholars for many decades, although a solid attempt was made in 1829 and 1830 by Curt Sprengel,[9] who also provided a Latin translation and some limited commentary. From Sprengel's Greek edition, J. Berendes produced a good German translation,[10] with firmly argued identifications of species and genera using Linnaean nomenclatures, and this translation has remained the best into a modern language, until Lily Beck's into English. Max Wellmann early realized that a full census of manuscripts was necessary in order to establish a reliable edition of the Greek, and with an article on Dioscorides' systematics,[11] Wellmann signaled his

---

[7] John Scarborough and Vivian Nutton, "The Preface of Dioscorides' *Materia Medica*: Introduction, Translation, Commentary," *Transactions & Studies of the College of Physicians of Philadelphia*, 4 (1982), 187-227 at p. 188 with n. 5.

[8] T. A. Osbaldeston, ed. ['a new English translation,' it is not], *Dioscorides. De materia medica*, with introductory notes by R. P. Wood. Johannesburg: Ibidis Press, 2000.

[9] Curt Sprengel, ed. and trans. [Latin], *Pedanii Dioscoridis Anazarbei De materia medica libri quinque* [in] C. G. Kühn, ed., *Medicorum Garecorum Opera quae exstant*, vols. 25 and 26 (Leipzig: Cnoblich, 1829-1830).

[10] J. Berendes, trans., *Des Pedanios Dioskurides aus Anazarbos Arzneimittellehre*. Stutt-gart: Ferdinand Enke, 1902; rptd. Schaan/Liechtenstein and Wiesbaden: Sändig Reprint Verlag, 1983.

[11] M. Wellmann, "Die Pflanzennamen des Dioskurides," *Hermes*, 33 (1898), 360-422.

intent to produce a freshly-edited Greek text of the *Materia medica*, published in three volumes from 1906 to 1914. It is this Greek text that Lily Beck has employed for her translation, and the striking differences between her Dioscorides in English, and that of the Goodyer-Gunther, are marked by the clarity of phrase, the precision of description, and the easy flow of the English mirroring the complete control of the Greek and of the field botany so essential to understanding the great Anazarban We are very fortunate, indeed, to have her English translation, and shortly to be added will be a full commentary, which will provide classicists, medical historians, and students of botany and pharmacology, with the first accurate English translation and commentary on Dioscorides of Anazarbus, perhaps the greatest medical figure of classical antiquity.

John Scarborough
School of Pharmacy and Department of Classics
University of Wisconsin

# PREFACE

Pedanius Dioscorides of Anazarbus wrote *De materia medica* during the second half of the first century A.D. and throughout the Middle Ages and Early Renaissance laymen and professionals alike used his work as a reference book for plants and disease. But when Carl Linnaeus (1707-1778) developped the modern botanical classifications, the popularity of *De materia medica* began to wane.

The edition and Latin translation of Curtius Sprengel, *Pedanii Dioscoridis Anazarbei De materia medica libri quinque*, 1829-1830, marks the beginning of the interest in Dioscorides in post-Renaissance times. In 1902, Julius Berendes issued a German translation that was based on the Greek text Sprengel had established, and between 1906 and 1914 Max Wellmann published a new critical edition of the Greek text. Subsequently, the scholarship of Vivian Nutton, John Scarborough, John Riddle, and Max Aufmesser kept this interest alive and added to our understanding of Dioscorides and his writings.

I was first attracted to *De materia medica* in graduate school, when I came across the interlinear English translation by the botanist John Goodyer, made between 1652 and 1655 but published only in 1934, Robert T. Gunther, editor. My interest was subsequently fanned by the translation with commentary of the "Preface of Dioscorides' *De materia medica*" by John Scarborough and Vivian Nutton (1982) and by John Riddle's *Dioscorides on Pharmacy and Medicine* (1985.) Furthermore, new discoveries in phytochemistry, modern studies in ethnobotany, researches into the curative practices of people all over the globe, the rise in the attention given to ancient pathologies, and the ever increasing appeal of natural remedies kept this interest alive and suggested that a modern English translation of Dioscorides was needed since the Gooodyer/Gunther edition is not only archaic in language, but as Gunther himself admits (p. VI,) it is "largely uncorrected." But it was not until my retirement that I could devote the time necessary for this task.

Ideally, this project should have been undertaken by a team of specialists including classical philologists, ethnobotanists, chemists, medical historians, and physicians, whose specialized knowledge and collaborative efforts could have answered many questions that this translation cannot address.

*De materia medica* is a major accomplishment, even though Dioscorides of course drew from his predecessors. First, because its vast scope includes plants, animals and animal products, minerals, manufacturing processes, and metallurgical procedures. Second, because its organization is original and its underlying principle is that therapeutic substances possess specific δύναμις/δυνάμεις = property/properties, capable of treating specific pathologies. These properties are of many different kinds. A property may be one of warming = θερμαντική or cooling = ψηκτική, of binding = στυπτική or of loosening = λυτική, of staunching = σταλτική or of dispersing = διαφορητική, of softening = μαλακτική or of hardening = σκληρυντική, of causing flatulence = φυσώδης or of relieving flatulence = ἐκκριτικὴ φυσῶν, etc. Drugs may also have other properties, such as escharotic, adhesive, detersive, diuretic, etc. that do not necessarily have opposites. Thus, knowing what properties are inherent in which materials is essential to the treatment of the sick and to avoiding illness or discomfort. Moreover, by grouping together substances of similar properties rather than listing them in the alphabetical order allegedly used by his predecessors, Dioscorides achieves two very happy results: the drugs are easier to remember and, since drugs with similar properties treat the same pathologies and bring about approximately the same results, possible substitutes are more or less on the same page.

Besides this organizational principle by properties, Dioscorides uses another structural feature within each chapter, namely the order of presentation which is as follows: morphology, habitat(s), relative qualities, methods of preparation, general properties and specific therapeutic applications, adulteration, compounding, and directions for storage. Of course not all these are applicable to all drugs, but the generally orderly presentation is the hallmark of a scientific mind.

**Style and Content**

Max Wellmann, in his article "Dioskurides," describes Dioscorides' language as "small-town Greek" and his writing style as "*schwer-*

*flüssig*" = sluggish (*P.W*., p. 1132.) The first part of this statement is gratuitous, the second subject to debate. This is not the place to discuss Wellmann's assessment of Dioscorides' literary merits, although one might point out that Dioscorides himself was very much aware that he was no stylist, and as if to anticipate Wellmann's criticism, he asks his readers in the Preface to judge his work not on form but on substance. One might add that *De materia medica* is a scientific treatise and that Dioscorides' style is no more "sluggish" than other scientific writings, then or now.

In the absence of index cards, punch cards, computers, or even ordinary scraps of paper, *De materia medica* contains few mistakes and fewer contradictions. Here and there one finds faults, e.g. III, 1 where he describes agaric this way: "Agaric is said to be a root resembling the laserwort; it is not compact on the surface as is the laserwort but of a loose texture throughout." He gives no morphology for laserwort, *Ferula tinginata,* L., III, 80 other than that it resembles giant fennel. Giant fennel, III, 77 is not described. Therefore, what we are told is that the roots of agaric, laserwort, and giant fennel resemble each other but we are not told what any of them look like. In III, 112, while discussing colt's foot, he says first that its root is useless, but toward the end of the chapter that it is useful for many things. In IV, 162, he says that the pith of the black hellebore is removed the same way as the pith of the white hellebore, but in the section on white hellebore, IV, 148, there are no directions for the removal of the pith. In IV, 178 he says that the seed of herb terrible is like that of *epithymon,* IV, 177, but the seed of *epthymon* is never described. In V, 104 he discusses yellow orpiment and in V, 105 sulfide of arsenic. He says that these two substances have the same properties. Yet, he describes yellow orpiment as being depilatory and sulfide of arsenic as treating bald spots. On the whole, however, imperfections or inconsistencies are few, and of course we cannot know whether these peccadillos are Dioscorides' or corruptions of the original text.

Dioscorides' tract contains few superstitions. When he discusses practices that today's western world generally dismisses as magic, nonsense, or humbug, he very commonly prefaces his remarks with "they say" or "it is reported," or "it seems." For instance, I, 93: "It is said that the root [of fiery thorn] can even effect miscarriages when the abdomen is struck with it gently three times or when it is anointed with it." II, 16,1: "Some add that eating vipers promotes longevity." II, 47: "The liver of a rabid dog, eaten roasted by those bitten by it, is believed to keep them safe from rabies. As a precaution, they also use the canine tooth of the dog that bit them, tied in a little pouch, and fastened onto their arm." Occasionally, a bit of the irrational insinuates itself into the text with no other authorship than that of Dioscorides. E.g. II, 171,4: "[Scilla] does ward off evil when hung whole on front doors." III, 150,2: "[Stinking bean trefoil] is an amulet for women whose labor is difficult, but immediately after giving birth the amulet must be removed and thrown away." IV, 24: "If someone after chewing [alkanet] spat it out into the mouth of the animal [that bit him,] it kills it." IV, 117: "The infusion of its root [i.e. oleander] has a property that tames wild animals when they drink it." Elsewhere he simply reports magical practices without either espousing or disavowing them, e.g. IV, 132: "[Sea starwort] is also cut for witchcraft." These statements are troublesome and do not sit well on modern ears, especially in view of his claim in the Preface to "experience" and to "personal observations."

**Translation and Transliteration**

It is not uncommon in ancient Greek, not just for Dioscorides, to use shrub for tree, fruit for seed, hair for leaves, leaves for needles, —to give but a few examples. The word λιπαρά = bright or smooth or sleek or shining or fat, proved difficult to deal with. When Dioscorides says that a plant has leaves that are λιπαρά, which of these meanings does he have in mind?

There are many other questions. For instance, does the word μῆνιγξ plural μήνιγγες, which Dioscorides uses almost formulaically in the expression αἱμορραγίας ἐκ μήνιγγος (μηνίγγων) ἐπέχει (I, 68,2; II, 49,1; 79,1; V, 84) mean membrane(s) in general or does it mean meninges? Hemorrhaging from eye or ear membranes may be visible but how does one know of meningeal bleeding? And no matter how one chooses to translate μήνιγξ, how exactly in II, 79 does "pigeon blood, in particular, stay hemorrhages from the μηνίγγες"? Another is Dioscorides' use of three terms: ἄσθμα = asthma, δύσπνοια =

dyspnea, and ὀρθόπνοια = orthopnea. All three refer to condition involving breathing difficulties to which modern science asssigns different causes. His references to them are numerous, 19 for orthopnea, 9 for dyspnea, 27 for asthma. In two instances, I, 73,3 and III, 83,1, he makes references to asthmatics and to sufferers from dyspnea within the same sentence, and in III, 25, 1, III, 36,2, III, 83, and III, 84,2 to orthopnea and asthma. Thus it is clear that he views these conditions as distinct and differing from each other, but it is not clear why.

*De materia medica* presents many other challenges to the translator. In *Webster's New International Dictionary* a sore is defined as "a place in an animal body where the skin and flesh are ruptured or bruised, so as to be tender or painful; an ulcer or a boil; strictly, a wound, bruise, or abrasion that has become infected or a suppurating ulcer or boil," LSJ defines ἕλκος as wound, festering wound, sore, or ulcer. Dioscorides uses ἕλκος, pl. ἕλκη without modifiers, with modifiers, such as παλαιά = old, νεμόμενα = spreading, κακοηθή = malignant, and with body parts, such as ἐν στόματι = in the mouth. Unless he used ἕλκος with a modifier, it has been difficult to know the exact meaning.

In transliterating Greek words into English I have tried to be consistent and only rarely did I sacrifice consistency to accepted usage. I do not indicate long and short quantities of vowels. Thus an "*o*" can be either an omicron or an omega, an "*e*" either an epsilon or an eta. I transliterated "υ" as "y" and the diphtongs "*αι*," "*ει* ," "*οι*, " "*αυ*," "*ευ*," and "*ου* " as "ai," "ei," "oi," "au," "eu," and "ou." I indicate no accents. I transliterate Greek "κ " with a "c" and I have resisted making exceptions, even though some familiar words containing a "κ" look odd when transliterated into English with a "c."

A few more final words about this edition, about the translation, about translation in general, and about the prescriptions in his books:

Errata in the earlier editions have been corrected. I am grateful to reviewers and to readers who have brought some of them to my attention.

Occasionally Dioscorides' sentences are very long. To provide some structure while staying faithful to the text, I have made generous use of punctuation.

The Italians have a saying, *traduttore traditore.* Wrestling with this text has reminded me that often there is no precise correspondence in meaning among languages and that the best one can hope for is only an approximation of the writer's intention.

The remedies contained in this book are only of historical interest and must not be used for self-medication.

**Indexes**

Several readers of the first edition suggested that, in addition to the English to Greek Indexes, Greek to English Indexes would have been helpful especially to those whose primary language is not English. Both the publishers and I agreed. Thus, the second edition as well as the third revised edition contain three additional indexes: Index of Plants and Plant Products: Greek-English, Index of Animals and Animal Products: Greek-English, and Index of Minerals and Inorganic Products: Greek-English. Following the suggestions of readers and reviewers, this fourth edition has an additional index: Index of Plants: Botanical Names-Greek-English.

For the botanical identifications of plants, I have relied primarily on Jacques André, *Les noms des plantes dans la Rome antique*, and secondarily on Liddell, Scott and Jones, *Greek English Lexicon.* In instances where Jacques André identifies a plant but not its synonym, I have given to the synonym the identification Jacques André gave to the plant.

Plants, animals, and minerals have been indexed only if they are the main topic of a chapter, but not if they are one of the ingredients of a complex preparation.

**Acknowledgements**

I am grateful to Professor John M. Riddle of North Carolina State University in Raleigh for his unfailing encouragement, for reading sample pages of this translation, and for his good advice. I am indebted to Professor John Scarborough of the University of

Wisconsin in Madison for giving unstintingly of his time by going through the entire translation; his copious and constructive comments have much improved this work. To Ryan Hart of the Office of Development at Vassar College I owe a large debt of gratitude for the many hours he devoted to my manuscript, scanning the entire text, eliminating formating inconsistencies, and elegantly solving problems that my deficiencies in word processing technology had created. And last but not least I am thankful to the Alexander S. Onassis Public Benefit Foundation for its generous grant in support of this project.

# BOOK I

## Preface

Dear Areios,

**1.** Even though many writers, not only ancient but also modern, have written about the preparation, properties, and testing of drugs, I shall try to show you that it is neither a vain nor a foolish impulse that possessed me to undertake the present work. I have done so because some of them did not give complete accounts, while others based their disquisitions for the most part on written sources. For instance, Iollas of Bithynia[1] and Heracleides of Tarentum[2] treated only a small part of the subject, ignoring completely the lore of herbal remedies, nor did they in fact mention minerals or spices at all. On the other hand, Crateuas,[3] the root cutter, and Andreas,[4] the physician, both of whom

---

[1] Iollas of Bithynia lived during the third century B.C. His preparations are mentioned both by Celsus, *De medicina*, V, 22.5 and by Pliny, *N. H.*, XX, 187 and 198 who also includes him in his list of authorities for books XII, XIII, XX-XXVIII, and XXXIII-XXXV. Neither Celsus nor Pliny faults him in any way. See "Iolas," *P.W.* 9, pt. 2 (1916): 1855; Max Wellmann, "Zur Geschichte der Medizin," p. 561; John Scarborough and Vivian Nutton, "The Preface," p. 202; John Riddle, *Dioscorides on Pharmacy and Medicine*, pp. 19-20.

[2] Heracleides of Tarentum was a physician of the first century B.C. who worked in Alexandria. Pliny uses him as a source for *N. H.*, XII and XIII. He was much esteemed by Galen for his integrity and for his medical knowledge. See Galen, *Commentary IV on Hippocrates' Joints*, 40; C. G. Kühn, ed. XVIII, part 1, 735, "Heracleides," *P.W.* 8, pt. 1 (1912): 493-496; John Scarborough and Vivian Nutton, "The Preface," p. 203; John Riddle, *Dioscorides on Pharmacy and Medicine*, pp 19-20; and J. Vallance, "The Medical System of Asclepiades of Bithynia," ANRW, II, 37, 1 (1993).

[3] Crateuas lived in the first century B.C. and was physician to Mithridates VI of Pontus (120-63 B.C.) Pliny uses him among other authorities for *N. H.*, XX-XXVII. Largely discredited is the theory of Charles Singer that Crateuas' illustrated herbals were directly ancestral to the Vienna MS (A.D. 512), Singer, "The Herbal in Antiquity and its Transmission to Later Ages," *JHS* 47 (1927), 1-52. See also Max Wellmann, *Krateuas;* John Scarborough and Vivian Nutton, "The Preface," p. 204; John Riddle, Dioscorides on Pharmacy and Medicine, pp. 5, 18, 181-191; and John Scarborough, "Crateuas," *OCD*, third edition, (1996), pp. 406-407.

[4] Andreas, third century B.C. physician of Ptolemy V Philopator. Pliny lists him as one of his sources for *N. H.*, XX-XXVIII and XXXII-XXXV. See John Scarborough

are reputed to have addressed themselves to this part of the subject more completely than the rest, left many highly serviceable roots and certain herbs unnoticed.

**2.** Yet one must give high marks to the ancient writers for being accurate, even though they were not comprehensive, and this certainly cannot be said of the modern ones, among whom are Julius Bassus,[5] Niceratus,[6] Petronius, Niger, and Diodotus,[7] all of them followers of Asclepiades.[8] They have seen fit to describe in great detail materials that are common and well known to everyone but handed us down slapdash accounts of the properties of drugs and methods for testing them. Nor did they judge the action of drugs empirically, but prattling about causes, they attributed to each of them differences in particles and, what is more, they confused one drug with another.

**3.** For instance, Niger, who is considered prominent among them, supposes that the resinous juice of the spurge is the juice of the spurge olive which grows in Italy, that perfoliate St. John's wort is the same as crispate St. John's wort, that aloe is mined in Judea, and propounds wrongly many other notions similar to these that are contrary to manifest facts, proving unequivocally that his account is based not on personal observations but on writings that he misunderstood. Niger and the rest of them have also blundered regarding organization: some have brought into collision disconnected properties, while others used

---

and Vivian Nutton, "The Preface," pp. 204-205.

[5] Julius Bassus flourished in the first half of the first century A.D. Pliny uses him for *N. H.*, XX-XXVII and XXXIII-XXXIV. See John Scarborough and Vivian Nutton, "The Preface," p. 205.

[6] Niceratus was a physician of the first century A.D. Although Pliny does not mention him in his list of sources, he does refer to him in *N. H.*, XXXII, 101. See John Scarborough and Vivian Nutton, "The Preface," p. 205.

[7] At issue here is whether Dioscorides criticizes three people, Petronius, Niger, and Diodotus, or two, Petronius Niger and Petronius Diodotus. See John Scarborough and Vivian Nutton, "The Preface," pp. 205-206 who support correctly the notion of three rather than two individuals, physicians of the first century A.D.

[8] Asclepiades of Prusa in Bithynia was a physician practicing in Rome in the first century B.C. Pliny lists him as one of his references for *N. H.*, XIV, XXIII-XXIV, and XXVI-XXVII. Epicurus influenced him. Health, according to him, was the unopposed movement of bodily corpuscles while sickness ensued when pores where blocked by too many particles. He believed in diet rather than in drugs. See John Scarborough and Vivian Nutton, "The Preface," pp. 206-208. John Riddle, *Dioscorides on Pharmacy and Medicine*, pp. 7 and 11-12.

an alphabetical arrangement, separating materials and their properties from those closely connected to them. The outcome of this arrangement is that it is difficult to commit to memory.

**4.** I, on the other hand, having had from a very young age, so to speak, an abiding interest in *materia medica* and having covered much territory—for you know that I have led a military life—have collected at your encouragement my findings in five books. It is to you that I dedicate this collection in gratitude for your kindness towards me. And while you are by nature friendly towards all men refined by education and especially towards those in your discipline, towards me, you have been particularly so. No trifling example of your perfect character is also the attitude of the most excellent Laecanius Bassus[9] towards you, which I noticed while living with you and seeing the enviable goodwill that each of you has for the other.

**5.** But I do beg you, as I also beg my future readers, not to scrutinize the vigor of my style, but rather to notice, along with my experience, the care I have bestowed upon the subject. For since I know, on the one hand, from personal observation in utmost detail most items, and, on the other hand, since I have a thorough understanding of the rest from accounts on which there has been unanimous agreement and previous examination in each case by natives, I shall try to use both a different arrangement and to list the materials according to the natural properties of each one of them. It is perhaps clear to everyone that there is a great need for a treatise on pharmacology, which, coupled with the entire art of healing, provides by itself in every section an invincible ally And because it can be expanded in the areas of preparation, compounding, and testing on diseases, as inquiries into each drug make additional contributions, I shall include traditional as well as related material, so that the account be complete.

**6.** So, first and foremost in order of importance is to pay proper attention to the storage and timely collection of each drug; for whether drugs are strong or weak depends strictly on whether the collection was made at the right time: one must assemble the material in clear weather. This, too, makes a great deal of difference: was the collection made after a dry or a rainy spell, as it does also matter whether the

[9] He was consul in 64 A.D.

sites from which it was made are mountainous, high-up, breezy, cold, or dry. For the properties of plants gathered from these places are stronger. By contrast, the properties of plants growing on plains, wetlands, shady or poorly aerated locations, on the whole, are weaker, and this is especially true of collections made out of season or that are decayed by reason of disease.

**7.** Also one must certainly not forget that plants often reach their peak either sooner or later, depending on the particular nature of the site and on climatic conditions, that some plants, because of their peculiar nature, bear flowers and leaves in winter, and that others bloom even twice a year. Anyone who wishes to gain experience in these matters must be present when plants sprout newly from the ground as well as when they are in their prime and past their prime. For neither the person who has come across a plant only at its seedling stage can point it out when at its prime, nor can the person who has seen plants in their prime recognize them as seedlings. Because of changes in the leaves, in the size of stems, blossoms, and fruits, and because of certain other characteristics, people who have not made their observations in this manner were greatly mislead regarding some plants.

**8.** This is certainly why some writers were wrong in saying that some plants bear neither bloom, nor stem, nor fruit, as in the case of dog's-tooth grass, coltsfoot, and cinquefoil. But the person who has come across plants often and in many places will most readily recognize them. One should certainly know that some herbal medicines, such as white and black hellebore, last for many years while others are good for up to three years. Plants resembling young shoots, such as French lavender, wall germander, hullwort, wormwood [*Artemisia arborescens*], worm seed, wormwood [*Artemisia absinthium*], hyssop, and their like, one must collect when big with seed, flowers before they begin to fall off, fruit when ripe, and seeds as they start to dry and before they drop to the ground.

**9.** Also one must extract[10] juice from herbs when their stems have newly sprouted; the same applies to leaves. One must catch saps and gums by cutting the stems when still at the peak of perfection, but

[10] Extractions are made either by infusion or decoction.

roots intended for storage, for extracting their juice, and for their outer layers must be dug up at the time the plants begin to shed their leaves. Clean roots must be dried immediately in places that are free of moisture, but roots containing earth or clay must be washed with water. Both blossoms and whatever aromatic parts there happen to be should be stowed in moisture-free limewood boxes and there are instances when they are wrapped to good avail in papyrus or in leaves to preserve their seeds. All silver, glass, or horn vessels will do nicely for liquid medicines, as will earthenware vessels, provided they are not thin, and of the wooden containers, all that are made of boxwood. Brazen receptacles are suitable for eye lotions and for all preparations that are made with vinegar, or raw pitch, or oil of Syrian cedar, but hard fats and marrows should be stored in containers made of tin.

**I, 1 ἶρις, *Iris florentina* L., *I. germanica* L., *I. pallida* Lam., Iris**

**1.** The Illyrian iris bears leaves like the corn flag, but larger, wider, and fatter, and flowers parallel on stems, curling, and in many colors: for one sees them either white or quince-yellow or purple or bluish. It is because of this diversity of color that it has been likened to the heavenly rainbow. The roots are below ground, articulated, firm, and aromatic. After cutting them, you must dry them in the shade, thread them with a linen string, and store them. Illyrian and Macedonian irises are superior and of these the best are matted and stunted, hard to break, yellowish in color, highly aromatic, rather spicy in taste, pure in scent, not clammy, and ptarmic when cut. The Libyan iris is both white in color and bitter in taste, <and> it ranks second in strength.[11] As irises age, they become worm-eaten, but it is then that they become more fragrant.

**2.** All irises have warming and attenuating properties that are suitable for coughs and for thinning fluids hard to bring up.[12] Seven *drachmai*[13]

[11] The geographic epithets of irises in medical treatises indicate origins, not different species, Jacques André, *Les noms des plantes dans la Rome antique,* p. 133.

[12] It is the rhizome of the iris that he uses and it is from the rhizome called orris or Florentine orris that now extracts are made for the food, cosmetic, wine, and liqueur industries. The rhizome is used also in folk medicine as expectorant, as demulcent, and to relieve dentition pains. Norman Grainger Bisset, *Herbal Drugs and Phytopharmaceuticals*, p. 279 and P. G. Gennadios, Φυτολογικόν Λεξικόν, p. 440.

in weight drunk in hydromel purge thick fluids and bile. They induce sleep, they cause eyes to tear, and they cure colic. When drunk with vinegar they help those bitten by wild animals, splenetics, people who have spasms, hypothermics or shiverers, and those who ejaculate prematurely, and when drunk with wine they draw down the menses. Their decoction, too, is suitable for women's vapor baths, softening and dilating the genitalia, it is a clyster for hip disease,[14] and it fleshes up both ducts and hollows.

**3.** Applied like a pessary with honey, the roots draw down embryos/fetuses,[15] and when used boiled as cataplasms they soften scrofulous gland swellings and old indurations. Dried, they fill up ulcers, they cleanse them with honey, and they flesh up bones stripped of flesh. Plastered on with vinegar and unguent of roses, they help for headaches and they clear away birthmarks and freckles when smeared with twice as much white hellebore. They are compounded with pessaries, emollients, and analgesics, and on the whole they are useful for many purposes.

### I, 2 ἄκορον, *Iris pseudacorus* L., Yellow flag

**1.** The yellow flag has leaves that resemble the leaves of iris but narrower, and it has roots that are not unlike those of iris, except they are entangled and they do not grow straight down but sideways and at

---

[13] See Weights and Measures.

[14] Dioscorides uses the word ἰσχίας, which LSJ defines as 1) "hip disease" and 2) as "sciatica." Sciatica in modern medicine means neuritis or neuralgia of the sciatic nerve. This term is commonly used also for a variety of pains in the area of the hip and adjoining parts. Throughout this work I shall translate ἰσχίας as "hip disease" or "hip ailment," the adjective ἰσχιαδικός as "subject to" or "pertaining to" or "good for hip disease," and the noun ἴσχιον, as "hip joint." See also Max Aufmesser, *Etymologische und wortgeschichtliche Erläuterungen zu De materia medica des Pedanius Dioscurides Anazarbeus*, henceforth cited as *Erläuterungen*, p. 363, where he objects to "sciatica" as being anachronistic.

[15] Ἔμβρυον in classical Greek refers either to an embryo or to a fetus. Its etymology comes from ἐν, "in" and βρύειν, "to swell," or "teem," or "grow luxuriant." The Greek scholiast Eustathius in his commentary on the *Odyssey*, 9, 245 defined ἔμβρυον as "that which grows in the womb" regardless of its stage of development. In English, however, in viviparous vertebrates, embryo and fetus refer to two distinct stages of development: embryo is applied only to the early stages of the development of a young organism within the mother's body. Later this young organism is called fetus (in human embryology, usually after the third month of development.)

the surface of the ground, being marked with knobs, and they are somewhat white, pungent in taste and not unpleasant in scent. Best is that which is thick and white, not worm-eaten, and full of scent. Such is the one in Colchis and the one from Galatia, called *asplenon*.[16]

**2.** The root has a warming property. Its decoction[17] is diuretic when drunk; it is suitable for pains in the side, chest, and liver, for colic, ruptures, spasms, and it reduces the spleen; it helps those suffering from strangury, those bitten by wild animals, and it is used in sitz baths for female complaints, just like iris. The juice of its root gets rid of those elements that cast a shadow over the pupils of the eyes.[18] The root is compounded beneficially also with antidotes.

**I,3 μῆον, *Meum athamanticum* Jacq., Spignel, Baldmoney**

The spignel called Athamantic[19] grows lavishly in Macedonia and Spain. In stalk and leaves it resembles the dill, but it is stouter than dill, shooting up to a height of about two cubits, spreading over its roots, which are delicate, horizontal and straight, long, aromatic, and warming the tongue. Boiled in water or even ground fine and drunk without previous cooking, the roots relieve dry conditions around the bladder and kidneys, they are suitable for difficult micturition, for stomach gas and for colic, for uterine conditions, and for pains in the joints. Ground up fine with honey, they are helpful, in lieu of a lozenge, for chest rheums; boiled for a sitz bath they draw down blood

---

[16] The etymology of ἄσπληνον is from alpha privative and σπλήν, "spleen" and Dioscorides recommends its use in this chapter for the reduction of enlarged spleens. See also n. 18 below for the use of alpha privative in the etymology of ἄκορον.

[17] The distinctions among (1) ἀπόζεμα, "decoction," (2) ὀπός, "vegetable juice, the milky substance that is drawn from a plant by tapping it," (3) χυλός, "juice of plants, decoction, flavor," (4) χυμός, much like χυλός though sometimes distinguished from it, "juice of plants, flavor," and (5) ἀφέψημα, "decoction," are often blurred. In this passage, because ἀπόζεμα (1) and χυλός (3) are used in contradistinction to each other, the task is easy, but as a rule there is a fuzziness of meaning associated with these words.

[18] The "shadow" may be cataracts, see Dsc. Bk. I, 54, 2 and n. 57 and the presumed capability of this plant to treat them is embedded in its name: ἄκορον, from alpha privative and κόρη, "eye-pupil."

[19] Pliny, *N. H.*, XX, 253 says that it is called Athamantic or Athamanic "because, as some think, it was discovered by Athamas, or according to others because the most esteemed variety is found in Athamania," a district in Epirus on or near Pindus.

through the menses and when plastered on the pubes of youngsters they set micturition going. But it does also cause headaches if drunk in amounts greater than recommended.

### I, 4 κύπερος, *Cyperus rotundus* L.,[20] Galingale

**1.** The galingale: some call it *erysisceptron* as they call the camel's-thorn. It has leaves resembling those of leek but longer and more slender, a stem a cubit tall or even taller, angular, like the stem of camel hay, at the top of which there is an outgrowth of small leaflets and of seed. Also the roots, for which the plant is used, grow below ground, just like elongated olives linked with each other, or they are even round, black, aromatic, and bitter. It grows in cultivated and marshy areas. Best is that which is very heavy and thick, bulky and hard to break, rough, aromatic with a touch of pungency. Such is the Cilician, the Syrian, and the one from the Cycladic islands.
**2.** It has properties that warm, open, and that are diuretic, operating on patients with kidney stones and edemata when drunk. It helps people stung by scorpions and it is good for uterine[21] chills and closings when used in vapor baths, drawing down the menses. Dried up and ground fine, it is effective in the treatment both of mouth sores and of spreading ulcers. It is mixed with heat-producing emollients and it is serviceable for thickening unguents.

### I, 5 ἕτερον εἶδος κυπέρου, *Curcuma longa* L., Another kind of galingale

It is reported that there is also another kind of galingale[22] that grows in India. It resembles ginger, it is saffron-colored and bitter when chewed, and it is a fast-acting depilatory when smeared on.

---

[20] J. Berendes, *Des Pedanios Dioskurides aus Anazarbus Arzneimittellehre in fünf Büchern*, (henceforth cited as J. Berendes,) p. 27, identifies it as *Cyperus rotundus, C. longus* (*Cyperaceae*,) and the "other kind of galingale" mentioned in ch. 5, below as *Curcuma longa* (*Zingiberaceae*;) Max Aufmesser, Pedanius *Dioscurides aus Anazarba*, pp. 25-26, identifies both plants as *Alpinia galanga (Zingiberaceae.*)

[21] Ancient Greek does not distinguish between the uterus and the cervix and ordinarily it is context that helps determine which of the two is meant.

[22] This other type of galingale is turmeric.

**I, 6 καρδάμωμον, *Elettaria cardamomum*, White and Maton, Cardamom**

Cardamom is best if it comes from Commagene, Armenia, and the Bosporus. It grows also in India and in Arabia. Be sure to choose that which is hard to break, full, closed—for if it is not closed, it is unsuitable—overpowering in scent, pungent in taste, and somewhat bitter.

It has a warming property. When drunk with water, it is good for epileptics, coughs, for patients suffering from hip disease, for paralysis, for ruptures, spasms, colic, and it gets rid of the intestinal flatworm. Drunk with wine, it is suitable for those suffering from kidney dysfunction, difficult micturition, scorpion stings, and for all animal venoms. One *drachma* drunk with the bark of the root of sweet bay breaks stones. When burned to produce smoke from below, it also destroys embryos/fetuses, and, when smeared on with vinegar, it gets rid of mange. It is also used to thicken perfumes.

**I, 7 νάρδος, *Nardostachys jatamansi* DC., *Patrinia scabiosifolia* Fisch., Spikenard**

**1.** There are two kinds of spikenard: one is called Indian spikenard and the other Syrian, not because it is found in Syria, but because one part of the mountain on which it grows faces Syria and the other India. And of the one called Syrian the best is fresh and light, abounding in down, yellow in color, highly aromatic, and besides resembling galingale in smell, it has a short spike, it is bitter in taste, it dries up the tongue, and its scent lingers on for a while.

**2.** Of the Indian spikenard, there is one called *Gangitis*, taking its name from a river called Ganges, which flows close to the mountain on which it grows. It is a rather weak plant, because it is found on wetlands, and it is somewhat tall, having several spikes growing from the same root that are full of down, entangled, and foul-smelling. But that which grows on higher elevations is more aromatic, its spikes are shorter, it smells like galingale, and it possesses all the qualities that the one called Syrian also possesses. There is also a spikenard called Sampharitic, named so from a district;[23] it has large spikes, it is lighter

---

[23] Oribasius calls it "Sappharetic." There is a locality called Saphar in southwestern

in color, and at times it has a middle stem smelling as rank as a he-goat; you must pick it out and reject it.
**3.** Spikenard is also sold soaked; one knows if it has been soaked because its spike is white, rough, and devoid of down. They adulterate it by blowing into it powdered antimony combined with water or date palm wine to compress it and to make it heavier. To use it, you must remove any earth that may adhere to the roots and sift it, separating the cloud of dust, which is very useful for hand washing.
They have warming, desiccative, and diuretic properties and so, when drunk, they bind the bowel, and, when applied as a pessary, they stem uterine excretions and serous discharges.
**4.** When drunk with cold water, they are helpful for nausea, heart-burn, flatulence, liver ailments, jaundice, and renal dysfunctions. Boiled down with water and used for vapors in a sitz bath, they heal uterine inflammations. They are good for purulent blepharitis, toning the eyelids and furthering the growth of eyelashes, and they are used as a scented body powder against excessive perspiration. They are mixed with antidotes, too. Triturated with wine and molded, they are stored in a new, unpitched vessel for eye medications.

**I, 8 κελτικὴ νάρδος, *Valeriana celtica* L., Celtic spikenard**
**1.** The Celtic spikenard grows in the Alps, around Liguria. The locals call it *saliunca*; but it grows also in Istria.[24] It is a small shrub that is pulled up with its roots in bundles that are as big as a handful. It has oblong and yellowish leaves and a quince-yellow flower. Only the stems and roots are useful and aromatic. Therefore you must lay them on the ground on top of moist papyrus, having doused the bundles with water the day before and removed the soil, and on the following day you must cleanse them. For its serviceable component is not washed off together with the chaffy and foreign matter on account of the vitality it gains from the moisture.
**2.** But it is adulterated with a similar herb that is plucked with it, called he-goat, because of its stench. Its identification is easy because this herb has no stalk, it has leaves that are lighter in color and shorter,

---

Arabia, which is probably the one meant here.
[24] A country in Italy, bordering on Illyria, at the head of the Adriatic.

and its root is neither as bitter nor as aromatic as the real one. After separating then the stems and roots and discarding the leaves, if you should wish to put them up, combine them ground up with wine and after shaping the mixture into disks, keep them in a new clay pot, sealing it carefully. Excellent is that which is fresh and aromatic, heavily rooted, not easily broken, and full.

**3.** It does accomplish everything that Syrian spikenard accomplishes, although it is more diuretic and better for the stomach. It helps for inflammations around the liver, the jaundiced, and for stomach gas when drunk with a decoction of wormwood *Artemisia absinthum*; it helps similarly the spleen, conditions associated with the bladder and kidneys, venomous bites when drunk with wine, and it is incorporated into emollients, draughts, and warming salves.

### I, 9 ὀρεινὴ νάρδος, *Valeriana tuberosa* L., Mountain spikenard

The mountain spikenard, which is called by some both *thylacitis* and *pyritis,* grows in Cilicia and Syria. It has leaves and stems resembling those of eryngo, but smaller and not in the least jagged or prickly. Its roots are below ground, black, aromatic, two or even more, like those of asphodel, although they are finer and considerably shorter. It bears neither fruit nor flower. Its root is good for all the things for which Celtic spikenard is good.

### I, 10 ἄσαρον, *Asarum europaeum* L., Hazelwort

**1.** The hazelwort, but some call it wild spikenard. It has leaves like those of ivy, although they are much softer and rounder, and a flower growing between its leaves, purple at the base, resembling the calyx of henbane, and whereon lies the fruit looking like a grape seed. Its numerous roots are underground, angular, delicate, oblique, resembling dogtooth grass, but they are much more delicate and they are aromatic, warming and biting the tongue a great deal.

**2.** Their properties are diuretic and warming, being suitable for those suffering from edemata and from chronic hip disease. They also draw down the menses. An amount of seven *oungiai* by weight drunk with hydromel is purgative just like white hellebore. They are mixed also with unguents. It grows on shaded mountains, abundantly so in the

Pontic region, in Phrygia, in Illyria, and in the territory of the Vestini of Italy.[25]

**I, 11 φοῦ, *Valeriana phu* L., Cretan spikenard**

**1.** Some call Cretan spikenard wild spikenard. It grows in the Pontic region. It has leaves nearly resembling the leaves of parsnip or of horse parsley, a stem about a cubit tall or taller, smooth, soft, somewhat purple, hollow, marked off by joints, and flowers that are comparable to those of narcissus, but bigger, pale-white, and shot with purple. The root that is higher up is about as thick as a small finger and it has secondary roots that extend sideways like those of camel hay or of black hellebore, which are entangled with each other, yellowish, aromatic, resembling in scent spikenard with a somewhat foul-smelling oppressiveness.

**2.** When drunk, the dry root can warm and activate micturition. Its decoction, too, can do the same thing and it is good for pain in the side; it also draws down the menses and it is mixed with antidotes.

It is adulterated with root of butcher's broom. But it is easy to recognize butcher's broom because its roots are tough, difficult to break, and devoid of scent.

**I, 12 μαλάβαθρον, ~ *Cinnamomum tamala* Nees, ~ *C. iners* Blume, ~ *C. zeylanicum* Blume, ~ *Pogostemon patchouli* Pell., Malabar[26]**

**1.** Some entertain the notion that malabar is the leaf of Indian spikenard, being misled by the similarity of their scent. But there are many plants similar to spikenard in scent, like Cretan spikenard, hazelwort, and iris. Malabar is definitely not the leaf of Indian spikenard but a distinct kind of plant that grows on the Indian marshes, a leaf suspended on water, just like duckweed, which they

---

[25] In Central Eastern Italy.

[26] P. G. Gennadios, Φυτολογικόν Λεξικόν, p. 508 says that these leaves are of cinnamon, *Cinnamomum malabathrum* or *C. tamala* native to Malabar and Java. Jacques André, *Les noms des plantes dans la Rome antique*, p. 151 adds *C. iners* Blume, C. *zeylanicum* Blume, etc. as possible additional sources and proposes that a more likely candidate may be patchouli, *Pogostemon patchouli* Pell., an East Indian shrubby mint yielding a fragrant essential oil. See also J. Innes Miller, *The Spice Trade of the Roman Empire, 29 B.C. to A.D. 641*, pp. 74-77.

collect, thread immediately with linen thread, and after drying it, store it. It is also said that during the summertime, after the water has dried up, they burn the earth with its undershrub and unless this procedure is followed, the leaf no longer grows.

**2.** Of fine quality is that which is fresh, off-white with a tinge of black, unbroken and whole, overpowering in scent and of a lingering sweet smell, resembling spikenard in taste, and not salty. But that which is weak and chopped fine, yielding an emanation of decay, is inferior. It has the same properties as spikenard except that spikenard accomplishes everything more effectively. On the other hand, malabar has more diuretic and more wholesome properties, and, when boiled in wine and plastered on ground up, it is suitable for eye inflammations. It is also placed under the tongue to make the mouth smell good and it is set among articles of clothing because it does keep them free of moths and fragrant.

### I, 13 κασσία, Cinnamomum *cassia* Blume, Cassia[27]

**1.** There are many kinds of cassia growing up and down spice-bearing Arabia. It has thick-barked shoots and leaves like those of the pepper. Choose it pale-yellow, healthy looking, resembling coral, narrow, smooth, long and thick-quilled, pungent in taste and astringent, somewhat burning, spicy, and smelling of wine. This kind of cassia is called by the locals *achy*[28] and by the merchants in Alexandria *daphnitis*. Superior to this cassia is the one that is dark, purplish, and thick. It is called *gizir*, it smells of roses, and it is especially well suited for the art of medicine. The one I spoke of first ranks second, and third is that which is called Mosylian[29] bramble.

**2.** But the rest are worthless, as are the cassia called *asyphe,* which is dark, unsavory, with a thin or even a broken bark, and the cassias called *citto* and *darca.*

---

[27] Both cassia and cinnamon, see ch.14 below, are species of *Cinnamomum cassia* Blume, commonly referred to as cinnamon. Cassia is the name of the Chinese species while cinnamon of the Malayan. It is the bark of these trees, stripped from the branches and sun-dried that is used. More on the subject, J. Innes Miller, *The Spice Trade of the Roman Empire, 29 B.C. to 641 A.D.*, pp. 42-47.

[28] A Hebrew word.

[29] I.e. from Mosylon, a coastal town on the Gulf of Eden, modern Somalia.

There is also a spurious cassia, which is uncannily similar and which is tested by its taste, being neither pungent nor spicy; moreover, its bark clings to the pith. And there is a broad quill, which is soft, light, lush, and is superior to the other. Reject that which is whitish and scabby smelling like leeks and that which has quills that are not thick but scabby and thin.

**3.** It has warming, diuretic, desiccative and mildly astringent properties. It is suitable for eye medicines directed at shortsightedness and for emollients. Smeared on with honey, it removes birthmarks; when drunk, it draws down the menses and it helps victims of viper bites; it is good to drink for all internal inflammations and for the kidneys, and it is used by women for sitz baths and for making thick smoke to dilate the cervix. Should cinnamon cassia be unavailable, twice the amount of cassia mixed with reagents has the same effect, and it is highly useful.

### I, 14 κινάμωμον, *Cinnamomum tamala* Nees, *C. iners* Blume, Cinnamon

**1.** There are many kinds of cinnamon that have names in local dialects. The best is the *Mosylon,* because it retains a certain resemblance to the cassia called *Mosylitis,* and of this, the best is fresh, dark in appearance, ash-colored tending towards the color of wine, with shoots that are slender and smooth, serially knotted, and highly aromatic. Deciding which is the finest very nearly revolves around the specific character of its aroma; for the scent of the finest along with its special character and sweetness is found to be like rue or like garden cress; moreover it is pungent, biting in taste, and somewhat salty with some heat; nor does it crumble quickly when rubbed together, and the portion between the knots is downy and smooth when broken into pieces.

**2.** In testing it, break off the young shoot from one root. Such a test is easy. For the fragments happen to have compounds and as soon as you begin the test, the best of them, releasing their scent and filling the nose, forestall the selection of the inferior. There is also a kind that grows on mountains; it is thick and stunted, very yellow in appearance. And there is kind that ranks third from the *Mosylon.* It is dark and smooth, fibrous and not highly articulated. A fourth kind is white, spongy, round in appearance and slight; it is easily broken, its root is large, and [it smells of cassia.] A fifth kind <smells> overpowering <like cassia, > it is yellowish, and its bark resembles a yellowish-red cassia; it feels solid to the touch, it is not entirely fibrous, and it is thick-rooted. Among all these cinnamons that which smells of frankincense or of myrtle or of cassia or of Nepal cardamom is inferior.

**3.** Pick out and reject that which is white, scabby, whose branches are shriveled, and not smooth; reject, too, as worthless, that which is woody toward the root. There is also another kind that resembles it, called *pseudocinamomon*. It is not a well-developed plant, it is not vigorous in scent, and it is faint in action. And there is also something that is called *zingiberi*,[30] which is wood of cinnamon and bears some likeness to cinnamon; it is detected by its looks and stench. As for the one called *xylocinamomon*, it, too, resembles cinnamon both in root and shoot, which is highly articulated, but it is a woody cinnamon having long and vigorous shoots and a much inferior scent. Some say that *xylocinamomon* is even generically different from cinnamon, being of a different nature.

**4.** All cinnamons have warming, diuretic, emollient, and digestive properties. When drunk and when applied with myrrh, they draw down both the menses and embryos/fetuses, they are suitable antidotes for venomous animals and for poisons, they clear away those elements that cast a shadow over the pupils of the eyes, and when smeared on with honey they remove birthmarks and freckles. They are also helpful for coughs, head colds, edemata, kidney diseases, and difficult micturition. They are combined with the most costly unguents and in general they are highly useful. Ground up, compounded with wine, and dried in the shade, they are stored for later use.

[There is also something called *cinnamon,* which some call *pseudocinamomon*. It is a well-sprouting plant and its shoots are thick, but it is much inferior to cinnamon, both in scent and in taste.][31]

---

[30] Perhaps "ginger."

[31] Wellmann remarks that this passage in the Saracenus edition of Dioscorides, Lyon, 1598, is bracketed as an interpolation and that it stems from the writings of Crateuas.

**I, 15 ἄμωμον, *Amomum subulatum* Roxb., Nepal cardamom**

**1.** Nepal cardamom[32] is a small shrub that resembles a wooden bunch of grapes and that is tangled up. It also has a small flower, like a gillyflower, and leaves similar to the bryony. The best is the Armenian, golden in color, having wood that is yellowish and quite aromatic. But the Median, because it grows on plains and on marshlands, is weaker; it is large, greenish-yellow, soft to the touch, with fibrous wood, and it smells like oregano. The Pontic is yellowish, neither tall nor hard to break, resembling grape clusters, full of fruit, and overpowering in scent. Choose that which is fresh and white or reddish, not compressed or entangled, but loose and slackened, full of seed resembling small clusters, heavy, very aromatic, free of any signs of rot, pungent, biting in taste, of one color and not pied.

**2.** It has warming, astringent, desiccative, soporific, and, when applied as a poultice on the forehead, analgesic properties. It also softens and dissipates boils, and it benefits victims of scorpion bites when used with basil as a cataplasm. It soothes inflammations of the eyes, of the internal organs with raisins, and it is useful for female disorders both in pessaries and in sitz baths. Its decoction, when drunk, helps those suffering from liver disease, kidney disease, and gout.[33] It is compounded both with antidotes and with very costly unguents.

Some adulterate Nepal cardamom with what is called *amomis*,[34] a plant that resembles Nepal cardamom but has neither scent nor fruit,

---

[32] ἄμωμον was often confused with cardamom, *Elletaria cardamomum* Maton. See J. Innes Miller, *The Spice Trade of the Roman Empire, 29 B.C. to A.D. 641*, pp. 67-68 and 71.

[33] Gout is metabolic disease characterized by painful inflammations around the joints caused by deposits of urate of sodium. Sometimes there is also an excessive amount of uric acid in the blood. Spencer, in his translation of Celsus, *De medicina*, vol. 1, pp. 463-465, says that dictionaries wrongly give gout as the only meaning of podagra and that in many classical writers and in Celsus these words mean pains in the foot or hand. Spencer suggests that the increased incidence of gout reported by Pliny and Galen was not necessarily caused by the rich diet of the affluent citizen, but perhaps by chronic lead poisoning brought about by use of lead in the construction of aqueducts in Imperial times. See more on gout in John Riddle, *Dioscorides on Pharmacy and Medicine*, pp. 44-47. Here and throughout this translation *podagra* is translated as gout.

[34] Not identified. Pliny, *N. H.*, XII, 49 says that there is something called *amomis,* which has fewer veins, it is tougher, and it is less aromatic. It seems to be either a

growing in Armenia, and having a flower that resembles that of oregano. In examining such plants always avoid broken pieces and choose those that have their shoots intact stemming from one root.

**I, 16 κόστος, *Saussurea lappa* Clarke, Costusroot**

**1.** The best costusroot is the Arabian, being white and light and having a very sweet smell. The Indian ranks second. It is strong, dark, and airy like fennel. The Syrian ranks third. It is heavy, colored like boxwood, and overpowering in scent. It is excellent when fresh, white, full throughout, compact, dry, not worm-eaten, free of a foul smell, biting and hot in taste.

It has properties that warm, that are diuretic, emmenagogic, and serviceable for uterine ailment when used in pessaries, vapor baths, and douches.

**2.** When drunk in the amount of two *oungiai*, it helps those bitten by vipers, with wine and wormwood *Artemisia absinthium*, it helps for chest pains, spasms, and flatulence, and, with honey, it is an aphrodisiac. With water, it also drives out intestinal flatworms and, when combined with oil, it is an ointment for shiverers that is applied prior to the onset of the shivering fit and for paralytics. Anointed with water or honey, it also removes freckles; it is compounded both with emollients and with antidotes.

In adulterating it, some mix it with very sturdy roots of Commagene calamint. But it is easy to find out if it has been adulterated, for calamint is neither hot in taste nor does it give off a vigorous and strikingly sweet smell.

**I, 17 σχοινος, *Cymbopogon schoenanthus* Spreng., Camel hay**

**1.** Camel hay: there is a kind that grows in Libya, another in Arabia, and another in that part of Arabia called Nabataia, which is the best. Second best is the Arabian, which some call *Babylonion* and others *teuchitis*; the Libyan is useless. Choose that which is fresh, reddish, and full of flowers, purplish and fine when split, smelling like roses when rubbed between the hands, and biting the tongue with a degree of burning. It is its flower, reeds, and root that are used.

---

different plant or else Nepal cardamon that was gathered unripe.

**2.** It has properties that warm, crush stones, promote digestion, soften, open up, are diuretic, emmenagogic, that relax breathing, cause headaches, and bind moderately. The flower is useful in draughts for expectorations of blood and for pains in the stomach, lung, liver, and kidneys; it is also mixed with antidotes. But the root is more astringent and this is the reason it is given for nauseous stomachs, also for edemata and spasms in the amount of one *drachma* with an equal amount of pepper for several days. Its decoction is serviceable in sitz baths for uterine inflammations.

**I, 18 κάλαμος ἀρωματικός, *Acorus calamus* L., Sweet flag**

The sweet flag grows in India. The best is orange-tawny, having frequent knots, and coming apart into many splinters when broken into pieces; its reed is full of whitish spider webs; it is sticky, astringent, and somewhat pungent when chewed.[35]

It can set micturition in motion when chewed. It is for this reason that having been boiled down with dogtooth grass or with celery seed and drunk, it is suitable for those having edemata, for kidney disease patients, for people suffering from strangury, and for ruptures. When drunk and when applied, it draws down the menses, and it treats coughs when burned by itself and with turpentine, the smoke being sucked with the mouth through a tube. It is also boiled down for women's sitz baths. It is compounded with emollients as well as with incense for fragrance.

**I, 19 βάλσαμον, *Commiphora opobalsamon* Engl., Mecca balsam**

**1.** Mecca balsam: the tree looks like dyer's buckthorn or fiery thorn in size, having leaves similar to those of rue, but they are much whiter and more evergreen; it grows only in Judea,[36] along a certain glen and it does vary in ruggedness, height, and slenderness. At any rate, the

---

[35] In modern pharmacopoeias the essential oils of its rhizomes are used internally as stomachics and carminatives and externally as rubefacients, Norman Grainger Bisset, *Herbal Drugs and Phytopharmaceuticals*, p. 116.

[36] Both J. Berendes, p. 19 and Max Aufmesser, Pedanius *Dioscurides aus Anazarba,* p. 33 translate this passage "it grows in India," misreading, perhaps, Ἰουδαία for Ἰνδία.

thin and hairy part of the shrub is called *eutheriston,*[37] perhaps because it is easily collected, since it is weak.
But the so-called *opobalsamon*[38] is extracted during the burning heat of the Dog Star by incising the tree with iron scrapers. However, only a small quantity of juice flows so that each year no more than six or seven *choes* are collected and a weight of it is sold locally for double the weight of silver.
**2.** The juice is of fine quality when fresh, when its scent is vigorous, pure, and not sharp, when it is easily diluted, when it is smooth, and when it is astringent and somewhat biting the tongue. But it is adulterated in a variety of ways. For some mix it with ointments as, for instance, terebinth, flower of henna, mastic, lilies, oil of ben tree nut, *metopion,*[39] honey, cerate of myrtle or very thin unguent of henna flowers. But this kind can easily be detected. For when dropped onto a woolen cloth and thoroughly washed out, that which is pure leaves neither stain nor spot, but the adulterated clings to it, and when sprinkled on milk it coagulates the milk, a thing that the adulterated juice does not do. Moreover, the unadulterated, when poured on milk or water, dissolving immediately, becomes milky, but the adulterated floats like oil, whirling and spreading out in a star-like manner. Yet, as time goes by, even the pure one deteriorates, thickening by itself.
**3.** But those who believe that the pure, when dripped on water, first sinks to the bottom then rises to the surface undissolved are mistaken. The wood called *xylobalsamon* passes muster when fresh, slender-stemmed, yellowish-red, fragrant, and smelling slightly like juice of Mecca balsam. But of the fruit—for it, too, is highly useful—choose that which is yellow, full, large, heavy, biting and burning in taste, and smelling slightly of juice of Mecca balsam. There is a seed brought from Petra resembling that of crispate St. John's wort with which

[37] "Easily harvested."
[38] This is the juice of Mecca balsam. Strabo, 16. 2. 41 says that it is a miracle cure for headaches, incipient cataracts, and dim sightedness and that it is very dear because it is produced only at Jericho. For a discussion on its species and habitats see J. Innes Miller, *The Spice Trade of the Roman Empire, 29 B.C. to 641 A.D.*, pp. 101-102.
[39] The term is used for an aromatic Egyptian ointment containing *metopon*, the resinous juice of allheal, *Ferula galbaniflua.* See Dsc. Bk. I, 59. It is also used for oil of bitter almonds. See Dsc. Bk. I, 33.

people adulterate the fruit. You will recognize it from the fact that it is bigger, empty, weak, and tasting like pepper.

**4.** It is the juice, however, that is the most efficacious, being capable of heating a great deal, of clearing off the elements that cast a shadow over the pupils of the eyes, and of counteracting uterine chills when applied with cerate of roses. It draws down both the afterbirth and embryos/fetuses and it dissipates fits of shivering when rubbed on. It also cleanses the sordid elements of sores. It is digestive as well as diuretic when drunk; it is suitable for those suffering from dyspnea, for those who have drunk leopard's bane with milk, and for those bitten by wild animals. It is compounded with analgesics, with emollients, and with antidotes, and, in general, the juice of Mecca balsam has the most efficacious properties, the fruit ranks second, and the wood is the least efficacious.

**5.** When drunk, the fruit is suitable for pleurisy, inflammations of the lungs, coughs, for patients suffering from hip disease, for epileptics, for dizziness, for those suffering for orthopnea, colic, difficult micturition, and for those bitten by wild animals; it is a good thing to use for making thick smoke from below to treat female problems and boiled down in sitz baths, dilating the cervix and absorbing moisture. As for the wood, it has the same properties as the fruit, except to a lesser degree. When boiled in water and drunk, it is helpful for indigestion, colic, venomous bites, and spasms, it is diuretic, and, with dried iris, it is suitable for head injuries; it also reduces epithelial waste. It is mixed also into the astringents of unguents.

### I, 20 ἀσπάλαθος, *Alhagi maurorum* L., Camel's-thorn[40]

Camel's-thorn, but some call it *erysisceptron,* others *sphagnos,* and the Syrians *diaxylon*: it is a woody shrub with many thorns growing in Nisyros, Syria, and Rhodes; perfumers use it as fixative. It is of fine quality when heavy and reddish or purplish after it has been stripped of its bark, dense, aromatic, and bitter in taste. There is also another

---

[40] See Jacques André, *Les noms des plantes dans la Rome antique*, p. 28 for a different identification by P. Fournier, R. PH, 24, 1950, pp. 172-178, who says that it is a kind of Astragalus.

kind of this plant, which is white, woody, devoid of taste, and decidedly inferior.
It has a warming property with astringency. It is for this reason that when boiled with wine and used as a mouthwash, it is suitable for thrush; when used as a wash, it is suitable for the filth around the genitalia, for spreading ulcers, and for fetid nose sores, and, when mixed in a pessary, it draws down the embryos/fetuses. Its decoction stays the bowels and the expectoration of blood when drunk, and it puts an end to difficult micturition and to flatulence.

### I, 21 βρύον, *Evernia* L., Tree moss

Tree moss, but some call it *splachnon*; it is found on trees of the cedar, white poplar, and oak families. The best grows on cedars and that on poplars is second best. It is good, if it is highly aromatic and light in color, but if it is somewhat black, it is inferior.
It has an astringent property that operates on uterine pathologies in decoctions for sitz baths. Because of the astringent element it contains, it is mixed both with unguents made from ben and with ointments, and it is well suited for making fragrant stuffs and analgesics.

### I, 22 ἀγάλοχον, *Aquilaria agallocha* Roxb., Aloewood/Eagle-wood

Aloewood is a wood brought from India and Arabia; it resembles thyine wood/citron wood. It is mottled, aromatic, rather astringent in taste with a degree of bitterness, and it has a leathery and somewhat variegated bark.
When chewed or when its decoction is used as a mouthwash, it sweetens the breath; it is a scented powder for the entire body, and it is burned in lieu of frankincense. A weight of one *drachma* of its root when drunk soothes excessive accumulation of stomach fluids, stomach limpness, and heartburn, and it helps people hurting in the side and liver, dysenterics, and the colicky when drunk with water.

### I, 23 νάσκαφθον, *Nascaphthon*

*Nascaphthon*, but some call it *narcaphthon*.[41] This one, too, is brought from India. It is like bast, resembling the bark of the mulberry tree. It

[41] In LSJ it is described as fragrant Indian bark, used as a spice, etc., perhaps the same as λάκαφθον, an aromatic bark, an ingredient of the Egyptian κῦφι, a compound

is burned for its sweet scent, it is mixed with man-made fragrances, and it helps for a constricted cervix when burned to produce thick smoke from below.

**I, 24 κάγκαμον, ~ *Commiphora kataf* Forsk., ~ *Styrax benzoin* Dryand., Bisabol**

Bisabol is the sap of an Arabian tree;[42] it looks somewhat like myrrh and it is foul tasting. People use it for incense; they also fumigate their clothing with it together with myrrh and storax.

It is reportedly capable of slimming obese people if a quantity of three *obols* is drunk with water or with vinegar and honey for several days. It is given to splenetics, epileptics, and asthmatics, and, when combined with hydromel, it draws down the menses. It quickly removes scars in the eyes, it treats dim-sightedness when diluted with wine, and for pyorrhea and toothache there is nothing better.

**I, 25 κῦφι, *Cyphi***

**1.** *Cyphi*[43] is an incense preparation that pleases the gods; the priests in Egypt use it lavishly. It is also mixed with antidotes and it is given to asthmatics in drinks. Many are the accounts proffered for preparing it and among them there is also this one: one-half *xestes* galingale, and an equal amount of ripe juniper berries, 12 *mnai* shiny seedless raisins, five *mnai* purified pine resin, one *mna* each of sweet flag, camel's-thorn, and camel hay, 12 *drachmai* myrrh, nine *xestes* old wine, and two *mnai* honey.

**2.** After removing the seeds from the raisins, cut and pound them in a mortar with the wine and myrrh, and, after pounding and sifting the other ingredients, mix them with the raisins and let them steep together for a day. Then boiling the honey until it reaches a viscous

---

incense. Jacques André, Les *noms des plantes dans la Rome antique*, p. 170, says that it is a spice of uncertain origin, the product of an Indian tree.

[42] Jacques André, ibid. p. 47 says that this is a gum of a poorly identified tree. See also J. Innes Miller, *The Spice Trade of the Roman Empire, 29 B.C. to 641 A.D.*, pp. 39 and 108-109.

[43] A compound incense that the Egyptians used as a drink to clean the inner parts of the body and as an ointment. Plutarch, *Moralia. Isis and Osiris,* 80, describes the composition of Egyptian *cyphi* (16 ingredients) and describes the ritual associated with its preparation.

consistency, mix carefully the melted pine resin; then rubbing in together carefully the remaining ingredients, stow in an earthenware vessel.

**I, 26 κρόκος, *Crocus sativus* L., Saffron**

**1.** The best saffron for medical purposes is the Corycian[44] and when it is fresh and well-colored, having a little bit of white on its pistil, longish, uniform, unbroken, intact, full, staining the hands when wet, neither moldy nor dried up, but attractive in scent and pungent. For if it does not fit this description, it is either old or it has been retted. Second to the Corycian is saffron that comes from Corycos that faces Lycia and the one from Lycian Olympus, and then that from Aigai in Aitolia. But the Cyrenaic and that from Centuripae in Sicily have no strength. All of them are vegetable-like. The inhabitants of Italy, however, use it to dye citron wood, since it is juicy and well colored and it is for this reason that it is sold for a great deal of money—but the one I mentioned first is used for drugs.

**2.** It is adulterated with a mixture of chopped saffron residuum and litharge or galena to give it weight, and it is daubed with concentrated must. The presence of dust and its musty smell give away these adulterants. It has digestive, emollient, somewhat astringent, and diuretic properties. It brings about a healthy complexion, it counteracts nausea when drunk with grape syrup and, when smeared on with woman's milk, it checks tearing of the eyes.

**3.** It is mixed advantageously with draughts for internal afflictions and with pessaries and poultices for the uterus and anus. It is aphrodisiac, it soothes inflammations caused by erysipelas when anointed, and it is useful for inflammations of the ears. But they say that it is also poisonous when an amount of three *drachmai* is drunk with water. To triturate it easily, it must be dried in the sun in a clean, warm, clay <vessel> and stirred rapidly. Even its root is diuretic when drunk with grape syrup.

---

[44] Corycos, a promontory in Cilicia, South Central Turkey. Strabo, *Geography*, 14.5.5, narrows the site even further and says, that the best saffron grows in the Corycian grotto, some twenty stadia from Corycos.

**I, 27 κροκόμαγμα, *Saffron* residuum**

One makes saffron residuum by squeezing the aromatics used in the preparation of unguent of saffron[45] then molding them. It is good when it is fragrant, smelling moderately of myrrh, heavy, dark, free of woody matter, decidedly saffron-colored when soaked, smooth, somewhat bitter, intensely coloring the tongue and teeth with color that lasts for several hours. The Syrian is of this sort.

It has properties that clean the elements that cast a shadow over the pupils of the eyes, are diuretic, emollient, aid digestion, and warm.

**I, 28 ἑλένιον, *Inula helenium* L., Elecampane**

**1.** Elecampane: but some call it *symphyton,* others *Persice*, others *Medice*, others *Orestion*, others *nectarion*, others *cleonion*, others *batos Idaia*, and others *phlomos Idaios*. It has leaves nearly resembling those of the narrow-leaved mullein but rougher and longish — and they are stemless; it has a root that is large, aromatic, somewhat pungent, and orange-tawny, from which off-shoots are taken for planting; they are just like the off-shoots on lilies and arums.

**2.** The root is dug up in the summer, and after it is cut up, it is dried. When drunk, its decoction sets micturition and the menses in motion. The root itself, consumed as a lozenge made with honey, is suitable for coughs, orthopnea, ruptures, spasms, flatulence, and bites of wild animals, being on the whole capable of heating. Its leaves boiled down with wine are plastered to good avail on people suffering from hip disease. Preserved in grape syrup, the root is also good for the stomach; vendors of pickled fruit dry it for a short time then, after boiling it down, sprinkle it with cold water, then place it in concentrated must and store it for use.

**I, 29 ἑλένιον ἄλλο, *Thymus incanus* L., Another elecampane**

Crateuas writes that there is a different elecampane[46] that grows in Egypt. It is an herb having twigs a cubit long lying flat on the ground like tufted thyme, but leaves that are similar to the lentil's, except they are longer and in profusion around the twigs; it has a pale root

---

[45] The aromatics are saffron and myrrh. See Dsc. Bk. I, 54.

[46] Jacques André, *Les noms des plantes dans la Rome antique*, p. 118 says that this is a species of thyme.

the thickness of a small finger, slender lower down, thicker higher up, having a dark bark. It grows by the seaside and on hillocks.

A single root can help those bitten by wild animals when drunk with wine.

### I, 30 ἔλαιον, Olive oil

**1.** For health purposes, the oil that was pressed from unripe olives is the best; it is called *omphacinon.* And of this oil the best is young, not pungent, and aromatic. This kind is also useful in the manufacture of unguents. Because of its astringency, it is good for the stomach, it both staunches the gums and firms the teeth when held in the mouth, and it is antiperspirant. But that which is shiny and aged is more suitable for preparations that soften. In general, however, all oils warm and soften the flesh, guarding the body from being easily chilled and making it better prepared for activity.

**2.** They ease and soften the bowel and they take the edge off abrasive medications. They are given also for poisons, being repeatedly drunk and vomited. A quantity of one *cotyle* drunk with an equal quantity of barley-water or plain water is purgative; a dose of six *cyathoi* boiled with rue is given to good avail to drink warm to the colicky; it ejects intestinal worms, and the same preparation is injected as a clyster in preference to all others for intestinal obstructions. Old oil warms more, it is more conducive to perspiration, and it is a salve for sharp-sightedness. But should old oil be unavailable, it is to be imitated as follows: pouring into a pot the strongest oil available, boil it down until it reaches the viscosity of honey and use it; for it has the same strength as the aforesaid.

**3.** Oil of the wild olive tree, on the other hand, is more astringent and while it ranks second for health use, it is more suitable for headaches than unguent of roses, and it checks both perspiration and the falling of hair. It also clears off dandruff, scurf, mange, and leprosy, and it delays the graying process when anointed daily.

Olive oil is made white this way: taking olive oil which is light-colored and no more than a year old, pour it into a new, wide-mouthed clay vessel — let there be a quantity of 100 *cotylai* — and setting it in the sun, stir it daily with a ladle from its center, using a downward

stroke from high up so that it may change and foam from the continuous mixing and beating.
**4.** On the eighth day, steeping 50 *drachmai* of clean fenugreek in warm water, drop it when softened, without squeezing out the water, into the oil afore mentioned. Add also an equal amount of burned out *pitys* pine chip; it should be as resinous as possible and splintered; leave it so for another eight days. At the end of this period, scoop up the oil with the ladle and, if the process has been successful, pour it out into a new vessel that was previously washed with aged wine and strewn with 11 *holcai* of dry melilot wreaths and an equal amount of iris and store. Otherwise, it must again be placed in the sun and worked until it becomes white.
**5.** From the oil described above, it is also possible to prepare Sicyonian oil this way: pouring into a wide-mouthed, tin-plated kettle one *chous* of white new olive oil, made from unripe olives, and one-half *chous* of water, bring to boil over a low fire, stirring gently. After it has come to a boil twice, withdraw the fire, and scoop out the olive oil when cool; then add fresh water, boil it with the olive oil, and after doing the rest as indicated above, store. This oil is made mostly in Sicyon and it is called Sicyonian. It has a moderately warming quality being suitable for fevers and for conditions affecting tendons. Women use it also as a cosmetic.
**6.** The <dirt>[47] that collects in bathrooms can warm, soften, and disperse; it is also <serviceable> in salves for chaps and callous lumps. Also the sweat from wrestling schools that has absorbed dust and that is like filth helps for chalkstones around the knuckles when plastered on them and those suffering from hip disease when applied hot instead of a softener or a hot compress. The filth both from the walls of gymnasia and from statues warms and disperses growths that refuse to be assimilated and is suitable for abrasions and old sores.

### I, 31 ἐλαιόμελι,[48] Olive tree sweet gum

Olive tree sweet gum flows from the trunk of olive trees throughout Palmyra, in Syria; it is thicker than honey and sweet in taste. A

---

[47] This dirt is a mixture of olive oil, moisture from the baths, and sweat.
[48] A compound word from ἔλαιον, "oil" and μέλι, "honey."

quantity of two *cyathoi* drunk with one *cotyle* of water removes undigested and bilious matter down the bowel. Those who take it, however, do become dazed and weak. No need to worry; but they must be forced to get up and not be allowed to fall asleep.
It is made also from the fat of their young branches. The best of it is aged, thick, rich, and not turbid. It heats, it is especially effective for the elements that cast a shadow over the pupils of the eyes when anointed, and it helps both for leprosy and pains around the tendons when rubbed on.

### I, 32 κίκινον ἔλαιον, Castor oil

**1.** Castor oil is prepared this way: taking as many ripe seeds of the castor oil tree as you think fit, and after drying them in the sun by spreading them out as one spreads grapes to dry in a sunny spot in the vineyard until the seed-coverings break and fall off, and after collecting their flesh, cast them into a mortar; then pounding them carefully, place them in a tin-plated pot containing water and boil applying heat from below. When they have released all the moisture they contain, lifting the pot from the fire, skim the floating oil with a spoon, and store.
**2.** But the Egyptians, because they use it in very large quantities, prepare it differently: having winnowed the seeds of the castor oil tree, place them in a mill and grind them carefully; then putting the grindings into baskets, press them with an utensil. Seeds of the castor oil tree are ripe when they detach themselves from the capsules that enclose them.
Castor oil is good for mange, scurf, boils on the buttocks, for uterine closings and twistings, also for unsightly scars and earaches; moreover, it makes the salves with which it is compounded more effective. It both drives watery matter down the bowel when drunk and it expels intestinal worms.

### I, 33 ἀμυγδάλινον ἔλαιον, Almond oil

**1.** Almond oil, which some call *metopion*, is prepared this way: after removing the skin and drying four *choinices* of bitter almonds, pound them lightly in a mortar with a wooden pestle until they form a ball, and, pouring over them two *cotylai* of hot water, let them absorb it for half an hour; then pound them again more vigorously. Then scraping them on a board, press them lightly and recover the paste from the fingers with a spoon; then again pouring over the mass one *cotyle* of water and allowing the paste to absorb it, repeat the process. One *tetrachoinicon* yields one *cotyle* of almond oil.

**2.** It is efficacious for uterine pains and uterine suffocation,[49] for twistings and inflammations in the same areas, moreover, for headaches, for earaches, for ringing and for singing in the ears. It does benefit kidney patients, people experiencing difficult micturition, those suffering from stones, from asthma, and from spleen disease. In combination with honey, root of white lily, and either henna cerate or rose cerate, it removes facial blemishes, freckles, and wrinkles, and it is curative of dim-sightedness. With wine, it clears scurf and dandruff.

### I, 34 βαλάνινον, Oil from the nut of the ben tree[50]

Oil from the nut of the ben tree is similarly prepared. It is capable of clearing blemishes, birthmarks, facial eruptions, black pigmentations

---

[49] The modern English term for uterine suffocation is hysteria, although it is no longer used in psychiatric parlance. It has been replaced by "conversion symptom" on the grounds that in states of hysteria there is conversion from emotional to physical manifestations, Ilza Veith, *Hysteria: The History of the Disease*, Preface p. VIII. In Ancient Egypt, the condition was referred to as the "wandering womb" and in the Georg Ebers papyrus, which dates back to the 16th c. B.C., the chapter on Diseases of Women is devoted largely on hysteria, Ilza Veith, ibid. pp. 2-4. Several Greek medical writers have described the condition as affecting the uterus, where it starts, the carotids, the heart, and the membranes of the brain. Languor, paleness, loss of speech, fear, then rigidity of limbs are some of its manifestations. When the attack abates so do the symptoms diminish and the patient slowly recovers her normal composure. See Soranus, *Gynecology*, III. 4. 26-30; Paulus Aegineta, III. 71, 1: 633. Plato, *Timaeus* 91c describes uterine suffocation this way: "…whenever the matrix, or womb, as it is called, — which is an indwelling creature desirous of child-bearing — remains without fruit long beyond the due season, it is vexed and takes it ill; and by straying all ways through the body and blocking up the passages of the breath and preventing respiration it casts the body into the uttermost distress and causes, moreover, all kinds of maladies; until the desire and love of the two sexes unite them." There is also a description of uterine suffocation in Celsus, *De medicina*, Bk. IV. 27. 1.

[50] For LSJ βαλάνινον is oil of zukkum, spelled also zachum, and derived from the bito tree, *Balanites aegyptiaca*. For Jacques André, *Les noms des plantes dans la Rome antique*, pp. 32-33, it is made from the nut of the ben tree. See further Dsc. Bk. IV, 157.

of scars, and of softening the stool. But it is bad for the stomach. Infused with goose fat, it is suitable for earaches, for ringing and for singing in the ears.
Similarly to the above oils are prepared sesame oil from sesame seed and walnut oil from walnuts. They have the same properties as oil from the nut of the ben tree.

**I, 35 ὑοσκυάμινον, Oil of henbane**

Oil of henbane is prepared this way: taking the white seed dry and pounding it while new, mix it with hot water as indicated above in the passage on almond oil; then after bringing to the top the parts at hand that are getting to be dry, mix them with the rest, and continue doing so until it becomes black and ill-smelling; then passing it through a sieve, put it up. It is good for earaches and it is mixed with suppositories since it is emollient.

**I, 36 Κνιδίου κόκκου, Oil from berries of spurge flax**

Oil from berries of spurge flax is prepared the same way with berries that were skinned and pounded. When drunk, it purges the bowel.
Safflower oil is also made the same way. Its property is the same as that of oil made from berries of spurge flax, although it is not quite as strong.

**I, 37 ῥαφάνινον, Oil of radish**

Oil of radish is prepared from its seed like the other oils. It is suitable for those afflicted by pediculosis and it clears roughnesses on the face. The people in Egypt use it, boiling it with their side dishes.
Oil of black cumin has the same properties and method of preparation as oil of radish.

**I, 38 σινάπινον, Mustard oil**

They make mustard oil by triturating mustard seed, wetting it with hot water, then mixing it with oil and straining it. It is efficacious for chronic ailments, since it alters the state of pores.[51]

---

[51] Asclepiades of Prusa is the originator of the theory that disease is the result of stopped pores. See Dsc. Bk. I, n. 8.

**I, 39 μύρσινον, Oil of myrtle**

**1.** Oil of myrtle is prepared this way: after collecting the tender leaves of the black myrtle, be they of the wild or of the cultivated kind, pound them, squeezing them vigorously; then mix with their juice an equal amount of oil of unripe olives and heat gently over coals until they boil together, removing the scum. But there is an easier method, which is to boil in water and oil the leaves that are tender, having first pounded them, and to skim the scum. Some individuals, however, drop the leaves into the oil and steep them in the sun. And some thicken the oil beforehand with pomegranate peels, cypress, galingale, and camel hay.

**2.** It is stronger when it is somewhat bitter and oily in taste, pale-green, translucent, and when it smells of myrtle.

It has astringent and hardening properties. It is for this reason that, having been mixed with healing substances, it is efficacious for burns, scurf, dandruff, pustules, abrasions, chaps, callous lumps, weak joints, perspiration, and for everything that needs either astringency or contraction.

**I, 40 δάφνινον, Oil of sweet bay**

**1.** Oil of sweet bay is made from tree-ripened bay berries cooked in water. For the membrane that surrounds them releases some grease, which, after it has been broken by hand, is scooped up with a spoon. But some, after thickening oil of unripe olives with galingale, camel hay, and sweet flag, throw on top sweet bay leaves and cook them together; others add also bay berries until the oil becomes quite aromatic, and others mix both storax and myrtle.

**2.** The mountain sweet bay and the broad-leaved sweet bay are best for making it; oil of sweet bay is of excellent quality when it is fresh, pale-green in color, very bitter, and pungent.

It has properties that warm, soften, open up, and lessen weariness. It is suitable for all afflictions of tendons, for shivering fits, earaches, catarrhs, and headaches. But it also causes nausea when drunk.

**I, 41 σχίνινον, Oil of mastic**

Oil of mastic,[52] prepared the same way from the ripe fruit <of the mastic tree or> pre-thickened like oil of sweet bay, cures the mange of herds and of dogs, and it is advantageously compounded with suppositories, analgesics, and medications for leprosy. It also checks perspiration. Oil of terebinth, too, is made the same way. It dries and contracts.

**I, 42 μαστίχινον, Mastic oil**

**1.** Mastic oil[53] is made from triturated mastic resin. It is good for all uterine complaints, warming gently, contracting, and softening, for indurations that spread over the stomach, for bowel ailments, for dysenteric diseases, and for facial blemishes, cleansing and achieving a fresh and healthy complexion. The best is made on the island of Chios.

**2.** And because unguents, too, are suitable for certain conditions, both when mixed with medicines and when rubbed on as lotions or when smelled, we think it reasonable to report also on them. In considering an unguent, it is essential to notice whether it smells of the unguent for which it is named. Such test is the best. However, because of the dominance of stronger compounds, some unguents do not keep their smell, as in the case of unguent of marjoram, saffron, fenugreek, and certain others that must be approved on the basis of one's experience with them.

**I, 43 ῥοδίνου σκευασία, Preparation of unguent of roses**

**1.** Preparation of unguent of roses:[54] five *litrai* eight *oungiai of* camel hay, 20 *litrai* five *oungiai* of olive oil. After chopping and softening the camel hay with water, boil while stirring, then strain, add into the

---

[52] Both oil of mastic, σχίνινον, and mastic oil, μαστίχινον, described in Dsc. Bk. I, 42, below, are products of the mastic tree, *Pistacia lentiscus*. The former is made from its fruit, the latter from its resin.

[53] See Dsc. Bk. I, n. 52.

[54] Beginning with ch. 43, Preparation of unguent of roses, through ch. 56, Thickening of unguent of iris, the style differs from the balance of the chapters. Not only are the quantities for each prescription very large but also the weights and measures are Sicelo-Greek as opposed to Attic, Goodyear, *The Greek Herbal of Dioscorides* p. 30.

20 *litrai* five *oungiai* of the oil the petals of 1,000 unmoistened roses, and having rubbed your hands with aromatic honey, stir several times applying gentle pressure. Then leaving it alone overnight, express it. After the dregs have settled, change the receiving vessel and lay it aside in a bowl that was coated with honey. Then placing the pressed petals into a washing tub, pour over them eight *litrai* three *oungiai* of the thickened oil and squeeze the liquid out again. This will be your second oil.

**2.** And if you so desire, after pouring over them up to a third or fourth moistening, squeeze out; and so is made the first, second, third, and fourth unguent. And as often as you do so, smear first the vessels with honey. But if you wish to make a second insertion of petals, throw into the oil which was first pressed out the same number of fresh, unmoistened rose petals and stirring with your hands, which you previously moistened with honey, press out, and make the second, third, and fourth unguent, expressing it as before. And as often as you do this, add fresh rose petals: for it does become stronger.

**3.** The oil accepts the addition of rose petals up to the seventh insertion and no more. Be sure also to rub the basin with honey. You must separate carefully the oil from the juice. For even the least amount of juice carried along ruins the unguent. But some crushing only the rose petals themselves, steep them in oil and, changing it every seven days until the third steeping, store it this way. Others first thicken the oil by adding sweet flag and camel's-thorn and others add also alkanet for good color and salt as preservative.

**4.** It has properties that are astringent and cooling suited for lotions and mixtures for poultices. When given to drink, it also loosens the bowel and abates heartburn; it causes hollow sores to heal up, it soothes malignancies, it is an unguent for scurf and cutaneous eruptions, a lotion for incipient headaches, and a mouthwash for toothaches. When anointed, it is good for hardened eyelids and, when used as a clyster, it is useful for intestinal irritations and uterine inflammations.

**I, 44 ἐλατίνου σκευασία, Preparation of unguent of date palm inflorescence**

Preparation of unguent of date palm inflorescence: after crushing and shredding the inflorescence of date palm, place it in a tub, pour over it oil of unripe olives, and leave it for three days; then lifting it into a sieve squeeze it out. But be sure that the two ingredients are of equal weight; then store tidily in a vessel and use. Its properties are analogous to those of unguent of roses, but it does not soften the bowel.

**I, 45 μελίνου σκευασία, Preparation of unguent of quince**

**1.** Preparation of unguent of quince: mixing six *xestes* of olive oil with 10 *xestes* of water, add three *oungiai of* crushed spathes of palm inflorescence and one *oungia of* camel hay, and, setting it aside for a day, boil; then straining the oil, put it into a wide-mouthed jar, place on top a reed mat or a loosely woven rush mat and on top of that lay quinces, and cover them with cloths; set aside for several days until the oil has absorbed the strength of the quinces.

**2.** But some having wrapped the quinces in cloths for ten days so that their sweet smell be contained and not dissipated into the atmosphere, steep them in olive oil for two days and nights, then strain and store.

It has astringent and cooling properties that are effective for scabby sores, dandruff, chilblains, shingles, and uterine ulcerations when injected; it controls urinary inflammations when used as a clyster and it stops sweating. It is also drunk against blister beetles, poisonous beetles, and the processional caterpillar.[55] It is of excellent quality if it smells of quinces.

**I, 46 οἰνανθίνου σκευασία, Preparation of unguent of wild vine inflorescence**

Preparation of unguent of wild vine inflorescence: after drying the aromatic inflorescence of the grape vine, place it into oil of unripe olives and stir turning it upside down. Leave it alone for two days, strain, and store.

---

55 πιτυοκάμπη a stinging and urticating caterpillar of the pinewoods. Its identification with the processional caterpillar is tentative.

It has an astringent property that corresponds to that of unguent of roses, except that it does not loosen nor soften the bowel. Of this unguent, too, the best smells decidedly of wild vine inflorescence.

**I, 47 τελίνου σκευασία, Preparation of unguent of fenugreek**

**1.** Preparation of unguent of fenugreek: nine *litrai* fenugreek, five *litrai* olive oil, one *litra* sweet flag, two *litrai* galingale. Steep well the dry ingredients in the oil for seven days, stirring three times daily, then strain and store. Some, however, steep together cardamom instead of sweet flag and Mecca balsam wood instead of galingale. And others first thicken the oil with these ingredients and then steep the fenugreek and strain.

**2.** It is capable of softening abscesses and of aiding digestion. It is especially well suited for all indurations in the area of the uterus, it is an instillation for women having difficulty giving birth, whenever the vagina becomes very dry after the fluids have been carried off, and for anal inflammations; it is also used successfully in clysters for tenesmus, it clears dandruff and scurf, in combination with wax it is beneficial for burns and chilblains, it clears freckles, and it is mixed into cosmetics.

Choose that which is fresh, smells faintly of fenugreek, cleanses the hands, and tastes bittersweet. For this kind is the best.

**I, 48 σαμψουχίνου σκευασία, Preparation of unguent of marjoram**

**1.** Preparation of unguent of marjoram: take tufted thyme, cassia, wormwood Artemisia *arborescens*, flowers of bergamot mint, myrtle leaves, and marjoram, taking into consideration the strength of each of these ingredients. Pound them all in the same container and pour over them enough oil of unripe olives as not to overpower the properties of the ingredients it soaks; leave it alone for four days and press; then soak again the same quantity of the same fresh ingredients for the same length of time, and press. For it is stronger this way. Choose it dark olive in color, smelling of much marjoram, and moderately sharp.

**2.** It has warming, attenuating, and sharp properties. It is efficacious for closings and twistings of the uterus, it draws down the menses and the afterbirth, it revives those in a state of uterine suffocation, and it soothes pains of the lower back and groin. But because it hardens the *pudenda muliebra* with its excessive astringency, it is best used with honey. Rubbed on, it also abates pain and it is advantageously mixed into poultices for patients suffering from tetanic recurvation and on those who for some reason or other have spasms.

### I, 49 ὠκιμίνου σκευασία, Preparation of unguent of basil

Preparation of unguent of basil: taking 20 *litrai* of olive oil scented with flowers of henna, as we will describe below (I, 55), and after stripping the leaves of 11 *litrai* eight *oungiai* basil, by weight, soak them for a night and a day in the oil, then strain and set aside. Then empty out the contents from the strainer and again pour over them the same quantity of the oil and squeeze. This is called *deutereion*; they do not tolerate a third soaking. Then taking again the same quantity of fresh basil, soak, as described in the chapter on unguent of roses (I, 43), pour over them the oil used in the steeping process, and letting them in it for the same length of time, strain and store. And if you like, you may add and soak basil three or four times, which should always be fresh. It can also be made with oil of unripe olives. But the other way is best.

It accomplishes the same things as unguent of marjoram, although less effectively.

### I, 50 ἀβροτονίνου σκευασία, Preparation of unguent of wormwood *Artemisia arborescens*

Preparation of unguent of wormwood Artemisia *arborescens*: cast into nine *litrai* five *oungiai* of oil scented for making unguent of henna flowers eight *oungiai* of leaves of wormwood *Artemisia arborescens* and after soaking them for a night and a day squeeze them out. But if you wish to infuse it several times, after removing the first leaves and adding new ones, soak and squeeze them out.

It has a warming property, which is effective for uterine closings and indurations and which draws down the menses and the afterbirth.

### I, 51 ἀνηθίνου σκευασία, Preparation of unguent of dill

Preparation of unguent of dill: eight *litrai* nine *oungiai* olive oil, 11 *litrai* eight *oungiai* dill flowers. Soak the dill flowers in the oil for a day and then squeeze them with your hands and store. But should you wish to prepare it with a double infusion, soak similarly new flowers of dill.

It is able to soften the areas around the uterus and to dilate. It is suitable for recurring shiverings, warming and abating weariness, and it is beneficial for pains in the joints.

**I, 52 σουσίνου σκευασία, Preparation of unguent of lily**

**1.** Preparation of unguent of lily, which some call *leirinon*: mixing nine *litrai* five *oungiai* olive oil, five *litrai* 10 *oungiai* sweet flag, and five *drachmai* myrrh with fragrant wine, boil; then filtering the oil, pour it over three *litrai* six *oungiai* cardamom that was chopped and soaked in rainwater and, after allowing it to become well soaked, strain. Then taking three and one-half *litrai* of the thickened oil and after stripping the leaves of 1,000 white lilies place them in a wide basin, not a deep one, and pouring the oil over them, stir with your hands having first coated them with honey. Leaving it alone for a day and night, in the morning, transfer into a strainer and press out.

**2.** Immediately strain and separate the oil from the water that was squeezed out with it. Because just like unguent of roses it does not tolerate it, but it heats up with it, bubbles up, and spoils. Decant several times into different vessels previously smeared with honey, sprinkling fine salt and removing carefully the dirt that collects. Transferring the pressed aromatic herbs from the strainer into the basin, pour over them again the same quantity of scented oil as before, and add 10 *holcai* chopped cardamom, stirring vigorously with your hands; and after a short while strain, removing impurities from the run-off.

**3.** Pouring over them scented oil a third time, repeat the process, adding the cardamom, too, and similarly salt, and daubing your hands with honey and pressing. The product of the first straining will be the best, that of the second straining will be the next best, and of the third will be rated the least good. Then, after taking again 1,000 white lilies, stripping their leaves, arranging them, and pouring over them the olive oil from the first straining, proceed according to the directions, doing the same things you did to the first batch, mixing in cardamom, then strain and do the same things to the second and third batch, as described, adding also the cardamom; and as often as you soak new white lilies, so often your unguent will be stronger.

**4.** Finally, when you think you have enough, mix into each batch two *drachmai* good myrrh, two *drachmai* cinnamon, and 10 *drachmai* saffron. But others recommend to make it this way: having chopped and sifted equal quantities of saffron and cinnamon, place them in the basin with water and pour over them the first batch of strained unguent; then allowing a short time to pass, transfer into dry vessels previously daubed with gum, myrrh, saffron, and honey diluted with water. Do the same to the second and third pressings.

**5.** Still others prepare the unguent uncompounded, using oil from the nut of the ben tree or some other oil and white lilies. The best is reputedly made in Phoenicia and Egypt. It is excellent if it smells of white lilies.

It has properties that warm, soften, open uterine closings and boils, and in general, it is the most useful of all substances for women's diseases. It is also good for scurf, cutaneous eruptions, dandruff, and eczemas; it diffuses quickly bruises and makes them uniformly colored and it is through and through rarefying. When drunk, it also draws the bile down the abdomen and it is diuretic. But it is bad for the stomach and it causes nausea.

**I, 53 ναρκίσσινον, Preparation of unguent of narcissus**

You will thicken unguent of narcissus this way: nine *litrai* five *oungiai* of washed oil; six *litrai* two *oungiai* of camel's-thorn, chopped and steeped in water. Mixing the camel's-thorn with one third of the oil, boil; then removing the camel's-thorn and after chopping up five *litrai* eight *oungiai* sweet flag and a lump of myrrh, and after passing them through a sifter, combine them with aged aromatic wine, and having mixed them, boil. When the oil has boiled up also with these ingredients, remove from the heat, filter the oil when cool, then taking of the oil[56] … pour into a basin and add as many narcissus flowers as you can, stirring for two days, as described

[56] By analogy, the lost words indicated by the dots may have been ἐξελὼν τὰ ἀρώματα, "removing the aromatics".

in the section on unguent of lily, then strain and decant several times. For this one, too, spoils.
It is good for uterine problems, softening indurations and closings in the area of the uterus. But it causes headaches.

**I, 54 κρόκινον, Preparation of unguent of saffron**
**1.** In preparing unguent of saffron you will first thicken the oil as described in the section on unguent of lily, using the same quantities and weights. Taking three and one-half *litrai* of olive oil, which was thickened for unguent of lily, add 50 *drachmai* saffron, and stir several times a day, doing so for five consecutive days. On the sixth day, filter off tidily the oil from the saffron, pour over the same saffron the same quantity of the oil, and stir for 10 days; then pouring the oil out, add 40 *drachmai* myrrh pounded and sifted, and stir well in a bowl, then store. But some use oil scented for making unguent of henna also for unguent of saffron. The best smells strongly of saffron and it is this kind that is fit for medicinal uses; second best is that which smells like myrrh.
**2.** It has heating and soporific properties, wherefore it is appropriately used often on patients suffering from phrenitis either in compresses, or as an inhalant, or smeared on their nostrils. It makes pus, it cleanses sores, it is good for uterine indurations and closings, and for malignancies within the uterus with wax, saffron, marrow, and with a double amount of oil. For it furthers maturation, softens, soothes, and moistens. Laid on with water, it is also efficacious for cataracts.[57] The unguents called *onychinon*,[58] *boutyrinon*,[59] and *styracinon*[60] are

[57] The word used here is ἀπογλαύκωσις, "formation of a γλαύκωμα," that is of a "cataract." Throughout *De material medica*, Dioscorides uses several different terms that appear to mean "cataract." In addition to ἀπογλαύκωσις, they are: ἀχλύς, νεφέλιον, λεύκωμα, ὑπόχυμα, ὑπόχυσις, and τὰ ἐπισκοτοῦντα ταῖς κόραις. Aufmesser, *Erläuterungen,* translates all these words as "cataract" and so have I, except as follows, where I have used the LSJ definitions: ἀχλύς, "mist over the eyes," νεφέλιον, "cloud-like opacity on the eye," and τὰ ἐπισκοτοῦντα ταῖς κόραις, "those elements that cast a shadow over the pupils." Throughout the text, I am translating ἄργεμον as "albugo."
[58] Made from the aromatic substance *onyx.* Not identified. See also Dsc. Bk. I, 67, I, n. 81, and Dsc. Bk. II, 8.
[59] Made of butter.

analogous to it, resembling it closely in preparation and efficacy; they differ only in their names.

### I, 55 κυπρίνου στύψις καὶ σκευασία, Thickening and preparation of unguent of henna

**1.** Thickening and preparation of unguent of henna:[61] one part clarified oil of unripe olives and one and one-half parts rainwater. Pour some water over the oil and mix the balance with the aromatics that will be added. Then taking five and one-half *litrai* camel's-thorn, six and one-half *litrai* sweet flag, one *litra* myrrh, three *litrai* nine *oungiai* cardamom, and nine *litrai* five *oungiai* oil, and after chopping the camel's-thorn and soaking it by placing it in water, cook it with the oil until they boil together. Then soaking the myrrh in aromatic old wine, mix the sweet flag chopped up with the myrrh, and, removing the camel's-thorn, add the mixture of sweet flag.

**2.** After it has boiled also with it, take it off the heat; strain the oil from the cauldron, pour it over the cardamom which was chopped and mixed with the remaining water, and stir non-stop with a spatula until it cools. Then after straining the oil, cast into every 28 *litrai* of oil, 46 *litrai* eight *oungiai* henna flowers, and letting them become well steeped, strain through a basket. But should you wish more, adding the same quantity of new flowers, express them the same way; also if you wish to prepare it with a double or triple infusion. For it does grow stronger.

**3.** You must select that unguent which is of good quality and overpoweringly aromatic. Some add also cinnamon.

It has heating, softening, and dilating properties, which are suitable for afflictions around the uterus and tendons, for sufferers from pleurisy, and for fractures, being used by itself as well as mixed with cerate. It is compounded with emollients suitable for tetanic recurvation, for sore throat, and for inflammation of the groin, as well as with analgesics.

---

[60] Made of storax.

[61] This recipe begins with ratios rather than fixed quantities: One part of clarified oil of unripe olives and one and one-half parts of rainwater; the oil is mixed with some water, reserving some for blending the aromatic. Then very large quantities of dry stuff, roughly 5,550 grams, are mixed with a rather small quantity of liquid, roughly 3,090 grams, an absurd ratio, as J. Berendes, p. 74, points out.

**I, 56 ἰρίνου στύψις, Thickening of unguent of iris**

**1.** Thickening of unguent of iris: after chopping as finely as possible six *litrai* and eight *oungiai* spathes and combining them with nine *litrai* and five *oungiai* of olive oil, mix with 10 *cotylai* of water then, placing the mixture into a cauldron, boil until the oil becomes scented, then strain into a bowl that has been smeared with honey. It is from this scented oil that the first unguent of iris is prepared, by steeping iris in the thickened oil, as indicated.

**2.** But others recommend the following procedure: boil nine *litrai* five *oungiai* olive oil with five *litrai* two *oungiai Mecca* balsam wood, chopped as specified; then removing the Mecca balsam wood, add nine *litrai* 10 *oungiai* chopped sweet flag and a lump of myrrh moistened with aged aromatic wine; then taking 14 *litrai* of the thickened and aromatized oil, steep in it an equal weight of chopped iris; leave it for two days and two nights and strain it by pressing hard and vigorously. And should you wish it to be stronger, steep in like manner two and three times the same weight of iris and strain.

**3.** The best smells only of iris and of nothing else. Such is the unguent of iris that is made in Perge of Pamphylia and that made in Elis of Achaia.

It has emollient and heating properties. It cleanses scabs, putrid humors, and filth; it is suitable for problems in the area of the uterus, for inflammations, and for stoppages; it aborts embryos/fetuses, and it opens up hemorrhoids. In combination with vinegar, rue, and bitter almonds, it is suitable for ringing ears, for chronic catarrh, the nostrils being anointed with it, and for fetid nasal polyps.

**4.** When an amount of one *cyathos* is drunk, it purges the bowel, it is good for intestinal obstructions, and it is diuretic. <It is fit> for those having difficulty vomiting, smearing it either on the fingers or on the emetics, for people who have a sore throat, either as an ointment or as a gargle combined with water and honey, and for roughness of the trachea. It is also given to those who have drunk hemlock or mushrooms or coriander.[62]

---

[62] See Dsc. Bk. III, 63, where the ingestion of too much coriander seed "dangerously disturbs the thinking process."

**I, 57 γλεύκινον, Unguent of new sweet wine**

The simple unguent of new sweet wine is made from oil of unripe olives and from camel hay, sweet flag, Celtic spikenard, spathe,[63] camel's-thorn, melilot, costusroot, and new sweet wine, masses of pressed grapes being placed around the vessel containing the aromatics, wine, and oil. It is stirred twice a day for thirty days, and then, after it has been expressed, it is stored.

It has heating, softening, and relaxing properties, which are good for shiverings and for all conditions relating to contracted tendons and the uterus. It is more effective than all other analgesics, being emollient.

**I, 58 ἀμαράκινον, Unguent of marjoram**

**1.** Unguent of marjoram that is made at Cyzicus is the best. Its is prepared both from oil of unripe olives and oil from the nut of ben tree, which are thickened with Mecca balsam wood, camel hay, and sweet flag and seasoned with marjoram, costusroot, Nepal cardamon, spikenard, cassia, fruit of the Mecca balsam, and myrrh. But some people make it more sumptuous by mixing also cinnamon. Honey and wine are also used for daubing the vessels and for mixing the chopped aromatics.

**2.** It has heating, soporific, softening, opening, burning, and diuretic properties; it is serviceable for putrefying sores, abscesses, and hydroceles ensuing from surgery; it breaks scabs and malignant sores; it is suitable for difficult micturition being smeared on the urinary orifice, for inflammations of it, and for opening hemorrhoids being smeared on them; it sets the menses going when applied to the cervix; it dissipates uterine indurations and swellings, and it is good for muscle pains and injured tendons when sprinkled on a loosely textured woolen cloth and applied.

**3.** As for the unguent called *Megalleion*,[64] it used to be made long ago, but it is no longer found. Yet it is not out of place to remark on it also, so as to make my account all-inclusive. <Its> preparation is the same

---

[63] See Dsc. Bk. I, 109.

[64] So named after its inventor Megallos. See T. Kock, ed., *Comicorum Atticorum Fragmenta,* Ar. *Fr.* 536, Stratt. 33. In Goodyer, *The Greek Herbal of Dioscorides*, p. 40, n. 1, however, it is suggested that it is named after Megale, near Syracuse.

as that of unguent of marjoram, but it abounds in pine resin and therein it differs. It is mildly emollient. It should be pointed out that pine resin is combined with unguents neither to preserve them nor to make them more pleasurable, but for color and viscosity. Resin of the terebinth tree boiled down until it becomes odorless is mixed therein. Boiling directions will be set forth in the section on pine resin (I, 71.) Also the unguent called *hedychroun*, which is made at Cos, has both the same properties and the same method of preparation as unguent of marjoram, but it smells sweeter.

**I, 59 μετώπιον, *Metopion***

**1.** In Egypt, they make an unguent which they call locally *metopion,* because they mix in it *chalbane*:[65] for the wood from which *chalbane* is made is called *metopon.* It is composed of bitter almonds, oil of unripe olives, cardamon, camel hay, sweet flag, honey, wine, myrrh, fruit of the Mecca balsam, resinous juice of allheal, and pine resin. It is of excellent quality when it is oppressive in scent and greasy, smelling more of cardamon and myrrh than of the resinous juice of allheal.

**2.** It intensely heats, it burns, it opens up, it draws and cleanses sores, and it is good for torn tendons and muscles as well as for septic hydroceles. It is mixed both with emollients and with cerates, and it useful for shivering fits and for those who suffer from tetanic recurvation. It is sudorific, it opens up what needs opening round the uterus, it loosens uterine indurations, and, on the whole, it has an emollient property.

**3.** The unguent called *Mendesion* is made with oil from the nut of the ben tree, cassia, and pine resin. Some, after weighing out the ingredients, add a small quality of cinnamon cassia, but to no useful purpose. For substances that have not been cooked together do not release their properties. Its activity is similar to that of *metopion*, although to a lesser degree, nor does it last as long.

---

[65] Χαλβάνη is the resinous juice of allheal, *Ferula galbaniflua.*

**I, 60 στακτή, *Stacte***

*Stacte* is called the oily substance from fresh myrrh,[66] pounded with a small quantity of water, and pressed with a tool. It is highly aromatic and very expensive, [and] being in its own right the unguent called *stacte.* It is of excellent quality when not mixed with oil and when even the tiniest amount possesses a great deal of strength, when it warms, and when it is comparable to myrrh and to those unguents that warm.

**I, 61 κιναμώμινον, Unguent of cinnamon**

**1.** Unguent of cinnamon is prepared from oil of nut of the ben tree, from astringents of Mecca balsam wood, sweet flag, and camel hay, and from aromatics of cinnamon, fruit of Mecca balsam, and four times more myrrh than cinnamon. Honey, too, is added when mixing them. Excellent is that which is not harsh, mild in scent, smelling of myrrh, viscous, highly aromatic, and bitter in taste. For this kind acquires its viscosity not from pine resin but from myrrh. For pine resin adds neither bitterness nor aroma.

**2.** It has exceedingly sharp, warming, and bitter properties. It does open up while warming, and it dissipates, disperses, and absorbs liquids and odors. But it causes headaches. Combined with a double amount of olive oil, wax, and marrow, it is also effective for ailments in the area of the womb. For when used this way it loses much of its sharpness and becomes emollient; otherwise it inflames and indurates more violently than all other viscous unguents. With cardamon, it is palpably effective for abscesses, putrid humors, hydroceles, carbuncles,[67] and gangrenes; it is also effective in salves for recurring shiverings, for tremblings, and for those bitten by poisonous animals, and it is applied with ground figs on those bitten by scorpions and poisonous spiders.

[66] See Dsc. Bk. I, 64.

[67] ἄνθρακες, translated here as "carbuncles", but according to some it means "smallpox". See LSJ s.v. ἄνθραξ.

**I, 62 νάρδινον μύρον, Unguent of spikenard**

Unguent of spikenard is prepared in different ways, with the leaf of Malabar[68] as well as without it. But by and large it is compounded with oil from the nut of the ben tree or of unripe olives. They add camel hay to thicken the oil, and costusroot, Nepal cardamom, spikenard, myrrh, and Mecca balsam to make it sweet smelling. It is of good quality when it is light, not sharp, and when it smells of dry spikenard or of Nepal cardamom.

It has attenuating, sharp, cleansing, and heating properties. But unless it contains pine resin, it is fluid and not glutinous. It is also prepared inexpensively with oil of unripe olives, camel hay, sweet flag, costusroot, and spikenard.

**I, 63 μαλαβάθρινον Unguent of the leaf of malabar**

Unguent of the leaf of malabar has the same thickeners as unguent of spikenard, but it contains more myrrh. It is for this reason that it warms, having the same properties as unguents of saffron and of marjoram.

**I, 64 σμύρνα, *Balsamodendron myrrha*, Myrrh**

**1.** Myrrh is the resin of a tree which grows in Arabia and which resembles the Egyptian acacia. When the tree is incised, the resin drips from it on mats spread beneath, but some of it congeals around the trunk. There is one kind of myrrh called *pediasios lipara*;[69] from it stacte[70] is obtained by pressing it; there is another kind called *Gabirea liparotate*,[71] growing on fertile and rich soils, which also yields a great deal of *stacte.* But the best is the Troglodytic,[72] named from the land that produces it; it is pale, biting, and translucent. There is also one kind called *lepte*,[73] ranking second to the Troglodytic; it is soft like bdellium, somewhat malodorous, and it grows in sunny spots.

---

[68] See Dsc. Bk. I, n. 26.
[69] "Field-grown fatty."
[70] See Dsc. Bk. I, 60.
[71] "Gabirea very fatty."
[72] Derived from the Troglodytes, name of an Ethiopian people.
[73] "Fine."

**2.** But the one called *causalis* is well past its prime, dark and dried up; and the worst of all is called *ergasime*, being dry and devoid of fatty substance, harsh; it resembles gum in appearance and efficacy; worthless, too, is that which is called Minaian.[74] They even make tablets from them. From fatty myrrhs, the tablets are aromatic and fatty, but from the dry, they are devoid of fatty substance and aroma and they are weak due to the addition of oil during the shaping process. Myrrh is adulterated by mixing it with gum that was soaked in an infusion made from myrrh.

**3.** Select that which is fresh, crumbling, light, uniformly colored and having white, nail-like, and smooth internal separations when broken; also choose it small-lumped, bitter, aromatic, pungent, and capable of warming. But if it is heavy and pitch-like in color it is useless.

It has heating, soporific, agglutinative, desiccative, and astringent properties. It both softens the uterus and opens it when closed,[75] and when applied with an infusion of wormwood Artemisia *absinthium* or lupine, or with the juice of rue, it also draws rapidly down both the menses and embryos/fetuses.[76] It is taken as a little pill the size of a bean for chronic coughs, orthopnea, pains of the side and chest, diarrhea, and dysentery.

**4.** It is also good for shivering fits, if two hours before their onslaught an amount the size of a bean is drunk with pepper and water, and it mends roughness of the trachea and hoarseness of voice when placed under the tongue and sucked. It kills intestinal worms, it is chewed against bad breath, and it is smeared with a liquid astringent to combat armpit odor. Used as a mouthwash with wine and oil, it strengthens teeth and gums. Dusted on head-wounds, it mends them. Smeared on with snail flesh, it heals bruised ears and exposed bones and in combination with opium poppy juice, castor, and horned poppy juice it heals pussy and inflamed afflictions of the ears.

---

[74] There are several different readings in the codices for *Minaia*, e.g. *aminnea*, *aminea*, etc. *Minaia* draws strength from Galen, XIV, 68 who writes "some call it Minaian from a place throughout which they say the most wonderful [myrrh] is produced."

[75] See Dsc. Bk. I, n. 21.

[76] See Dsc. Bk. I, n 15.

**5.** It is applied with cassia and honey for facial eruptions, it wipes off lichen-like skin eruptions with vinegar, and it strengthens falling hair when smeared on with gum ladanum, wine, and unguent of myrtle. It also soothes chronic catarrhs when smeared on the nostrils with a feather brush. It fills out sores in the eyes and it cleanses both leucomas[77] and the elements that cast a shadow over the pupils of the eyes; it also clears off trachomas. There is also soot made from it in the same manner as soot from frankincense, as we shall demonstrate below (I, 68,) which is suitable for the same purposes.

**I, 65 Βοιωτικὴ σμύρνα, Boiotian myrrh**

Boiotian myrrh,[78] on the other hand, is the chopped root of a certain tree that grows in Boiotia. Choose that which resembles myrrh in scent. It has warming, emollient and relaxing properties. It is also compounded profitably with fragrant stuffs.

**I, 66 στύραξ, *Styrax officinalis* L., Storax**

**1.** Storax is the sap of a tree that resembles the quince tree. The best is yellow, fatty, and resinous; it has whitish lumps, its scent lasts for a very long time and, when softened, it releases some honey-like moisture. Such are the Gabalitic, Pisidian, and Cilician storaxes, but storax that is black, friable, and bran-like is inferior. There is also a sap resembling gum and which is translucent and myrrh-like; this, however, is scarce. They adulterate storax by mixing wood dust from its tree that is produced by worms with honey, dregs of iris, and certain other ingredients.

**2.** Some, after odorizing wax or suet, soften it thoroughly with storax when the days are very hot and sunny, squeeze it through a strainer with wide holes into cold water forming little worms, and sell it, calling it *scolicites.*[79] Those who are inexperienced regard this kind as

---

[77] See Dsc. Bk. I, 55 and n. 57.

[78] Robert Gunther, the editor of Goodyer, *The Greek Herbal of Dioscorides*, p. 43, n.1, says that "It has been suggested that this is ἱπποσέλινον, alexanders, *Smyrnium Olusatrum* because Theophrastus notes that it produces tears like myrrh." On alexanders see Dsc. Bk. III, 67.

[79] I. e. worm-like.

genuine, paying no attention to its scent. For storax that has not been adulterated has a penetrating smell.
It has warming, emollient, and digestive properties. It is effective for coughs, catarrhs, discharges from the nostrils, hoarseness of voice, loss of voice, and ringing in the ears.
**3.** It is suitable both for cervical stoppages and indurations, it draws down the menses when drunk and when applied, and it gently softens the bowel when a small amount is swallowed with turpentine. It is combined profitably both with emollients and analgesics. It is burned, toasted, roasted and made into soot just like frankincense, and its soot is suitable for the same purposes as that of frankincense. The ointment that they manufactured from it in Syria warms and softens a great deal. It does, however, cause headaches and it is heavy and soporific.

### I, 67 βδέλλιον, *Commiphora mukul* Engl., Bdellium

**1.** Bdellium — which some call *maldacon* and others *blochon* — is the sap of an Arabian tree.[80] It is excellent when bitter in taste, translucent, resembling bull's-hide glue, greasy in its interior and easily molded, free of wood and dirt, sweet smelling when passing into fumes, and resembling *onyx*.[81] There is also a kind, which is greasy and black, chunky, *palathe*-like,[82] and which is imported from India. Bdellium is also brought dry, resinous, and somewhat black, from Petra; it ranks second in strength. People adulterate it with gum; however, the kind that has been adulterated leaves a different sort of bitterness on the taste buds and it is not as sweet smelling when passing into fumes.
**2.** It is able to heat, soften, and dissolve indurations, tumors of the throat, and hydroceles when applied with the saliva of someone fasting. Applied directly or burned for fumigations, it opens up the cervix,[83] and it draws out the embryos/fetuses[84] and all moisture. It

[80] See J. Innes Miller, *The Spice Trade of the Roman Empire, 29 B.C. to A. D. 641*, pp. 69-71.
[81] *Onyx* here is the lid of a cockle which feeds on spikenard and which smells nice when burned. See Dsc. Bk. II, 8.
[82] *palathe* is a cake of preserved fruit.
[83] See Dsc. Bk. I, n. 21.
[84] See Dsc. Bk. I, n. 15.

both shatters stones and draws down the urine when drunk, and it is given successfully to those who cough and to those bitten by wild animals. It is good for ruptures, spasms, pain in the side, and intestinal rumblings. It is also mixed with emollients that are suitable for indurations and for mending tendons. It is prepared for use by pounding it while pouring over it wine or hot water.

**I, 68 λίβανος, *Boswellia* sp.,[85] Frankincense**

**1.** Frankincense is produced in Arabia, the land called "frankincense-bearing". The male, which is called *stagonias,* ranks first; it is naturally round. This kind is uncut and white; when crumbled, it is greasy inside, and when set afire, it burns quickly. The Indian is both yellowish and dull in color and it is even made artificially round. For they cut it into square shapes and after placing them into earthenware vessels roll them around until they acquire the round shape; but as time goes by, this kind, which is called *Syagrios*,[86] becomes yellow. *Orobias*[87] ranks second as does also *smiliotos*, which some call *copiscos*, being smaller and more yellow.

**2.** There is also one called *amomites*;[88] it is otherwise white and when worked on, it becomes malleable like mastic. All frankincense is adulterated being treated with *pitys* pine resin and gum. But it is easy to determine whether it has been adulterated, because gum does not blaze up when set afire and the resin vanishes into smoke, but frankincense flares up. Smell, too, betrays frankincense that has been adulterated.

It can contract, heat, cleanse the elements that cast a shadow over the pupils of the eyes, fill and cicatrize ulcerated cavities, mend bloody wounds, and keep in check all hemorrhages including from membranes.[89] Used ground up in a dressing with milk, it soothes

[85] I am grateful to Otta Wenskus for suggesting in his review of the first edition that λίβανος might have been best identified as *Boswellia* sp. instead of *B. carterii* on the grounds that frankincense derives from a variety of Boswellias. See Bibliography.

[86] Deriving its name from a promontory by the same name in Arabia, present day Ras Fartak.

[87] Deriving from ἐρέβινθος, "chick-pea."

[88] ἀμωμίτης, " like Nepal cardamom."

[89] The term μῆνιγξ/μήνιγγες means "membrane/membranes" and "meninges," LSJ. For Max Aufmesser, *Erläuterungen,* μῆνιγξ means only meninges, the membrane that

malignancies around the anus and elsewhere, and when anointed with vinegar and pitch, it removes incipient warts that spread under the skin[90] and lichen-like eruptions.

**3.** With goose or pork fat, it treats both burns and chilblains; applied as a cleansing ointment with soda, it treats dandruff, with honey, whitlow, and with pitch, broken ears; but for the rest of ear ailments it helps being poured into the ears with sweet wine; it also helps breasts inflamed in consequence to giving birth if smeared on them with Cimolian earth and unguent of roses. It is mixed profitably with medications for the trachea as well as for the bowels, and when drunk it benefits patients who cough up blood. But it does cause madness when drunk by the healthy and it is even lethal when too much is drunk with wine.

**4.** They burn frankincense by placing it on a clean earthen vessel and setting it afire from below with a morsel of frankincense lit with a candle until it burns. But it must bc covered with some type of lid after it is fully burning until it goes out; for this way it does not burn to ashes. But some place around the container a hollow, brazen vessel, perforated in the middle, to capture the soot, as we shall show below in the discussion on soot of frankincense.[91] Others, however, placing it in an unfired earthen pot and plastering it all over with clay, burn it in the oven. It is also parched on a new earthenware container on top of red-hot coals until it no longer bubbles nor emits any greasiness or any moist vapor. It brakes easily when fully burned.

**5.** The best bark of frankincense is thick, greasy, aromatic, fresh, smooth and neither rough nor fibrous. It is adulterated, however, by

---

surrounds the brain and spinal chord. This membrane includes the pia mater, arachnoid and dura mater. Dsc. uses μῆνιγξ/μήνιγγες five times, I, 68, 2. 11, 49, 1, 72, 2; 79, 1, and 87; V, 84, 2 and ὕμην, "membrane" once, in V, 139. I suggest that in all six passages, the application of the cure is upon an external "membrane" rather than on the "meningeal membrane."

[90] Throughout *De materia medica* Dioscorides uses several terms for warts. 1) μυρμηκία, "wart that spreads under the skin;" it is also the "irritation" it causes, which was compared to the creeping of ants, μύρμηκες. 2) ἀκροχορδών, which differs from μυρμηκία in that it has a thin neck. 3) ἧλος, "wart" but it also means "callus." Throughout this translation I have translated ἧλος as "wart." 4) θύμιον, "large wart." 5) θύμος, "warty excrescence." All definitions are from LSJ.

[91] At the end of this chapter.

mixing it with bark of *strobilos* pine or of *pitys* pine.[92] But for these, too, the test is fire. For the rest of the barks when burned do not ignite, but vanish into smoke without a sweet scent, but the bark of frankincense lights up and passes off into sweet smelling fumes. It, too, is burned exactly like frankincense.

It has the same properties as frankincense, although it is more effective and more astringent; wherefore it is better suited for people who cough up blood when drunk and for women suffering from fluxes when used in a pessary. It is also good for scars in the eyes, corneal ulcers, and filth. Parched, it is effective also for ulcerative blepharitis.

**6.** Powder of frankincense is of excellent quality when white, clean, and granular. It has the same properties as frankincense but to a lesser degree. Some, however, in adulterating it, mix with it sifted resin of pitys pine and fine meal, or bark of brayed frankincense. Here, too, fire puts these to the test, because it will not smolder evenly nor with the same intensity, the vapor being thin as air, sooty, and impure, and the scent has a compounded effluvium.

**7.** Make soot of frankincense this way: grasping with a pair of tweezers one lump of frankincense at a time and after holding it close to a flame, place it in a hollow, new pan; cover it with a concave brazen lid perforated in the middle and carefully cleaned, and place under one of its sides or under both sides small stones four fingers high to reveal whether it burns and to create a space for adding ever more lumps; before the first lump is completely burned add another until you think enough soot has been collected. But make sure to wipe continuously all around the external parts of the brazen lid with a sponge of cold water; this way all soot settles on the lid, because it is not very hot; otherwise it falls down on account of its lightness and it gets mixed with the ash of the frankincense.

---

[92] The identification of pines is hopelessly confusing. Thus, in LSJ, πίτυς is pine, especially Corsican pine, *Pinus laricio*, but it is also Aleppo pine, *Pinus halepensis*, as well as the stone pine, *Pinus pinea. Strobilos*, too, is rendered as stone pine, but with the botanical identification Pinus *cembra,* and *peuce* is another name for Corsican pine, *Pinus laricio.* In view of these difficulties pines will not be translated but rendered only in transliteration. See also Jacques André, *Les noms des plantes dans la Rome antique,* p. 200 where he says that πίτυς ever since Ennuis and Cato referred to different kinds of pines.

**8.** Therefore, scraping off the first soot, repeat the process as long as you think that you need to and move aside the ash of the frankincense that was thoroughly burned. It is capable of soothing inflammations of the eyes, checking discharges, cleansing sores, filling cavities, and stemming erosive sores. Soot of myrrh, of resin, and of storax is similarly prepared. They are suitable for the same purposes. In a like manner obtain soot also from the rest of the saps.

**I, 69 πίτυς, *Pinus*, *Pitys* pine**[93]

**1.** The *pitys* pine is a familiar tree. Of the same kind is also the pine called *peuce,* although it differs in form. The bark of both is astringent; ground up, it is a suitable plaster for abrasions, and, with litharge and frankincense powder, for superficial sores and third degree burns. When made up with cerate of myrtle, it cicatrizes sores on tender skin and keeps in check spreading ulcers when applied ground with a solution of copper sulfate;[94] burned to produce thick smoke from below, it expels embryos/fetuses[95] and the afterbirth and when drunk it checks diarrhea and sets micturition going.

**2.** Their leaves,[96] too, ground up and plastered on, assuage boils and keep wounds free of inflammations; triturated and boiled in vinegar they soothe toothaches when used as a warm mouthwash; one *holce* of leaves drunk with water or with a mixture of hydromel is suitable for sufferers from liver disease. Both the bark and leaves of *strobilos* pine do the same when drunk; also when a small piece of their wood is finely splintered and boiled in vinegar, it stops a toothache if the decoction is held against the infected tooth; even spatulas are made from them, which are handy for preparing analgesics and pessaries.

---

[93] See n. 91 above.

[94] Blue vitriol.

[95] See Dsc. Bk. I, n. 15.

[96] The "leaves" here are pine needles. There is no word in ancient Greek for pine needle and Theophrastus, *H. P.*, 1. 10. 4 in describing the various differences of greenery, writes "there are various other differences between leaves; some trees are broad-leaved, as vine fig and plane, some narrow-leaved, as olive pomegranate myrtle. Some have, as it were, spinous leaves, as fir, Aleppo pine, prickly cedar..." and later in 1. 10. 6 he writes "Leaves differ also in their shapes; some are round, as those of pear, but some are divided and like a saw, as those of the silver-fir..."

**3.** While they burn, their soot is collected for writing ink; it is also good for painting the eyelashes and eyelids, for eroded corners of the eyes, for loss of eyelashes, and for tearing eyes.
*Pityides* are called the nuts found in the cones of *pitys* and of *peuce* pines. They have an astringent and somewhat warming property; taken either by themselves or with honey, they help for coughs and for chest ailments.
**4.** Shelled nuts of *strobilos* pine when eaten or when drunk with grape syrup and cucumber seed are diuretic and apt to dull burning sensations around the bladder and kidneys; taken with juice of purslane, they assuage gnawing stomach pains, they tone up flaccid bodies, and they decrease loss of liquids. *Strobilos* pine nuts, gathered intact from the tree, ground fresh, and boiled in grape syrup, are good for persistent coughs and tuberculosis when an amount of three *cyathoi* of their liquid is drunk daily.

**I, 70 σχῖνος, *Pistacia lentiscus* L., Mastic**
**1.** The mastic is a well-known tree, astringent in its entirety; for its fruit, leaf, bark of its branches and of its root have the same properties. Juice is made from its bark, root, and leaves boiled in water for a long time, then after cooling, the leaves are discarded and the liquid is boiled again until it reaches a honey-like consistency.
Being astringent, it is effective for coughing up blood, diarrhea, and dysentery when drunk; also for uterine bleeding and for uterine and anal prolapses. And in general, it is possible to use it instead of shittah tree or hypocist.
**2.** The juice of its pressed leaves also effects the same results. Their decoction, when poured over unfilled cavities, fills them, mends bones which do not form a callus, checks uterine discharges, prevents spreading ulcers, and is diuretic. Used as a mouthwash, it also firms up loose teeth. Small, green pieces of its wood, rubbed against the teeth instead of toothbrushes, clean them. From its fruit, they also make astringent oil, which is suitable for things that need thickening.
**3.** This tree produces also a resin, which is called *schinine*, but others call it *mastiche*. When drunk, it is useful for blood coughing and for old coughs. It is good for the stomach and it promotes eructation; it is mixed with dentifrices as well as with unguents for the face because it

makes it shine; it also glues on eyelashes, it sweetens the breath when chewed, and it staunches the gums. It is produced of excellent quality and in abundance on the island of Chios. It is outstanding when it shines and when it is like Tyrrhenian wax in whiteness, when it is thick, air-dried, brittle, and sweet smelling; but that which is pale-green is inferior. They adulterate it by mixing it with frankincense and resin of the *strobilos* pine.

**I, 71 τέρμινθος, *Pistacia terebinthus* L., Terebinth**

**1.** The terebinth is a well-known tree. Its leaves, fruit, and bark, being astringent, are well suited for the same purposes as the mastic tree when similarly prepared and used. Its fruit is edible, difficult to digest, warming, and diuretic. It is an excellent aphrodisiac and when drunk with wine, it is good for bites of venomous spiders.[97]

Its resin is brought from that part of Arabia that is near Petra; but it is also produced in Judea, Syria, Cyprus, Libya, and the Cycladic islands. It is, indeed, of good quality, if it is quite translucent, clear, glassy in color, aromatic, and smelling of terebinth.

**2.** Terebinth resin surpasses all resins; resin of mastic is ranked below it, then *pitys* pine and fir resins, among which are also ranked both *peuce* pine and *strobilos* pine resins.

All resins are capable of warming, softening, relaxing, and provoking vomiting. They are suitable to use in lozenges for coughs and for tuberculosis either by themselves or with honey, and they thoroughly cleanse impurities from the chest. They are both diuretic and further digestion, they also soften the stool; they are suitable, too, for attaching eyelashes, for leprosy with verdigris, a solution of copper sulfate,[98] and soda, for ears running with serous matter with honey and oil, and for itching of the genitalia.

**3.** They are blended with plasters, emollients, and analgesics, and they help for pains in the side when rubbed on by themselves or when plastered on.

Liquid resins are produced from *pitys* pine and *peuce* pine; they are brought from Gaul and Etruria; formerly, liquid resin was also

[97] Specifically, the *lathrodectus and malmignatte.*

[98] Blue vitriol.

imported from Colophon, whence it was surnamed *Colophonia* and from that part of Galatia that boarders the Alps; the inhabitants there call it in their language *larica*;[99] it is an excellent remedy in a lozenge and by itself for chronic coughs. These resins, too, differ in color; for there is one which is colorless, another is of the color of oil, another resembles honey as does Venice turpentine.

**4.** Liquid resin is also made from the cypress tree; it is efficacious for the same conditions. But of the dry resins, one is made from *strobilos* pine, another from fir, another from *peuce* pine, and another from *pitys* pine. Choose among all of these that which is most fragrant and translucent, neither brittle nor very moist, wax-like, and easily broken. The best among them is the resin of the *pitys* pine and of the fir; for they are aromatic and smell like frankincense. A variety of resins are imported from the island of Pityousa, which lies along the coast of Spain.[100] Those from *peuce pine*, *strobilos* pine, and cypress are rather inferior and do not have the same properties as the others but they are taken for the same purposes as the others. The resin of the mastic tree definitely corresponds to that of the terebinth tree.

**5.** All liquid resins are heated in a vessel four times as large as the amount of liquid poured into it; for after placing in a brazen cauldron one *chous* of resin and two *choes* of rainwater, you must boil gently over coals, stirring constantly until it becomes odorless, easily breakable, and dry enough to give to the touch; then after cooling, you must store it in an unpitched earthenware vessel. It does become extremely white. But you must first strain all resins by melting them down to separate the dirty element.

**6.** They are also heated without water over coals, at first gently; then, when they are at the point of congealing, you must place underneath them much coal all at once and boil continuously for three days and three nights until they acquire the unique feature already mentioned. Then store as described. But to store the dry ones, it will really be sufficient to boil them for an entire day. Burned resins are useful for scenting emollients, for analgesics, and for coloring unguents. They

---

[99] Venice turpentine, *terebinthina veneta* from the larch, *Larix decidua.*

[100] There are two islands by the name of Pityousa off the coast of Spain: Ebesus (Ibiza) and Ophiussa (Fementera). See Strabo, 3. 5. 1, where they are described.

also collect soot of resin the same way as from frankincense, which is useful for paints of the eyelids and eyelashes, for ulcerated corners of the eyes, for damp eyelids, and for tearing eyes. Ink, with which we write, is also made from it.

### I, 72 πίσσα, Pitch

**1.** Raw pitch, which some call *cona,* is collected from very greasy wood of *peuce* pine and of *pitys* pine. It is good when it shines, when it is smooth, and when it is clean.

A quantity of one *cyathos* taken as a lozenge with honey is effective for deadly poisons, consumptives, patients with internal abscesses, coughs, asthma, and for severe congestion in the chest; it is also effective for inflammations of the tonsils, of the uvula, and for sore throats when smeared on, for serous discharges from the ears when applied with unguent of roses, and for snake bites when plastered on with fine grains of salt.

**2.** Mixed with an equal amount of wax, it removes psoriatic nails and it dissipates uterine growths and anal indurations. Boiled with barley meal and a child's urine, it breaks scrofulous swellings in the glands;[101] smeared on with sulfur or with the bark of *pitys* pine or with bran, it keeps in check shingles; mixed with frankincense powder and a salve, it glues draining passages; smeared on, it is suitable for fissures both on the feet and anus; with honey, it fleshes out and cleans sores, and, with raisins and honey, it detaches carbuncles and dead flesh. It is combined advantageously also with septic medications.

**3.** There is also pitch oil made from pitch by separating the liquid element of pitch. For it stands on the surface pretty much like whey and it is removed by means of a clean woolen cloth suspended during the boiling process over the pitch; when the cloth becomes drenched by the rising steam, it is squeezed out into a vessel, and this is done as long as the pitch boils. It is good for as many conditions as is liquid

---

[101] Dioscorides uses several terms to signify swellings of glands: φύγεθλον, "swelling of the glands, esp. of the groin and armpit; " χοιράς, "scrofulous swelling of the glands of the neck, etc.," φλεγμονὴ βουβώνων, "inflammation of groin [glands];" παρωτίς, "tumor of the parotid gland."

pitch. Plastered on with barley meal, it restores hair on bald spots. This pitch oil and raw pitch treat both animal sores and mange when smeared on.

**4.** And there is also soot that is made from raw pitch as follows: placing a small amount of the pitch in a new lamp that has been outfitted with a wick, light it; then covering the lamp with a new earthenware vessel that is shaped like a *clibanos*,[102] on top being round and narrow, below having holes as do the *clibanoi*, let it burn. When the first moisture is expended, pour more, until you have accumulated enough soot, and use it. It has sharp and binding properties. It must be used for paints for the eyelids and eyelashes, for ointments, whenever hair needs to grow on eyelids that have been afflicted by purulent blepharitis, for weak eyes, for eyes that do not tear, and for ulcerated eyes.

**5.** Dry pitch is made from boiling raw pitch. Some call it *palimpissa.*[103] Some of it is sticky, called *boscas,* and some dry. It is good when clean, greasy, aromatic, somewhat yellow, and resinous. The Lycian and <the> Bryttian are of this kind, laying claim to two natures, to that of pitch and at the same time to that of resin. It is capable of warming, softening, suppurating, dispersing growths and swellings of glands, and fleshing out sores. It is also profitably mixed with wound medications.

Some say that *zopissa* is the resin that is scraped with the wax from ships, which some call *apochyma*,[104] being able to dissolve, because it is bathed in seawater; others, however, call by this name the resin of the *pitys* pine.

### I, 73 ἄσφαλτος, Asphalt

**1.** Asphalt from Judea far surpasses the rest. It is of fine quality when shining purple, lively in scent, and heavy; but that which is black and dirty is poor, for they adulterate it, mixing it with pitch. It is produced also in Phoenicia, Sidon, Babylon, and Zacynthos. Up and down the

---

[102] κλίβανος is a covered clay vessel wider at the bottom than at the top used for baking bread by putting hot embers around it, LSJ.

[103] I. e. "pitch boiled again."

[104] "That which is poured off."

land of the Agrigentes of Sicily, a liquid floats on wells which people use in their lamps instead of oil and which they call incorrectly Sicilian oil, for it is a type of liquid asphalt.
And there is something called pitch-asphalt, produced in Apollonia, near Epidamnos; it is carried down from the Ceraunian Mountains by the rush of the river and it is cast on the shores in condensed lumps, smelling of pitch mixed with asphalt.
**2.** There is also a kind called naphtha; it is the filtrate of Babylonian asphalt, being white in color, although it is also found in black. It is highly flammable so that it can catch fire even from afar; it is useful for cataracts and leucomas.
All asphalts have properties that are anti-inflammatory, agglutinative, dispersive, emollient, and beneficial for uterine suffocations and prolapses when applied, smelled, or burned to produce thick smoke from below. They also check epileptic attacks just as lignite stone does when burned to produce thick smoke.
**3.** When drunk with wine and castor, they set the menses going, and they are helpful for chronic coughs, asthma, tics, dyspnea, snakebites, and for pains of the hip joints and of the side. They are given as a small pill to those with bowel ailments; drunk with vinegar, they dissolve blood clots; melted down with barley gruel, they are administered as a clyster to dysenterics; when burned to produce thick smoke, they cure catarrhs and they soothe toothaches when plastered around the aching tooth. Dry asphalt heated in an ear spoon,[105] glues on hairs,[106] and when combined with bruised meal of raw corn, wax, and soda and applied as a cataplasm, it helps the gouty and arthritic. Pitch-asphalt, however, is capable of all the things that pitch and asphalt combined are capable of doing.

### I, 74 κυπάρισσος, *Cupressus sempervirens* L., Cypress

**1.** The cypress binds and cools. Its leaves when drunk with grape syrup and with a small amount of myrrh are good for bladder

---

[105] The instrument used is a μελωτίς, "probe." It often has a concavity at one end very much like a spoon. Tiny μελωτίδες were used for the removal of earwax and were common articles associated with women's toiletries.
[106] Hair, here, is most likely eyelashes.

incontinence[107] and for difficult micturition. Its small pale-green berries, chopped up and taken in a drink with wine, are good for coughing up blood, dysentery, diarrhea, orthopnea, and coughs. Their decoction, too, does the same. Chopped up together with a fig, they soften indurations and they treat polyps in the nostrils.

**2.** Boiled with vinegar and triturated with lupines, they remove scaly nails, applied as a plaster, they draw in intestinal hernias, and the leaves do the same. Its small berries, when burned with the foliage, are reputed even to repel mosquitoes. The leaves ground up and plastered over wounds mend them and are antihemorrhagic, and when triturated with vinegar dye hair. They are plastered on by themselves as well as with barley groats to treat erysipelas, shingles, carbuncles, and inflammations of the eyes. Mixed with a cerate, they strengthen the stomach when placed on it.

### I, 75 ἄρκευθος, *Juniperus* L., Juniper

Juniper: there is one kind that is tall and another that is dwarf. Both heat and attenuate; they are also diuretic and when burned so as to produce smoke they drive away wild animals. As for its berry, one kind is of the size of filberts and the other is like small beans, round, and aromatic, sweet when chewed, and yellowish. The berry is called *arceuthis*; it is moderately warming and astringent, good for the stomach, effective for chest diseases, coughs, flatulence, colic, and malignant ulcers when drunk. It is also diuretic. It is for this reason that it is suitable for spasms, ruptures, and for uterine suffocations.

### I, 76 βράθυ, *Juniperus Sabina*, L., Savin

The savin which some call *boraton.* There are two kinds of this tree: one kind resembles the cypress in foliage, but it is thornier and oppressive in smell and, as far as trees are concerned, it is stunted, spreading itself considerably sideways; its leaves are used for incense. The other has leaves that resemble those of the tamarisk.

---

[107] I am in agreement with Max Aufmesser, *Pedanius Dioskurides aus Anazarba,* p. 63, who translates κύστει ῥευματιζομένῃ, as *Blaseninkontinenz* bladder incontinence, For his discussion on ῥεῦμα, ῥευματίζομαι, ῥευματικός, ῥευματισμός, ῥέω see his Erläuterungen, pp. 437-438 where he separates the instances where ῥεῦμ- refers to 'flow' from those where it refers to 'rheumatism of the joints.'

The leaves of both kinds halt spreading ulcers and assuage inflammations when pasted on; they remove black spots when laid on with honey, and they loosen dirt and carbuncles. When drunk, they draw down blood through the urine and they expel embryos/fetuses. Used topically or burned to produce thick smoke from below, they do the same. They are also mixed with unguents that warm and, in particular, with the unguent that is made with sweet new wine.

### I, 77 κέδρος, *Juniperus* L., Cedar

**1.** The cedar is a tall tree[108] from which the so-called *cedria*[109] is collected. It has berries just like the cypress, but considerably smaller. There is also another cedar that is dwarf, thorny, producing berries just like the juniper, of the size of a myrtle-berry, and round. The best *cedria* is that which is thick and translucent, robust, heavy in scent, and when dribbled remains globular and does not spread out. It has properties that on the one hand promote decay of live organisms and on the other hand preserve corpses. It is for this reason that some called it also "life of the dead". It also destroys both clothing and leather goods due to the intensity of its heating and drying action.
**2.** It is suitable for eye medications, bringing about sharp-sightedness when anointed, and it clears both leucomas and scars. Used as a rinse with vinegar, it kills earwigs, injected with a decoction of hyssop, it stops ringing and hissing in the ears, and, when instilled into a tooth's cavity, while it does shatter the tooth, it also stops the pain. It accomplishes the same result also as mouthwash with vinegar. Anointed all around the genitalia prior to sexual intercourse, it causes barrenness, it is an ointment for sore throats, it helps for inflammations of the tonsils, it destroys lice[110] and their eggs when smeared on, it is a helpful plaster with salt for bites of the horned serpent,[111] and when taken with grape syrup it is an antidote to drinking sea-hare.[112]

---

[108] This is the Syrian cedar, κέδρος μεγάλη *Juniperus excelsa* L. as opposed to the κέδρος μικρά, *Juniperus communis* L.
[109] I. e. resin.
[110] The medical term for infestation of lice is pediculosis.
[111] *Cerastes cornutus.*
[112] *Aplysia leporina.*

**3.** Taken in lozenge form or when smeared on, it helps those afflicted by elephantiasis; when one *cyathos* is gulped down, it clears and treats lung sores; used as a clyster, it destroys grubs and intestinal worms and it draws down embryos/fetuses.
There is also an oil which is separated from *cedria* by means of a woolen cloth suspended over it during the boiling process, as described in the chapter on pitch;[113] it is good for all the things that *cedria* is good. This oil, when rubbed on vigorously, is a singularly effective treatment for the mange of quadrupeds, both dogs and cattle, it destroys their ticks when applied, and it cicatrizes wounds that are the result of shearing.
**4.** Its soot, which has the same properties as soot of pitch, must be collected the way one collects soot of pitch.
The berries of the Syrian cedar are called *cedrides*. They have properties which warm and which are bad for the stomach. But they do help for coughs, spasms, ruptures, and strangury. They both draw down the menses when ground fine and drunk with pepper and they are taken with wine as an antidote to drinking sea-hare. They even ward off wild animals if they are rubbed on the body with deer fat or marrow. People mix them also with antidotes.

**I, 78 δάφνη, *Laurus nobilis* L., Sweet bay**
**1.** The sweet bay: one kind is narrow-leaved and another has broader leaves. Both warm and soften and it is for this reason that their decoctions in sitz baths are well suited for ailments around the bladder and uterus. Of their leaves, those that are freshly sprouted are mildly astringent; ground fine, they are beneficially plastered on wasp and bee stings and they are capable of assuaging all inflammations if daubed on with bread and barley meal, but they weaken the stomach and cause vomiting when drunk.
**2.** The bay berries, on the other hand, warm more than the leaves. Ground fine they are efficacious for tuberculosis, orthopnea, and rheums in the chest area when taken as a lozenge with honey or grape syrup. They are drunk with wine for scorpion bites and they clear dull-white leprosies. The juice that is pressed out of them, injected into the

---

[113] See Dsc. Bk. I, 72.

ears with aged wine and unguent of roses, helps for earaches, ringing in the ears, and hardness of hearing; it is also mixed with analgesics, with ointments that warm, and with resolvent medications. The bark of their root breaks stones, kills embryos/fetuses, and helps those suffering from liver disease when a quantity of a *triobolon* is drunk with aromatic wine.

**I, 79 πλάτανος, *Platanus orientalis* L., Plane**

The leaves of the plane tree that are tender, boiled in wine and plastered on, stem discharges from the eyes and they do relieve both their swellings and inflammations. Its bark, boiled with vinegar, is a mouthwash for toothaches. Its globular catkins, drunk when fresh with wine, help those bitten by snakes and they treat burns when smeared on with suet. But should the fine down of the leaves and of the globular catkins creep into the eyes and ears, it inflicts damage to sight and hearing.

**I, 80 μελία, *Fraxinus ornus* L., Manna ash**

The manna ash is a well-known tree. The juice of its leaves as well as the leaves themselves when drunk with wine and when applied as a plaster help those bitten by vipers. Its bark removes leprosies when burned then smeared on with water. But they say that its wood-shavings are poisonous, if one drank them.

**I, 81 λεύκη, *Populus alba* L., White poplar**

The bark of white poplar helps for hip diseases and strangury when an amount of one *oungia* is taken in a drink; it is reported that it also causes barrenness[114] when drunk with the kidney of a mule, and it is said that the leaves do the same when taken with vinegar following

---

[114] Dioscorides uses the following expressions relating to conception: σύλλη(μ)ψις, "conception, pregnancy;" ἀσυλληψία, "inability to conceive, barrenness;" ἀσύλληπτος, "not conceiving, preventing conception;" ἀτόκιος, -ον, "causing barrenness." All definitions are from LSJ. I have followed them here and throughout this translation. These definitions, however, will have to be reexamined because in today's English to be barren means to be incapable of producing offspring, to be sterile, and I do not believe that Dioscorides directives aim at sterility but rather at preventing pregnancy.

menstruation. Instilled tepid, the juice of the leaves helps also for earaches. The globular catkins that appear during the sprouting of the leaves, ground up and anointed with honey, treat dim-sightedness. Some report that the bark of the white and of the black poplar, cut up into small pieces and strewn on garden-plots previously fertilized with manure causes edible mushrooms to grow in all seasons.

**I, 82 μάκιρ, *Holarrhena antidysenterica* Wall., Mace**

Mace is a bark brought from abroad; it is yellowish, thick, and very astringent in taste. It is drunk for coughing up blood, dysentery, and diarrhea.

**I, 83 αἴγειρος, *Populus nigra* L., Black poplar**

The leaves of black poplar, plastered on with vinegar, help for gout pains. Its resin is compounded with emollients. Its fruit, when drunk with vinegar, is reported to help epileptics. It is said that the sap of black poplars, as it runs down on the river Eridanus,[115] congeals and becomes the so-called amber, which some call it *chrysophoron*.[116] It is aromatic when rubbed and golden in color. When drunk ground up, it checks diarrhea and fluid discharges from the stomach.

**I, 84 πτελέα, *Ulmus glabra* L., Elm**

**1.** The leaves, branches, and bark of the elm are astringent. The leaves are effective for leprosy when plastered on ground up with vinegar and they close up wounds; but the bark is even more effective when wrapped around wounds instead of a bandage because it is fibrous. An amount of one *oungia* of rather thick bark, when drunk with wine or cold water, brings up phlegm. A decoction of its roots or leaves poured over fractures knits them quickly. The liquid found in its seed-capsules when it begins to bud, if applied on the face, cleanses it, but as this liquid dries up, it resolves itself into gnat-like creatures.

**2.** The leaves that are tender are even used as cooked vegetables for side dishes.

---

[115] Originally a mythical river and only later identified with the Po.

[116] "Wearing gold."

The decaying matter that is compacted from its dead wood and stumps, sprinkled like meal, cleanses and cicatrizes sores. Mixed with an equal amount of anise oil, burned on a linen cloth, and plastered on smoothly controls spreading ulcers.

### I, 85 κάλαμος, *Arundo* L., Reed

One kind of reed is called *nastos* from which arrows are made, another *thelys*[117] from which tongues for flutes are made, another is called *syringias*; it has stout fibers, frequent knots, and it is suitable for writing books, another is thick and hollow, growing by river beds; it is called *donax*,[118] some, however, call it Cyprian, and there is yet another called *phragmites*,[119] which is somewhat white, slender, and familiar to all; its root draws out thorns and splinters when ground and plastered either by itself or with the eyes of the reed's root stock, and it soothes sprains and pains in the lower part of the back when plastered on with vinegar. Its leaves cut up when pale-green and applied cure erysipelas and the other inflammations. The bark, when burned and plastered on with vinegar, treats bald spots. But the silky flower tuft of the reeds will cause deafness if it should fall into the ears. The so-called Cyprian reed, too, can do the same.

### I, 86 πάπυρος, *Cyperus papyrus* L., Papyrus

Papyrus, from which papyrus roll is made, is familiar to all and highly useful in medical practice for opening fistulas.[120] It is prepared, after it has been soaked, by wrapping it with a linen thread until it dries. For as it is inserted compressed, it becomes filled with moisture and, as it swells, it opens the fistulas. Its root, moreover, has something that is even nutritive: for the people in Egypt, after chewing it, extract its juice and spit out the chewed matter. They also use these reeds for timber. Papyrus that is burned to ashes keeps in check sores in the mouth and everywhere else; but papyrus roll that was set on fire does this kind of thing better.

---

[117] "Female."
[118] "Pole-reed."
[119] "Hedge-reed."
[120] Also "ducts" or "channels" in the body.

**I, 87 μυρίκη, *Tamarix tetrandra* Pall., Tamarisk**

**1.** The tamarisk is a well-known tree growing close to lakes and stagnant waters, bearing fruit as it were a flower, catkin-like in structure. And there is one kind of tamarisk which is cultivated in Egypt and in Syria, resembling the wild tamarisk in all other respects, except that it bears fruit like an oak gall, irregular in shape, and astringent in taste; it is serviceable instead of oak galls for eye and mouth afflictions, and in a drink for coughing up blood, for those suffering from bowel ailments, for women suffering from fluxes, for jaundice, and for those bitten by venomous spiders; it also reduces swellings when plastered on.

**2.** The bark, too, accomplishes the same results as the fruit. The decoction of its leaves reduces the size of the spleen when drunk with wine and, as mouthwash, it helps for toothaches; it is serviceable for sitz baths for women suffering from fluxes as well as a washing liquid for those who breed lice[121] and bugs. The ash of its timber, too, if applied as a pessary, checks discharges from the uterus. Some make even cups from its stump for spleen disease patients to use as drinking cups, on the ground that they are helped when drinking from them.

**I, 88 ἐρείκη, *Erica arborea* L., Tree heath**

The tree heath is a shrubby tree resembling the tamarisk, although it is a great deal smaller; bees use its flower to make a honey, which is not particularly good.

Its foliage and flowers, plastered on, treat snakebites.

**I, 89 ἀκακαλλίς, *Acacallis***

*Acacallis* is the gall of a shrub that grows in Egypt[122] and that resembles somewhat the fruit of tamarisk. Its infusion is incorporated into eye salves that are serviceable for sharp-sightedness.

**I, 90 ῥάμνος, *Rhamnus cathartica* L., Boxthorn**

The boxthorn is a shrub that grows around hedges, having upright twigs and thorns like those of the fiery thorn, but leaves that are

[121] See Dsc. Bk. I, n. 109.

[122] This shrub is the oriental tamarisk.

longish, less shiny, and soft. Besides this one, there is also another boxthorn that is lighter in color, and even a third one having darker and broader leaves turning somewhat red, long twigs, about five cubits long and more thorny; its thorns, however, are weaker and blunter. The fruit is broad, thin, like a little sac, resembling a vertebra.
The leaves of all of them are effective for erysipelas and shingles when plastered on. It is said, moreover, that its branches when laid on gates or windows ward off the ill effects of spells.

**I, 91 ἅλιμον, *Atriplex halimus* L., Tree purslane**
The tree purslane is a shrub that grows in hedges; it is similar to boxthorn, although it does not have thorns, and its leaves are very much like those of the olive tree, but broader; it grows along coastal areas and fences. Its leaves are used as vegetables boiled for eating. One *drachma* of its root taken in a drink with honey and milk assuages spasms, ruptures, and colic; it also draws out the milk.

**I, 92 παλίουρος, *Paliurus australis* Gaertn. = *P. spina Christi* Mill., Christ's-thorn**
Christ's-thorn is a well-known shrub, thorny and sturdy; its seed is greasy and glutinous; when drunk, it helps for coughs, it brakes up bladder stones, and it operates on snakebites. The leaves and root are astringent and their decoction controls diarrhea when drunk, it draws down the urine, and it helps for poisons and for bites of wild animals. The root, ground up and applied, dissipates all new growths and swellings.

**I, 93 ὀξυάκανθα, *Cotoneaster pyracantha* Spach., Fiery thorn**
The fiery thorn: but some call it *pyren and* others *pyracanthe.* It is a tree that nearly resembles the wild pear, but it is smaller and very prickly; it bears fruit that resembles a myrtle-berry, full, red, easily broken, and containing seeds; it has a root much cloven and deep.
Its fruit checks diarrhea and leucorrhea when drunk and when eaten. Its root, plastered on ground up, draws out splinters and thorns. It is said that the root can even effect miscarriages when the abdomen is struck with it gently three times or when it is anointed with it.

**I, 94 κυνόσβατος, *Rosa sempervirens* L., White rose**

The white rose: but some call it *oxyacantha*. It is a tree-like shrub, much bigger than a bramble. It bears leaves broader than the myrtle's, strong thorns around its twigs, a white flower, and fruit that is oblong, resembling an olive pit, growing red as it ripens and having its insides woolly. The fruit dried and stripped of its wooly interior — for it is harmful to the trachea — checks diarrhea when boiled in wine and drunk.

**I, 95 κύπρος, *Lawsonia inermis* L., Henna**

The henna is a tree having leaves around its young shoots that nearly resemble those of the olive tree, although they are broader, tenderer, and of a paler-green color; it has aromatic white flowers, clustered like a bunch of grapes, and black seed, similar to the seed of the elder tree. The best grow in Ascalon and in Canopus.

The leaves have an astringent property; it is for this reason that they treat the thrush when chewed and they are good for carbuncles and for the other fiery inflammations when plastered on. Their decoction is a rinse for burns. Ground up, the leaves even dye the hair brown when soaked in quince juice and smeared on. The flower stops headaches if it is laid ground up on the forehead with vinegar. The henna unguent made from it warms and softens tendons, it is aromatic, and it absorbs compounds that heat.

**I, 96 φιλύρα, *Phillyrea* L. sp., Lime tree**

The lime tree resembles the henna tree in size and its leaves are like those of the olive tree, but they are wider and darker. It has fruit that resembles the mastic's, dark, somewhat sweet, and disposed in clusters. It grows in rough places. Its leaves are astringent like the leaves of the wild olive. They are effective for conditions in need of astringency especially for mouth sores when chewed and when their decoction is used as a rinse; also when the decoction is drunk, it draws down the urine and menses.

**I, 97 κίσθος, *Cistus* L. sp., Rock rose**

**1**. The rockrose, which some call *cistharos* or *cissaros*, is a shrub growing on rocky places; it has many branches, it is woody, and it is not tall; it has leaves that are rounded, stiff, dark, and rough; its flowers are like those of the pomegranate tree, red on the male, white on the female.

The flowers, ground up, have an astringent property when drunk with dry wine. It is for this reason that they are well suited for dysenterics when taken twice a day. Laid on all by themselves they stop spreading ulcers and with a salve they heal burns and old sores.

**2.** Hard by the roots of the rockrose grows the so-called hypocist, but some call it *orobethron* or *cytinos*; it resembles somewhat the flower of the pomegranate tree; part of it is orange-tawny and part white;[123] juice is extracted from it just as from the shittah tree. But some, after drying and crushing it, soak and boil it, and perform the other operations as on dyer's buckthorn. It has the same properties as the shittah tree, but it is more astringent and more desiccative; when drunk or when injected, it is good for sufferers from bowel ailments, dysenterics, people who spit up blood, and for leucorrhea.

**3.** And there is also another kind of rockrose, called by some *ledon*; it is a shrub with the same growth habits as the rockrose, but it has longer and darker leaves that gain some greasiness in the spring; the property of these leaves is astringent operating on as many conditions as the rockrose. It is from this shrub that the product called gum-ladanum is made. For this greasiness, as is well known, attaches its self on the beards and thighs of he- and she goats as they graze on its leaves, because it happens to be sticky. After it is removed, it is filtered then stored in the shape of small lumps. Some even drag ropes over the shrubs and after scraping off the grease that was formed on them shape it.

**4.** The best of it is aromatic, pale, easily molded, greasy, free of sand or dirt, and resinous. Such is the one made in Cyprus, but the Arabian and Libyan are less valuable.

---

[123] This is a parasitic plant with orange-tawny and white scales covering its stalk. Its etymology reveals its parasitic nature: *hypo-*, "underneath" and cist- from κίσθος, "rockrose." See Berendes, p. 112.

It has properties that warm, soften, and open. Mixed with wine, myrrh, and oil of myrtle, it stops hair from dropping off; smeared on with wine, it improves the appearance of scars, and when poured into the ears with a mixture of water and honey or with unguent of roses, it treats earaches. It is burned to produce smoke from below for ousting the afterbirth, it treats uterine indurations when mixed with a pessary, it is compounded profitably with analgesics, with cough preparations, and with emollients, and it stays the bowels when drunk with aged wine. It is also diuretic.

**I, 98 ἔβενος, *Diospyrus ebenum* Koenig and *D. melanoxylon* Roxb., Ebony**

**1.** The best ebony is the Ethiopian, being black and free of fissures, resembling wrought horn in its smoothness, compact when crushed, somewhat biting in taste and astringent, and when placed on coals, it smolders aromatically and without smoke. Because of its greasiness, ebony that is fresh even goes up in flames when it comes near a fire, and when scraped against a whetstone it becomes somewhat yellow. There is also an Indian ebony that has white and yellow divisions and equally frequent knots; but the one mentioned first is better. Some try to sell wood of the shittah tree or even the wood called *sycamina*[124] as ebony since they are similar; but their ploy is discoverable both because these woods are loosely-grained and split apart into small splinters of a purplish color and because they are not at all biting in taste or aromatic when burning.

**2.** It is capable of cleaning the elements that cast a shadow over the pupils of the eyes and it is a potent remedy both for old rheums and for burn blisters. And after making a very fine powder from it, if one used it in salves, the salves will be more effective. It is also made into eye medicines: its shavings or filings are soaked in Chian wine for a day and night, then they are carefully triturated and shaped into eye salves. But some, reducing first the ebony into powder, sift it, and then do the rest the same way, and others use water instead of the wine. It is also burned in an unfired earthen pot until it turns into ashes, then it

---

[124] Wood from the mulberry tree.

is washed like burned lead. Prepared in this manner, it is suitable for blepharitis and blepharitis sicca.

**I, 99 ῥόδα, *Rosa*, L. sp., Roses**

**1.** Roses cool and contract, but the dried ones contract more. You must extract the juice from roses that are young, cutting off with shears the so-called *onyx*;[125] this is the white part on the petal, then you must squeeze and pound in a mortar the rest until compressed into a ball, and thus store for eye ointments. The petals are dried in the shade, being turned frequently lest they become moldy.

The expressed juice from dried roses that were boiled in wine is effective for headaches, hurting eyes, earaches, hurting gums, anal pains, and for pains of the uterus when smeared on with a feather brush and when used as a wash.

**2.** The roses themselves, chopped up without being squeezed, are good when plastered on for inflammations of the hypochondrium, for excess of fluids in the stomach, and for erysipelas. Ground up fine when dry, they are sprinkled on the inside of thighs,[126] and they are mixed with lip salves, with wound medications, and with antidotes. They are also burned to use in paints for eyelids and eyelashes. The flower found in the middle of the roses, dried and laid on, is good for discharges from the gums. Rose hips control diarrhea and spitting of blood when drunk.

**3.** The so called *rhodides* are prepared this way: 40 *drachmai* fresh roses, free of moisture and withered, five *drachmai* Indian spikenard, and six *drachmai* myrrh, ground up, are molded into small disks of three obols and are dried in the shade; they are stored in an unpitched earthen jar sealed tightly all around. But some add also two-*drachmai* costusroot and an equal amount of Illyrian iris, mixing them with honey and Chian wine. Because they take away the edge of perspiration, women use them hung around their neck instead of fragrant wreathes. They use them also ground up in after-the-bath

[125] I. e. the white part at the end of the rose-petals by which they are attached to the stalk.

[126] Their use here is as dusting powder, since they contract (pores), to fight perspiration and as deodorant.

powders, also in ointments, and they wash themselves out with cold water after they have dried.

**I, 100 λύκιον, *Rhamnus petiolaris, Rh. Lycoïdes, Rh. punctata* Boiss., Dyer's buckthorn**

**1.** Dyer's buckthorn, which some call *pyxacantha*, is a thorny plant, having shoots three cubits long or even longer that are surrounded by dense foliage similar to that of boxwood. It has fruit like pepper, black, firm, very bitter, and the bark is pale-colored, like diluted *lycion*, and it has many wide and woody roots. It grows abundantly in Cappadocia, Lycia, and in many other places. It favors rough terrains.

**2.** Juice is extracted by crushing the roots together with the shrubbery, and after soaking them for several days then boiling them, the woody elements are discarded and the liquid is again boiled until it reaches a honey-like consistency. But they adulterate it during the boiling process by mixing it with *amorge*[127] or with juice of wormwood *Artemisia absinthium* or with bile of ox. Taking then away the foamy substance that floats on top during the boiling, store it for eye medications and use the rest for other purposes. Juice is extracted also from its fruit, which is similarly crushed and baked in the sun. Best and most efficacious is dyer's buckthorn that burns, that its foam is somewhat reddish when quenched, that is black on the outside but orange-tawny inside, that is devoid of smell, astringent, and bitter, and that is saffron-colored; such is the Indian, which is superior and stronger than the rest.

**3.** It has an astringent property, it cleanses the elements that cast a shadow over the pupils of the eyes, and it treats blepharitic itches, irritations, and discharges of long standing. It is also good smeared on for ears oozing with pus, inflammations of the tonsils, ulcerated gums and chapped lips, anal fistulas, and abrasions caused by friction. It is fit both for those suffering from bowel ailments and for dysenterics when drunk and when used as a clyster. It is given with water to people who spit blood and who cough, and to those who were bitten by a mad dog it is given either in a small pill or as a drink with water.

---

[127] See Dsc. Bk. I, 102 below.

It even dyes hair blond and it treats whitlow, shingles, and putrefying sores. It also halts leucorrhea when applied.
**4.** It is said that Indian *lycion* is made from a shrub called *lonchitis*. It is a kind of prickly plant, having erect shoots, three cubits long or even longer, many rising from its trunk, thicker than the shoots of bramble. Its bark when cracked open is somewhat red and its leaves are similar to those of the olive tree. Boiled in vinegar and drunk, its greenery reportedly treats inflammations of the spleen and jaundice and brings on the periods of women. It is said that it accomplishes the same even when taken in a drink ground up raw and that two *mystra* of its seed when drunk purge off watery elements and help for poisons.

**1, 101 ἀκακία, *Acacia* sp., Shittah tree**
**1.** The shittah tree grows in Egypt. It is a tree-like, thorny plant, shrubby and crooked, having a white flower, fruit just like the lupine's, white and lying in pods, from which, too, the juice is extracted when dried in the sun; it is black from ripe fruit but somewhat yellow from unripe. Choose it slightly yellow and sweet smelling as when on the shittah tree. Some extract juice also from the leaves together with the fruit. Gum Arabic comes from this thorny plant.
**2.** It has astringent and cooling properties. The juice is suitable for eye diseases and for erysipelas, for shingles, chilblains, membranous growths over the eyes,[128] mouth sores, and it corrects prolapses of the eyes. It stops leucorrhea, it draws in prolapses of the uterus, and when drunk or when used as a clyster, it stops diarrhea. It also dyes hair black. It is washed for conditions affecting the eyes by working <the juice> with water and continuously pouring off the film that collects on top until the water appears clean and so it is made up into small troches.
**3.** The fruit is burned with the pod in an unfired earthen pot and it is roasted over coals that are fanned. The decoction of this thorny plant when poured over weak joints firms them. Its gum is best if worm-

[128] πτερύγιον, an eye condition whereby a membrane grows over the eye from the inner corner.

shaped, green like glass, translucent, and free of woody matter. Then ranks that which is white; but the one that is resinous and greasy is useless.
It has properties that stop the pores and that take off the edge of sharp drugs with which it is mixed, and when smeared on with egg, it prevents the formation of blisters on burns.
**4.** There is also another shittah tree that grows in Cappadocia and in Pontus that resembles somewhat the Egyptian, yet it is considerably smaller, low-growing, and more delicate; moreover, it is quite full of thorns, which are pointed like pales. It has leaves like the rue's. In the fall, it bears seed, smaller than a lentil in little capsules that are joined together; each capsule is composed of three or four cells. This one, too, is astringent, the juice being extracted from the entire plant, except that it has been proven to be of less value since it is unserviceable for eye medications.

### I, 102 ἀμόργη, *Amorge*

*Amorge* is the sediment of pressed olives. It binds when boiled in a Cyprian copper vessel to the point of a honey-like consistency, it is effective for the same conditions as dyer's buckthorn, and there is nothing like it for toothaches and for wounds when smeared with vinegar or wine or honey mixed with wine. It is mixed both with eye medications and with substances that cause adhesion, it improves with age, and it is a useful rinse for ulcerated genitalia, seat, and uterus. Boiled with oil of unripe olives until it reaches the consistency of honey and plastered on, it ejects decayed teeth and treats the mange of domestic animals when smeared with an infusion of lupines and chameleon.[129] *Amorge* that was not boiled and that is fresh helps sufferers from gout and arthritis when embrocated warm, and it reduces the swellings of those suffering from edemata when daubed on a fleece and applied.

---

[129] The name given to various plants because their leaves change color, Theophrastus, *H. P.*, 6.4.3 and elsewhere. χαμαιλέων λευκός, pine-thistle, *Atractyllis gummifera*, is discussed in Dsc. Bk. III, 8; χαμαιλέων μέλας, chameleon-thistle, *Cardopatium corymbosum,* in Dsc. Bk., III, 9; he also calls it ἰξίας.

**I, 103 ἄγνος ἢ λύγος,[130] *Vitex agnus-castus* L., Chaste tree**

**1.** The chaste tree is a tree-like shrub which grows by the side of rivers and on rough terrains and gullies, having shoots that are hard to break and leaves like those of the olive but softer. Some bear a white flower with a touch of purple and others a purple flower; the seed is like pepper.

It has warming and softening properties. When drunk, its fruit helps those bitten by wild animals, those with spleen disease, and those with edemata.

**2.** It draws down milk and it brings on the menses when a quantity of one *drachma* is drunk with wine; but it also slackens the organ of generation[131] and it affects the head inducing deep sleep. The decoction of the plant itself and of its fruit helps in sitz baths for conditions and inflammations around the uterus. Its seed sets the menses in motion when drunk with pennyroyal, when burned to produce thick smoke from below, and when inserted; it also stops headaches when plastered on, and it is soaked with vinegar and oil for those affected by lethargic fever and phrenitis.

**3.** Its leaves chase away wild animals when burned as to produce smoke or when scattered about; when plastered on, they help people who were bitten by wild animals, they soften testicular indurations with butter and grape leaves, and the seed soothes anal fissures when smeared on with water and treats sprains and wounds when plastered on with the leaves. It seems also to prevent abrasions incurred while walking should one hold in hand one of its shoots.

---

[130] ἅγνος, "pure" or "chaste," λύγος, akin to λυγίζω, "bend" or "twist" as one does with a withe. Women used the shrub, as stated at the end of this chapter, symbolically during the Thesmophoria, a festival in Athens and elsewhere in Greece in honor of Demeter *thesmophoros* (the law-giver).

[131] Here Dioscorides uses the expression ἐκλύει γονήν; it slackens the organ of generation and in III, 45,1 on Rue, in III, 58, on Dill and in III, 148 on Hemp he uses σβέννυσι γονήν, "it quells the organ of generation." Pliny, *N. H.*, XX, 259 on Hemp says *"semen eius extinguere genitura dicitur,"* which the Loeb translator renders "its seed is said to make the genitals impotent." And Gal. XII 8 (under Paul. Aeg VII 3 s.v.) writes that "the fruit of hemp causes the organ of generation to whither," (my translation). See also Dsc. Bk., III, 132,2 where the white water lily effects a slackness of the genitalia, ἀτονίαν ἐργάζεται αἰδοίου.

It was named *agnos* because women make it a point of religion during the Thesmophoria to use it as bedding, and *lygos* because of the yielding quality of its shoots.

### I, 104 ἰτέα, *Salix* L. sp., Willow

The willow is a well-known tree; its fruit, leaves, bark, and juice have astringent properties. The leaves, ground up and drunk with a little pepper and wine, are suitable for intestinal obstructions and they cause barrenness when taken by themselves with water. The fruit helps people who spit blood when drunk. The bark, too, does the same things and it removes warts and calluses when plastered on them burned and mixed with vinegar. The juice of the leaves and of the bark, heated with unguent of roses in the shell of a pomegranate, helps for earaches, their decoction is an excellent rinse for gout, and it washes off dandruff. They even collect its sap by incising the bark at blossom time, for it is found within congealed. It has the ability to clean the elements that cast a shadow over the pupils of the eyes.

### I, 105 ἀγριελαία, *Olea europaea* L., var. *silvestris* Miller, Wild olive tree

**1.** The wild olive tree, which some call *cotinos* and others Ethiopian olive, has astringent leaves. When laid on ground up, they can check erysipelas, shingles, pustules that are most painful at night, carbuncles, spreading ulcers, whitlow, and, when plastered on with honey, they can cause tissues to form a line of demarcation around scabs. They clean filthy sores, dissipate swellings of the glands and inflammations when plastered on with honey, glue on skin detached from the head, and, when chewed, treat both mouth sores and thrush. Both their juice and their decoction do the same.

**2.** When applied, the juice controls hemorrhaging and leucorrhea, as do also the leaves control defects in the eyes inside the cornea and pustules. Moreover, they keep in check sores and old rheums. It is for this reason that they help for erosions of the eyelids when mixed with eye salves. Those extracting the juice must chop up the leaves, then pouring wine or water over them, squeeze out the liquid, and after drying it in the sun, mold it. Juice that is extracted with wine is more potent and more suitable for storage than juice extracted with water. It is good for ears that discharge matter and that suppurate.

**3.** The leaves are also suitable for people with bowel ailments when plastered on with bruised meal of raw corn. The leaves together with the flowers are used instead of vegetable ashes; they are burned in an unfired earthen vessel luted all around the mouth with clay until the clay is baked, then they are quenched with wine and after they have been kneaded again with wine they are similarly burned. Then they are washed like white lead and molded. For eye medications, it seems that this kind of ash is every bit as good as ashes from minerals; therefore, it must be thought to have the same strength.

The leaves of the cultivated olive tree can also accomplish the same results, but they want in strength; it is for this reason that they are more suitable for eye medications, seeing that they are milder.

**4.** The liquid that is secreted from its green wood as it burns, when smeared on, treats dandruff, mange, and the lichen-like eruptions on the skin of animals. Also their fruit treats dandruff and spreading ulcers when plastered on. The inside of olive-pits, combined with animal fat and flour, drives out nails afflicted by psoriasis.

The olives that swim in pickling brine ground up and plastered on, prevent burns from forming blisters and cleanse dirty sores. The juice of the brine, used as a mouthwash, reduces swollen gums and strengthens loose teeth.

**5.** The olive that is somewhat yellow and fresh is costive and good for the stomach, but the black and ripe olive spoils easily, it is bad for the stomach, it is unsuitable for the eyes, and it causes headaches. But when roasted and plastered on, it halts spreading ulcers and causes carbuncles to break away.

The oil from the wild olive is a mouthwash for purulent gums, it can bind loose teeth, and by itself it is suitable as a warm compress for discharging gums; one must, however, dip into the oil a probe wrapped with wool and apply it to the gums until they look white.

**6.** The sap of the Ethiopian olive tree is somewhat like scammony, pale-yellow, composed of small beads, and pungent. But the kind that is like gum, somewhat black, and not pungent is useless. Both the olive that grows in our land and the wild olive tree produce that sort of sap. It is good for the dim-sighted, it wipes off both scars and leucomas[132] when smeared on, it sets micturition and the menses going, and it is good for toothaches when placed into the cavity. But it is also registered among the deadly poisons, it draws down embryos/fetuses, and it treats lichen-like eruptions on the skin and leprosy. The wild olive tree is called Ethiopian olive.

**I, 106 δρῦς, *Quercus* L. sp., Oak**

**1.** The entire oak tree has an astringent property, but its membranous part between the bark and the trunk is most astringent; the same is also true of that part beneath the shell surrounding the acorn. Their decoction is given to those suffering from bowel ailments, to dysenterics, to those who spit blood, and they are added ground up in pessaries for women suffering from fluxes.

The acorns, too, accomplish the same; they are diuretic and cause headaches when eaten and they produce gas. They are good to eat for venomous bites and both their decoction and the decoction of their husks are antidotes for arrow poisoning when drunk with cow's milk.

**2.** Ground up raw and plastered on, they soothe inflammations, and, with salt pork, they are suitable for malignant indurations and pernicious sores. The acorns of the holm oak are more potent than those of the oak.

Both the Valonia oak and the holm oak, being species of oak, are efficacious for the same things. The bark of the holm oak boiled in water until it becomes soft and plastered all night long on hair that had been smeared with Cimolian earth, dyes it black. The leaves of all oaks, chopped up fine, are suitable for swellings and they firm up areas lacking tonicity.

As for the Sardian acorns,[133] which some call *lopima* or *castaniai* or *mota* or Zeus' acorns, they, too, are astringent and efficacious for the same conditions, especially the membrane between the flesh and the peel. Their flesh is suitable also for those who drank poison that kills on the same day.

---

[132] Caused by the thickening of the cornea.

[133] "Sweet chestnuts."

### I, 107 κηκίς, *Cecis*

**1.** *Cecis* is the fruit[134] of the oak tree. One kind of this fruit is called *omphacitis*; it is small, knobby, heavy, and lacking an aperture, and another is smooth, light, and perforated. You must choose the *omphacitis*, since it is more effective.

Both, however, are considerably astringent and when ground up control overgrown flesh, discharges from the gums and uvula, and the thrush in the mouth. Their inner part, when placed on the cavity of teeth, stops toothaches. They also become styptic when heated on coals until they catch fire then quenched with wine or vinegar or brine-vinegar.

**2.** Their decoction is good in sitz baths for uterine prolapses and discharges. Soaked in vinegar or water, they also dye hair black. They are suitable for dysenterics and for those with bowel ailments ground up, sprinkled with water or wine, and drunk; also when combined with side dishes or boiled whole in the water in which some food appropriate for them will be cooked. And in general, it is appropriate to adopt their use wherever there is a need to contract, to stop, or to dry something.

### I, 108 ῥοῦς ὁ ἐπὶ τά ὄψα, *Rhus coriaria* L., Sumac

**1.** The sumac that is sprinkled on prepared foods,[135] which some call *erythron*, is the fruit of the sumac called *byrsodepsice rhous*.[136] It was so named because tanners use it to steep hides. It is a small tree, growing on rocks, about two cubits tall, whose leaves are elongated, reddish, and incised in a saw-like manner around the periphery; the

---

[134] Dioscorides uses the word καρπός, "fruit, seed, with seed vessel" and seems to consider κηκίς, "oak-gall" as an integral part of the oak and not as it is, in actuality, an excrescence produced by the presence of parasitic organisms, both vegetable (fungi, mold) and insects, mites or worms. Usually the insect pierces the bark or leaf and lays its eggs in the incision where the gall is produced and the larvae live and feed. The galls of certain oaks produced by the cynipoid gallflies contain much tannic acid, as does the Aleppo gall of *Quercus infectoria* referred to in this chapter as *omphacitis*.

[135] LSJ defines ὄψον as "cooked" or otherwise "prepared food, a made dish" eaten with bread and wine; also as a "delicacy" or a "relish" and at Athens, especially, as "fish" the chief delicacy of the Athenians; προσόψημα as "anything eaten with or besides" the regular meal. For a detailed discussion on ὄψον and on ὀψοφαγία, the act of eating an ὄψον, see James Davidson, *Courtesans and Fishcakes*, pp. 20-34.

[136] Meaning "tanning sumac."

fruit is like grape clusters, close-packed, corresponding in size to the fruit of the terebinth tree, and somewhat flat; the bark-like membrane that surrounds it is very useful.

**2.** The leaves have an astringent property that is efficacious for the same purposes as the shittah tree. Their decoction dyes hair black, it is a clyster as well as a drink and a sitz bath solution for dysentery, it is an infusion for ears discharging pus, and the leaves, when plastered on with vinegar or honey, keep in check membranes which grow over the inner corner of the eyes and cankers. The juice of the dry leaves, boiled with water like dyer's buckthorn to a honey-like consistency, is suitable for all the conditions that dyer's buckthorn is suitable.

**3.** Its fruit, too, does the same, being suitable, in side dishes, for people with bowel ailments and for dysenterics; it keeps free of inflammations bruises, abrasions, and black eye when plastered on with honey, it also cleanses roughness of the tongue with honey, it stays leucorrhea, and it treats hemorrhoids when applied with ground up oaken charcoal. Its infusion, too, thickens as it boils; to some degree, it is more effective than the fruit. It bears also a gum that is inserted into the cavities of teeth to allay pain.

### I, 109 φοῖνιξ, *Phoenix dactylifera* L., Date palm

**1.** The date palm grows in Egypt. Its fruit is harvested half-ripe in late summer; it is somewhat like the nut of the ben tree and it is called *ptoma*. It is greenish-yellow and it smells of quince. But if it should be allowed to ripen fully, it becomes *phoinicobalanos*.

It is sour and astringent; it is for this reason that if drunk with dry wine it is effective for diarrhea and leucorrhea; it also checks hemorrhoids and it closes wounds when plastered on them. Dates that are fresh are more astringent than the dry ones, but they cause headaches and if eaten in large quantities they inebriate.

**2.** Dry dates, ground up and plastered on with quince and with cerate made from flowers of wild vines, help those spitting blood, those with stomach ailments, dysenterics, and sufferers from bladder disorders; but above all the *caryotides* dates treat roughness of the bronchial tubes when eaten. The decoction of Theban dates abates heartburn when drunk and restores one's strength when taken with aged hydromel. Also the Theban dates themselves do the same when eaten.

There is also a wine made from them, which is as effective as the fruit; their decoction strongly contracts and binds both when drunk neat and when used as a gargle.

**3.** Date pits are burned in an unfired earthen vessel, like everything else, and then after they have been quenched with wine, they are washed and used as vegetable ash. They are suitable for paints of the eyelids and eyelashes and if burned insufficiently the process is repeated.

They have properties that are astringent and that stop the pores, operating on eye pustules, on defects in the eye within the cornea, and on falling eyelashes with spikenard; with wine, they control overgrown flesh and cicatrize wounds. The dates from Egypt, the ones from the dwarf palms, are most appropriate.

**4.** The date palm frond, which some call *elate* or *spathe*, is the hood of the fruit of date palms when they are still blooming. Perfumers use it for thickening unguents. The best of it is aromatic, binding, heavy, closed, and internally greasy.

It has an astringent property that controls the expansion of ulcers and that draws together dislocated joins when ground up and mixed with emollients and poultices. It benefits slackened hypochondria, the stomach, and liver conditions when mixed with the appropriate plasters.

**5.** Its decoction, used frequently as a rinse, dyes hair black, it is a suitable drink for kidney disease, for ailments associated with the bladder, and for the inner organs, and it checks diarrhea and uterine flux. Applied when soft with pine resin and wax and left on for 20 days, it treats the mange. The fruit it encompasses is also called *elate*; but some call it *borassos* and since it, too, is astringent, it is capable of the same things as *spathe* but without its usefulness in unguents. Even the white core of its stem is good for as many things as is *borassos* when eaten fresh or boiled.

### I, 110 ῥόα, *Punica granatum* L., Pomegranate

**1.** All pomegranates are juicy, good for the stomach, and lacking in nutrients. Among them, the pomegranate that is sweet is certainly tastier, creating a degree of warmth in the stomach, and causing flatulence; consequently, it is unsuitable for people running a fever;

but the pomegranate that is sour helps for heartburn and is diuretic. It is tasteless, however, and astringent; the one that has a wine-like flavor is of moderate action.

**2.** The pips of the sour pomegranate, when dried in the sun and sprinkled on side dishes or when boiled with them, stay diarrhea and fluid discharges from the stomach, they help those who spit blood, if drunk after they were soaked in rainwater, and they are suitable for sitz baths for dysenterics and for women suffering from fluxes. The juice of the pips boiled and mixed with honey, is useful for sores in the mouth, the genitalia, the seat, for fleshy excrescences on the digits, for spreading ulcers, for excrescences, for earaches, and for afflictions in the nostrils; this is especially true of the juice of the sour pomegranate.

Its flowers, which are also called *cytinoi*, are themselves also astringent, they dry, they are capable of stopping bleeding wounds and for gluing them together, and they are suitable for the same purposes as the pomegranate. Their decoction is a mouthwash for flaccid gums and loose teeth and an adhesive plaster for intestinal hernias when used in a poultice.

**3.** Some say that should healthy people swallow as few as three *cytinoi*, they will be free of ophthalmia for the entire year. Juice is extracted from them the way it is extracted from the hypocist.

Even the peels of the pomegranate, which some call *sidia*, are adapted for the same purposes as the *cytinoi,* because they, too, have an astringent property. The decoction of the roots ejects and destroys intestinal flatworms when drunk.[137]

## I, 111 βαλαύστιον, Flower of the wild pomegranate

*Balaustion* is the flower of the wild pomegranate. There are several kinds of it: for it is found in white, red, and pink, and it resembles the flower of the cultivated pomegranate. Juice is extracted from it just as from the hypocist.

It has an astringent property, efficacious for the same purposes as the hypocist and the flower of the cultivated pomegranate.

---

[137] The peels contain tannic acids but the antihelminthic property rests on the presence (4-6%) of pelletierine alkaloids, J. Berendes, p. 132.

## I, 112 μυρσίνη ἡ ἥμερος, *Myrtus communis* L., Cultivated myrtle

**1.** The cultivated myrtle that is black is more suitable for medical use than the white, and of this, the one growing on mountains is best, although it has a more insipid fruit.

Its property and that of its fruit are astringent. The fruit is given to eat both fresh and dry to people who spit blood and to those experiencing a burning sensation in the bladder. Also the juice from pressed fresh myrtles does the same, being good for the stomach, diuretic, and suitable with wine for those stung by venomous spiders and scorpions. The decoction of its fruit colors hair; boiled with wine and laid on, the fruit treats sores on the extremities, plastered on with very fine barley groats, it assuages eye inflammations, and it is plastered on for lachrymal fistulas. It clears off dandruff, scurf, and pustules, and it stays falling hair. It is also mixed with oily plasters, as is also the oil that is made from its leaves. The decoction of its leaves is suitable for sitz baths and it is poured to advantage over joints that are loose, not mended, and weakened.

**2.** Also the wine made from it by pressing the fruit and boiling it for a while—for unless it was prepared this way it becomes sour—if drunk beforehand counteracts nausea, it is effective for as many purposes as is the fruit, and it is an appropriate sitz bath for uterine and anal prolapses and for feminine discharges. It clears off dandruff, scurf, and pustules, and it stays falling hair. It is also mixed with oily plasters, as is also the oil that is made from its leaves. The decoction of its leaves is suitable for sitz baths and it is poured to advantage over joints that are loose, not mended, and weakened. It clears dull-white leprosy and it is used as an infusion for ears that exude pus and for dyeing hair black. Their juice also does the same.

**3.** The leaves themselves, ground up and plastered on with water, are suitable for those sores that contain a great deal of moisture, for all areas that are afflicted by rheums, for people suffering in the bowels, and when combined with oil of unripe olives or with a little unguent of roses and wine, for shingles, erysipelas, testicular inflammations, pustules that are most painful at night, and callous lumps. Dried, they are advantageously sprinkled ground up on whitlows, on membranous growths over the eye, on very wet armpits and thighs, and they stay the sweats of heart patients. Burned and even raw, they treat burns, in combination with a cerate, membranous growths over the eyes, and whitlows.

**4.** Juice is extracted from the leaves by pouring over them old wine or rainwater and then squeezing them. It is used while fresh, for after it has dried it is moldy and weak.

But the so-called *myrtidanon* is an irregular, tuberous, and uniformly colored excrescence, as if it were hands around the trunk of the myrtle. It is more astringent than the myrtle. After it has been chopped, mixed with harsh wine, and shaped into troches, it is dried in the sun then stored. It is more effective than either the leaf or the fruit, being combined with cerate and with pessaries, also with sitz baths and poultices in need of astringency.

### I, 113 κεράσια, *Prunus avium* L., Fruit of the cherry tree

Cherries, too, ease the bowel if consumed fresh, but they constipate if eaten dried. The gum of cherry trees, taken with diluted wine, treats a chronic cough and brings about healthy looks, sharp-sightedness, and good appetite. It helps also those suffering from stones when drunk with wine.

### I, 114 κεράτια, *Ceratonia siliqua* L., Fruit of the carob tree

The fruit of the carob tree when consumed fresh is bad for the stomach and diarrheic, but when consumed dry, stems the bowel flow, being better for the stomach and diuretic, especially fruit which was put up from the pressings of fresh grapes.[138]

### I, 115 μηλέα,[139] *Pirus malus*, Apple tree

**1.** The leaves, flowers, and shoots of all fruit trees are astringent but especially those of the quince tree. The fruit, too, is astringent when unripe, but not so after it has ripened. Fruit that ripens in spring produces bile, is unfit for all sinewy parts, and causes flatulence.

κυδώνια. Quinces are good for the stomach, diuretic—they become more palatable when cooked—they are useful to patients with bowel

---

[138] This passage seems to be corrupt. See LSJ s.v. στέμφυλον, "mass of pressed grapes." It is suggested that in the pl. it may be a drink.

[139] This chapter begins with μηλέα, "apple tree" but the discussion that follows is about μῆλα, "apples" (the fruit) or "tree-fruits."

ailments, dysenterics, people who spit blood, and to those suffering from cholera, especially when raw. Their infusion, too, is suitable for suffering from fluid discharges from the stomach or from diarrhea.
**2.** Juice taken from raw quinces helps those suffering from orthopnea and their decoction is a lotion for anal and uterine prolapses. As for the quinces from honey,[140] they, too, are diuretic, and the honey acquires the same properties, for it becomes costive and astringent. Quinces cooked with honey, while good for the stomach and tasty, are less costive. Raw quinces are mixed with poultices for diarrhea, upset stomach and heartburn, inflamed breasts, indurated spleens, and callous lumps. They also make a wine from them by chopping and pressing them and mixing one *xestes* honey with 12 *xestes* juice to preserve it; otherwise it does turn sour.
**3.** It suits all the purposes that have been mentioned. There is even an ointment that is made from quinces, the so-called *melinon,* which we use whenever we need astringent oil. But one must choose the right quinces; these are small, round, and aromatic. Those that are called *strouthia* and that are big are less useful. Their blossoms, both dried and fresh, are suitable to use in poultices for conditions needing astringency and for inflammations of the eyes; they are also suitable to drink for blood spitting, for diarrhea, and for the flow of menstruation.
*μελίμελα.* Summer apples soften the bowel and expel intestinal organisms; they are bad for the stomach and cause heartburn. Some call them sweet apples.
**4.** *Ἠπειρωτικά.* The apples called *Epeirotica* and in Latin *orbiclata,*[141] are good for the stomach; they are capable of staunching the bowel and of stimulating micturition; on the other hand, they are less effective than quinces.
*τὰ ἄγρια [μῆλα].* Crab apples resemble the spring apples in binding. You must use the least ripe among all of them for things needing astringency.

---

[140] These are quinces preserved raw in honey.
[141] These are "rose apples," *orbiclata,* from Lat. *orbiculata sc. mala*, rounded apples. Pliny, *N. H.*, XV, 51 says that they are called *Epeirotica* from Epirus where they were first produced.

*τὰ Περσικὰ μῆλα*. Peaches are good for the stomach; the ripe ones ease the bowel, but the unripe constipate and, if they have been dried, they constipate more; also the decoction that is made from the dry ones stems fluxes from the stomach and bowel.

**5**. *Ἀρμένικα*. The smaller ones, which are called Armenian,[142] are tastier than the above. In Latin they are called *brecoccia.*

*Μηδικὰ ἢ Περσικὰ ἢ κεδρόμηλα, Ῥωμαιστὶ κίτρια*. Everybody knows the ones called Median or Persian or *cedromela* and in Latin *citria*;[143] for it is a tree bearing fruit repeatedly throughout the year and the fruit itself is oblong, wrinkled, golden in color, somewhat oppressively aromatic, and has a pear-shaped seed.

These fruits have the power of counteracting the effects of poisons and of purging the bowel when drunk with wine, and both their decoction and their juice are rinses for good breath. They are eaten especially by pregnant women to abate the craving they have for strange foods; placed into small chests, they seem to keep even clothing free of moths.

### I, 116 ἄπιος, *Pirus communis* L., Pear

Pears are of many kinds. All of them are astringent and it is for this reason that they are suitable for poultices that are able to disperse. The decoction of dried pears and the pears themselves when taken raw stop diarrhea; they are harmful, however, if eaten on an empty stomach.

The wild pear is a kind of uncultivated pear that ripens slowly. It has a more astringent property than the pear; it is for this reason that it is suitable for the same purposes; its leaves, too, are astringent. The ash of its wood is an effective remedy for those choking from mushrooms. Some say that mushrooms become harmless when cooked with wild pears.

---

[142] These are apricots.
[143] "Citrons."

**I, 117 λωτός, *Celtis australis* L., Nettle tree**

Nettle, the tree,[144] is a plant of a good size; it bears fruit bigger than pepper, sweet, edible, good for the stomach, and binding the bowel. The decoction of the sawdust of its wood helps dysenterics and women who are having fluxes when drunk and when used as a clyster; it also colors hair blond and prevents it from falling.

**I, 118 μέσπιλον, *Mespilus germanica* L., Medlar tree**

Medlar, the tree,[145] which some call *aronia*, is thorny and similar in its leaves to the fiery thorn. It bears small <round> fruit, resembling an apple, which is sweet and contains three kernels. It is for this reason that some also call it "three-kernelled." It is astringent and wholesome, binding the bowel.

There is also another kind growing in Italy which some call *epimelis* and others *setanion*. It is a tree resembling the apple tree even in foliage, except that it is smaller; it, too, has a round and edible fruit with a wide base, it is somewhat astringent and slow to ripen.

**I, 119 κρανία, *Cornus mas* L., Cornelian cherry tree**

Cornelian cherry is a vigorous tree, bearing fruit like olives, longish, pale-green at first, but on ripening, yellow or wax-colored, edible, and astringent; it is suitable for intestinal flux and dysentery being added both into concentrated must and into food; it is also pickled like olives. The juice that runs from its green wood as it burns is efficacious for lichen-like eruptions of the skin when smeared on.

**I, 120 οὖα, *Sorbus domestica* L., Sorb apples**

Sorb apples[146] that are quince-yellow and that have not yet ripened, sliced, and dried in the sun, are capable of staunching the bowel when eaten; their meal, which is made by grinding them, taken in lieu of barley groats, and their decoction when drunk do the same.

---

[144] "Tree" is used with "nettle" and in the next chapter with "medlar" to distinguish them from non-trees of the same name.

[145] See n. 143 above.

[146] Also known as serviceberries and the tree that produces them as service tree.

### I, 121 κοκκυμηλέα, *Prunus domestica* L., Plum tree

The plum tree is well known. Its fruit is edible, bad for the stomach, and laxative; but the fruit of the Syrian plums, and especially of those grown in Damascus, having been dried, is good for the stomach and capable of staunching the bowel. The decoction of its leaves, prepared with wine and used as a gargle, controls discharges from the uvula, from the gums, and from the tonsils. The fruit of the wild plum trees, dried after it has ripened, produces the same results, and when boiled with concentrated must becomes better for the stomach and more capable of staunching the bowel. The gum of the plum tree is adhesive and lithotritic when drunk with wine; it treats lichen-like eruptions on children when anointed with vinegar.

### I, 122 κόμαρος, *Arbutus unedo* L., Strawberry tree

The strawberry tree resembles the quince tree. It is thin-barked. Its fruit is as big as a plum, stoneless, called *memaicyla*, somewhat yellow when ripe, chaffy when eaten, bad for the stomach, and causing headaches.

### I, 123 ἀμυγδάλη, *Prunus Amygdalus* Stokes, esp. var. *sativa* Asch., Almond

**1.** The root of the bitter almond ground up and boiled removes facial freckles; the almonds themselves also do the same when plastered on. Applied as pessaries, they bring on the menses, plastered on the forehead with vinegar and unguent of roses, they help for headaches, with wine, they help for pustules that are most painful at night, and they are suitable with honey for decaying sores, for shingles, and for dog bites. When eaten they allay pain, they soften the bowel, they are soporific, and they are diuretic. They are taken with starch and mint for blood spitting, they are drunk with water or licked as a lozenge with turpentine for kidney disease and inflammations of the lungs, with grape syrup, they help those having difficult micturition and those who suffer from stones, and, when taken as a lozenge the size of a filbert made up with honey and milk, they help for liver disease, for coughs, and for flatulence in the colon.

**2.** They also prevent drunkenness if about five almonds are consumed before drinking; they do even kill foxes if they should eat them with something else.[147] Its gum binds, warms, and helps for spitting blood when drunk, and it removes the superficial lichen-like eruptions of the skin when anointed with vinegar. Taken in a drink with diluted wine, it treats chronic coughs, and it benefits people who suffer from stones when drunk with grape-syrup. The sweet and edible almond tree is far less effective than the bitter; but it, too, thins and is diuretic. And its almonds settle heartburn when eaten fresh with their skin.

**I, 124 πιστάκια, *Pistacia vera* L., Pistachio nuts**

Pistachio nuts that grow in Syria are like the nuts of *strobilos* pine; they are good for the stomach. When eaten and when drunk ground up in wine, they help those bitten by snakes.

**I, 125 κάρυα βασιλικά, *Juglans regia* L., Walnuts**

**1.** Walnuts, which some call Persian nuts, when eaten, are hard to digest, bad for the stomach, produce bile, cause headaches, and they are not recommended for people who cough. But when consumed by a fasting person, they are useful for vomiting; eaten beforehand together with dried figs and rue, they counteract deadly poisonings, and when eaten in large quantities, they expel the intestinal flatworm. They are also plastered with a little honey and rue on inflamed breasts and on sprains. They are effective with onion, salt, and honey for dog and human bites and they stop colic when roasted in their shell and placed on the navel.

**2.** Their husk, burned, kneaded with wine and oil, and smeared on children, produces luxuriant hair and restores hair on bald patches; also its inside, ground up, burned, and applied as a pessary with wine, stems the menses. The meat of old walnuts demarcates gangrenes and carbuncles when plastered on, and it treats lachrymal fistulas and baldness when chewed and used topically. They also make oil from them by chopping and pressing them. Fresh walnuts are better for the stomach since they are sweeter; and it is for this reason that they are mixed with garlic to remove its edge; they also remove livid spots when plastered on.

---

[147] Namely, bait.

**3.** *Ποντικά.* Filberts, which some call *leptocaria*,[148] are harmful <to the head> and bad for the stomach. They, too, treat an old cough when ground up and drunk with hydromel, and they assuage a catarrh when baked and consumed with a bit of pepper. Fully burned whole, ground up, and smeared on with lard or with bear fat, they restore hair on bald spots. Some say that their shells blacken the pupils and hair of grey-eyed children if after being burned and emulsified with oil the emulsion is used to drench the front part of their heads.

### I, 126 μορέα ἢ συκάμινον, *Morus nigra* L., Mulberry tree

**1.** The mulberry is a well-known tree; its fruit loosens the bowel, it is perishable, and it is bad the stomach. Its juice does the same, but it becomes more astringent when boiled in a brazen pot or fermented in the sun. Mixed with a little honey, it is effective for rheums, spreading ulcers, and inflamed tonsils. It becomes stronger when split alum,[149] oak-gall, galingale, myrrh, and saffron have been added; also fruit of the tamarisk, iris, and frankincense. Chopped up when dry, the unripe mulberries are mixed instead of with the fruit of sumac with prepared foods and help those with bowel ailments.
**2.** The bark of its root, boiled with water and drunk, loosens the bowel, expels the intestinal flatworm, and helps those who drank leopard's bane. Ground up and plastered with oil, the leaves treat burns, and they color hair when boiled in rainwater with leaves of grape vine and of black fig. The juice of its leaves, drunk in the amount of one *cyathos*, helps those bitten by venomous spiders, and the decoction of its bark and leaves is a good mouthwash for toothaches. Around the time wheat is harvested, juice is extracted from its root, after it has been dug up and chopped; for on the following day, one finds a congealed substance that acts on toothaches, dissipates growths, and cleanses the bowel.

---

[148] "Thin-shelled nuts."
[149] See Dsc. Bk. V, 106.

**I, 127 συκόμορον, *Ficus sycomorus* L., Sycamore fig**

**1.** Sycamore fig: but some call this tree, too, mulberry. Its fruit, too, is called *sycomoron*[150] because it is unpalatable. It is a large tree, like the fig tree, extremely juicy, with leaves like those of the mulberry tree. It bears fruit three or four times a year not from its branches, as it is borne on the fig tree, but from its trunk; it resembles the fruit of the wild fig tree, it is sweeter than the wild fig, seedless, and it does not ripen unless scratched with the nail or a knife.

**2.** It grows abundantly in Caria, in Rhodes, and in lands not rich in grains. It does help in time of famine because it bears fruit continuously; but the fruit is diarrheic, devoid of nutritional value, and bad for the stomach. The tree is tapped in the spring, before fruiting, by scratching its bark superficially with a stone, because if it is scratched too deeply, it releases nothing. The sap is collected with a sponge or with wool, and after it is dried and shaped, it is stored in a clay vessel.

**3.** The sap has properties that soften, that cause wounds to adhere, and that disperse indigestible substances. It is drunk and it is rubbed on for snakebites, indurated spleens, stomach pains, and for shivering from shock. But this sap quickly grows worms.

In Cyprus grows also a different sycamore fig. For its leaves are like the leaves of the elm and not like the sycamore's and it produces fruit about the size of plums and sweeter. Everything else is the same as described above.

**I, 128 σῦκα, *Ficus caria* L., Figs**

**1.** Ripe figs that are soft[151] are bad for the stomach, loosen the bowel — but the flow they cause is easily checked — provoke pustules and perspiration, serve to quench thirst, and cool. Dry figs are nutritious, they warm, they are thirst-making, they ease the bowel, they are unfit for fluid discharges of the stomach and diarrhea, but they are suitable for the throat, trachea, bladder, kidneys, for those who have bad color due to a lingering illness, for asthmatics, epileptics, and for those suffering from edemata. Boiled with hyssop and drunk, they clear up

[150] Deriving from σῦκον, "fig" and μορόν, "insipid."

[151] As opposed to the ripe ones but tough, from which the dried figs are processed.

chest conditions; they are suitable for old coughs, for chronic conditions of the lungs, and they soften the bowel when eaten chopped up with soda and safflower.

**2.** Their decoction is a serviceable gargle for inflammations of the trachea and tonsils, it is mixed both with bruised meal of raw corn and with fenugreek or barley gruel for women's vapor baths, and with rue it is a clyster for colic. Plastered on, after they have been ground up and boiled, they dissipate indurations and tumors of the parotid glands, they soften small abscesses, and they ripen swellings of the glands, especially when combined with iris or with soda or with unslaked lime; but they accomplish the same results even when brayed raw with the ingredients mentioned above. With pomegranate peel, they completely clear membranous growths over the eyes, and with a solution of copper sulfate, they treat sores in the shanks that are hard to cure, pussy, and malignant.

**3.** Boiled in wine, mixed with wormwood *Artemisia absinthium* and barley flour, and plastered on, they help those people with edemata. Burned and mixed with cerate, they treat chilblains, and when ground raw, made up with liquid mustard, and instilled, they treat ringing and itching in the ears.

The milky substance[152] of the wild and of the cultivated fig trees causes milk to curdle just like rennet; it also dissolves curdled matter, as does vinegar, it causes ulcerations on bodies and it dilates, it loosens the bowel and it relaxes the uterus when drunk with very fine meal, it draws down the menses when applied with egg yolk or Tyrrhenian wax, and it is useful with flour of fenugreek and vinegar in poultices for the gouty. It clears both leprosy and lichen-like eruptions of the skin, freckles, dull-white leprosy, and, with barley groats, itching.

**4.** It helps those stung by scorpions when dribbled on the stroke, those afflicted by venomous animals, and those bitten by dogs; it helps for toothaches when taken up in wool and instilled into the decayed tooth, and it removes the warts which spread under the skin, the flesh surrounding them having been coated with suet. The juice of the tender shoots of the wild fig tree also accomplishes the same things. It

---

[152] That is the juice drawn from the fig trees by tapping and used as rennet.

is extracted when the shoots are as if pregnant, and when the buds are not yet open. After they are chopped, they are pressed and the juice is dried in the shade and stored. Both the milky substance and the juice are used in ulcerating drugs.

**5.** The soft branches, when boiled with beef meat, tenderize it and make the milk more laxative if they should be used to stir it during the boiling process instead of a spatula.

The wild figs, which some call *erineoi*, plastered on boiled, soften all deposits and scrofulous swellings in the glands and they remove warts that spread under the skin and warty excrescences when plastered on raw with soda and flour. The leaves can also do the same things, and they treat scurf, dandruff, and pustules that are most painful at night when laid on with vinegar and salt. Eyelids that are fig-like in texture and rough are rubbed with them, and *leuce*[153] is plastered with the leaves or the branches of the black fig tree. They are also good for dog bites with honey and for impetigo contagiosa.[154]

**6.** Wild figs together with leaves of the corn poppy restore also bones; with wax, they dissolve small abscesses, and when plastered on with bitter vetch and wine, they are suitable for bites of the field mouse and of the millipede.

They also make a powder from the ashes of the burned branches of the wild and cultivated fig trees. It must be washed, however, many times and it must be aged. It is suitable for caustic medications and gangrenous conditions; it cleans and it absorbs superfluous matter. To use it a sponge must be repeatedly drenched with it and applied; in some instances it is used in a clyster, for instance, for dysenterics, for fluxes of long standing, and for large fistulous ulcers which spread under the skin: for it does clean, it glues, it fleshes up, and it glues together in the same manner as the medications for staunching blood.

**7.** It is also given to drink for blood coagulation and for injuries due to falls, for ruptures, for spasms, dissolved with one *cyathos* fresh water and mixed with a little oil, and it helps people with bowel ailments

---

153 λεύκη, a cutaneous disease so called from its white color.

154 LSJ describes κηρίον = μελικηρίς as "cyst" or "wen." Here and throughout this translation I shall translate these words as impetigo contagiosa following Aufmesser, *Erläuterungen* s.v. κηρίον.

and dysenterics when a quantity of one *cyathos* is given by itself; it is a serviceable ointment with wine for those suffering from contracted tendons and spasms since it is sudorific, and it is drunk as an antidote to drinking gypsum and to bites of venomous spiders. The other soap powders, too, offer the same advantages, especially the soap powder that is made from oak. All of them are astringent.

### I, 129 περσαία, *Mimusops Schimperi* L., Persea

Persea is a tree in Egypt, bearing fruit that is edible and good for the stomach and on which the venomous spiders called *cranocolapta* are found, especially in the territory of Thebes.

Ground up and sprinkled dry, its leaves can stop hemorrhages. Some reported that this tree is poisonous in Persia and that it changed and became edible[155] after it was transplanted in Egypt.

[155] Apparently Persea was confused with *Sodanum sodomeum*, Goodyer, *The Greek Herbal of Dioscorides*, p. 92, n. 1.

# BOOK II

Dear Areios,
In the previous book, which was the first I compiled on *Materia medica*, I discussed spices, oil, unguents, and trees, including their juices, saps, and fruits. In this book, which is the second, I shall discuss living creatures, honey, milk, animal fats, and the so-called grains; also vegetables, to which I have subjoined those vegetables that have sharp properties since they are closely related, such as garlic, onion, and mustard in order to group together items of similar properties.

**II, 1 ἐχῖνος θαλάσσιος, Sea urchin**
The sea urchin is salubrious, eases the bowel, and it is diuretic. Its raw shell is compounded advantageously with soaps suitable for mange and, when burned, cleanses filthy sores and reduces sores that grow fungous flesh.

**II, 2 ἐχῖνος χερσαῖος, Hedgehog**
The skin of the hedgehog, when burned, is suitable to smear with liquid pitch on bald spots. Its flesh, dried up and taken with oxymel, helps people with kidney disease, internal edemata, spasms, elephantiasis, and those whose body is deteriorating; it also dries up rheums in the area of the inner organs. Also its liver, dried on an unbaked potsherd and stored, helps for the same conditions when similarly given.

**II, 3 ἱππόκαμπος, Sea horse**
The sea horse is a small marine animal. Having been burned, its ash, in combination with liquid pitch or lard or unguent of marjoram, restores hair on bald spots when rubbed on them.

**II, 4 πορφύρα, Murex**
**1.** Calcined murex has properties that dry, cleanse the teeth, check the overgrowth of flesh, and clean and cicatrize wounds. The same is also true of calcined trumpet shells, although they are rather caustic. But if

one after filling them with salt burned them again in an unbaked vessel, they are suitable for cleaning the teeth and for plastering on fiery inflammations. It is necessary, however, to allow the medication to become dry like a potsherd: for after the fiery inflammation has developed a scab, the plaster falls off automatically.

**2.** One can even make unslaked lime from them, as I shall demonstrate below in the section on unslaked lime (V, 132.)

*Cionia* are called the central columns in the interior of murex and trumpet shells that are surrounded by the convolutions of the shells. They are similarly calcined, having a more caustic property than trumpet shells or murex because it is their nature to exert pressure. As for the flesh of trumpet shells, it is tasty and wholesome but it does not soften the bowel.

### II, 5 μύακες Ποντικοί, Pontic sea mussels

The Pontic sea mussels are the best. When calcined, they produce the same result as do trumpet shells but when washed like lead they are especially useful with honey for eye preparations because they melt out thicknesses of the eyelids and cleanse leucomas and those elements that for some reason cast a shadow over the pupils of the eyes. Their meat is beneficially applied over dog bites.

### II, 6 τελλῖναι, *Tellinai*[1]

Young *tellinai* ease the bowel but their broth eases the bowel the most. Pickled and burned, then ground up and dripped with oil of Syrian cedar, they prevent hair that was plucked from the eyebrows from growing back.

The juice both of clams and of the other cockles, cooked with a little water, moves the bowel. It is taken with wine.

### II, 7 πορφύρας πώματα, Opercula of murex

Opercula of murex, boiled with oil and smeared on, halt the loss of hair; when drunk with vinegar, they reduce a swollen spleen and,

---

[1] Small bivalve shell-fish.

when burned to produce smoke from below, they waken women who are in a state of uterine suffocation[2] and expel the afterbirth.

**II, 8 ὄνυξ, *Onyx***

*Onyx* is the lid of a cockle that resembles the murex and that is found in the spikenard-bearing lakes of India; it is for this reason that it has a spicy flavor, given the fact that the cockles feed upon the spikenard. It is collected during droughts when the lakes have dried up. The best is that brought via the Red Sea, being off-white and shiny; but the Babylonian is black and smaller. Both, however, are aromatic when burned to produce smoke, smelling somewhat like castor.

These, too, when burned to produce smoke from below, awaken women who are in a state of uterine suffocation and epileptics, and they soften the bowel when drunk. The cockle itself, when burned, accomplishes all the things that both the murex and the trumpet shell accomplish.

**II, 9 κοχλίας χερσαῖος, Land snail**

**1.** The land snail is salubrious and hard to destroy. Excellent are those found in Sardinia, Libya, Astypalaia, Sicily, Chios, and the snail called *pomatias*, found in the Alps throughout Liguria. The marine snail, too, is wholesome and easy to excrete, but the riverine snail is foul smelling as is also the field snail that attaches itself on thorny plants and on small shrubs and that some call *sesilos* or *seselita*; it upsets the belly and stomach and it causes vomiting.

**2.** The shells of all of them when calcined are capable of warming, burning, and cleaning leprosies, dull-white leprosies, and teeth. Calcined whole together with their flesh, triturated, and smeared on with honey, they clear away eye scars, leucomas, freckles, and dim-sightedness. Plastered on raw with their shells, they draw out moisture from hydropic swellings and they are not peeled off until all the moisture has been drawn. They assuage gouty inflammations, they draw thorns when similarly plastered, and, when ground up and applied as a pessary, they bring on menstruation.

---

[2] See Dsc. Bk. I, n. 49.

**3.** Their flesh, ground up and plastered on with myrrh and frankincense, closes wounds, especially wounds that are along tendons, and when triturated with vinegar stops nosebleeds. Their live flesh, especially that of the Libyan land snail treats pains of the stomach when swallowed. Pounded whole with its shell and drunk with a little wine and myrrh, it cures the colicky and pains in the bladder. The land snail even glues on hair, if one pushed a needle through its flesh then touched the hair with the glutinous substance.

**II, 10 καρκίνων ποταμίων καέντων ἡ τέφρα, Ash of calcined riverine crabs.**

The ash of calcined riverine crabs, when drunk for three days in the amount of two spoonfuls with one spoonful of gentian root and with wine, is very helpful to those bitten by a mad dog and, with boiled honey, it assuages fissures on the feet and anus, chilblains, and ulcers. Riverine crabs, ground up raw and drunk with ass's milk, help for snakebites and for strokes of venomous spiders and scorpions. Eaten boiled with broth, they benefit tuberculars and those who have drunk sea-hare. Pounded together with basil and applied on scorpions, they kill them. Even sea crabs are capable of the same results but they are less efficacious than the riverine.

**II, 11 σκόρπιος χερσαῖος, Land scorpion**

The land scorpion, ground up raw and plastered on, is a remedy for its own stroke; it is also eaten roasted for the same purpose.

**II, 12 θαλασσίου σκορπίου χολή, Bile of sea scorpion**

The bile of the sea scorpion[3] is suitable for cataracts, leucomas, and dim-sightedness.

**II, 13 δράκων θαλάσσιος, Greater weever**

The greater weever,[4] cut open and applied, is a remedy for the wound that its prickle causes.

---

[3] A saltwater fish, probably *Scorpaena scrofa.*

[4] There are many species of the weever family whose long dorsal fin is supported by many sharp venomous spines that cause painful wounds. The British species are the greater weever, *Tracinus draco,* and the lesser weever, *Tracinus vipera.*

**II, 14 σκολοπένδρα θαλασσία, Sea scolopendra**
The sea scolopendra,[5] cooked in oil and rubbed on, is depilatory; but it causes itching when touched.

**II, 15 νάρκη θαλασσία, Electric ray**
The electric ray, plastered on chronic pains around the head, assuages the intensity of the pains and when placed on an everted or prolapsed anus reverts it to its original position.

**II, 16 ἐχίδνη, Viper**
**1.** Flesh of viper, boiled and eaten, sharpens the sight, is suitable for contracted tendons, and it stops scrofulous swellings of the glands from growing bigger. However, one must after skinning it, chop off the head and tail since they are devoid of flesh—for cutting the extremities with precision is apocryphal—and, < having removed the entrails>, after washing it, and cutting into pieces what is left, one must boil it with oil, wine, a little salt, and dill. They say that those to whom it is offered grow lice, which is patently false, and some add that eating vipers promotes longevity.
**2.** They also make salts from them for the same purposes, but they are not as effective. A live viper is put into a new pot and with it one *xestes* each of salt and of dry figs that were pounded together with six *cyathoi* of honey; then the lid of the pot is covered with clay and it is baked in the oven until the salts turn into coal. Then they are triturated and stored. Sometimes spikenard or a bit of leaf of Malabar is added to make them palatable.

**II, 17 ὄφις, Serpent**
The slough of a serpent boiled with wine is a remedy for earaches when instilled and for toothaches when used as a mouthwash. They mix it even with eye medications and especially the slough of viper.

**II, 18 λαγωὸς θαλάσσιος, Sea hare**
The sea hare resembles a small squid. Ground up and plastered on either by itself or with sea anemone can depilate.

---

[5] Perhaps of the genus *Nereis* or *Aphrodite*.

**II, 19 τοῦ δὲ χερσαίου λαγωοῦ ὁ ἐγκέφαλος, The brain of the land hare**

The brain of the land hare, broiled and eaten, is beneficial for trembling that comes from shock also for teething when rubbed on children and when eaten. Its head burned and anointed with bear's fat or with vinegar treats bald spots. If drunk three days after menstruation, its rennet is said to cause barrenness. It stops both uterine running and diarrhea, it is good for epileptics, also for poisons when drunk with vinegar, and it is especially good for the curdling of milk and for bites of vipers. When smeared on hot, its blood treats freckles, dull-white leprosy, and birthmarks.

**II, 20 τρυγόνος θαλασσίας τὸ κέντρον, Stingray sting**

The sting of the stingray that grows from its tail curling up[6] toward the scales assuages a toothache, for it shatters the tooth and ejects it.

**II, 21 σηπίας ἑψηθείσης τὸ μέλαν, Ink of boiled cuttlefish**

When consumed the ink of boiled cuttlefish is difficult to digest and softens the bowel. Its shell, fashioned into eye salves, is suitable for abrading rough eyelids; burned in its own shell until its laminated part separates and used ground up, it cleans dull-white leprosy, dandruff, teeth, and freckles. After it is washed, it is also mixed into eye medications. It is effective for leucomas of domestic animals when blown unto them, and, when ground up with salt and applied, it reduces the membranes that grow over the eyes from the inner corners.

**II, 22 τρίγλα, Red mullet**

A steady diet of red mullet seems to cause dim-sightedness. Split open raw and applied as a plaster, it treats the stings of the greater weever, scorpion, and spider.

**II, 23 ὄρχις ἱπποποτάμου, Testicle of hippopotamus**

Dried and triturated testicle of hippopotamus is drunk with wine for bites of reptiles.

---

[6] The meaning here is unclear, and Max Wellmann, *Pedanii Dioscuridis Anazarbei de materia medica*, Bk. II, p. 128, says that it is suspect.

**II, 24 καὶ ὁ τοῦ κάστορος ὄρχις, Testicle of beaver**

**1**. Also the testicle of the beaver[7]— this animal is amphibian, feeding mostly in the water on fish and crabs—is effective for bites of reptiles but it also induces sneezing, and, on the whole, it has many uses. For if drunk with two-*drachmai* pennyroyal, it sets the menses going and it expels both embryos/fetuses and the afterbirth. It is drunk with vinegar for flatulence, colic, hiccups, deadly drugs, and for pine thistle.[8] Sprinkled with vinegar and unguent of roses and smelled, it arouses both those affected by lethargic fever and those who suddenly fall asleep,[9] and it does the same when burned so as to produce smoke. When drunk and when anointed, it is a fit remedy for tremors, for spasms, for every problem that has to do with the tendons, and, in general, it has a warming property.

**2.** Always choose testicles that are joined together at one end—for it is not possible to find two sacs joined together in one membrane— and whose interior is waxy, oppressive in scent, foul smelling, harsh, biting, crumbly, and partitioned frequently with natural membranes. Some adulterate it by pouring into the pouch gum ammoniac or gum kneaded with beaver's blood then drying it. But the story that the animal when pursued tears off its testicles and throws them away is utter nonsense. For it is impossible for it to reach them since they lie flat like the hog's. After cutting open the skin, you must remove the honey-like liquid with the membrane that surrounds it and thus dry and store.

**II, 25 γαλῆ κατοικίδιος, Domesticated weasel**

The domesticated weasel, charred all around, salt-dried without its entrails, and desiccated in the shade is a very effective remedy for every kind of serpent when a quantity of two *drachmai* is drunk with wine; it is also an antidote for poisons when similarly taken. Its belly, filled with coriander and dried, helps those bitten by wild animals and epileptics when taken in a drink. Burned whole in a pot, it helps the

---

[7] J. Berendes, p. 161, says that the discussion here is not about the testicles of the male beaver but of an internal gland of the beaver identified by Bondeletius [sic] in the 16th century.

[8] See Dsc. Bk. III, 8 and n. 11.

[9] I.e. narcoleptics.

gouty when its ash is smeared on them with vinegar. Its blood, smeared on scrofulous swellings of the glands, benefits them as it also benefits epileptics.

**II, 26 βάτραχοι, Frogs**

Frogs are an antidote for all reptiles when boiled with salt and oil and their broth is consumed. Being similarly taken, they are also a remedy for chronic inflammations of tendons. Burned and sprinkled on, they staunch bleeding and, when smeared on with liquid pitch, they treat bald spots. The blood of pale-green frogs, when let fall in drops, prevents hair plucked from eyebrows from growing back. Boiled with water and vinegar and used as a mouthwash, they are also serviceable for toothaches.

**II, 27 σίλουρος, Sheatfish**

Sheatfish[10] when eaten fresh is nutritious and eases the bowel but when pickled it lacks nutritive value although it cleanses the trachea and makes the voice melodious. The flesh of pickled sheatfish draws out splinters when plastered on. Its brine is suitable to use in a sitz bath for dysenterics at the onset of their disease, removing the discharges to the outside, and treats patients suffering from hip disease when used as a clyster.

**II, 28 σμαρίδος ταριχηρᾶς ἡ κεφαλὴ καεῖσα, Head of salted *smaris***

The head of salted smaris [11] baked and <ground up> checks sores that grow a fungous flesh, stays the growth of spreading ulcers, and wipes out warts and warty excrescences. The flesh is suitable for people bitten by scorpions or dogs, as is all salted fish.

---

[10] The identification of *silouros* with sheatfish is tentative.

[11] A small sea-fish, *Smaris vulgaris.* In Modern Greek, too, it is called *smaris* or *marida,* the latter being a more colloquial word. Today it is found routinely on the menu of seashore restaurants, deep-fried and eaten whole, including spine, head, and tail. LSJ describes it as a "poor" fish, but the Greeks and many foreigners who are fish aficionados love it.

**II, 29 καὶ ἡ τῆς μαινίδος κεφαλὴ, Head of *Mainis***

Also the head of *mainis*,[12] burned, ground up, and sprinkled on hardened anal fistulas, removes them. The sauce[13] that is made from them when used in a mouthwash stops putrid humors in the mouth.

**II, 30 κωβιός, Goby**

If after placing a fresh goby[14] into a pig's tripe, you sewed the tripe up and boiled it in 12-*xestes* water until reduced to two-*xestes* then, after straining the liquid and setting it out in the sun and air, gave it to drink, you would gently purge the bowel. Applied as a cataplasm, it is also good for those bitten by dogs or snakes.

**II, 31 ὠμοτάριχος, *Omotarichos***

The so-called *omotarichos*[15] is the flesh of pickled tuna. When consumed it helps those bitten by the viper called *prester*— but one must offer them a great deal of it and force them to drink much wine and to vomit—and it is especially suitable for counteracting the ingestion of acrid foods. It is plastered successfully also on people bitten by dogs.

**II, 32 γάρος, Garum**

Every kind of garum[16] of pickled fish or meat arrests spreading ulcers and treats dog bites when used as a fomentation. It is also injected as a clyster into dysenterics and into those suffering from hip disease either to draw suppurated sores or to bring to head non-suppurated sores.

**II, 33 ζωμὸς ἰχθύων, Fish broth**

Broth made from fresh fish purges the bowel, being drunk either neat or with wine. For this purpose, the broth is properly prepared from

---

[12] A small sprat-like fish, *Maena vulgaris*.

[13] See Dsc. Bk. II, n. 16 below.

[14] Also referred to as gudgeon.

[15] ὠμοτάριχος is a compound word from ὠμός, "uncooked," and ταριχός, "salted, cured, or preserved fish or meat." This is the *lakerda* of modern Greeks, a delicious appetizer.

[16] Garum is ordinarily a fish paste or sauce. Here it is also made with meat. For a thorough understanding of fish garum, its commercial value as food in the daily diet of Mediterraneans, and its importance as a therapeutic see Robert I. Curtis, *Garum and Salsamenta*.

*phycis,*[17] *scorpions,*[18] rainbow-wrasse, perch, and other rockfish that are soft and free of foul smells simply with water, salt, oil, and dill.

**II, 34 κόρεις οἱ ἀπὸ κλίνης, Bed-bugs**

Seven bedbugs placed inside beans and swallowed before the onset of a quartan fever help those having an attack of quartan fever; they also help those bitten by asps when drunk without the beans, and when smelled they revive those in a state of uterine suffocation. Drunk with vinegar, they get rid of leeches and, when inserted ground up into the urethra, they bring an end to difficult micturition.

**II, 35 ὄνοι οἱ ὑπὸ τὰς ὑδρίας, Wood lice**

The wood lice that are found under water pitchers—they are polypeds that curl themselves up at the touch of hands—are helpful for difficult micturition and jaundice when drunk with wine. Anointed with honey, they help people with sore throats and, if they have been ground up, heated with unguent of roses in a pomegranate shell, and instilled, they help for earaches.

**II, 36 σίλφη, Cockroach**

The insides of the cockroach that is found in bakeries, pounded with oil or boiled and dropped into the ears, stop earaches.

**II, 37 πνεύμων θαλάσσιος, Jellyfish**

Fresh jellyfish triturated and plastered on, helps the gouty and those having chilblains.

**II, 38 ὁ δὲ χοίρειος καὶ ἄρνειος [καὶ ἄρκειος] πνεύμων, Pig, lamb, [and bear] lung**

The lung of pig, lamb, and bear applied to abrasions that were caused by shoes, maintain them free of inflammations.

---

[17] The female of a fish, probably a species of wrasse.

[18] Probably the sea-fish *Scorpaena scrofa*, used like the *mugilis* in Catull.15.19, Juv.10.317 to punish adulterers.

**II, 39 ἀλώπεκος πνεύμων, Lung of fox**
The lung of fox dried and taken in a drink helps asthmatics. Fat of fox also stops an earache when melted and poured into the ear.

**II, 40 ἧπαρ ὄνειον, Ass's liver**
Roasted ass's liver helps epileptics when eaten. They should take it, however, on an empty stomach.

**II, 41 αἰδοῖον ἄρρενος ἐλάφου, Genitalia of stag**
The genitalia of stag ground up and drunk with wine help those bitten by vipers.

**II, 42 ὄνυχες ὄνων, Asses' hooves**
Asses' hooves, burned and drunk in the amount of two spoonsful for several days, are reported to help epileptics. Made into a paste with oil, they dissipate scrofulous swellings of the glands and when sprinkled on they treat chilblains.

**II, 43 λειχῆνες ἵππων, Chestnuts of horses**
Chestnuts of horses—they are horny calluses molded in outline on their knees and hooves—are reported to help for epilepsy when drunk ground up with vinegar.

**II, 44 οἱ δὲ τῶν αἰγῶν ὄνυχες, Hooves of she-goats**
The hooves of she-goats burned and smeared on with vinegar treat bald spots.

**II, 45 τοῦ δὲ ἥπατος τῆς αἰγὸς ἰχώρ, Juice of she-goat liver**
The juice that runs off the liver of a she-goat, as it is roasted, is suitable to anoint for night blindness. And should one receive steam of boiling she-goat liver into his open eyes, he would benefit. And it is suitable also to eat the liver roasted for the same purposes. And they say that even epileptics are put very much to the test when they eat goat liver.

**II, 46 τὸ δὲ τοῦ κάπρου ἧπαρ, Boar's liver**
Fresh as well as dried boar's liver ground up and drunk with wine is good for snakebites.

**II, 47 κυνὸς δὲ λυσσῶντος ἧπαρ, Liver of rabid dog**
The liver of a rabid dog, eaten roasted by those bitten by it, is believed to keep them safe from rabies. As a precaution, they also use the canine of the dog that bit them, tied in a little pouch, and fastened onto their arm.

**II, 48 κασσυμάτων παλαιὰ δέρματα, Leather of shoe soles**
Old leather of shoe soles, burned ground up, and sprinkled on treats burns, scrapings, and shoe abrasions.

**II, 49 ἀλεκτορίδες, Hens**
**1.** Hens, ripped up open and applied while warm, help for bites of reptiles; but it is necessary to keep on changing them. Their brain, too, is given to drink with wine to those bitten by wild animals and it stops meningeal bleedings. But the cock's horny element that lies in the inside of its gizzard and that is scraped off when it is boiled, dried up and ground up, is an appropriate drink with wine for those with stomach ailments. Pullet broth, prepared without additives, is very commonly given to temper states of bad health and to those suffering from heartburn.
**2.** But the broth of old chickens is given as a cathartic. It is necessary, however, to remove the entrails, salt the cavity, and, after sewing it up, boil it with 20-*xestes* water, reducing it to three-*cotylai*. After it has been set outdoors to cool, the entire quantity is given. Some boil with it sea cole or mercury or safflower or polypody.[19] It drives out thick, raw, glutinous, and black masses, and it is suitable for chronic fevers, for periodic shiverings, asthma, arthritis, and for those who suffer from stomach gas.

**II, 50 ᾠόν, Egg**
An egg that is soft-boiled is more nutritious than an egg that can be sipped and a hard-boiled egg is more nutritious than a soft-boiled. Its boiled yolk is useful with saffron and unguent of roses for acute eye pains and with melilot for inflammations and callous lumps around the

---

[19] All four plants are described as being cathartic. See Dsc. Bk. II, 122, IV, 186, 188, and 189.

anus. Fried with the fruit of sumac or with oak-galls and eaten, the yolk checks diarrhea, also when it is offered by itself.
When raw its albumen cools, causes adherence, soothes when poured onto inflamed eyes, prevents burns from blistering when smeared on them immediately, guards faces from sunburns, it is an adhesive plaster for people who have a running nose when applied with frankincense on the forehead, and it abates inflammations of the eyes when a wool-pad that was soaked with it, unguent of roses, and wine-honey is applied to them. Sipped raw, it helps for bites of *haimorrhois*[20] but lukewarm it is suitable for stinging in the bladder, for kidney ulceration, for roughness of the trachea, for coughing up blood, for catarrhs, and for chest rheums.

**II, 51 τέττιγες, Cicadas**
When eaten roasted cicadas help pains around the bladder.

**II, 52 ἀκρίδες, Locusts**
Locusts that are burned so as to produce smoke from below are beneficial for difficult micturition, especially in women. The locust called *troxallis* or *onos*—it is wingless and large-limbed—newly caught, dried, and drunk with wine is very helpful to those stung by scorpions. The Libyans who live throughout Leptis use it extensively.

**II, 53 φήνη, *Phene***
The stomach of the bird *phene,*[21] called *ossifragus* in Latin, when given to drink in small sips is said to cause stones to pass with the urine.

**II, 54 κορυδαλλός, Lark**
The lark is a small bird that has on top of its head a crest like that of the peacock. This bird benefits the colicky when eaten roasted.

**II, 55 αἰθυίας ἧπαρ, Liver of shearwater**
The liver of shearwater,[22] cured and drunk with hydromel in the amount of two spoonsful, ousts the afterbirth.

[20] The bite of this serpent causes blood to flow from all parts of the body.
[21] A kind of a vulture.

**II, 56 χελιδὸνος νεοσσοί, Swallow's nestlings**

If when the moon waxes you cut open a swallow's nestlings from the first hatching, you will find stones in their belly. If you took two of them, one mottled and one plain, and before coming in contact with the soil you tied them in heifer's or deer's skin and hang them around the arm or neck of epileptics, you will help them; often you will even effect their complete recovery. When eaten like beccaficos, these nestlings are a medicine for sharp-sightedness, and both their ash and the ash of their mothers cause sharp-sightedness when burned in a clay pot and anointed with honey. The ash is also suitable to smear on those with sore throats and for inflammations of the uvula and tonsils. The swallows themselves and their nestlings, air cured and drunk in the amount of one *drachma* by weight with water, help those with sore throats.

**II, 57 ἐλέφαντος ὀδούς, Elephant's tooth**

The filings of elephant's tooth when plastered on treat whitlow. They have an astringent property.

**II, 58 ἀστράγαλος ὑός, Hog's hock**

Hog's hock, burned until from being black it becomes white again, ground up, and drunk, relieves colon flatulence and chronic colic.

**II, 59 ἐλάφου κέρας, Hart's horn**

An amount of two spoonsful of hart's horn burned and washed is a suitable drink for people who spit blood, dysenterics, people who suffer in the bowels, for the jaundiced, for bladder pains with tragacanth, and for women who are having discharges when taken with a liquid that is appropriate for their condition. After it has been placed in an unbaked clay pot and chopped up, the pot is sealed with clay and burned in an oven until the horn becomes white. It is washed like calamine. This type of preparation is suitable for eye rheums and sores on the eyes, and it cleans the teeth when rubbed against them. Burned raw to produce thick smoke, it drives away serpents, and when boiled with vinegar and used as a rinse, it assuages toothaches.

---

[22] The identification of this bird is tentative.

**II, 60 κάμπαι, Caterpillars**

The caterpillars that breed on vegetables, when smeared on with oil, are said to protect people from being bitten by venomous animals.

**II, 61 κανθαρίδες, Blister beetles**

**1.** Blister beetles that come from grain are suitable for storage. After placing them in an unglazed vessel and tying its mouth all around with a clean loosely woven cloth, turn it upside down over the steam of boiling, very strong vinegar and keep it until the blister-beetles are stifled; then threading them with a linen thread store them. Most effective are the ones that are mottled, that have quince-yellow, oblique stripes on their wings, and that are oblong in body, thick, and fat like the cockroaches; but the monochrome are ineffective. Similarly stored are the *bouprestis*, which are a kind of blister beetle, and the caterpillars found on the *pitys* pine. These, too, are stored, after being cooked briefly in a sieve hanging over hot ashes.[23]

**2.** They all share septic, warming, and ulcerating properties; it is for this reason that they are mixed with medicines for cancerous sores and they treat both leprosies and virulent lichen-like eruptions of the skin. They also draw down the menses when mixed with softening pessaries. Some reported that blister beetles, combined with remedies, help also those with edemata, on the theory that they set micturition in motion. Others have written that their wings and legs are an antidote for those who have drunk these beetles.

**II, 62 σαλαμάνδρα, Salamander**

Salamander is a kind of lizard that is sluggish, colorful, and wrongly thought to be incombustible. It has septic, ulcerating, and warming properties. It is mixed with medications that are putrefactive, ulcerating, and good for leprosy, just like the blister beetle, and it is similarly stored. Liquefied in oil, it is also depilatory. Disemboweled, dismembered, and decapitated, it is preserved also in honey for the same uses.

---

[23] All these beetles contain a vesicating element. Druggists call them Spanish flies. βουπρέστης apparently also causes cattle that eat it to swell up and die. Its pernicious action on cattle is embedded in its etymology, βούς, cattle and πρῆσις, distention. For a discussion on the Greeks' notion on the medicine-poison see John Riddle, *Dioscorides on Pharmacy and Medicine*, pp. 139-140.

**II, 63 ἀράχνη τὸ ζῷον, Spider, the insect**[24]

Spider, the insect, which some call *holcos* or *lycos,* kneaded on a linen pad, plastered onto a linen cloth, <and> applied to the forehead or the temples, cures fits of tertian fever. When plastered on, its web staunches the blood and maintains the surfaces of sores free of inflammations.

There is also another type of spider that spins its web white and dense. It is reported that this web cures fits of quartan fever when packed in a pouch and hung from the arm. And it helps for earaches when boiled with unguent of roses and the liquid is instilled into the ears.

**II, 64 σαύρας ἡ κεφαλὴ, Head of lizard**

The head of the lizard, ground up and plastered on, draws up splinters and all sorts of embedded objects; it also removes warts that spread under the skin, thin-necked warts, and warts. Its liver stops pain when inserted into the cavities of decayed teeth. The entire lizard split open and applied brings relief to those bitten by scorpions.

**II, 65 σήψ, Seps**

The *seps,* which some call Chalcidian lizard, treats those bitten by it when drunk in wine.

**II, 66 σκίγκος, Skink**

The skink: there is an Egyptian skink, an Indian, which is indigenous to the Indian Ocean, and another that is found in Gaetulia of Mauritania. It is a land crocodile, peculiar in kind, preserved in garden cress.

They say that a quantity of one *drachma* of the part that surrounds its kidneys when drunk with wine heightens one's sexual drive and that the intensity of the yearning is brought under control if one drank lentil broth with honey or lettuce seed with water; it is also mixed with antidote.

---

[24] The use of the generic article with ζῷον, in this instant "insect," is to distinguish ἀράχνη, "spider" from ἀράχνη, "a kind of pulse."

**II, 67 γῆς ἔντερα, Earthworms**

Earthworms ground up and laid upon severed tendons mend them, but they must be removed every other day; boiled with goose fat and instilled, they cure ear conditions. Boiled with oil, they assuage toothaches if injected into the ear situated above the aching tooth. They also set micturition in motion when drunk ground up with grape syrup.

**II, 68 μυογαλῆ, Shrewmouse**

The shrewmouse split open and laid on is a remedy for its own bite.

**II, 69 μύες, Mice**

It is commonly agreed that split mice are beneficially applied on those stung by scorpions and that roasted mice dry the saliva in the mouth of children who eat them.

**II, 70 γάλα, Milk**

**1.** In general, all milk is wholesome, nutritious, softens the stool, and produces stomach and intestinal gases. Spring milk is more watery than summer milk, and milk from green pastures softens the bowel more. Milk is of good quality when it is white, evenly thick, and if it congeals when dropped on *onyx*.[25] Goat milk has a lesser effect on the bowel because, by and large, goats eat food that binds the bowel, such as mastic, oak, young shoots of the olive tree and it is for this reason that it is good for the stomach. Sheep's milk is thick, sweet, fat, and not so good for the stomach. As for ass's, cow's, and horse's milk, they ease more the bowel and they upset the stomach.

**2.** All milk disturbs the bowel and the stomach wherever the pasture is scammony or hellebore or mercury[26] or *clematis*,[27] as we personally witnessed in the Vestini Mountains. For when the goats graze on the leaves of white hellebore, not only do they vomit as soon as they first

---

[25] See. Dsc. Bk. I, n. 81.

[26] This is the plant mercury.

[27] Dsc. uses κληματίς for periwinkle, *Vinca herbacea*, in IV, 7 and for traveller's joy, *Clematis Vitalba* in Bk. IV, 180. There is a third κληματίς listed in LSJ conjectured to be bearbine, *Convolvulus arvensis*. It is a pasture plant and this may be the *clematis* meant here.

taste the plant, but the milk they produce upsets the stomach and causes nausea. All boiled milk binds the bowel, especially milk that has been evaporated with very hot pebbles. In general, however, it seems to help for internal ulcerations, especially those of the throat, lung, intestines, kidneys, bladder, and for skin irritations, for pustules, and for unhealthy state of humors.

**3.** It is given fresh combined with raw honey and a little water; salt is also added. It causes less flatulence if it is boiled once. Boiled with pebbles until reduced by half, it comes to the rescue of discharges from an ulcerated bowel.

All milk contains whey, which, once it is separated, is suitable for thorough purging; it is given to those we wish to purge gently, for instance, melancholiacs, epileptics, leprotics, people who have elephantiasis, and for pustules that cover the entire body.

**4.** Milk is separated by boiling it in a new clay vessel and stirring it with a freshly cut branch of fig tree; after it has come to a boil two or three times, one *cyathos* of oxymel is sprinkled on each *cotyle* of milk. For this is the way that whey is separated from the cheesy element. It will be necessary during the boiling process, however, to wipe off continuously the rim of the vessel with a sponge dipped in cold water and to lower into the milk a silver cup full of cold water to prevent the milk from boiling over. The whey is given to drink at intervals in amounts ranging from one *cotyle* to five *cotylai* and during the intervals the people who drink it should keep walking.

**5.** Fresh milk is good also for the gnawing pains and inflammations from deadly substances, as from the blister beetle or the processional caterpillar or the *bouprestes* or the salamander or henbane or *dorycnion*[28] or leopard's bane or *ephemeron*.[29] To this end, cow's milk is most useful, being singularly suitable; it is also used as a rinse for mouth sores and for the tonsils as a gargle. Ass's milk, in particular, when used as a mouth rinse strengthens gums and teeth, butsheep's or cow's or goat's milk boiled with pebbles stops ulcerating diarrhea and tenesmus. It is also used as a clyster by itself as well as with either

[28] *Convolvulus oleofolius* Dsr.

[29] A poisonous plant, *Colchicum* L. sp. See Dsc. IV, 83.

barley-water or gruel, soothing considerably the gnawing of the intestines. It is administered as a clyster also for an ulcerated uterus.

**6.** Woman's milk is very sweet and highly nutritive. When suckled it is good for the gnawing of the stomach and for tuberculosis, and it is fit to give to anyone who has drunk sea-hare. Mixed with ground frankincense, it is dripped on eyes that are bloody from a blow, and when smeared on with hemlock juice and cerate it benefits the gouty. No milk, however, is appropriate for spleen and liver disease patients, for those affected in the nervous system, for people who have a fever, for those suffering from a headache, for those who are dizzy, and for epileptics, unless one offered them first the whey for purging purposes, as indicated. Some say that the milk of a primipara bitch thins hair when smeared on and that when drunk it is an antidote to deadly medicines and a means for expelling dead embryos/fetuses.

**II, 71 τυρός, Cheese**

When eaten without salt, new cheese is nutritious, good for the stomach, easy to digest, fattening, and it softens moderately the bowel. One cheese differs from another of the same kind according to the nature of the milk from which it is made. But if it has been boiled and pressed then baked, it binds the bowel; plastered on, it is also good for inflammations of the eyes and for black eye. Since cheese that has been freshly salted is less nutritious, it is suitable for reducing, it is unwholesome, and it distresses the stomach and intestines. Aged cheese tightens the bowel and its whey is highly nutritious for dogs.

The so-called *hippace* is horse cheese; it is foul smelling, highly nutritious, and equivalent to cow cheese. But some called *hippace* equine rennet.

**II, 72 βούτυρον, Butter**

**1.** Good butter is made from very fat milk; such milk is that of sheep. But it is made also from goat's milk; the milk is stirred in vessels and the fat is separated.

It possesses emollient and oily properties. It is for this reason that it loosens the bowel when a great deal of it is drunk and that in the absence of oil it is used in counteracting poisons. Mixed with honey and brushed on, it helps for teething, for the itching of children's gums, and for thrush, and it keeps the body in thriving condition and free of pimples when applied externally.

**2.** If it is neither ill-smelling nor old, it is good for inflammations and indurations of the uterus, it is used in clysters for dysentery and ulceration of the colon, it is compounded to good avail with suppurating preparations, and it is especially good for injuries along the tendons, the membranes, and the neck of the bladder. The same fills, cleanses, and fleshes up, and it benefits those bitten by an asp when laid on. Fresh butter is also mixed into side dishes instead of oil and into sweetmeats instead of suet.

**3.** Soot is collected from butter this way: pouring the butter into a new lamp, light it up and covering it with a clay vessel, pipe-shaped on top and perforated below like the *clibanoi*,[30] let it burn. When the first butter is spent, pour more and do the same until you have as much soot as you wish, then remove it with a feather and use it. Used in eye medications, it can dry and bind, it stops discharges, and it quickly fleshes up and <cicatrizes> sores.

### II, 73 ἔρια οἰσυπηρά, Greasy wool

**1.** Greasy wool is excellent when soft and when it comes from the neck and thighs; soaked in vinegar and oil or wine, it is good for fresh wounds, bruises, abrasions, livid spots, and bone fractures, for it absorbs the liquids and it softens due to the grease it contains. It is also good with vinegar and unguent of roses for a headache, for stomachaches, and for pains everywhere.

Burned wool has properties that heat, cicatrize, control fleshy excrescences, and heal sores. After it has been cleaned and carded, it is burned in an unbaked clay vessel like the other substances. The same way are burned also tufts of wool dyed in purple dye. But some, after carding the wool together with its filth and drenching it in honey, burn it the same way.

**2.** Others, however, dispose small skewers on a wide-mouthed clay vessel arranging them at a distance from each other, then they set on top of them thin splinters of pine wood and on top they place the

---

[30] κλίβανοι are covered earthen vessels wider at the bottom than at the top in which bread was baked.

wool, carded and soaked in oil but not dripping of it, then after placing again on top alternately splinters of wood and wool, they set the wool on fire gently from below the pine. After it has burned, they remove it and if there is either grease or pitch that drips down from the pine it is collected and stored. It is washed for eye medications in a clay platter into which water is poured and stirred vigorously with the hands; after it has come to rest, the liquid is decanted, fresh liquid is added, and again stirred, and the process is repeated until it does not bite but is mildly astringent when placed on the tongue.

**II, 74 οἴσυπος, Fat from greasy wool**

**1.** The fat from greasy wool is called *oisypos*; you will prepare it this way: taking soft greasy wool that was not cleaned with soapwort, wash it in warm water squeezing out all its filth. Placing this filth into a wide-mouthed vessel and pouring over it water, keep scooping it up vigorously with a ladle until it foams, or stir it vigorously with a spatula until a great deal of greasy foam gathers; then sprinkle it with seawater and when the floating grease comes to a stop, scoop it up into another clay vessel, and pouring water into the vessel, stir it again, sprinkle the foam with the seawater, scoop it up, and repeat the process until there is no longer any foam that forms on top, since the grease was spent.

**2.** Then kneading by hand the *oisypos* that you scooped up, remove immediately any impurity that it may contain, strain the first water, pour on new, and stir by hand, until it appears to be clean and white, and so store it in a clay vessel. Make sure that the whole process takes place when the weather is hot. But some, after straining the grease wash it in cold water, rubbing it with their hands as women rub the cerate. Prepared this way, it becomes whiter.

**3.** Others, after washing the wool and squeezing out its filth, gently boil it with water in a cauldron, then after removing the grease that floats on top, wash it with water as has been described; then straining it into a clay platter containing warm water and covering it with a linen cloth, set it in the sun until it becomes sufficiently thick and white; others pour out the first water after two days and pour on new. The best is that which has not been washed with soapwort and which is smooth, smells of greasy wool, becomes white when rubbed with

cold water in a shell, and is devoid of any hard or compacted matter as is that which is adulterated with cerate or with animal fat.
**4.** It has properties that warm, fill sores, and soften, especially the areas around the anus and the uterus with melilot and butter. It draws both the menstrual period and embryos/fetuses when applied as a pessary on wool, and it is good with goose fat for ear problems and for afflictions in the genitalia. It is also effective for corners of eyes that have been eroded by ulcers or that are scabby, and for eyelids that are calloused or that shed their lashes. It is burned on a new clay vessel until having been reduced to ashes it lets go of its fat. Also soot is collected from it the way we demonstrated above (I, 68,) which is suitable for eye medications.

### II, 75 πιτύα, Rennet

**1.** A weight of three *oboloi* of hare's[31] rennet taken with wine is suitable for those bitten by wild animals, for dysenterics, for women who suffer from discharges, for blood clots, and for coughing up blood from the chest; applied to the cervix with butter after menstruation, it aids conception, but if drunk after menstruation, it causes barrenness. The curdled milk of the horse, called by some *hippace*, is particularly good for the colicky and the dysenteric.
**2.** The rennet of kid, lamb, fawn, roe deer, flat-horned deer, gazelle, deer, calf, and antelope have the same properties; taken with wine they are suitable to treat the ingestion of hemlock and with vinegar for curdling of milk. But fawn's rennet, in particular, when applied for three days following menstruation causes barrenness. Seal's rennet seems to have the same property as that of beaver and to be especially good to drink for epileptics and for uterine suffocation.
**3.** This is the way one proves whether it comes from a seal: taking the rennet of some animal or other, most likely of a lamb, and after pouring water over it, let it stand for a short while, then pour the infusion over the seal's rennet: that which is genuine quickly becomes watery, but the spurious stays the same. Rennet is taken from the seal

[31] Although the text reads simply πιτύα λαγωοῦ, "hare's rennet," one must assume that the hare is a suckling, since rennet is found only in the stomach of animals that are at suckling stage or in the stomach of ruminants.

when the cubs are not yet able to swim. In general, all rennets congeal substances that have been dissolved and dissolve substances that have been congealed.

**II, 76 στέαρ, Fat**

**1.** Well suited for uterine conditions are goose fat and chicken fat that are fresh and that were not treated with salt; but if they were exposed to the sun or if they have turned rancid from age they are harmful to the womb. Take some fresh fat from these birds and, after removing its membrane, place it on a new clay platter that can accommodate twice as much fat as you intend to prepare, then cover carefully the container, place it under a very hot sun, and at once filter the fat that is melting into another clay vessel until all the fat is spent. Store it in a very cold place and use it.

**2.** But some instead of setting the platter in the sun rest it over hot water or over gentle and slow-burning embers. There is also another way of preparing it which is this: after the fat has been stripped of its membrane, it is triturated then placed in a pan and rendered together with a little fine salt; then it is strained through a fine linen cloth and stored. Prepared in this manner, it is suitable for medicinal preparations.

Swine fat and bear fat are cured this way: taking fat that is fresh and very rich, such is the fat that comes from the kidneys, dip it into a large quantity of very cold rainwater, remove its membrane, and rub it carefully with your hands, rubbing it as if you were scraping it.

**3.** Then washing it repeatedly with new water, place it in a clay pot large enough to accommodate twice the amount of fat and after pouring enough water to cover the fat, place it on slow-burning embers, stirring it with a spatula. When it has melted, straining it through a strainer into water and, after letting it cool, straining it again, place the strained product carefully into the pot that had been already washed clean, and pouring water over it melt it slowly; then remove it from the fire, wait for a while for the dregs to settle, and decant into a mortar moistened with a sponge. When it has hardened pick it up, remove the impurities from the bottom, melt it for a third time without water, then pour it out into a mortar, clean it, put it into a clay vessel, and store it well-sealed in a very cold place.

**4.** He-goat, sheep or deer fat is cured this way: taking any one of the fats mentioned and after washing it and removing its membrane as prescribed above in the paragraph on swine fat, place it in a mortar to soften and knead it, adding a small quantity of water over it until no bloody clot is secreted, no scum floats upon it, and until it becomes shiny. Then after placing it into a clay pot and adding enough water to cover it, set it on gently burning coals and stir. When all of it has been rendered, pour over it water, cool it, and, after washing the vessel, melt it for a second time and repeat the steps mentioned above.
**5.** Then melting it for the third time without water in a moistened mortar, strain it and after it has cooled, following the directions on the chapter on swine fat, store it.
Beef suet that is taken from the kidneys must also have its membrane removed and must be washed in seawater from the open sea, then it must be placed in a mortar and chopped up carefully while being sprinkled with seawater. When all of it has dissolved, it must be put in a clay pot, seawater must be poured on top to cover it by at least a span, and it must be boiled until it throws off its characteristic smell.
**6.** Then for every one Attic *mna* of suet four *holcai* of Tyrrhenian wax must be added and strained, the dirt from the bottom must be removed, and the rendered suet must be placed in a new platter; then it must be carried out daily to the sun, covered all around, until it becomes white and loses its bad smell.
But bull suet must be cured this way: taking of this suet, too, that which is fresh and from the area of the kidneys, wash it in the current of a river, and, after removing its membrane, place it in a new clay pot, sprinkle on it a little salt, and melt it.
**7.** Then straining it into clear water, when it begins to solidify wash it again by hand, pounding it vigorously and changing the water repeatedly until it is well washed. Then placing it again in a pot, boil it with an equal amount of aromatic wine. When it has boiled twice, remove the vessel from the fire and let the suet stand there overnight; the following day, if any bad smell lingers on, transferring the aforementioned into another new pot, pour over it aromatic wine, and repeat the steps mentioned above until it casts off all its foul smell.
**8.** For certain conditions where salt is counter-indicated, it is also melted without salt. If it has been prepared this way it does not

become very white. Fat of leopard, lion, wild boar, camel, horse, and the like must be prepared similarly.

Calf and bull suet as well as deer fat and the marrow of this animal must be scented this way: having removed the membrane of the fat you intend to scent and after washing it as prescribed above, boil it with wine that does not contain seawater and that is fragrant; then after lifting it and leaving it alone overnight, pour over it more fresh wine of the same kind and in the same quantity as given earlier, and, after melting it and scooping it out carefully, add to every nine *cotylai* of suet seven *holcai* of Arabian camel hay.

**9.** But should you wish to make it smell even sweeter, add 40 *holcai* of its flowers and an equal quantity of date-palm and sweet flag, and one *holce* each of camel's-thorn and balsam wood; mix also one *oungia* each of cardamom, spikenard, cassia, and cinnamon—make sure that all of them are roughly chopped—then, after adding aromatic wine, cover and place the vessel on coals and bring to boil three times; then removing it from the fire, let it stand overnight; the following day, pour out the wine, add new wine of the same kind, bring to a boil similarly three more times, and set it aside.

**10.** In the morning, after taking up the fat, pour out the wine, wash the vessel, clean the dirt at the bottom of the fat, then melt, strain, store, and use it.

Even if it has been cured, it is scented the same way. This is how the fats mentioned above are thickened beforehand to receive more easily the strength of the aromatics: taking whichever of these fats you may choose boil it with wine, adding a branch of myrtle, tufted thyme and galingale, also camel's-thorn, all of them chopped coarsely together. Some are content with a single one of these ingredients. When it has come to a boil for a third time, lifting it gently and after straining it through a linen cloth scent it as shown.

**11.** Furthermore, you may even thicken animal fats this way: having chopped whichever of these fats you may wish—it should be fresh and free of blood and it should have the other characteristics spoken of repeatedly—and after placing it in a new pan and pouring over it enough aged aromatic white wine to cover it by about eight fingers, boil, using a gentle fire, until it has lost its natural scent and smells rather winy. Then removing the vessel from the fire and cooling it, scoop up two *mnai* of the fat, and after placing it in a pan and adding four *cotylai* of the same kind of wine and four *mnai* of chopped fruit of nettle tree, the wood of which is used by flute-makers, boil over a gentle fire stirring constantly.

**12.** When it has cast off its entire animal fat effluvium, strain, and cool; then taking one *mna* chopped camel's-thorn and four *mnai* marjoram flowers, mix them with aged wine and let them soak overnight. On the following day, pour them and the fat into a new clay pot that has the capacity of three *choes*, and, after adding one half *chous* wine, boil everything together at once. When the fat acquires the strength and scent of all the astringents, remove it from the fire, strain, solidify, and store. But should you wish to make it more aromatic, mix it with eight *holcai* of very fatty myrrh dissolved in old wine.

**13.** Chicken fat and goose fat should be scented this way: taking four *cotylai* of cured fat from either of these and putting it into a clay pot, mix it with 12 *drachmai* each of roughly chopped *erysisceptron*[32] and balsam wood, also spathe of the date inflorescence and sweet flag, then adding one *cyathos* of old Lesbian wine, place it over coals and let it come to a boil three times; then lifting the vessel from the fire and letting the contents grow cold for a day and a night, on the following day melt them and strain through a clean linen cloth into a silver receptacle.

**14.** When it has set, scoop up the aforesaid with a shell, put it into a clay pot, cover tightly with a lid, and set it aside in a very cold place. These things must be done in winter, for in summer the fat does not congeal. Some mix it with a little Tyrrhenian wax to make it dense and solid. In a similar manner one must scent pork and deer fat and the like.

Suet is scented with marjoram this way: taking one *mna* of well-cured suet—it should be preferably bull's suet—and one *mna* and a-half of mature, carefully crushed marjoram, mix and shape into little cakes, pouring over them plenty of wine; then place them into a vessel, cover, and leave them for the night.

---

[32] Name given to several plants, e.g. ἀσπάλαθος "camel's-thorn," κύπερος "galingale."

**15.** In the morning, setting them into a clay pot and pouring water over them boil gently. When the fat has lost its characteristic smell, strain it and let it stand all night long well-covered; the following day, lifting the little wheel and scraping the impurities from the base, again mix an additional *mna* and a-half of chopped marjoram, as indicated, and similarly turn it upside down, shape it into little cakes, and do the other things that were mentioned; finally, after boiling it, straining it, and removing any impurity there may be at the bottom, store in a very cold place.

**16.** If you wish to prevent uncured goose or chicken fat or calf suet from spoiling, you must do this: taking whichever fresh fat you prefer, wash it carefully, and after air-drying it on a sieve in the shade, place it after it has dried into a linen cloth and press it hard with your hands; then string a linen thread through it and hang it in a shady place. Many days later, store it in a very cold spot wrapped in new papyrus. They do not spoil if they are also stored in honey.

**17.** All fats have a warming property. However, bull, beef, and calf suet are somewhat costive and lion's fat is like them; they say, moreover, that the last also protects against those who plot harm. Elephant and deer fat put snakes to flight when smeared on; she-goat fat is more costive; it is for this reason that it is given with barley-groats and cheese to dysenterics and it is used boiled with juice of peeled barley as a clyster. Their broth is also suitable to use in porridges for tuberculars and it is given with success to people who drank blister beetle.

**18.** He-goat fat, being more relaxing, helps the gouty when mixed with she-goat dung and saffron, and applied. Sheep fat, too, does the same. Swine fat is suitable for conditions in the area of the uterus and seat, and for burns; cured swine fat that is very old warms and softens, and when washed with wine it is appropriate for people suffering from pleurisy; combined with either ashes or unslaked lime, it is appropriate both for swellings and for inflammations. They say, moreover, that ass's fat makes scars uniform in color. Goose fat and chicken fat are suitable for female conditions, for chapped lips, for the care of the face, and for earaches, and bear's fat seems to be good for growing hair on bald spots; it is also suitable for chilblains.

**19.** Fat from the fox is good for earaches, fat of riverine fish promotes sharp-sightedness when melted in the sun, mixed with honey, and anointed. Viper's fat is used for dim-sightedness, moreover, it operates on cataracts when mixed with Syrian cedar oil, Attic honey, and aged oil in equal parts and it eradicates hair plucked from armpits, if it is rubbed on the roots fresh, without any additives.

**II, 77 μυελός, Marrow**

**1.** The best marrow is that of deer, then that of calf, after this that of bull, then of she-goat and sheep. It becomes firm when summer nears fall: for during the other times of the year, it has the appearance of clotted blood and it is found in the bones like brittle flesh. It is difficult to know it, unless the person who removes it from the bones also puts it up.

All marrows soften, rarefy, warm, and fill up wounds. But deer marrow even routs wild animals when smeared on.

**2.** Fresh marrow that has been softened is treated like suet: pour over it water, remove the bones, then strain it through a linen cloth and wash it this way until the water is clean; then melt it in a bain-marie, remove the impurities which float on top with a feather brush, strain it into a mortar, and after it has set, store in a new clay vessel having scraped off carefully the sediment. But should you wish to store it untreated, do everything just as I have described in the section on chicken and goose fat (II, 76.)

**II, 78 χολή, Bile**

**1.** All biles are stored in this manner: taking a bile that is fresh and after tying its mouth with a linen thread, drop it in boiling water, leaving it for as long as it takes one to complete a race of three stades;[33] then taking it out, dry it in a place that is shady and free of moisture. Place biles intended for ophthalmologic uses, tied with a linen thread, into a glass jar containing honey, and, tying the end of the linen thread around the opening of the jar, store covered with a lid.

**2.** All biles are sharp and warm and differ more or less from each other according to their strength. For the bile of the sea scorpion and

[33] One stade = 606 3/4 English feet, about 1/8 of a Roman mile.

of the fish called *callionymos,*[34] of the sea turtle and of the hyena are thought to be strong, also that of partridge, eagle, white hen, and of the wild she-goat which is particularly suitable for incipient cataracts and for mist over the eyes,[35] albugo[36] and rough eyelids.
Bull's bile is much more efficacious than sheep's or he-goat's or pig's or even bear's. All biles bring about a desire to evacuate, especially in children, if one soaked a woolen wad in bile and placed it in their anus.
**3.** Bull's bile with honey is smeared especially for sore throats, it cures anal sores to the point of cicatrization, and it treats purulent ears and their fissures when instilled with milk of goat or a woman. It is good with leek juice for singing in the ears, and it is mixed into plasters for keeping wounds free from inflammations and into ointments for poisonous bites. It is effective with honey for cancerous sores, for pains of the genitalia and of the scrotum, and it is an excellent cleanser with soda or Cimolian earth for leprosy and dandruff.
**4.** Both sheep and bear biles are good for the same conditions, but they are weaker. Bear's bile, taken as a lozenge, benefits epileptics; that of the turtle, sore throats, sores that spread in children's mouths, and epileptics when inserted into their nostrils; but wild she-goat bile, smeared on, treats particularly those suffering from night blindness. He-goat bile, too, does the same; it also removes large warts, and it shrinks the prominences of people who suffer from elephantiasis when anointed. Swine's bile is used successfully for ear sores as well as for all other sores.

### II, 79 αἷμα, Blood

**1.** Goose, kid, and duck blood are beneficially mixed with antidotes; fresh blood of wild pigeon, turtledove, pigeon, and partridge is smeared on for eye injuries, for contusions, and for night blindness. Pigeon blood, in particular, stays hemorrhages from membranes. Baked blood of he-goat, she-goat, deer, and hare consumed straight

---

[34] *Uranoscopus scaber.*
[35] See Dsc. Bk. I, 55 and n. 57 on ἀχλύς used here.
[36] ἄργεμον, "albugo." See also Dsc. Bk. I, 55 and n. 57.

out of the pan stops dysentery and diarrhea and it is effective against poisons when drunk with wine. Hares' blood when smeared on warm treats freckles and birthmarks, and dogs' blood is a suitable potion for people bitten by rabid dogs or for those who drank a poisonous substance.

**2.** Blood of the land turtle is reportedly a suitable drink for epileptics, and blood of the sea turtle, when drunk with wine, hare's rennet, and cumin, is suitable for bites of wild beasts and for ingesting ranunculus.[37] Bull's blood dissipates and softens indurations when plastered on with groats. Blood of stallions is mixed with septic medications, that of chameleons is believed to thin hair on the eyelids, and the same is true of the blood of green frogs. Menstrual blood, when smeared all over and when stepped over, is believed to prevent women from conceiving, and it relieves gout pains and erysipelas when anointed.

---

[37] The Greek text reads "πρὸς ... πόσιν φρύνου." φρῦνος = φρύνη, "toad," and a synonym for φρύνη is βατράχιον, "frog." Greek does not seem to distinguish between toads and frogs. Βατράχιον, however, also means ranunculus, "buttercup," "crowfoot," of the family Ranunculacaea, "nearly all of which contain poisonous substances," see P. G. Gennadios, Λεξικόν Φυτολογικόν, pp. 186-187. Gennadios adds that "the βατράχιον ἕτερον of Dioscorides…[Dsc. Bk. II, 175,] which the Roman writers call *herba sardonica* is … (*R. sceleratus,* in French Herbe sardonique, or Mort aux vaches, or Grenouillette des marais,) indigenous to Western Europe, where even though it is highly poisonous, people eat it as a vegetable, because it loses its toxicity when cooked." See J. André, p. 215 where he suggests for this plant *R. lanuginosus* L. and *R. sardous* Crantz. See also Pausanias, *Description of Greece*, X, xvii, 13 where he refers to this herb as "deadly." As far as I was able to ascertain, poisonous frogs and toads are not native to Europe, but to China and to Central and South America. In John Goodyer, *The Greek Herbal of Dioscorides*, p. 121, this passage is translated "for the drinking of toad," Max Aufmesser, *Pedanius Dioscurides aus Anazarba*, p. 114, translates it "…gegen eingenommenes Krötengift," and J. Berendes, p. 191 "… und den Genuss des Krötengiftes." To be sure, the passage in Pliny, *N. H.* XXXII, 33 "et contra serpentium omnium et araneorum ac similium et ranarum venena auxiliatur" which parallels this one and which W. H. S. Jones translates "For the poisons of all serpents, spiders and similar creatures, and of frogs, it is of service" tempts to translate φρῦνος as frog. However, in the Pliny passage the damage is from a stroke, a sting, or a bite. Here the poison has been drunk.

**II, 80 ἀπόπατος, Dung**

**1.** Fresh dung of grazing cattle assuages inflammations from injuries when plastered on: it is wrapped in leaves, warmed up on hot ashes, and thus applied; this kind of application offers relief also for hip disease. Plastered on with vinegar, it dissolves scrofulous swellings of glands, indurations, and swellings of glands. The dung of male cattle, in particular, when burned so as to produce smoke restores a prolapsed uterus, and when burned for fumigation it repels mosquitoes. Trottles of goats, especially of mountain goats, clear away jaundice when drunk with wine, and when drunk with spices they are emmenagogic and expel embryos/fetuses.

**2.** Dried, ground up, and applied with frankincense in a wool wad they stop the feminine flow and, with vinegar, they stem the other hemorrhages. Burned and smeared on with vinegar or with oxymel, they treat bald spots, and they benefit the gouty when plastered on with lard. Boiled with vinegar or wine, they are applied for bites of vipers, shingles, erysipelas, and tumors of the parotid glands. The intense heat issuing from them is also used advantageously on patients of hip disease this way: having placed as a foundation on the space between the index finger and the thumb, where the hollow approaches the wrist, wool soaked in oil, set upon it one by one very hot trottles until the sensation reaches the hip through the arm and the pain stops. This method of using intense heat is called Arabian.

**3.** Sheep's trottles applied with vinegar treat pustules that are most painful at night, warts, warty excrescences, thin-necked warts, and they treat burns when combined with rose cerate. The dung of wild swine dried and drunk with water or with wine, controls coughing of blood, assuages chronic pain on the side, and with vinegar it soothes ruptures and spasms. Made up with rose cerate, it treats sprains. Raw as well as burned ass's dung and horse manure, mixed with vinegar, staunch bleeding. The dried manure of a herd donkey that grazes on grass converted into juice in wine and drunk is extremely helpful to those stung by scorpions.

**4.** Pigeon dung, since it warms and burns more, is mixed profitably with bruised meal; with vinegar, it dissipates scrofulous swellings of glands, with honey and linseed, it breaks off carbuncles all around, and when triturated with oil, it treats burns. Chicken dung, too, does the same, but less effectively, except that it is particularly good when drunk with vinegar or wine for poisonous mushrooms and for pain in the colon. Stork's dung, drunk with water, is believed to be good for epileptics and it is reported that the dung of the vulture, burned as to produce smoke, expels embryos/fetuses.

**5.** Mice droppings, ground fine with vinegar and smeared on, treat bald spots, and when drunk with frankincense and wine mixed with honey, they remove stones. Used as children's suppositories, mouse dung provokes a bowel movement. Dog's dung collected during the dog days, dried, and drunk with water or wine, binds the bowel. Fresh human feces, plastered on wounds, maintain them free from inflammation and glue them together, and when smeared with honey on people with sore throats, it has been reported that they help them.

**6.** Lizard dung is suitable to use on women for healthy coloration and for a glowing complexion. The best is very white and friable, it is light like starch, it is quickly converted with water into chyle, and when rubbed hard it is somewhat sour and yeasty in scent. They counterfeit it by feeding starlings rice and selling their dung, which resembles it. Others, after mixing starch with Cimolian earth and coloring it a bit with alkanet, sift it through a wide-meshed sieve on planks, and after drying the little worms sell them as lizard dung.

### II, 81 οὖρον, Urine

**1.** Man's own urine is a suitable potion for viper bites, for deadly poisons, for incipient edemata and a rinse for the stinging of sea urchins, sea scorpion, and greater weever. Any urine is a fomentation for dog bites and a cleanser with soda for leprosy and itching. Old urine is a rather effective cleanser for scurf, dandruff, mange, and eczema; it stems spreading ulcers, especially those in the genitalia when used as a clyster, and it dries up purulent ears; it also drives out the worms[38] that are in them when boiled in the rind of a pomegranate.

---

[38] The earwig and its Greek equivalent, σκώληξ ὁ ἐν τοῖς ὠσί, is so named from the belief that these creatures crawl into ears. They are actually harmless and this notion is patently false. See Max Aufmesser, *Erläuterungen* p. 446 and his *Pedanius Dioscurides aus Anazarba*, p. 116 where he suggests that here σκώληξ ὁ ἐν τοῖς ὠσί may mean earwax. In Dioscorides' time, people probably believed that earwigs crawl into ears, just as some believe so even today.

**2.** When sipped, the urine of an uncorrupted child is suitable for orthopnea and it wipes off scars, albugo, and misty eyes when boiled with honey in a brazen pot. From it and copper, they make a glue that is suitable for gold. The sediment of urine when smeared on abates erysipelas. Boiled with unguent of henna and applied, it soothes uterine pain, it relieves uterine suffocation, it cleanses the eyelids, and it clears scars on the eyes. Bull's urine, triturated with myrrh and instilled into the ears, assuages earaches; the urine of wild swine possesses the same property, but when drunk it is particularly efficacious for breaking and expelling stones from the bladder.
**3.** A quantity of two *cyathoi* of goat's urine drunk daily with spikenard and water reduces internal edemata eliminating urine and abdominal humors, and when instilled into the ears it treats earaches. The urine of lynx, which is called *lyngourion,* is believed to petrify as soon as it passes; but that is nonsense. For *lyngourion* is what some people call "feather-attracting amber" which when drunk with water is suitable for the stomach and for diarrhea. Tradition has it that ass's urine cures kidney disease when drunk.

### II, 82 μέλι, Honey

**1.** The best honey is the Attic, and of this the one called Hymettan ranks first; honey from the Cyclades and from Sicily—which is called Hyblaean—are second best. It is excellent if it is very sweet and sharp, very aromatic, blondish, not watery but ductile and strong, and when drawn, if it runs backwards, as if toward the finger.
It has properties that cleanse, open up, and stimulate the rise of humors. This is why it is a suitable rinse for filthy sores and hollows.
**2.** Boiled and applied, it glues together separated components, it treats the lichen-like eruptions on the skin when boiled with *stypteria*[39] and smeared on, it treats noises in the ears and earaches when dripped tepid into the ears with salt that was roasted and finely ground, it destroys both lice and their eggs when smeared on, and it repairs the foreskin of those whose lack of it is not due to circumcision: it is rubbed on their penis with honey, especially after the bath, for thirty

[39] Στυπτηρία sc. γῆ according LSJ is the name of any of group of *astringent substances* containing a) alum or b) ferrous sulfate.

days. It cleanses those substances that cast a shadow over the pupils of the eyes, and as an ointment or as a gargle it treats conditions of the trachea, the tonsils, and sore throats.

**3.** It stimulates micturition, it is a fit remedy for coughs, for snake bites, for drinking opium when taken warm with unguent of roses, for mushrooms, and for those bitten by rabid animals taken either as a lozenge or drunk. Raw honey, however, causes abdominal flatulence and touches off a cough, wherefore it must be used despumated. Spring honey ranks first, then that of summer; winter honey, being more viscous, is inferior and causes pimples.

**4.** The honey that is made in Sardinia is bitter because the bees feed on wormwood *absinthium*; applied as an ointment, it is suitable for freckles and facial blemishes.

In Pontic Heraclea, at certain times of the year, a honey is made, which, due to the peculiarity of the flowers on which the bees feed, drives those who eat it besides themselves with perspiration. But they are helped if they eat rue and salt meat and if they drink honey mixed with wine, and as often as they vomit they are offered the same things.

**5.** It is sharp, its smell causes sneezing, it treats freckles when smeared on with costusroot, and it lifts livid spots when smeared on with salt.

There is also something called sugar, which is a kind of crystallized honey found on reeds in India and in blessed Arabia; it resembles salt in consistency and it breaks like salt when subjected to the pressure of teeth. It softens the bowel, it is wholesome, and it benefits an ailing bladder and kidneys when dissolved in water and drunk. Used as a lotion, it also cleanses the elements that cast a shadow over the pupils of the eyes.

### II, 83 κηρός, Wax

**1.** Wax is excellent when it is yellowish and somewhat greasy, fragrant, and smelling ever so slightly of honey; also when it is pure, and when it is either of Cretan or Pontic origin. Wax that is naturally quite white and greasy ranks second. Wax must be bleached this way: having cut and cleaned white and very greasy wax, place it in a new vessel and after pouring over it enough seawater from the open seas, boil it briefly adding a little soda. After it has come to a boil two or three times, removing the vessel from the fire and allowing it to cool,

lift the wheel of wax, and after scraping any impurity that may surround it, boil it anew adding a second charge of seawater.
**2.** After the wax has come to a boil again, as indicated, lift the vessel from the fire and taking the base of a small new pot that you previously moistened with cold water, gently lower it into the wax, dipping it just enough to attract a very small quantity of wax and to set by itself. Lifting it up, remove the first round cake of wax, and for a second time let down the base of the pot, cooled with water, and repeat the process until you shall have taken up all the wax. Then after stringing the little wax cakes with a linen thread, suspend them at a distance from each other, misting them frequently during the day in the sun, and at night set them out under the moonlight until they become white. But if one wished to make the wax extremely white, he should do everything else the same way but he should boil it many times.
**3.** Some, however, instead of using seawater from the open seas, boil it once or twice in very strong brine, as stated above, then scoop it up with an ansate flask that is thin and round, then placing the small round wax cakes on thick grass, sun them until they become very white. They advise to embark on this project in the spring, at which time the sun is both weaker and allows for moisture to develop so that the wax cakes do not melt.
All waxes have the ability to warm, soften, and moderately fill up. They are also mixed with porridges for dysenterics and will prevent the milk of wet nurses from curdling, if they should swallow as much wax as ten millet grains.

### II, 84 πρόπολις, Bee glue [40]

You must choose bee glue that is yellow, aromatic, resembling storax, soft when very dry, and that is drawn the way mastic is drawn. It warms a great deal, it attracts substances to itself, and it extracts splinters. It both helps for old coughs when burned as to produce smoke and it removes lichen-like eruptions on the skin when plastered

---

[40] Propolis or bee glue is resinous material, which bees collect from various plants and use to reinforce their hives. Modern studies have proven that it has antibiotic properties. See Jean Langenheim, *Plant Resins*, pp. 427-429.

on. It is found around the openings of beehives and it is naturally waxy.

**II, 85 πυροί, *Triticum* L., Wheat**

**1.** Wheat[41] is excellent for health use if it is new, fully ripe, and quince-yellow in color; next to this one ranks the "three month"[42] wheat, which some call *setaneios.*[43] When eaten raw, wheat breeds round intestinal worms, but if chewed then plastered on, it benefits those bitten by dogs. Bread made with the finest wheat flour is more nutritious than bread made from coarse meal, and bread made from *setaneios* meal is lighter and easy to digest. *Setaneios* meal is plastered on with juice of henbane as a remedy for rheums of the tendons and for intestinal flatulence, and it removes birthmarks with vinegar and honey.

**2.** Its bran, when boiled with sharp vinegar and plastered on warm, gets rid of leprosies and it is a useful plaster for all incipient inflammations; when boiled with rue broth, it stops breasts from swelling with clots of milk and it is suitable both for those bitten by vipers and for the colicky. Dough made from its meal, being able to warm and to draw, thins especially the calluses on the soles of the foot and with salt it ripens and opens the other growths and abscesses. Meal made from *setaneios* wheat, plastered on with either vinegar or wine, is a fit remedy for venomous animals; boiled as one boils glue then used a lozenge, it benefits those who spit blood and when boiled with green mint and butter it is good both for coughs and for roughness of the trachea. Also the fine meal of this wheat, when boiled with a mixture of hydromel or with water mixed with oil, disperses all inflammations.

**3.** The bread, too, boiled with hydromel or even not boiled, relieves all inflammations when plastered on because it softens a great deal and it gently cools when mixed with herbs or some juices. As for bread that is old and dry, either by itself or combined with something or other, controls diarrhea, but fresh wheat bread, soaked in brine and applied

---

[41] πυροί, "wheat" *Triticum vulgare* L.
[42] σητάνειοι πυροί is wheat that is sown in the spring so as to ripen in three months.
[43] I. e. "this year's."

as a plaster, treats old lichen-like eruptions of the skin. A spoonful of thinned down and tepid glue, the kind they make from fine wheat-flour and very fine meal for gluing books, is a suitable drink for people who spit blood.

**II, 86 κριθή, *Hordeum* L., Barley**

**1.** Barley is excellent when it is white and clean but it is less nutritious than wheat; gruel made from barley groats is rather nutritious because during the boiling process the liquid thickens; it is beneficial for harshness, roughness, and ulcerations of the trachea, conditions for which wheat-gruel, too, is an appropriate prescription, being more nutritious and more diuretic. It also draws down the milk when boiled together with fennel seed and sipped.

**2.** Barley is diuretic and purgative, it causes flatulence, it is bad for the stomach, and it dissolves swellings. Its meal, boiled with figs and with a mixture of honey and water, dissipates swellings and inflammations; in combination with pitch, pine resin, and pigeon dung, it brings to a head indurations, and, with melilot and poppy capsules, it relieves those hurting on the side. It is also plastered on with linseed, fenugreek, and rue for intestinal flatulence, and, with liquid pitch, wax, the urine of an uncorrupted child, and oil, it brings to a head scrofulous swellings of the glands. With myrtle or wine or wild pears or bramble or pomegranate peel, it stems diarrhea and, with quince or vinegar, it benefits gouty inflammations.

**3.** Boiled with harsh vinegar, in the manner that a poultice of bruised meal of raw corn is boiled, and applied warm, it cures leprosies. Converted into chyle with water and cooked with pitch and oil, its meal makes pus, and it is a fit application for rheums of the joints when converted into chyle with vinegar and cooked with pitch. Barley groats bind the bowel and assuage inflammations.

**II, 87 ζῦθος, Beer**

Beer[44] is made from barley. It is diuretic, it affects the kidneys and tendons, it is especially hurtful to the membranes, it is apt to cause

---

[44] Beer made from barley is of Egyptian origin.

flatulence, to engender an unhealthy state of humors, and to cause elephantiasis. Ivory becomes malleable when soaked in it.

### II, 88 κοῦρμι, *Courmi*[45]

The so-called *courmi*, which is made from barley and which they often use as a drink instead of wine, causes headaches, is unwholesome, and does damage to sinewy parts. In Spain to the west and in Britain such drinks are also made from wheat.

### II, 89 ζέα, *Triticum* L., *Zea*

There are two kinds of *zea:*[46] one is called one-seeded, the other two-seeded, having its seed joined together in two flowering glumes. It is more nutritious than barley and it is tasty, but it is less nutritious than wheat when made into bread.

### II, 90 κρίμνον, *Crimnon*[47]

They process *crimnon* coarser than meal and they make it both from *zea* and from wheat. They make porridge from it. It is quite nutritious and easy to digest, but when made from *zea*, it does bind the bowel, especially if the *zea* was first roasted.

### II, 91 ὄλυρα,[48] Rice-wheat

Rice-wheat is of the same kind as *zea* but it is somewhat less nutritious than *zea*. It, too, is used to make bread and it is also used to make *crimnon*.

### II, 92 ἀθήρα, Gruel

Gruel is made from finely milled *zea*. It is a concoction resembling liquid porridge and it is a suitable thing to give to children. It is also used for poultices.

---

[45] A kind of beer.

[46] ζέα, too, is wheat, *Triticum monococcum*, one-seeded wheat. It is a wild wheat, indigenous to Greece, Yugoslavia, Asia Minor and Syria, while *Triticum dicoccum*, two-seeded wheat, is a descendant of a wheat native to Mesopotamia, P. G. Gennadios, Φυτολογικόν Λεξικόν, pp. 878 and 880.

[47] *Crimnon* is probably semolina.

[48] A cultural variety of *zea*, see Dsc. Bk. II, 89.

**II, 93 τράγος, *Triticum* L. sp., Spelt**
Spelt nearly resembles groats in shape; it is considerably less nutritious than *zea* because it has a great deal of chaff; it is for this reason that it is both difficult to digest and softens the bowel.

**II, 94 βρόμος, *Avena sativa* L., Oats**
Oat is a grass similar to wheat even in foliage; it is divided at intervals by joints. On top it bears fruit that resembles two-footed little grasshoppers and that contains seed that is used for poultices the way barley is used. They even make gruel from it that binds the bowel. Its juice when sipped is suitable for people who cough.

**II, 95 ὄρυζα, *Oryza sativa* L., Rice**
Rice is a kind of grain that grows in marshes and wetlands. It is moderately nutritious and it binds the bowel.

**II, 96 χόνδρος, Groats**
Groats are made from the wheat called two-seeded; they are more nutritious than rice, they bind the bowel more, and they are easier to digest. They clear away leprosies when boiled with vinegar and plastered on, they remove psoriatic nails, they treat incipient lachrymal fistulas, and their decoction is a useful clyster for those suffering from painful dysentery.

**II, 97 κέγχρος, *Panicum miliaceum* L., Millet**
Millet is less nutritious than the other cereals. But when used to make bread or when made into porridge, it checks the bowel and it provokes micturition. Toasted and placed into sacks while hot, it helps for colic and for the other pains.

**II, 98 ἔλυμος, *Setaria italica* P. B., Italian millet**
Italian millet, too, which some call *meline,* belongs to the cereal seeds. It is like millet, it is similarly made into bread, and it is suitable for the same conditions as millet, but it is less nutritious and less binding than millet.

### II, 99 σήσαμον, *Sesamum indicum* L., Sesame

Sesame is bad for the stomach and causes bad breath should it remain between the teeth after it has been eaten. Used as a poultice, it dissipates the thicknesses in tendons and it treats bruised ears, inflammations, burns, colon pains, and the bite of the asp. In combination with unguent of roses, it assuages headaches produced from heatstroke. The plant, boiled in wine, accomplishes the same things and it is especially well suited for inflammations of the eyes and for intense pains. They also make oil from it, which the people in Egypt use.

### II, 100 αἶρα, *Lolium temulentum* L., Darnel

The darnel that grows among wheat, ground and applied with horseradish rind and salt, can cause tissue to form a line of demarcation around spreading ulcers, mortifications, and gangrenes, and with native sulfur and vinegar it treats wild lichen-like eruptions of the skin and leprosies. Cooked in wine with pigeon dung and linseed, it dissolves scrofulous swellings of the glands[49] and it breaks up substances that refuse to ripen, and, when boiled with hydromel and applied as a poultice, it benefits those suffering from hip disease. Burned with barley groats or myrrh or saffron or frankincense to produce smoke from below, it aids conception.

### II, 101 ἄμυλον, Starch

**1.** Starch has been named *amylon*[50] because it is made without a mill. The best is made from *setanios* wheat,[51] be it either Cretan or Egyptian. It is made from *setaneios* wheat that is clean, soaked, and washed in fresh water; the water is poured off five times a day and if possible also five times at night. When the wheat has softened, you must decant the water gently and without stirring, lest the valuable part is washed out. When it appears to be very soft, removing the water, you must thresh it with your feet, then after pouring <again> water over it, you must thresh it, then you must remove the bran that

---

[49] See Dsc. Bk. I, n.100.

[50] ἄμυλον, from alpha privative and μύλος, "mill."

[51] I.e. "spring-wheat."

stands on top with a skimmer, clean the rest, place it into a strainer, and after straining it, you must dry it right away on new tiles under a very strong sun: for should it remain moist even briefly, it turns sour.
**2.** It is effective for running eyes, hollows, and blisters; it stems blood spitting, and it assuages the roughness around the trachea when drunk; it is mixed both with milk and with side dishes. They also make it from *zea*[52] soaked and washed for a day or two then pressed by hand, as one presses suet, and dried under a very hot sun, as indicated above. This sort of starch is unsuitable for medical use but it is fine for all other uses.

### II, 102 τήλεως ἄλευρον, Meal of fenugreek

**1.** Meal from fenugreek, a plant that some called *bouceron,* others *aigoceras,* others *carphos,* others *lotos,* and others *ceras aigeion,* has an emollient property. Finely ground, cooked with hydromel, and plastered on, it is good for internal and external inflammations and it reduces the spleen when it is applied finely ground with soda and vinegar. Its decoction is used as a sitz bath for female disorders that stem either from an inflammation or from a stoppage.
**2.** Having been cooked in water, its solid residue cleanses hair, washes off dandruff and scurf, and it is inserted with goose fat instead of a pessary, softening and dilating the areas around the uterus. Fresh fenugreek with vinegar is suitable for people whose stomach lacks elasticity or is ulcerated, and its decoction is suitable for tenesmus and for foul smelling dysenteric evacuations. With myrtle, its oil cleanses hair and scars on the genitals.

### II, 103 λινόσπερμον, *Linum usitatissimum* L., Linseed

Linseed has the same properties as fenugreek, dispersing and softening all internal and external inflammations when made up raw with honey, oil, and water. Applied as a poultice with soda and fig, it removes freckles and facial pimples; with ashes, it dissipates tumors of the parotid gland and indurations; boiled with wine, it clears out shingles and impetigo contagiosa, and, with equal parts of garden cress and honey, it removes psoriatic nails. It both brings up matter

[52] See Dsc. Bk. II, 89.

from the chest when taken as a lozenge with honey and it assuages coughs. Mixed with honey and pepper and taken often as a lozenge, it also disposes a person toward sexual activity. Its decoction, too, is used in clysters for intestinal and uterine pains, for purging the bowels, and it is useful for uterine inflammations in a sitz bath just like the decoction of fenugreek.

### II, 104 ἐρέβινθος ὁ ἥμερος, *Cicer arietinum* L., Cultivated chick-pea

The cultivated chick-pea softens the bowel, is diuretic, causes flatulence, produces a healthy complexion, draws forth the menstrual period and embryos/fetuses, and generates milk. It is plastered on with honey, especially the *orobias*[53] that has been boiled, for testicular inflammations, scurf, lichen-like eruptions of the skin, mange, warts that spread under the skin, and for cancerous and malignant ulcers. The other kind of chick-pea is called *crios*. Both are very diuretic and their decoction is given with rosemary for jaundice and edemata—but they do harm an ulcerated bladder and the kidneys. Some people recommend that for warts that spread under the skin and for thin-necked warts to touch each wart tip, when the moon is new, with a different chick-pea, then to wrap the chick-peas in a linen cloth and throw them backwards so that the warts would fall off.

There is also a wild chick-pea that is similar in foliage to the cultivated. It is sharp in scent, dissimilar in fruit, and good for all the things for which the cultivated chick-pea is also good.

### II, 105 κύαμος Ἑλληνικός, *Vicia faba* L., Greek bean

**1.** The Greek bean causes distension and flatulence, is difficult to digest, and causes bad dreams, but it is good for coughs and it is fattening. Boiled in sour wine mixed with water and eaten with its shell, it stays dysenteries and diarrhea and it is good to eat against vomiting. It causes less flatulence if the first water in which it was boiled is poured off. When it is green, it is worse for the stomach and causes more flatulence. Bean meal, plastered on either by itself or with barley meal, assuages inflammations from a blow, makes scars

[53] A type of chick-pea.

uniformly colored, benefits swollen and inflamed breasts, and dries up milk.

**2.** When combined with honey and with meal of fenugreek, it dissipates small abscesses, tumors of the parotid glands, and black eye, and, with roses, frankincense, and egg white, it stems prolapses of the eyes and corneal defects. Kneaded with wine, it repairs injuries and blows to the eyes; having been chewed without its shell, it is placed on the forehead as an adhesive plaster for discharges and it treats testicular inflammations when boiled in wine. Plastered on the pubes of children, it keeps them child-like for a long time and it also clears up dull-white leprosies.

**3.** Plastered on, the shells make plucked hair grow weak and thin; they dissipate scrofulous swellings of the glands[54] when laid on with barley meal, alum, and aged oil, and their decoction dyes wool.

Hulled and separated into two where the two parts of the bean grew together, it is laid on for hemorrhages caused by leeches and it stops the bleeding when the flat side of the bean is pressed against them.

### II, 106 Αἰγύπτιος κύαμος, *Nelumbo nucifera* Gaert., Egyptian bean

**1.** The Egyptian bean, which some call Pontic, grows abundantly in Egypt and it is found both in Asia and in Cilicia, in the marshes. It has a large umbellate leaf, a stalk that is a cubit long and thick as a finger, and a rose-colored flower which is twice as large as a poppy and which, after it has finished blooming, bears a little sack that resembles a wasp's nest. It contains the bean, which projects slightly beyond the cover, as if it were a bubble. It is called *ciborion*[55] or *cibotion*[56] because it is planted in moist lumps of earth and left this way in the water.

**2.** The root is below, thicker than a reed. The root, which is called *colocasion*, is eaten both boiled and raw. This bean is eaten even green, but after it has been dried, it becomes black and it is larger than the Greek bean. It has astringent and wholesome properties. Their

---

[54] See Dsc. Bk. I, n. 100.

[55] "Seed-vessel."

[56] "Small box."

meal is suitable for people with colic and dysentery when sprinkled on their drinks instead of barley meal and it is also given as porridge. But the shucks boiled in wine and honey and offered to drink in the amount of three *cyathoi* are more effective. Their green part in the middle is good for earaches; it is bitter in taste and it is instilled finely ground with unguent of roses.

**II, 107 φακός, *Ervum lens* L., Lentil**

**1.** Lentils, as a steady diet, dull the vision, are hard to digest, bad for the stomach, produce stomach and intestinal gas, and soften the bowel when cooked with their hulls. They are best boiled and when they release no blackness in the water. They have an astringent property, wherefore they bind the bowel if they are first hulled then boiled carefully, pouring off the first water in which they were boiled; for their broth loosens the bowel. They do cause, however, bad dreams and they are unsuitable for ailments associated with the tendons, lungs, and head.

**2.** They will do their job on fluxes from the bowel better, if along with vinegar either chicory[57] is mixed with them or endive or plantain or purslane or dark beet or myrtle berries or pomegranate rind or dried sorb-apples or medlars or quinces or pears or Theban dates or whole oak-galls, which are discarded after boiling, or sumac, the kind that is added on prepared foods; but one must boil them carefully with the vinegar, otherwise they surely upset the belly. Thirty lentils, hulled and swallowed, also calm an upset stomach. Boiled with barley meal and plastered on, they also comfort gout and, with honey, they glue together hollows, they cause scabs to break off, they cleanse sores, and when boiled with vinegar they dissolve indurations and scrofulous swellings of the glands.

**3.** With melilot or with quince, they treat eye and anal inflammations, unguent of roses being mixed therein; but for more severe anal inflammations and large hollows, they are used with cooked pomegranate rind or with dry roses mixed with honey; they are

---

[57] σέρις. Dsc. Bk. II, 132, distinguishes two types of this plant, the wild, which is chicory, also known as κιχόριον, *Cichorium intybus* L., and the cultivated, the endive, *Cichorium endivia* L.

similarly used for spreading gangrenes, or even mixing them with seawater; for pustules, shingles, erysipelas, and chilblains, they are used as described above, and when boiled in seawater they are a suitable plaster for breasts that have clots of milk and that are swollen.

**II, 108 ὄροβος, *Vicia ervillia* Willd., Bitter vetch**

**1.** The bitter vetch is a small, narrow-leaved, slender shrub that has small seed in pods. They make from it the so-called meal of bitter vetch, which is suitable for medicinal use. But if one ate it, it gives headaches, it disturbs the abdomen, and it draws blood through the urine. Offered to cattle boiled, it fattens them.

Meal of bitter vetch is made from it this way: choosing viable, white seeds, sprinkle them with water and stir them, and after allowing them enough time to soak up the water, roast them until their skin cracks all around; then after grinding and sifting them through a fine sieve, store the meal.

**2.** It softens the stool, it is diuretic, and it gives nice color; but consumed in too large quantities either in food or drink, it causes, along with colic, hemorrhaging through the bowel and bladder. With honey, it cleanses sores, birthmarks, blemishes, freckles, and the rest of the body; it stays spreading ulcers and gangrenes, it softens indurations in the breasts, and it breaks off all around malignant ulcers, carbuncles, and impetigo contagiosa. Kneaded with wine and used as a plaster, it treats dog, viper, and human bites; combined with vinegar, it puts an end to difficult micturition, colic, and tenesmus, and an amount the size of a nut taken with honey benefits also the malnourished. Its decoction, used as a rinse, treats chilblains and itching on the body.

**II, 109 θέρμος, *Lupinus* L., Lupine**

**1.** The cultivated lupine is a familiar plant the meal of which, combined with honey and taken as a lozenge or drunk with vinegar, destroys intestinal worms. Also the seeds themselves, well-soaked and eaten bitter, do the same; their decoction accomplishes the same when drunk with rue and pepper, it benefits patients with spleen disease, and it is a fomentation for gangrene, malignant ulcers, incipient mange, dull-white leprosies, blemishes, pustules, and scurf. The seed also

draws menstrual period and embryos/fetuses in a pessary with myrrh and honey. The meal cleanses the skin and livid spots, it assuages inflammations with water and barley meal, and with vinegar it soothes hip diseases and tumors.
**2.** Boiled in vinegar and applied as a plaster, it dislodges scrofulous swellings of the glands and breaks off all around carbuncles. Lupines, boiled in rainwater until the water thickens, cleanse the face, and when boiled with the root of chameleon-thistle[58] they cure the mange of sheep, if one washed them with the tepid decoction. The root, boiled with water and drunk, provokes micturition. Ground up, sweetened, and drunk with vinegar, lupines abate nausea and cure lack of appetite.
There is also a wild lupine that resembles the cultivated in every respect, but it is smaller; it accomplishes all the things the cultivated lupine accomplishes.

### II, 110 γογγύλη, *Brassica rapa* L., Turnip

**1.** When boiled, the root of the turnip is nutritious, causes flatulence, makes the flesh flabby, and is aphrodisiac. Its decoction is a fomentation for gout and chilblains and the root itself, ground up, is a beneficial plaster. The root is effective for ulcerated chilblains if one hollowed it out and melted rose cerate in it over hot ashes. Its shoot is eaten boiled and it is diuretic. Its seed is suitable for remedies and for antidotes that allay pain from poisonous bites; it helps also for deadly poisons and it is aphrodisiac when drunk. Pickled, it becomes less nutritious when eaten but it does restore the appetite.
**2.** ἀγρία γογγύλη. Eastern cress grows in fields. It is a shrub that is a cubit tall; it has many branches, it is smooth on top, it has smooth leaves, <a root> thick as a thumb or even thicker, and seed in cup-shaped pods. The pods, having been opened, contain another head-shaped pod in which there are little black seeds that are white inside when crushed. They are mixed with facial cleansers and with cleansers for the rest of the skin, such as are made from meal of lupines or wheat or bruised beans or bitter vetch.

---

[58] See Dsc. Bk. III, 9.

**II, 111 βουνιάς, *Brassica napus* L., French turnip**

The French turnip: its root also causes flatulence and it is less nutritious when boiled. Drunk before hand, its seed renders poisons ineffective and it is also mixed with antidotes. The root of this plant, too, is pickled.

**II, 112 ῥαφανίς, *Raphanus sativus* L., Radish**

**1.** The radish, too, causes flatulence, it is tasty, it is not good for the stomach, and it causes belching. It is diuretic and warms, and it eases the bowel if taken after meals, helping digestion rather nicely; but if eaten before meals it buoys the food. Eaten before meals, it is suitable also for people who plan to vomit and it sharpens the senses. Taken boiled, it helps those with a chronic cough and those who produce a thick substance in their chest. But its peel, taken with vinegar and honey, is more emetic, it is suitable for those with edemata, and when used as a poultice it is suitable also for spleen disease. With honey it stops spreading ulcers, it removes black eye, it helps those bitten by vipers, it restores hair on bald spots, and with meal of darnel it clears birthmarks. It does also help people who choke from mushrooms and it draws down the menses.

**2.** Its seed is emetic, diuretic, reduces the spleen when taken as a drink with vinegar, helps people with sore throats if they use it in a gargle boiled with warm vinegar and honey, helps for the bite of the asp when drunk with wine, and strongly demarcates gangrenes when plastered on with vinegar.

The wild radish, which the Romans call *armoracium*, has leaves resembling those of the cultivated, tending rather towards the leaves of charlock, but its root is thin, long, and somewhat sharp. Both the root and the leaves are boiled to eat as potherbs. It warms, it is diuretic, and it is very hot.

**II, 113 σίσαρον, *Pastinaca sativa* L., Parsnip**

The parsnip is a well-known plant. When boiled, its root is tasty, diuretic, and stimulates the appetite.

**II, 114 λάπαθον, *Rumex* L. sp., Monk's rhubarb**

**1.** One kind of this plant is called *oxylapathon*; it grows in marshes, it is tough, and it tapers toward the tips; another is cultivated and it is not dissimilar to the first. But there is a third kind which is wild, small, resembling plantain, soft, and low growing. And there is even a fourth kind of this plant, which some call *oxalis* or *anaxyris* or *lapathon agrion*; its leaves are similar to the leaves of the wild and small monk's rhubarb; the stem is not large and it tapers, and the seed is red and sharp, growing on the stem on off- shoots.

**2.** The greens of all of them when boiled soften the bowel. The plant itself used raw as a poultice with unguent of roses or with saffron dissolves impetigo contagiosa. The seeds of the wild, of *oxylapathon,* and of *oxalis* are beneficially drunk with water or wine for dysentery, to settle the stomach, for nausea, and for the stroke of scorpion; and if a person drank the seed before being struck, he will suffer no harm when struck. Their roots treat leprosies, chilblains, and psoriatic nails when plastered on either boiled or raw. One must, however, rub first the afflicted area out in the sun with soda and vinegar. Their decoction assuages also itching either when poured all over or when mixed with the bath water.

**3.** Boiled in wine and used as a mouthwash, they comfort toothaches; boiled in wine and plastered on, they dissipate scrofulous swellings of glands and tumors of the parotid glands, and with vinegar they reduce the spleen. Some use the roots also as amulets against scrofulous swellings of the glands, hanging them around their neck. Ground up fine and applied as a pessary, they also stop leucorrhea. Boiled in wine and drunk, they cure people who have jaundice, they break up stones in the bladder, they draw down the menses, and they help those struck by scorpions.

**II, 115 ἱππολάπαθον, *Rumex aquaticus* L., Dock sorrel**

The dock sorrel is a large monk's rhubarb that grows in marshes. It has the same properties as the above.

**II, 116 λαμψάνη, *Raphanus raphanistrum* L., Charlock**

The charlock is a wild green that is more nutritious and more wholesome than monk's rhubarb. Its leaves and stalk are eaten boiled.

**II, 117 βλίτον, *Amaranthus blitum* L., Blite**

The blite also is used as a potherb. It softens the bowel without having any medicinal property.

**II, 118 μολόχη, *Malva silvestris*, Mallow**

**1.** The mallow: the cultivated mallow is more edible than the wild. It is bad for the stomach, it eases the bowel, especially its stems, and it is beneficial to the intestines and the bladder.

Its leaves, chewed raw and used as a poultice with a small amount of salt, can remove lachrymal fistulas, but to cicatrize them, one must use the mallow without salt. It is also good to plaster on wasp and bee stings, and if a person smeared himself with raw leaves ground up with olive oil, he will be immune to stings. Plastered on with urine, they cure scurf and dandruff.

**2.** Boiled, ground up, and applied with olive oil, the leaves benefit burns and erysipelas. The decoction of this plant is an emollient sitz bath for the uterus and an appropriate clyster for gnawing pains of the intestines, uterus, and anus. The broth, cooked with the roots, helps for all deadly poisons: but the people who drink it must keep vomiting. It does also benefit those bitten by venomous spiders and it draws out milk. The fruit, mixed with seed of wild fenugreek and drunk with wine, abates pains around the bladder.

**II, 119 ἀνδράφαξυς, *Atriplex hortensis* L., Orach**

The orach is a well-known potherb. It is of two kinds, one wild and the other cultivated; it is used boiled like potherbs. It softens the bowel and it dissipates swellings of the glands when plastered on raw or boiled. Its seed treats jaundice when drunk with hydromel.

**II, 120 κράμβη ἥμερος, *Brassica oleracea*, Cultivated cabbage**

**1.** The cultivated cabbage eases the bowel when eaten blanched, but it constipates if it was boiled, especially if it was thoroughly boiled and cooked in lye. Summer cabbage is bad for the stomach and rather harsh, and the cabbage that grows in Egypt is inedible due to its bitterness. It helps the dim-sighted and quiverers when eaten, and it quells the ills of carousing and drinking when taken afterwards. The young sprout is more wholesome and more diuretic, but it is bad for the stomach and it upsets the bowel when pickled.

**2.** The juice of raw cabbage taken in a drink with iris and soda softens the stool, it helps those bitten by vipers when drunk with wine, and with meal of fenugreek and vinegar it helps the gouty and the arthritic; it is a fit application for filthy and old sores, and it clears the head when poured all by itself into the nostrils. Applied with meal of darnel, it draws down the menses. Its ground leaves, plastered on either by themselves or with barley groats, are effective for all inflammations and swellings and they cure erysipelas, pustules which are most painful at night, and leprosies. With salt, they demarcate all around carbuncles; they also stay the falling of hair from the head.

**3.** Eaten raw with vinegar, they benefit patients with spleen disease, they restore loss of voice when chewed and their juice is swallowed, and the broth of the cabbage sets into motion bowel movement and menstruation when drunk. Its flower, applied in a pessary after birthing, causes barrenness. The seed, especially of the cabbage that grows in Egypt, expels intestinal worms when drunk; it is also mixed with antidotes for poisonous bites, and it clears the face and birthmarks. The green stalks burned with the roots, combined with old lard, and plastered on stop chronic pains on the side.

**II, 121 κράμβη ἀγρία, *Brassica oleracea* L. ~ var. *silvestris*, ~ *B. cretica*, Wild cabbage**

The wild cabbage grows to a great extent on coastal and craggy areas; it resembles the cultivated but it is whiter, denser, and bitter; its sprout, boiled in lye, is not unsavory.

Its leaves, applied as a plaster, have the ability to close wounds and to disperse swellings and inflammations.

**II, 122 κράμβη ἡ θαλασσία, *Convolvulus soldanella* L., Sea cole**

The cabbage called sea cole is completely different from the cultivated cabbage, having long leaves that resemble those of the birthwort. Each of them grows on reddish little stalks from one leaf-stem, just like ivy, and their juice is white and scant. It is slightly salty and somewhat bitter in taste.

The entire plant is extremely laxative when eaten boiled. On account of its bitterness, some boil with it the fatty parts of meats.

**II, 123 σεῦτλον, *Beta maritima* L., Beet**

Beets are of two kinds: the dark binds somewhat the bowels when boiled with lentils, especially its root, while the white eases the bowel. Both, however, are unwholesome due to their content of soda; it is for this reason that their juice clears the head and is beneficial for earaches when poured into the nose with honey. The decoction of its roots and leaves, used as a rinse, washes off dandruff and eggs of lice and assuages chilblains. One must plaster with its raw leaves dull-white leprosies that were cleaned with soda, bald spots that were trimmed, and ulcers that spread. But the boiled root treats pustules, burns, and erysipelas.

**II, 124 ἀνδράχνη, *Portulaca oleracea* L., Purslane**

**1.** The purslane has astringent and cooling properties. Plastered on with barley groats, it helps for headaches, for eye and other inflammations, for heartburn, for erysipelas, and for pains in the bladder. When eaten, it eases the sensation of having one's teeth on edge, heartburn, intestinal inflammations and rheums; it is a good treatment for the burning sensation in the kidneys and bladder, and it unleashes impulses for sexual intercourse.

**2.** Its juice, too, acts very nearly like it when drunk and it is effective for fever, round intestinal worms, blood spitting, dysentery, hemorrhoids, and for the bites of the serpent *seps*.[59] It is also mixed profitably with eye medications, it is a clyster for intestinal fluxes and for a painful uterus, it is a lotion with unguent of roses for headaches caused by heatstroke, it is a cleanser with wine for head pustules, and it is plastered on with barley groats for gangrened injuries.

**II, 125 ἀσπάραγος πετραῖος ἢ μυάκανθος, *Asparagus officinalis* L., Asparagus**

Asparagus or *myacanthos*. Some call it *horminon*. Its small stem softens the bowel and provokes micturition when eaten boiled. The

[59] *Seps*, a serpent, the bite of which causes intense thirst.

decoction of its roots when drunk helps those who have difficulty micturating, the jaundiced, and those suffering from hip disease; boiled down with wine, it helps those bitten by venomous spiders also those who have a toothache when the decoction is held against the aching tooth. Its seed also accomplishes the same when drunk. They say, moreover, that if dogs should drink its decoction they would die. Some have reported that should one bury chopped ram's horns, asparagus shoots up.

**II, 126 ἀρνόγλωσσον, *Plantago* L. sp., Plantain**

**1.** The plantain, but some call it *heptapleuron* and others *polypleuron*. There are two kinds: one is small and the other is larger. The small one has narrower, smaller, and smoother leaves, a knobby stem that is leaning as if to the ground, pale green flowers, and its seeds are at the top of the stem. The larger sprouts better, it is broad-leaved, and it is like a vegetable. Its stem is knobby, reddish, a cubit tall, and surrounded from the middle to the top by delicate seeds. The roots are below ground, soft, dense, white, and thick as a finger. It grows around marshes, hedges, and wetlands. The large is more useful.

**2.** The leaves have astringent and desiccative properties on account of which they are fit to apply as a poultice on all malignancies, on people who have elephantiasis, and on sores that are running and foul. They also control hemorrhages, spreading ulcers, carbuncles, shingles, and pustules that are most painful at night. They cicatrize both chronic and irregular sores, they cure Cheironian[60] sores, they glue together hollows, and when plastered on with salt they are beneficial for dog bites, burns, inflammations, tumors of the parotid glands, scrofulous swellings of the glands, and lachrymal fistulas. The greens, boiled and taken with salt and vinegar, are suitable for dysenterics and the colicky; they are also given boiled with lentils instead of with beets, and the plant, having been boiled, is given halfway through a meal of dry food for anasarca; it is also good to give to epileptics and asthmatics.

---

[60] I.e. like Cheiron's sores. Cheiron was the wise and kind old centaur that was versed in medicine. Cheiron's sores may also refer to sores needing his aid, malignant.

**3.** The juice of the leaves used at frequent intervals as a mouthwash clears out completely spreading ulcers in the mouth. With Cimolian earth or with white lead, it cures erysipelas, and when employed as a rinse it is beneficial for fistulous sores. It is beneficial for earaches and ophthalmia when either instilled or mixed with eye salves; also for bleeding gums and for coughing up blood when drunk, and for tuberculars and dysenterics when used as a clyster. It is also drunk for tuberculosis and it is applied on a wool wad as a pessary for uterine suffocation and for uterine discharges.
**4.** Its seed, too, stops diarrhea and blood spitting when drunk with wine. The root, boiled down, stops toothaches when its broth is used as a mouthwash or when the root itself is chewed. Both the leaves and the root are given with grape syrup for bladder and kidney ulcers. It is said that three roots drunk with three *cyathoi* of wine and an equal quantity of water help for tertian fever and that four roots help for quartan fever. Some even use the roots as amulets to disperse scrofulous swellings in the glands.

**II, 127 σίον, *Sium angustifolium* L., Water parsnip**
Water parsnip grows in water. It is a small, oily, and upright shrub, having leaves that resemble the leaves of alexanders, but smaller and aromatic; when eaten either boiled or raw, they break and remove stones, provoke micturition, draw out menses and embryos/fetuses, and they are useful to dysenterics when eaten. Crateuas reports on it as follows: it is a small and shrubby herb, having many round leaves which are bigger than the green mint's, dark, smooth, resembling the rocket's.

**II, 128 σισύμβριον, *Nasturtium officinale* R. Br., Watercress**
The watercress: but some call it *cardamine* and some call this plant, too, *sion*. It is a water plant that grows in the same places as water parsnip. Some call it *cardamine* because of its likeness in taste to *cardamon*.[61] Its leaves are at first round, but as they grow bigger they split like those of rocket. They warm, they are diuretic, and they are

[61] LSJ, καρδάμων, "nose-smart."

eaten even raw. Applied as a plaster all-night long and washed off in the morning, they remove birthmarks and freckles.

**II, 129 κρῆθμον, *Crithmum maritimum* L., Samphire**

The samphire is a shrubby little herb; it is lush, about a cubit tall, growing on stony and on coastal areas, it is laden with oily, whitish leaves that resemble the leaves of purslane, although they are wider, longer, and somewhat salty in taste. It has white flowers and its fruit is like that of rosemary, soft, sweet smelling, and round. When it has dried, it opens up, and inside it has its seed as if it were wheat. It has three or four roots that are thick as a finger, sweet smelling, and pleasant in taste.

The fruit, leaves, and root, boiled in wine and drunk, can help those with difficult micturition and people with jaundice; they also set the menses in motion. It is eaten as vegetable either boiled or raw. It is also preserved in brine.

**II, 130 κορωνόπους, *Plantago coronopus* L., Hartshorn**

The hartshorn is an oblong little herb that lies low upon the ground; its leaves are split. It, too, is used as a boiled vegetable. When eaten, its root is good for the colicky.

**II, 131 σόγχος, *Sonchus asper* L. and *S. oleraceus* L., Sow thistle**

There are two kinds of sow thistle: one kind is more wild and more prickly, the other is more tender and more edible; the stem is angular, reddish, and hollow; it has leaves that are split at intervals at the curvature.

They can cool and they are mildly astringent. It is for this reason that they are appropriate to use as cataplasms for heartburn and for inflammations; their juice stops gnawing in the stomach and draws down milk when sipped, and when applied with a wool wad, it helps for anal and uterine inflammations. Plastered on, the herb and the root help those bitten by scorpions.

**II, 132 σέρις, *Cichorium intybus* L., *Cichorium endivia* L., Chicory or Endive**

**1.** There is a wild and a cultivated. The wild is called bitter or chicory and it is both more wide-leaved and more wholesome than the one grown in the garden. The one that grows in the garden, too, is of two kinds: for one kind is more lettuce-like and broad-leaved, the other is narrow-leaved and rather bitter.

**2.** All of them are astringent, they cool, and they are wholesome. They also stay the bowel when taken boiled with vinegar and the wild endives are very much more wholesome. For they comfort a weak stomach and heartburn when eaten and when plastered on with barley groats or by themselves and they are a plaster for heart patients. They are useful for gout and they help for eye inflammations. The herb and the root help those struck by scorpions and for erysipelas when plastered on with barley groats. Their juice is smeared with white lead and vinegar on areas in need of chilling.

**II, 133 χονδρίλη, *Chondrilla juncea* L., *C. ramosissima* L., Gum succory**

**1.** Gum succory: it has leaves, stalk, and flowers like those of chicory, wherefore some say that it, too, is a kind of wild chicory, but the entire plant is more delicate. One finds gum around its little twig, which resembles mastic and which is as big as a bean; it draws down the menses when applied ground up with myrrh as pessary the size of an olive, on a linen cloth. The herb, chopped up with the root, is shaped into little lozenges to which honey is added; these lozenges, dissolved and mixed with soda, clear away dull-white leprosies. The gum even glues hair back.

**2.** The fresh root, too, accomplishes the same when a needle is dipped into it and applied to the hair. Drunk with wine, it is also suitable for the bite of vipers and its juice, when boiled with wine and drunk or even when drunk all by itself, stays the bowel.

There is also another kind of gum succory; its leaves are eroded all around, elongated, and lie on the ground; it has a stalk that is full of juice and a root that is delicate, sharp-edged, light, round, somewhat yellow, and full of juice.

The stalk and leaves have digestive properties and the juice glues back eyelashes. It grows in earthy soils and in cultivated fields.

**II, 134 κολόκυνθα ἐδώδιμος, *Lagenaria vulgaris* Ser., Edible bottle gourd**

The edible bottle gourd, ground up raw and plastered on, assuages swellings and abscesses. Its shavings are profitably plastered on the front part of the head of children suffering from heatstroke; similarly for eye inflammations and for gouty inflammations. The juice from the shavings is of service for earaches when instilled into the ears either by itself or with unguent of roses and it benefits a burning surface when smeared on it. The juice squeezed from a gourd that has been boiled whole is mildly diarrheic when drunk with a little honey and soda. And if one hollowed the gourd raw, poured into it wine, exposed it to the sun and air, then offered the wine diluted to drink, it does gently soften the stool.

**II, 135 σίκυς ἥμερος, *Cucumis sativus* L., Cucumber**

**1.** The cucumber eases the bowel, it is wholesome, it cools if it is not spoiled, it is appropriate to use for the bladder, and it revives those who fainted if they should smell it. Its seed, too, is mildly diuretic and it is suitable for ulcerations of the bladder when taken with milk or grape-syrup. Its leaves, used as a poultice with wine, treat dog bites, and with honey they also treat pustules that are most painful at night.
The flesh of the *pepon*[62] is digestive and diuretic when eaten and it assuages inflammations of the eye when used as a cataplasm.
**2.** Its rind is applied on top of the head of children suffering from heatstroke and on the forehead as an adhesive plaster for running eyes. The juice with the seed, mixed with meal and dried in the sun, is a cleansing suspension and makes the face brightly clean. An amount of one *holce* of dry root drunk with hydromel is emetic; but should one

[62] Jacques André, *Les noms de plantes dans la Rome antique*, p. 192, says that the L. *pepo* is borrowed from the Gr. πέπων "ripe", which in early Greek was more fully expressed as σίκυος πέπων, "ripe cucumber" while σίκυος "cucumber" without the qualifier πέπων was eaten unripe.

wish to vomit gently after dinner, two *obols* will be sufficient. It even cures impetigo contagiosa when plastered <ground up> with honey.

**II, 136 θρίδαξ ἥμερος, *Lactuca sativa* L., Cultivated lettuce**

**1.** The cultivated lettuce is wholesome, somewhat cooling, soporific, it softens the bowel, and it draws down milk. It becomes more nutritious when boiled, and it is good for people with stomach ailments when eaten unwashed. When its seed is drunk, it helps those who frequently emit their semen during sleep and it is a deterrent to sexual intercourse. A steady diet of lettuce causes dim-sightedness.

**2.** It is preserved in brine. After it has run to stalk, it has something that resembles the properties of the juice and of the milky liquid of the wild lettuce.

ἀγρία θρίδαξ. The wild lettuce resembles the cultivated, but it is leggier; also, its leaves are lighter in color, thinner, rougher, and bitter in taste. To some degree its activity is very similar to that of the poppy; this is why some mix even its milky juice with the milky juice of the poppy. Its milky juice, drunk with sour wine mixed with water in the amount of two *obols,* washes off watery matter; it clears both albugo and misty eyes, and it is good for sunburn when smeared on with a woman's milk.

**3.** In general, it is soporific and analgesic; it also brings on menstruation, and it is given to drink to those struck by scorpions and to those bitten by poisonous spiders. The seed, when drunk just like the seed of the cultivated lettuce, prevents frequent emission of semen during sleep and it is a deterrent to sexual intercourse; the juice, too, is able to accomplish the same, but more weakly. The milky juice is stored in clay vessels after it has been exposed to sunlight like the other plant extracts.

**II, 137 γιγγίδιον, *Malabaila sekakul* Russ., *Gingidium***

*Gingidium* grows plentiful in Cilicia and Syria. It is a small herb resembling the wild carrot, but it is more slender and bitterer, having a whitish and bitter root. It is used as a vegetable raw as well as boiled and it is also eaten pickled. It is wholesome and diuretic.

**II, 138 σκάνδιξ, *Scandix pecten-Veneris* L., Wild chervil**
The wild chervil: this plant, too, is a wild green, somewhat harsh and rather bitter, edible, and when eaten either boiled or raw it eases the bowel, it is wholesome, and it is diuretic. Its decoction when drunk is useful for the bladder, kidneys, and liver.

**II, 139 καυκαλίς, ~ *Caucalis grandiflora* L., *Caucalis***
Some call the *caucalis* wild *daucos*. It is a small stem, a span long, somewhat hairy, with leaves similar to the leaves of the fennel, narrowly incised and downy, and at its tip it has a white and aromatic umbel. This plant, too, is used as a vegetable, being eaten boiled as well as raw. It is diuretic.

**II, I40 εὔζωμον, *Eruca sativa* Lam., Rocket**
The rocket is aphrodisiac when eaten in large quantities; its seed, too, does the same, and it is diuretic, digestive, and laxative. The seed is used also as seasoning for boiled foods. To preserve it for a long time, they wet it with milk or vinegar, shape it into small wheels, and store it.
There grows also a wild rocket, especially in the western part of Spain, the seed of which the locals use also instead of mustard. It is much more diuretic and much sharper than the cultivated.

**II, 141 ὤκιμον, *Ocimum basilicum* L. sp., Basil**
**1.** The basil when eaten in large quantities causes dim-sightedness. It softens the bowel, it sets gases in motion, it is diuretic, it stimulates lactation, and it is hard to digest. When plastered on with very fine meal, unguent of roses, and vinegar, it helps for inflammations, for the stroke of the sea dragon and scorpion when plastered by itself, and for pains in the eyes when plastered with Chian wine. Its juice clears away misting of the eyes and dries their rheums.
**2.** The seed is suitable for black bile, for those who have difficulty micturating, and for the flatulent when drunk; it also stops excessive sneezing when inhaled through the nose; the plant, too, does the same; but one must close tightly his eyes at the approach of the sneeze. Some avoid it and do not eat it because basil that has been chewed and set out in the sun breeds worms. The Libyans believe in addition that

those who have consumed it and who were struck by a scorpion cannot be saved.

**II, 142 ὀροβάγχη, ~ *Orobanche crenata* Forsk., Chokefitch**

The chokefitch: some call it *cynomorion,* some *leon,* and the Cypriots call it *thyrsitis.* It is a small, reddish stalk, about two spans tall, sometimes even taller, leafless, somewhat greasy, soft, hairy, covered with either whitish or quince-yellow flowers. Its root is below ground, thick as a finger, having holes when the stalk dries. It seems to choke certain pulses among which it grows, whence its name.[63] It is used as a vegetable both raw and boiled, being eaten out of a flat dish just like asparagus and when added to pulses it is reputed to cook them faster.

**II, 143 τραγοπώγων, *Tragopogon porrifolius* L., Salsify**

The salsify, but some call it *come.* It has a short stalk, leaves that are similar to the leaves of saffron, and a root that is long and sweet. On the stalk there is a large calyx from the top of which grows a great deal of down whence it took its name.[64] The herb is edible.

**II, 144 ὄρνιθος γάλα, *Ornithogalum umbellatum* L., Starflower**

The starflower is a tender little stalk, delicate, whitish, about two spans tall, having at the top three or four soft offshoots from which grow flowers that are outwardly greenish but after they have opened they are milky in appearance, and in their midst there is a small head, which is incised like the fruit of rosemary and which is baked with bread like black cumin. The root is bulb-like; it is eaten raw, boiled, or baked.

**II, 145 ὕδνον, *Tuber cibarium* L. sp., Truffle**

The truffle is a globular root that has no leaves, no stalks, and that is dug up in the spring. It is edible. It is consumed raw as well as boiled.

---

[63] The etymology of ὀροβάγχη is from ὀροβός, "bitter vetch" and ἄγχω, "strangle," i.e. "that which strangles the bitter vetch," Jacques André, *Les noms des plantes dans la Rome antique,* p. 181.

[64] τραγοπώγων, from τράγος, "goat" and πώγων, "beard."

**II, 146 σμῖλαξ κηπαία, *Vigna sinensis* Endl., Cowpea**[65]

Its fruit is called *lobia*, but some call it *asparagos*. It has leaves like the ivy's but softer, slender stalks, and tendrils that wrap themselves around the surrounding shrubbery and that grow tall enough to form a canopy. It bears fruit like the fenugreek but longer and bulkier and within it the seeds resemble kidneys; they are not uniformly colored but partly reddish. It is grown for food. The fruit with the seed is boiled like asparagus; it is diuretic and it causes nightmares.

**II, 147 Μηδική, *Medicago sativa* L., Alfalfa**

Alfalfa[66] looks like the clover in the meadows when it begins to sprout, but as it grows it becomes more narrow-leaved, sending up stalks similar to the stocks of clover on which grow seeds the size of lentil, curved like small horns. The seed, after it has been dried, is mixed with flavored salts, as seasoning, but when plastered on green, it benefits conditions in need of cooling. Cattle farmers use the entire plant instead of dogtooth grass.

**II, 148 ἀφάκη, *Vicia sativa* var. *angustifolia* L., *V. articulata* Hornem., Tare**

The tare is a shrub that grows in fields; it is taller than the lentil, narrow-leaved, and the little sacs on it, which are bigger than those of the lentil, contain three or four black seeds, smaller than the lentil's.
The little seeds have an astringent property; it is for this reason that when roasted or boiled just like lentils they stem diarrhea and fluid discharges from the stomach.

**II, 149 πράσον κεφαλωτόν, *Allium porrum* L., Leek**

**1.** The leek causes flatulence, it is unwholesome, it causes nightmares, it is diuretic, it eases the bowel, it attenuates, it causes dim-sightedness, it draws down the menses, and it is harmful to a suppurated bladder and kidneys; but when boiled with peeled barley

---

[65] In the first edition, I translated σμῖλαξ κηπαία as kidney bean, which, Otta Wenskus, in Anzeiger für die Altertumswissenschaft, LXIII, Band, Juli/Oktober 2010, 3./4. Heft, p. 159, says is a New World plant and adds that cowpea is the most common English name for this plant.

[66] Also known as lucerne.

and eaten, it brings up matter from the chest. Its foliage, boiled in seawater and vinegar, is used in sitz baths for occlusions and indurations of the uterus. It becomes sweet and less flatulent when boiled in two waters then dipped in cold water.

**2.** The chopped leaves of leeks are rather sharp, they have even some astringency; this is why their juice with vinegar stems hemorrhaging, especially nosebleeds; combined with frankincense or frankincense powder, it is aphrodisiac, and when mixed with honey it is good as a lozenge for all chest conditions and for tuberculosis. The chopped leaves also cleanse the trachea when consumed. But a steady diet of chopped leaves causes dullness of sight and is bad for the stomach.

**3.** The juice, drunk with hydromel, helps those bitten by wild animals, as does the leek itself when used as a poultice; the juice helps both for earaches and for noises in the ears when instilled with frankincense and vinegar or with milk or with unguent of roses. The leaves remove facial pimples when plastered on with the fruit of the sumac that is used on prepared foods, treat pustules that are most painful at night, and cause scabs to break off all around when plastered on with salt. Moreover, two *drachmai* of the seed drunk with an equal amount of myrtle-berries keep in check chronic bringing up of blood.

**II, 150 ἀμπελόπρασον, *Allium ambeloprasum* L., Wild leek**

The wild leek, <on the one hand>, is worse for the stomach than the cultivated, on the other hand, it warms more, it is more diuretic, and it draws down the menses. It is suitable to be eaten by those bitten by wild animals.

**II, 151 κρόμυον, *Allium cepa* L., Onion**

**1.** The onion: the long onion is sharper than the round, the yellow sharper than the white, the dry sharper than the fresh, and the raw sharper than either the cooked or the pickled. All onions are pungent and apt to cause flatulence; they stimulate the appetite, they attenuate, they are thirst-making, they cause nausea, they cleanse, they ease the bowel, they are good for opening outlets for various secretions as well as for hemorrhoids, and they are used as suppositories peeled and dipped in olive oil. Their juice smeared on with honey helps for dim-sightedness, albugo, cloud-like opacities that begin to become

suffused,[67] and for sore throats when daubed on. It moves menstruation, it clears the head when poured down the nose, and in combination with salt, rue, and honey it is used as a poultice for people bitten by dogs.
**2.** Rubbed on in the sun with vinegar, it cures dull-white leprosies; combined with an equal amount of ashes, it stops blepharitis, and with salt it checks pimples. Combined with chicken fat, the juice is useful for abrasions caused by shoes as well as for hardness of hearing, for singing in the ears, for purulent ears, for water in the ears, and for bald spots when rubbed on. For it challenges hair to grow faster than bastard-sponge. But it also causes headaches. Onions make the sick lethargic if they should eat too many, and having been boiled they become more diuretic.

### II, 152 σκόρδον, *Allium sativum* L., Garlic

**1.** There is a kind of garlic that is cultivated and that grows in gardens; in Egypt, this one is single-headed and white. They call the cloves inside it *aglithes*. There is also another kind, which is wild, called *ophioscordon*.
It has properties that are sharp, warm, tend to relieve flatulence, to upset the bowel, to dry the stomach, to make one thirsty, and to cause ulcerations on the surface of bodies.
**2.** When eaten, it expels the flat intestinal worm, it is diuretic, and there is nothing better than it for people bitten by vipers and for those who hemorrhage if they should drink wine continuously or if it is triturated with the wine then drunk. It is also used as plaster for the same purposes as well as on people bitten by a mad dog; it even helps them when they eat it and it is suitable to use against the injurious effects of change. It clears bronchial tubes and it assuages chronic coughs when eaten raw, baked, or boiled, and it kills lice and their eggs when drunk with a decoction of oregano.
**3.** Burned, mixed with honey, and smeared on, it treats black eye and bald spots, but on the bald spots it should be used with unguent of spikenard. With salt and oil, it treats pustules; with honey, it removes birthmarks, lichen-like eruptions, scurf, dandruff, dull-white leprosies,

[67] See Dsc. Bk. I, 55 and n. 58.

and leprosies. Boiled down with a splinter of pinewood and with frankincense and held in the mouth, it relieves toothaches, and it is used as a poultice with fig leaves and cumin for the bite of the shrewmouse. The decoction of its foliage used as a sitz bath brings on menstruation and the afterbirth; it is also burned to produce smoke from below for the same purposes. The paste made with garlic and black olives, which is called *myttotos*,[68] sets the urine in motion and opens passages when eaten; it is also useful to those with edemata.

**II, 153 σκορδόπρασον, *Allium descendens* L., Garlic leek**

The garlic leek grows like a large leek, partaking of the properties of the leek and of the garlic; it is for this reason that it has compounded properties that accomplish everything that both the leek and garlic accomplish, except more mildly. It is used as a potherb for food, just like the leek, boiled and sweetened.

**II, 154 σίνηπι ἢ νᾶπι, *Sinapis alba* L., Mustard**

**1.** Choose it not dry and brittle but round and green inside when crushed, as if juicy, and gleaming. For this kind is fresh and in its prime.

It is capable of warming, attenuating, drawing, and of purging away phlegm when chewed. Its juice when mixed with hydromel or with wine and honey is a suitable rinse for tonsillitis and for chronic and callous roughness of the trachea.

**2.** Brought close to the nostrils after it has been ground up, it causes sneezing, it resuscitates epileptics and women suffering from uterine suffocation, and it is plastered on the shaven head of people who suffer from lethargic fever. Combined with figs and applied until it begins to irritate the skin, it is suitable for hip diseases, afflictions of the spleen, and, in general, for all chronic pains, whenever we wish to transfer something from deep inside the body to the surface in order to cause a counter-irritation. Plastered on, it also treats baldness, and with honey or animal fat or cerate it cleanses the face and clears away black eye.

---

[68] A savory dish of cheese, honey, garlic, etc.

**3.** It is smeared on with vinegar for leprosies and for wild lichen-like eruptions of the skin. It is also drunk for fits of intermittent fever when sprinkled dry like barley groats on top of the drink; it is mixed advantageously with absorbing plasters and with itch salves, and it is beneficial with fig for hardness of hearing and for ringing in the ears when ground fine and instilled into the ear. Combined with honey and smeared on, its juice is suitable for dim-sightedness and for rough eyelids. Juice is extracted when the seed is still green then the extract is dried in the sun.

**II, 155 κάρδαμον, *Lepidium sativum* L., Garden cress**

**1.** The garden cress that grows in Babylon is considered to be the best. The seed of all of them warms, is sharp, bad for the stomach, upsets the bowel and expels intestinal worms, reduces the spleen, destroys embryos/fetuses, moves the menstruation, and is aphrodisiac; it is like mustard and rocket, and it clears away leprosies and lichen-like eruptions of the skin.

**2.** Combined with honey and applied as a plaster, it reduces the spleen and clears away impetigo contagiosa; boiled with porridges and drunk, it brings up matter from the chest and it is a remedy for snakebite when drunk. Used as a fumigant, it chases away snakes; it stems the loss of hair and it breaks all around carbuncles, making pus. Plastered on with vinegar and barley groats, it is beneficial for patients suffering from hip disease, it dissipates both swellings and inflammations, and when applied with brine it causes small abscesses to suppurate. Even its greenery accomplishes the same results, although to a lesser degree.

**II, 156 θλάσπι, *Capsella bursa pastoris* L., Shepherd's-purse**

**1.** Shepherd's-purse[69] is a little herb with narrow leaves, about a finger's length, bending on the ground, cloven at the end and somewhat greasy. It sends up a small stalk, two spans tall that has a few side-shoots, and all around it there is fruit that is somewhat wide at the top; it encloses small seed like the seed of garden cress, quoit-shaped, looking as if it had been bruised; it is from its appearance that

[69] Shepherd's-purse, θλάσπι is akin to θλάω, "bruise, crush."

it received its name; the flower is whitish. It grows on roads, copings, and walls.

**2.** Its seed is sharp, warms, and purges bile both upwards and downwards when an amount of one *oxybaphon* is drunk. It is used in clysters for people with hip disease, it brings forth blood, and it breaks internal suppurative inflammations when drunk; it does also set the menses going and it destroys embryos/fetuses.

Crateuas tells also of another shepherd's purse which some call *Persicon sinepi*; it is broad-leaved and large-rooted. It, too, is mixed in clysters for hip disease.

### II, 157 δράβη, *Lepidium draba* L., Arabian mustard

Arabian mustard is an herb, a cubit tall, having delicate twigs; both sides of its leaves are like those of pepperwort but softer and whiter, and on top there is an umbel like that of the elder, having white blossoms. Its greenery is boiled together with peeled barley, especially in Cappadocia. Its dried fruit is mixed into the side dishes instead of pepper.

### II, 158 ἐρύσιμον, *Sisymbrium officinale* Scop., *S. irio* L., Hedge mustard

Hedge mustard grows around cities and building lots and in gardens. It has leaves similar to those of wild rocket, fibrous stalks, and quince-yellow flowers. At the tips there are horn-shaped pods which are thin, like those of fenugreek, and which contain seeds very similar to the seeds of garden cress. They are hot in taste and effective for chest rheums, abscesses, coughs, jaundice, and hip disease when taken as a lozenge with honey. They are also drunk for deadly poisons. Plastered on with either water or honey, they are beneficial for latent ulcers, indurations, tumors of the parotid glands, inflammations of the testicles and of the breasts, and, in general, they thin and warm. They become milder for lozenges after they have been soaked in water then roasted, or tied in a small piece of linen cloth then baked wrapped up in dough.

**II, 159 πέπερι, *Piper nigrum* L., Pepper**

**1.** The pepper is said to be a tree that grows in India. It produces fruit, which is at first oblong like pods; this is <the> long pepper, the contents of which nearly resemble millet; it will eventually become mature pepper. Unfolding at the right time, it makes clusters that bear peppercorns like the ones we know; some of them are even like unripe grapes, which are the white pepper, highly useful for eye medications, antidotes, and preparations for poisonous bites.

**2.** The long pepper, because it is unripe, is more suitable to use in antidotes and for medications against poisonous bites; the black pepper, on the other hand, is sharper than the white, tastier, and more aromatic because it is ripe. It is also more useful in dressings. The white pepper, being unripe, is weaker than the one mentioned before. Choose that which is very heavy, full, black, not very wrinkled, fresh, and not bran-like. Among the black pepper, one finds something that is devoid of nutritional value, empty, and light. It is called *bregma*.

**3.** In general, it can warm, further digestion, promote the production of urine, attract, promote the production of perspiration, and cleanse those elements that cast a shadow over the pupils of the eyes; when drunk or when smeared on, it is suitable for recurring shivering fits, it helps those bitten by wild animals, and it draws embryos/fetuses. Applied after sexual intercourse it is thought to cause barrenness, taken in lozenges and in drinks it is fit for all conditions associated with the chest, smeared on with honey it is suitable for sore throats, and when drunk with tender leaves of sweet bay it ends colic. Chewed with raisins it purges away phlegm, it is analgesic and good for the health, it stimulates the appetite, and it helps digestion when mixed in sauces.

**4.** Made up with pitch it dissipates scrofulous swellings of the glands and with soda it clears away dull-white leprosies. It is roasted over coals in a new clay pan, being stirred like lentils.

But its root is not ginger, as some supposed it to be, as we shall demonstrate forthwith. On the contrary, the root of pepper is like that.

But its root is not ginger, as some supposed it to be, as we shall demonstrate forthwith. On the contrary, the root of pepper is like that of costusroot, warming the taste and stimulating salivation; it reduces the size of the spleen when plastered on with vinegar or when drunk, and when chewed with stavesacre it cleanses away phlegm.

**II, 160 ζιγγίβερι, *Zingiber officinale* Rosc., Ginger**

The ginger is a distinct plant growing extensively in Troglodytic Arabia, where people use its greenery for many purposes, just as we use rue, boiling it for draughts and mixing it into boiled foods. It has small rootlets, like the root of galingale, which are off-white, taste like pepper, and are aromatic. Choose them not worm-eaten. Because ginger decays easily, some preserve it and ship it to Italy in clay vessels, being useful for flavoring. It is consumed with the preserving medium.

It has warming and digestive properties. It gently softens the bowel and it is wholesome. It acts on the substances that cast a shadow over the pupils of the eyes, it ins mixed with antidotes, and, in general, its properties resemble somewhat those of pepper.

**II, 161 ὑδροπέπερι, *Polygonum hydropiper,* L., Smartweed**

The smartweed grows mostly near stagnant waters and gentle streams; it sends out a knobby stalk that is surrounded by branches and leaves resembling those of mint, but they are bigger, whiter, more tender, sharp in taste like pepper, and completely devoid of a spicy scent. The fruit, which grows on small twigs near the leaves, is dense and botryoid; it, too, is sharp. It has a small and useless root.

The leaves with the fruit used as a poultice can dissipate swellings and chronic indurations and can clear away black eye. Dried and brayed, they are mixed with salt and with side dishes instead of pepper.

**II, 162 πταρμική, *Achillea ptarmica* L., Sneezewort**

The sneezewort is a little shrub that has many small, round branches like those of wormwood, surrounded by many longish leaves resembling the leaves of the olive tree. At the top, there is a tiny little head as of the chamomile, round, sharp in scent, and provoking sneezing, whence its name.

The leaves can clear black eye if they are plastered on with the flowers. But the flowers do cause a great deal of sneezing. It grows on mountainous and rocky terrains.

**II, 163 στρούθιον, *Saponaria officinalis* L., Soapwort**
The soapwort, which wool-cleaners use to clean wool, is well known; its root is sharp and diuretic; it helps liver disease patients, for coughs, orthopnea, and jaundice when a spoonful is taken with honey; it also purges the bowel. Taken with allheal and with the root of the caper, it breaks stones, it is diuretic, and it softens an indurated spleen. Used topically, it draws down the menses, it thoroughly destroys embryos/fetuses, and when plastered on with barley groats and vinegar it removes leprosies. Boiled with barley meal and wine, it dissipates growths. It is mixed both with eye salves for sharp-sightedness and with emollients. It also causes sneezing and cleanses through the mouth when poured ground up with honey into the nostrils.

**II, 164 κυκλάμινος, *Cyclamen graecum* Link., Cyclamen**
**1.** The cyclamen has leaves similar to those of ivy, but they are mottled on top and at the bottom with whitish spots; the stem is four-fingers long and leafless; on it grow rose-like, purplish flowers. It has a black root that resembles a turnip and it is somewhat flat. It drives phlegm and water downwards when drunk with a mixture of water and honey, and it sets the menses going when used topically or when drunk. They say that should a pregnant woman step over its root she miscarries; it also promotes quick birthing when worn. It is drunk with wine for deadly poisons, especially for the sea hare, it is an antidote for snakes when used topically or when drunk, and it causes drunkenness when mixed with wine.
**2.** Drunk in the amount of three *drachmai* with grape syrup or with a mixture of hydromel, it also cures jaundice; but the person drinking it must stay in bed, in a warm house, covered with several layers of clothing that he may perspire; as for the sweat that is secreted, it is found to be distinctly bilious in color. Their juice is instilled into the nostrils with honey to purge the head and it is applied with a wad of wool to the anus for the removal of excrements. Rubbed on the navel, on the lower part of the belly, and on the hip joint, it softens the bowel and it causes miscarriages; anointed with honey, the juice is suitable for people who have cataracts and for the dim-sighted. It is also mixed

with abortifacients and it restores a prolapsed anus when smeared on with vinegar.

**3.** Juice is extracted from the root by braying it and squeezing it; the extract is boiled until it reaches a honey-like consistency. The root cleanses the skin, stems the growth of pimples, and heals injuries with vinegar as well as by itself or with honey. Plastered on, it softens the spleen, it eliminates both freckles and baldness, and it is suitable for sprains as well as for gout. Its decoction is an effective rinse for small festering head-wounds and chilblains, and the root itself cicatrizes them if it is boiled in old olive oil and the oil is rubbed on them. Having been hollowed, it is filled with olive oil and placed on hot ashes; sometimes a little Tyrrhenian wax is added so as to become glutinous. It is an outstanding salve for people who develop chilblains. After it has been cut up, the root is stored like squill. They say that it is also used burned and shaped into small discs for love charms. It grows in thickly shaded places, especially under the trees.

### II, 165 κυκλάμινος ἑτέρα, *Lonicera periclimenum* L., Another cyclamen

Another cyclamen, which some call *cissanthemon,* has leaves like those of ivy but smaller; thick and knobby stems wrapping themselves spirally around the nearby trees, and white fragrant flowers. The fruit is like grapes in a bunch, similar to that of the ivy, soft, slightly sharp in taste and sticky; the root is useless. It grows on rough terrains.

A quantity of one *drachma* of its fruit drunk with two *cyathoi* white wine for 40 days reduces the spleen as it is eliminated through the urine and the excrement; it is also drunk for orthopnea and it cleanses the substances associated with childbirth when drunk.

### II, 166 δρακόντιον, *Arum dracunculus* L., Dragon arum

**1.** The dragon arum[70] has large ivy-like leaves that have white spots, and a stem that is upright, two cubits tall, pied, zigzag, shot with purple spots and thick as a wand. The fruit at the top is like a bunch of grapes, at first, grass green in color then after it has ripened saffron-colored and pungent in taste. The root is somewhat round, bulb-

[70] Also known as green dragon and as edderwort.

shaped, similar to the root of the cuckoopint, and it has a thin skin. It grows in densely shaded places, around hedges and walls.
The juice of the fruit can stop an earache when instilled into the ear with olive oil, it can destroy morbid excrescences when placed on a woolen wad into the nostrils, and it can even stem cancers when anointed.
**2.** A quantity of thirty seeds, drunk with sour wine mixed with water, causes miscarriages and they say that the smell of its fading flowers is destructive to newly conceived embryos. Having a warming property, the root helps for orthopnea, ruptures, spasms, coughs, catarrh, and it makes humors in the chest easy to bring up when eaten either boiled or raw with honey or all by itself; dry and ground up, it is taken with honey as a lozenge.
**3.** It is diuretic and aphrodisiac when drunk with wine, it cleanses and cicatrizes malignant and cancerous sores when triturated with bryony and honey, and it is fashioned into probes for fistulas and for the removal of embryos. And they say that should one rub his hands with the root, no viper would bite him. It also clears away dull-white leprosies if smeared on with vinegar. The leaves are suitable to apply ground up on fresh wounds instead of pledgets, they are also suitable for chilblains when boiled in wine and applied, and cheese wrapped in its leaves does not spoil.
**4.** The juice of the root is good for cloud-like opacities on the eyes, leucomas, and misting eyes. The root is cultivated also to use for good health, being eaten either boiled or raw. The inhabitants of the Gymnesian islands, which are called Balearics, mix the boiled root with a great deal of honey and serve it instead of flat cakes to dinner guests. The root must be stored at the time wheat is harvested; having been dug up, washed, and cut into pieces, it must then be threaded with a linen thread and dried in the shade.

### II, 167 ἄρον, *Colocasia antiquorum* Schott., Cuckoopint

The cuckoopint, which the Syrians call *loufa*. It sends out leaves similar to those of dragon arum, but smaller and without spots, a stem one span tall, purplish and pestle-shaped, upon which the saffron-colored fruit grows; the root is white tending toward the root of dragon arum; it, too, is eaten boiled, although it is less pungent. Its leaves are cured for eating; they are also eaten boiled after they have dried by themselves.

The seed, leaves, and root have the same properties as dragon arum. The root, plastered on, is efficacious for the gouty. It is stored the same way as the root of dragon arum and, in general, it is edible because it is not very pungent.

**II, 168 ἀρίσαρον, *Arisarum vulgare* Targ.-Tozz., Hooded arum**

The hooded arum is a small herb that has a root like an olive; it is more pungent than the root of cuckoopint, wherefore it stops spreading ulcers when plastered on. They also make from it salves which are effective for fistulas. The root destroys the genitalia of all living things when inserted.

**II, 169 ἀσφόδελος, *Asphodelus* L. sp., Asphodel**

**1.** The asphodel: it is a plant with which most people are familiar, having foliage like that of a large leek and a smooth stem, at the top of which there is a flower called *anthericon*. The roots are below ground, longish, round, similar to acorns, having a pungent taste and a warming property. Taken in drink, they provoke both micturition and menstruation, and one *drachma* of root, drunk with wine, treats pains on the side, coughs, spasms, and ruptures.

**2.** An amount the size of a vertebra, when eaten, makes people happier, and three *drachmai* are given with success to people bitten by snakes. But one must also plaster the bites with its leaves, root, and flowers combined with wine; on the other hand, sordid sores, spreading ulcers, breast and testicular inflammations, growths, and small abscesses must be plastered with the root boiled with wine lees, but newly-sprung inflammations with barley groats. The juice of the root, combined with sweet old wine, myrrh, and saffron, and boiled, becomes a medicinal ointment for the eyes; it is suitable to use warmed up all by itself as well as with frankincense, honey, wine, and myrrh for suppurating ears, and the juice assuages a toothache when instilled all by itself into the ear of the opposite side.

**3.** Plastered on, the ash of the root restores hair on bald spots; olive oil that was boiled in hollowed out roots benefits chilblains and burns when plastered on them, it helps those suffering from earaches when poured into the ear, and the root, smeared on dull-white leprosy that was first abraded in the sun with a linen cloth, clears it. Drunk with wine, its fruit and flowers are the antidotes *par excellence* for scolopendra and scorpions; they are also powerful purgatives.

**II, 170 βολβὸς ἐδώδιμος, *Muscari comosum* Miller, Purse tassels**

**1.** Purse tassels: the red is wholesome and it is brought from Libya, but the one that is bitter and like squills is more wholesome and it furthers digestion. All of them are pungent and warming, aphrodisiac, roughening the tongue and tonsils, highly nutritious and fattening, and causing flatulence. Plastered on either by themselves or with honey, they are beneficial for sprains, bruises, splinters, pains in the joints, and gout, and they similarly benefit swellings of those afflicted by dropsy and dog bites when used with honey; they also repress perspiration.

**2.** Plastered on with ground pepper, they stop stomach pains; with baked soda, they clear dandruff and scurf; either by themselves or with egg yolk, they clear away black eye and facial pimples, and with a mixture of vinegar and honey, birthmarks; they are used with barley groats for bruised ears, also for contused nails. Roasted on hot ashes and applied with the heads of burned *Maenae vulgares*,[71] they remove excrescences on the body and they remove freckles and black scars if one <should burn> them, mix them with bastard sponge, and smear them on in the sun. Boiled with vinegar and consumed, they are good for ruptures; but one must guard against eating too many because they attack the nervous system.

**II, 171 σκίλλα, *Urginea maritima* Baker = *Scilla maritima* L., Squill or Scilla**

**1.** The squill has sharp and heating properties; it becomes extremely useful after it has been baked. It is wrapped in dough or clay then placed in an oven or buried in coals until the surrounding dough is well baked. Removing the dough, if the squill did not become tender, it is wrapped in new dough or clay and we shall repeat the process. For unless it was baked this way it is harmful to give, especially if

[71] Small sprat-like fish that were salted.

offered for intestinal ailments. It is also baked in a lidded clay pot set in the oven. It is its core that is used, the outer parts being stripped off.
**2.** It is also boiled cut up, the first water is poured out and fresh water is added until the water is neither bitter nor pungent, then the squill is dried in the shade, sliced, and the slices are kept separated with linen thread so as not to touch each other. We use the slices for wine, vinegar, and oil of squill; the core of raw squill, boiled with olive oil or sodden with pine resin, is applied to fissures on the feet, and it is a poultice for viper bites when boiled in vinegar.
**3.** To soften the stool, we give on an empty stomach one or two spoonsful of one part baked squill with eight parts triturated baked salt; we also give it in draughts and in fragrant prescriptions to those whose micturition we wish to set in motion, to those with edemata, to people with stomach ailments whose food remains crude in the stomach, to the jaundiced, the colicky, to people who have chronic coughs, to asthmatics, and to people who bring up either blood or phlegm. It is enough to take in lozenge form with honey an amount of one *triobolon*.
**4.** It is also boiled with the honey and eaten for the same purposes, assisting digestion very nicely; it does drive the glutinous element down the bowel. It is good boiled for the same purposes being taken the same way; one must not give it, however, to people who have any kind of internal ulceration; baked and smeared on, it is also good for thin-necked warts and for chilblains. Its seed, ground, compounded with dry figs or honey, and eaten, softens the bowel. It does also ward off evil when hung whole on front doors.

**II, 172 παγκράτιον, *Pancratium maritimum* L., Sea daffodil**

The sea daffodil: some call this plant also squill. It has a root like that of large purse-tassels, reddish, bitter and burning in taste; its leaves are like those of the white lily, but longer.

It has the same properties as the squill, it is prepared the same way, and it is given in the same dose, affecting the same conditions. Its activity, however, is more moderate than that of the squill; it is for this reason that juice extracted from the root, mixed with bitter vetch flour, and shaped into little pastilles is profitably given with hydromel to people with spleen disease and to those with edemata.

**II, 173 κάππαρις, *Capparis spinosa* L., Caper**

**1.** The caper: but some call it *cynosbaton,* others *capria*, others *coracos melon*, others *ophioscordon*, others *ophiostaphylon*, others *thallia*, others *petraia*, others *holophyton*, others *ionites,* some *aeichloron*, others *hippomanes*, and others *trichomanes.* It is a thorny shrub, lying on the ground in a circular fashion. It has hook-like thorns like the bramble, round leaves that resemble those of the quince-tree, and fruit[72] as of the olive. After the fruit has opened, it puts out a white flower, and after the flower has fallen one finds something that resembles an elongated acorn which, when opened, contains seeds like those of the pomegranate that are small and red.

**2.** It has many large woody roots. It grows for the most part on rough ground, poor soil, on islands, and in building lots. Both its fruit and stem are cured for food.

It disturbs the belly, it is bad for the stomach, and it is thirst making, but when eaten boiled, it is more wholesome than raw. Its fruit reduces the spleen when drunk with wine for thirty days in the amount of two *drachmai*, it is diuretic, it draws bloody excrement, it helps for hip disease and for paralysis when drunk, it is also used for ruptures and spasms, it draws down the menses, it purges away phlegm, and when its fruit is boiled with vinegar and used as a mouthwash it stops a toothache.

**3.** When dry, the skin of the root is suitable both for all the above conditions and cleanses all chronic, sordid, and calloused sores; it is also plastered with bruised meal of raw corn on people with spleen disease, it helps for toothaches if one bit on it, and when ground up it wipes off with vinegar dull-white leprosies. Triturated, the leaves and root dissipate indurations and scrofulous swellings of the glands, and the juice destroys earwigs when instilled. But the Libyan caper, which grows in the region of the people called Marmarides, causes a great deal of flatulence, that of Apulia causes vomiting, and that from the Red Sea and Arabia is indeed extremely sharp, causing blisters in the mouth and putrefying the gums to the point of stripping them from the teeth; this is why it is unfit to eat.

---

[72] This is actually the bud.

**II, 174 λεπίδιον, *Lepidium latifolium* L., Pepperwort**

The pepperwort, which some call *gingidion,* is a familiar little herb that is preserved in brine with milk. Its leaves have sharp and ulcerating properties, wherefore they are a highly irritating plaster for people with hip disease when applied for a quarter of an hour ground up with root of elecampane; it is similarly applied also on patients with spleen disease; it wipes out even leprosies. Its root is believed to relieve toothaches if suspended around the neck.

**II, 175 βατράχιον, *Ranunculus* L., sp. Ranunculus**

**1.** Ranunculus: some call it *selinon agrion.* There are many kinds of this plant but they all have the same properties: they are sharp and highly ulcerative. One kind has leaves similar to the leaves of coriander, but wider, off-white, and greasy, a quince-yellow flower, although sometimes purple, a stem that is not thick, a cubit tall, and a small, white, and bitter root that has side-shoots just like the side-shoots of hellebore. It grows near streams. There is also another kind that is downy, longer stemmed, and it has more notches on its leaves. It grows extensively in Sardinia and it is very sharp; they call this one *selinon agrion.*[73] And there is a third kind that is very small and ill smelling; its flower is like gold, and a fourth kind that resembles the last one, with flowers that seem milky.

**2.** Used as a plaster, the leaves and tender stems have painfully ulcerative and escharotic properties, wherefore they remove psoriatic nails and mange; plastered on for a short time, they get rid of marks, warts that spread under the skin, warts with thin necks, and bald spots; and after they have been boiled, their decoction is used warm to rinse chilblains. The root, dried, ground fine, and brought near the nostrils, provokes sneezing; it also relieves toothaches when used topically; but it does shatter the teeth.

**II, 176 ἀνεμώνη, *Anemone coronaria* L., Poppy anemone**

**1.** The poppy anemone: some call it *argemonion* and some *eremion.* It is of two kinds: one kind is wild[74] and the other cultivated. And of the

---

[73] See Dsc. II, n. 37.

[74] This is the scarlet windflower, *A. fulgens* which J. Berendes, p. 252, identifies as *A.*

cultivated, some have red flowers and others whitish, somewhat milky in appearance or purple. It has leaves like those of coriander, the ones towards the ground having rather narrow slits, little stems that are downy and thin, on top of which the flowers are as of the poppy, and the center of the little heads are black or dark in color; the root is about as big as an olive or bigger, divided at intervals as if by joints. The wild is in every respect larger than the cultivated: not only does it have leaves that are broader and tougher but it also has a more oblong head; it has a red flower and many delicate rootlets. And there is one with darker leaves,[75] which is sharper.

**2.** Both kinds have a sharp property, wherefore the juice of their root when instilled into the nostrils is suitable for clearing the head; also when chewed, the root brings up phlegm; boiled in grape syrup and used as a plaster, it treats inflammations of the eyes and wipes off eye scars; it also cleanses the sordid elements of sores. Both the leaves and stems boiled together with barley gruel and eaten draw forth milk; used in a pessary, they draw down the menses and when plastered on they remove leprosies.

**3.** Some people, however, being unable of distinguish from the wild poppy anemone the so called wind-rose[76] and the corn poppy—regarding the latter we shall report in the chapter on poppies (IV, 63) —because their flowers are of the same red, mistakenly call the wind-rose poppy anemone. But the red color of the wind-rose is less deep as is also the red of the corn poppy; both it and the wind-rose bloom later; also, the wind-rose yields juice that is saffron-colored and very sharp in taste but the juice of the corn poppy is whiter and sharp. Both have in the middle a little head very nearly like that of the wild poppy, except that the head of wind-rose is somewhat broad on top and that of the corn poppy somewhat narrow. But poppy anemones neither yield juice nor have capsules, but a tip like that of asparagus, and for the most part those grow in fields.

---

*hortensis.*

[75] J. Berendes, p. 253, identifies this as *Anemone apennina.*

[76] ἀργεμώνη, *Papaver argenone* L. See Dsc. II, 177, below.

**II, 177 ἀργεμώνη, *Papaver argemone* L., Wind-rose**

The-wind rose: generally speaking, it is like a wild poppy, but its leaf is similar to the leaf of poppy anemone and it is split; its flower is red, the head resembles a corn poppy, but it is more elongated and broad at the upper parts, and it has a round root; it yields juice that is saffron-colored and pungent.

It clears albugo and cloud-like opacities in the eyes, and when plastered on the leaves soothe inflammations.

**II, 178 ἀναγαλλίς, *Anagallis arvensis* L., *A. caerulea* Schreb., Pimpernel**

**1.** The pimpernel, but some call it *cichorion*. There are two kinds of this plant differing in their flower: for the one with a dark-blue flower is called female and the other with the red flower male. They are little shrubs, heaped on the ground, having small, somewhat round leaflets on four-cornered stems, tending toward the leaves of *helxine*,[77] and fruit that is round.

Both kinds are used for wounds, they relieve inflammations, they extract splinters, and they are able to check spreading ulcers.

**2.** Their juice, used as a gargle, purges phlegm from the head; it is also infused into the nostrils; additionally, it stops a toothache if you should pour it into the nostril above the aching tooth. With Attic honey, it also clears albugo and it helps for dim-sightedness; when drunk with wine it is beneficial for viper bites, kidney disease, liver disease, and edemata. Some say that the one that has the dark-blue flowers stems prolapses of the anus when applied as a plaster and that the red-flowered aggravates them.

**II, 179 κισσός, *Hedera helix* L., Ivy**

**1.** The ivy has many characteristics that distinguish one species from the next, but the principal characteristics are three: there is one kind called white, another black, and another spiral. And the white has

[77] In Dsc. Bk. IV, 39 and Bk. IV, 85, two different plants called *helxine* are discussed. The one in Bk. IV, 39 is the bindweed, *Convolvulus arvensis.* The plant of Bk. IV, 85 is pellitory, *Parietaria officinalis.* Compare also the description in Bk. IV, 85 with that of Bk. II, 183.

white fruit, the black has black or saffron-colored fruit, which some call *Dionysion*, and the spiral not only does not bear fruit, but it also has delicate twigs as well as delicate, angular, and graceful leaves.
All ivies are pungent, astringent, and act on the nervous system. A pinch of their flowers[78] drunk with wine is good for dysentery, but one must take the drink twice a day; they are also suitable for burns when triturated with a cerate.
**2.** The leaves that are tender, boiled with vinegar or triturated raw, treat the spleen; the juice of the leaves and of the berry clusters is poured into the nose with unguent of iris or honey or soda for chronic headaches; it is also sprinkled on the head with vinegar and unguent of roses, and with olive oil it treats purulent ears. But the juice of the leaves of the black ivy and of its berry clusters when drunk cause sterility, and if consumed to excess confuse the mind; five of the berries triturated, heated with unguent of roses in the shell of a pomegranate, and instilled into the ear on the opposite side of an aching tooth, assuage the toothache and the berries also dye hair black.
**3.** The leaves boiled in wine are applied as a poultice on every kind of sore, and when plastered on boiled, as indicated, treat burns, malignancies, and freckles. The berries, ground up and drunk or burned so as to produce smoke from below, set the menses going and an amount of one *drachma* taken in a drink at the end of the menstrual period causes barrenness. The leafstalk, too, smeared with honey and placed in the uterus, draws menstrual period and embryos/fetuses, and the juice when instilled clears off the bad smells and putrid humors of the nostrils. Its sap when smeared on thins the hair and destroys lice, and the juice of the roots when drunk with vinegar helps those bitten by venomous spiders.

### II, 180 χελιδόνιον μέγα, *Chelidonium majus* L., Celandine

**1.** The celandine: some call this plant *othonna* and others *crimnon*. It has a thin stem, about a cubit tall or even taller that has offshoots full of leaves like those of ranunculus; the leaves of celandine, however, are tender and somewhat grey in color; also along each leaf there is a

---

[78] The 'pinch' here is defined by "the flowers one can pick up using three fingers."

flower as of the gillyflower. The juice is saffron-colored, sharp, somewhat biting, bitter, and foul smelling. The root in the upper part is single, but in the lower multiple. The fruit is like that of the horned poppy, delicate, long like a cone, containing little seeds bigger than the poppy's.

**2.** Its juice, mixed with honey and boiled in a brazen cauldron over coals, is good for sharpening the vision; at the beginning of the summer, the root, leaves, and fruit are converted into juice; it is then dried in the shade, and molded. Drunk with anise and white wine, the root treats people who have jaundice; plastered on with wine it treats shingles and when chewed it stops toothaches. It seems that it was named *chelidonion*[79] because it grows when the swallows appear and withers when they leave. Some have also reported that should any of the fledglings of a swallow be blind, mother swallows in offering this herb cure its blindness.

### II, 181 χελιδόνιον τὸ μικρόν, *Ficaria verna* Huds., Pilewort

The pilewort: some call it *pyros agrios*. It is a small herb, hanging loose from leafstalks, stemless, enveloped by ivy-like leaves, but rounder, smaller, tenderer, and less shiny. It has many small roots coming out of the same place like wheat that has been heaped up together; there are three or four of them that grow long. It grows near waters and marshlands.

It has a sharp property, nearly resembling that of poppy anemone, ulcerating the skin, and it removes the mange and nails affected by psoriasis. Juice extracted from the root is useful for pouring into the nose with honey to purge the head.

### II, 182 ὀθάννα, *Othonna*

**1.** Some say that *othonna* is the juice of celandine, others that it is the juice of the horned poppy, others that it is the juice of the flowers of the horned poppy, others that it is a mixture of the juices of dark-blue flowered pimpernel, henbane, and poppy, others that it is the juice of some Troglodytic herb which is called *othonna* and that this herb grows also in that part of Arabia which is towards Egypt. It has leaves

---

[79] χελιδόνιον, "swallow."

that resemble the leaves of rocket, full of holes as though moth-eaten, rough, and not very juicy. It puts out a saffron-colored flower that has broad petals on account of which some thought that it is a kind of a poppy anemone.

**2.** It is converted into juice for eye medications whenever there is need to clean, stinging and clearing all things that cast shadows over the pupils of the eyes. They say also that from this herb flows some sort of moisture, which, after washing and removing the stones, they shape into little discs for the same purposes. Some say, however, that it is an Egyptian stone, native to Thebes, copper-colored, small in size, biting the taste with burning and binding.

### II, 183 μυὸς ὦτα, *Asperugo procumbens* L., Madwort

The madwort: but some call it *myos otis*. It sends out many reddish stalks from one root that are hollow at the lower end; the leaves are narrow and longish, having their mid-rib raised, dark in color, growing two by two at intervals, ending in a sharp point, and from the axils grow delicate stems on which there are small dark-blue flowers like the pimpernel's. The root is thick as a finger and has many shoots. Generally, this herb is similar to *scolopendrion*,[80] although it is softer and smaller. Its root cures lachrymal fistulas when plastered on. Some call also the *helxine*[81] madwort.

### II, 184 ἰσάτις, *Isatis tinctoria* L., Woad

The woad, which the dyers use, has foliage like the plantain's, but shinier and darker, and a stem over a cubit long.

When used as a poultice, its leaves are able to dissipate every swelling and growth; they close bloody wounds, stem hemorrhages, and treat cancerous sores, shingles, and erysipelas.

### II, 185 ἰσάτις ἀγρία, *Isatis agrestis* L., Wild woad

The wild woad, which closely resembles the one dyers use, has leaves that are larger in relation to the leaves of the lettuce and many delicate and much-cloven reddish stalks. From their tip, as if hanging, there are

---

[80] This name is given to several different plants, e.g miltwaste, polypody, etc.

[81] See Dsc. Bk. II, 178 and II, n. 77.

many tongue-like little sacks containing the seed; the flower is quince-yellow and delicate.

It is capable of the same results as the previous one; it also helps people with spleen disease when drunk and when plastered on.

**II, 186 τηλεφώνιον, *Andrachne telephioides* L., *Telephonion***

*Telephonion*, but some call it *aeizoon agrion*, others *andrachne agria*, and others *bryon.* It resembles the purslane both in foliage and stem, having two hollows that develop at each <joint> of leaves from the base of which grow six or seven little branches full of coarse, fleshy, and sticky leaves; the flowers are white. It grows in vineyards and in cultivated fields.

The leaves treat *leuce*[82] when applied as a poultice for six hours; afterwards, however, bruised meal of raw corn must be used. Rubbed on with vinegar in the sun, they also remove dull-white leprosy, but they must be wiped off after they have dried.

---

[82] A cutaneous disease so-called from its color.

# BOOK III

Dear Areios,
In the previous books I have discussed aromatics, oils, unguents, trees and their fruits and saps, also animals, cereals, vegetables, and pungent herbs. In this book, which is the third, I shall deal with roots, extracts, herbs, and seeds, both wholesome and harmful.

## III, 1 ἀγαρικόν, *Polyporus* sp., Agaric

**1.** Agaric is said to be a root resembling the laserwort; it is not compact on the surface as is the laserwort but it is of loose texture throughout. One kind of this plant is male and the other female, the difference between them being that the female contains straight gills while the male is globular and growing entirely as a single unit; both, however, taste the same, at first they are sweet, then after shooting up they are rather bitter.[1] It grows in Agaria[2] of Sarmatica.[3]
**2.** Some say, however, that it is the root of a tree and others that it sprouts on Valonia oaks from rot, exactly as mushrooms. It also grows in Asiatic Galatia[4] and in Cilicia[5] on cedar trees but it is brittle and weak.
**3.** It is astringent, it warms, it is good both for colic and indigestion, for ruptures and falls; an amount of two *obols* is given with wine to those who are fever free but with wine and water to those who have a fever. About one *drachma* is given to those with liver disease, asthma, difficult micturition, kidney disease, jaundice, uterine suffocation, and bad complexion; to the tuberculars it is offered with grape syrup; to those with spleen disease with oxymel; to people with stomach

---

[1] In modern pharmacy, the male, agaric of the larch, *Polyporus laricis*, was used as cathartic, and the female, agaric of the oak, *Polyporus igniarius*, as a styptic, for dyeing, and for tinder, as its scientific name indicates. Dioscorides has considerably many more uses.
[2] Suspect reading; unknown location.
[3] Designating an area extending from eastern Germany to the Caspian Sea.
[4] In the center of modern Turkey.
[5] On the southern coast of modern Turkey, opposite Cyprus.

ailments to chew and swallow just as is, without drinking any water with it; it is given similarly for heartburn.

**4.** A weight of three *obols* taken with water stops blood spitting. Taken with an equal amount of oxymel, it is good for pains of the hips, of the joints, and for epilepsy. It also draws down the menses and the same amount is given successfully to women inflated in the uuterus. It prevents shivering if given before its onslaught and it even cleanses the bowel when one or two *drachmai* are drunk with hydromel.

**5.** A dose of one *drachma* taken with diluted wine is an antidote for deadly poisons, a dose of three *obols* drunk with wine helps for strokes and bites of vipers, and on the whole it is suitable for all internal disorders, being given according to the strength and age of the recipients, to some with water and to others with wine or with oxymel or with hydromel.

### III, 2 ῥᾶ, *Rheum ribes* L., Rhubarb[6]

**1.** The rhubarb: but some call it *rheon.* It grows in the lands above the Bosporus from where it is brought. The root is black, resembling that of centaury, but it is smaller and somewhat redder, odorless, spongy, and somewhat light. It is best when it is not worm-eaten, when it tastes slimy, releasing a great deal of astringency, and when it is yellowish and somewhat like saffron in color when chewed.

**2.** When drunk, it is good for flatulence in the stomach, for lack of energy, for all sorts of pains, spasms, and ruptures, for patients with spleen, liver, and kidney disease, for the colicky, for disorders associated with the bladder and chest, for tension in the general area of the stomach, and for disorders in the area of the uterus, for hip ailments, blood-spitting, asthma, hiccups, dysentery, for bowel conditions, for fits of intermittent fever, and for bites of wild animals.

**3.** You will administer it the same way as agaric, for each condition using the same quantity and the same liquids. When rubbed on with

---

[6] Identified in LSJ as *rheum officinale*, but D. J. Mabberley, *The Plant Book s.v. rheum officinale* says that the habitat of *rheum officinale* is W. China and Tibet. For Jacques André, *Les plantes dans la Rome antique*, p. 217, whose identifications I follow, it is *rheum ribes* L.

vinegar, it removes livid spots and lichen-like eruptions of the skin and when plastered on with water, it disperses all chronic inflammations. Its primary property is astringency with a degree of heating.

**III, 3 γεντιανή, *Gentiana lutea* L., *G. purpurea* L., Gentian**

**1.** The gentian: it seems that it was first discovered by Gentian, king of the Illyrians, for whom it was named. Its leaves near the root resemble nut tree or plantain leaves and they are reddish; the ones in the middle of the stem and especially those near the top are slightly jagged. Its stem is hollow, smooth, one-finger thick, two-cubits tall, divided by joints, and surrounded at large intervals by leaves. It has broad fruit that is in capsules, it is light, chaffy, somewhat like the fruit of cow parsnip, and a long root resembling that of <the long> birthwort, thick, and bitter; it grows on very high mountain ridges and in shady and wet spots.

**2.** The root has warming and astringent properties; an amount of two *drachmai* given to drink with pepper, rue, and wine helps people hbitten by wild animals, and an amount of one *drachma* of extracted juice helps for pains in the sides, falls, sprains, and ruptures; drunk with water, it is also good for people with liver and stomach ailments. Applied as a pessary, the root expels embryos/fetuses, it is a wound medication when plastered on like dyer's buckthorn, it is a remedy for ulcers that undermine, especially its juice, and it is an unguent for inflamed eyes. The juice is mixed instead of opium with eye salves that are harsh, and the root is a cleanser for dull-white leprosies.

**3.** Juice is extracted by crushing it and soaking it in water for five days; then after boiling it in the water until the roots float and after the water has cooled down, it is strained through a linen cloth; then it is boiled until it becomes of honey-like consistency and stored in a clay vessel.

**III, 4 ἀριστολοχεία, *Aristolochia rotunda* L., *A. longa* L., *A. clematitis* L., Birthwort**

**1.** The birthwort: it was given its name from the belief that it is very helpful to women during childbirth. There is a kind which is round, called female; it has ivy-like leaves that are pungently aromatic,

somewhat round, and soft, and that surround many shoots rising from one root; its twigs are long, its flowers white, resembling little caps, and the red part in them is ill-smelling.
**2.** The long birthwort is called male as well as *dactylitis*; it has more elongated leaves than the round and its little branches are slender, about a span in size; the flower is purple, ill smelling, becoming pear-shaped after it has withered. The root of the round is globular like a turnip, but of the long it is thick as a finger, a span long or even longer; both are for the most part like boxwood inside, bitter in taste, and foul smelling.
**3.** There is also a third kind; it is long and it is called also *clematitis*. It has slender twigs, laden with leaves that are somewhat round and they resemble the leaves of houseleek, flowers like the rue's, and very long thin roots that have a thick and aromatic bark and that are singularly useful to perfume-makers for thickening their unguents.
**4.** The round is efficacious for the rest of the poisons, but for snakes or for deadly poisons it is the long birthwort that is efficacious when one *drachma* is drunk with wine and when it is plastered on; it also draws out all parturient matter compacted in the uterus, the menses, and embryos/fetuses when drunk with pepper and myrrh. It does the same also when applied in a pessary.
**5.** The round helps for all the conditions for which the one previously mentioned is helpful but when drunk with water it helps especially for asthma, hiccups, shivering, the spleen, ruptures, spasms, and pains in the side. Plastered on, it lifts up thorns, it removes needles <and> splinters from bones, it outlines flesh mortifications, it cleanses all around sores that are sordid, and with iris and honey it fills up hollow sores. It also cleanses gums and teeth. It is thought that the *clematitis*, too, is good for the same conditions; however, it is less potent than the ones mentioned first.

### III, 5 γλυκύρριζα, *Glycyrrhiza glabra* L., G. echinata L., Licorice

**1.** Licorice: some call it *Pontice rhiza*, others *gentiane*, others *Scythion*, others *adipson*, <and others *symphyton*>. It grows abundantly in Cappadocia and Pontus. It is a small shrub having two-cubit long shoots surrounded by closely growing leaves which resemble the leaves of mastic and which are shiny and sticky to the touch; but its flower is like a hyacinth,[7] the fruit is as big as the globular catkins of the plane tree, rather rough, having pods like the lentil's that are reddish and small; the roots are long like the roots of gentian, somewhat astringent, and sweet; juice is extracted from them like from dyer's buckthorn.

**2.** The juice is good for hoarseness of the trachea; it must be placed under the tongue to melt it.[8] Drunk with grape syrup, it is suitable for heartburn, chest and liver ailments, itching of the bladder, and for kidney ailments; allowed to melt in the mouth, it quenches thirst; smeared on, it is good for wounds, and it is good for the mouth when chewed. The decoction of fresh roots is also suitable for the same purposes. Dried and pounded fine, the root is suitable to use as a powder on membranes that grow over the eyes from the inner corners.

### III, 6 κενταύριον τὸ μέγα, *Centaurea centaurion* L., Centaury

**1.** The centaury, but some call it *narce* and others *gentiane*: it has leaves similar to the leaves of the walnut tree, oblong, pale in color like the leaves of the cabbage; their margin is serrated like a saw; it has a stem like that of monk's rhubarb, two-cubits tall or even three, having many offshoots rising from the root, on which there are heads resembling poppies that are somewhat long in circumference. The flower is dark blue; the seed is similar to that of safflower, nestled as if among flowers made of wool; the root is thick, solid, heavy, about two-cubits long, full of juice that is sharp with a degree of astringency and sweetness, and reddish; the juice, too, is similarly red.

**2.** It likes a rich soil, a sunny location, thickets, and hillocks. It grows in abundance in Lycia and, within Peloponnesos, in Elis, Arcadia, Messene, and around Pholoe, Lycaion, and Cyllene.[9]

The root, taken with wine, is suitable for ruptures, spasms, people with pleurisy, dyspnea, for an old cough, and for those who spit blood, provided they are free of fever; but to those who run a fever an amount of two *drachmai* of root is given with water.

---

[7] Variously interpreted either as the wild hyacinth, bluebell, *Scilla bifolia* or as the blue larkspur, *Delphinium Ajacis* L.

[8] Presumably a lozenge made from the juice is placed under the tongue and left there to dissolve slowly.

[9] The last three are mountains on Peloponnesos.

**3.** It is similarly given both for colic and for pains in the uterus. It draws down the menses and embryos/fetuses when whittled, shaped like a pessary, and applied to the uterus. The juice accomplishes the same. The root is also good for injuries, chopped up if moist, but if it is dry, it is first moistened and then chopped up. For it does draw matter together, it agglutinates, and it contracts meats that are boiling if one chopped it up and cooked it with the meats. People in Lycia use its extracted juice instead of a decoction of dyer's buckthorn.

**III, 7 κενταύριον τὸ λεπτὸν ἢ μικρόν, *Erythraea centaurium,* L., Feverfew**

**1.** Feverfew, which some people call *limnesion* because it likes marshlands. This plant resembles St. John's wort and oregano, having a stem that is over a span tall and angular, flowers faintly purple like those of rose campion, small and longish leaves like the rue's, fruit like grains of wheat, and a small useless root that tastes bitter.

**2.** This plant[10] brayed while fresh and plastered on mends injuries, and it both cleanses and cicatrizes old wounds; boiled and drunk it dispels through the bowels matter that is bilious and thick; its decoction is a suitable clyster for those with hip ailments, delivering blood and relief. The juice is useful for eye conditions, cleansing with honey those elements that cast a shadow over the pupils of the eyes, and it induces menstruation and abortion when used in a pessary; when drunk it is especially good for ailments around the tendons.

**3.** Juice is extracted from the greenery, which is collected when big with seed, soaked for five days then boiled until it sticks out above the water; then after it has cooled, it is strained through a woolen cloth, the greens are discarded, and the liquid is again boiled until it reaches a honey-like consistency. But some, chopping the herb while green and full of seed, squeeze out the juice, then place it in an unpitched clay vessel in the sun, condense it, stirring it continuously with a stick, scraping the substance that congeals all around and mixing it with the liquid, and cover it up carefully at night; for dew is proven to prevent the thickening of liquid juices.

---

[10] In the First edition, I incorrectly translated αὕτη as "This root."

**4.** Juices extracted from roots or herbs that are dry are prepared by cooking them like gentian, but those extracted from moist barks, roots, or herbs are concentrated in the sun as described above. Juice is similarly extracted from the deadly carrot, mandrake, unripe grape, and the like; but dyer's buckthorn, wormwood, hypocist and plants that are like them are concentrated by boiling as previously described.

### III, 8 χαμαιλέων λευκός, *Atractylis gummifera* L., Pine thistle

**1.** Pine thistle,[11] which some people call *ixia*[12] because in some places a sticky substance is found near its roots, which women use also instead of chewing gum.[13] It has leaves similar to those of the thistle or of the golden thistle but they are rougher, more pointed, and stronger than the leaves of chameleon thistle; it has no stalk, but it sends forth from its center a prickle resembling a sea urchin or an artichoke; it has purplish flowers resembling downy hair, seed very much like the safflower's, a root that is thick when growing in fertile hillocks but rather slender when in mountainous locations, white inside, slightly aromatic in flavor, oppressive in smell, and sweet; it expels the flat intestinal worm when drunk.

**2.** It is taken in the amount of one *oxybaphon* in dry wine with a decoction of oregano; one *holce* is given successfully to drink with wine to those with edemata — for it does reduce their swelling — and its decoction is drunk for difficult micturition. Taken with wine, it is

---

[11] P. G. Gennadios, Φυτολογικόν Λεξικόν p. 466 says the root of pine thistle, was considered to be therapeutic not only in antiquity, as attested here, but also in many localities among common modern day Greek folks. Yet, the plant in all its parts contains atractyline, a highly toxic substance. Frequent ingestion of it or of its decoction can induce poisoning. Gennadios reports that at Marousi, in the northern outskirts of Athens, in 1905, three youngsters were given a decoction of the root as an antidote to measles and all three children died, and that in 1908, at Meleai on Mount Pelion, youngsters died from ingesting pine thistle heads. He adds that in Algeria the shoots of pine thistle and its heads are used as edible greens. See also J. Mabberly, *The Plant Book*, p. 146, who says that it contains atractyloside, the effects of which on mammals are like strychnine.

[12] Akin to ἰξός, any sticky substance.

[13] According to P. G. Gennadios, op. cit. n.11 above, the practice continues among women of modern Greece and the notion of "chewing" is imbedded in the etymology of some of its colloquial Modern Greek names: μαστιχομάραθο, "chewing gum fennel," μαστιχάγκαθα, "chewing gum thorn," ἀγριομαστιχιά, "wild chewing gum."

also an antidote for poisonous bites, and it kills dogs, boars, and mice when mixed with barley groats, water, and oil and strewn about.

**III, 9 [χαμαιλέων] ὁ μέλας, *Cardopatium corymbosum* L., Chameleon thistle**

**1.** Chameleon thistle, which some called *oulophonon* or *ixia* or *cyno<zolon* or *cyno>mazon* or *ocimoeides*: it, too, resembles the golden thistle in its leaves, although they are fewer, more delicate, and shot with red. It sends up a stalk thick as a finger, a span tall, and reddish, on which grow an umbel and prickly flowers, which are thin, hyacinth-like, and variously colored. Its root is thick, dark, compact, at times even worm-eaten, somewhat yellow when split open, and pungent when chewed. It grows in dry plains, in mountainous regions, and in coastal areas.

**2.** Ground and mixed with a little copper sulfate, cedar oil, and lard, the root can get rid of mange; blended with sulfur and asphalt, boiled with vinegar, and smeared on it cleanses lichen-like eruptions on the skin; its decoction when used as a rinse stops toothaches, and the root when plastered on with an equal amount of pepper and wax helps aching teeth. They also foment teeth with it after boiling it down with vinegar and pouring it over them; but if it is applied hot with a brush on an aching tooth it shatters it.

**3.** With sulfur, it also clears away leprosy and dull-white leprosies. It is mixed with septic medications and when plastered on cancerous and malignant sores it removes and cures them.

It is called chameleon on account of the diverse coloring of its leaves: for they are either very pale green or whitish or deep-blue or red, depending on the differences of the regions.

**III, 10 κροκοδείλεον, *Eryngium maritimum* L., Sea holly**

The sea holly: it resembles the thistle chameleon. It grows in woody regions, having a long, light and somewhat thick root, and a pungent smell like that of garden cress.

The root, boiled in water and drunk, can drive out much blood through the nostrils. It is also given to people with spleen disease, benefiting them greatly.

**III, 11 δίψακος, *Dipsacus fullorum* L. and *D. silvestris* L., Teasle**

**1.** Teasel: it, too, belongs to the group of plants that are thorns. It has a tall and thorny stem and leaves that encircle the stem like the lettuce, two on each joint, and they are somewhat long; they, too, are thorny, having, as it were, some prickly bubbles on their mid-rib both inside and out, and hollows near the junction of the leaves that collect water from rains and dew, whence the plant derived its name.[14] At the end of the stem of each side-shoot there is a head like a sea urchin, longish and prickly which when dried appears to be white; taken apart, the head contains worms in the middle of its innermost part.

**2.** Its root, boiled in wine and pounded so as to become thick as cerate, treats anal fissures and fistulas when inserted; this medication must be stored in a copper box. They say that it is a remedy both for warts that spread under the skin and for warts that have a thin neck. The worms contained within the head, wrapped up and worn around the neck or arm are said to cure quartan fevers.

**III, 12 ἄκανθα λευκή, ~ *Cnicus ferox* L. or ~ *C. acarna* L., Fish thistle**

**1.** Fish thistle grows on mountains and in wooded areas; it has leaves that resemble the leaves of pine thistle but they are narrower, whiter, somewhat hairy, and prickly; it has a stem that is over two-cubits long, thick as the thumb or even thicker, whitish, and hollow; at its tip there is a prickly head resembling a sea urchin but smaller and longish; the flowers are purple containing seed like the safflower's, except that it is rounder.

**2.** Its root helps those who spit blood and people who suffer from stomach and abdominal ailments; it provokes micturition and it is plastered on for swellings. Its decoction is beneficial for toothaches when used as a mouthwash and its seed when drunk helps children who have spasms and people bitten by snakes. And they say that it automatically chases away wild beasts when hung upon a person.

---

[14] δίψακος cognate with δίψα, "thirst."

**III, 13 ἄκανθα Ἀραβική, *Notobasis syriaca* Cass. = *Cirsium syriacum* Gaertn., Smaller milk thistle**

Smaller milk thistle: it seems that it is of similar nature as the fish thistle and that it is astringent. Its root is more or less equally suitable for leucorrhea, for spitting of blood, and for the other fluxes.

**III, 14 σκόλυμος, *Scolymus maculatus* L. and *S. hispanicus* L., Golden thistle**

Golden thistle: its leaves fall between the leaves of chameleon and of the so-called fish thistle except that they are darker and thicker; it sends up a long stem teeming with leaves, on which there is a thorny head. The root, from which the value of the plant stems, is below ground, black, and thick.

Boiled in wine and drunk, it helps those whose armpits and the balance of their body are ill smelling. It removes much stinking urine. The herb when newly growing is used as a boiled vegetable just like asparagus.

**III, 15 ποτίρριον, *Astragalus poterium L.*, Goat's thorn**

**1.** Goat's thorn: but some call it *phrynion,* the Ionians *neuras*, and others *acidoton*. It is a large shrub, having long, soft, fibrous, and slender twigs resembling those of the tragacanth, small round leaves, — the entire shrub is shrouded by much wooly down, although it is prickly — small, greenish-yellow flowers, and fruit which, although it tastes savory and pungent, is useless. It grows in sandy and hilly areas.

**2.** The roots are below ground, two- or three-cubits long, strong, and sinewy; they release a sap that is like gum when cut close to the ground.

Brayed and plastered on, they mend severed tendons and wounds; the decoction of this root also is suitable to drink for conditions relating to tendons.

**III, 16 ἀκάνθιον, *Onopordum acanthium* L., *O. illyricum* L., Cotton thistle**

Cotton thistle: it has leaves similar to those of the fish thistle and prickly excrescences on top that are covered by cobweb-like down.

They say that after harvesting this down they make from it a cotton-like thread.
Its root and leaves help for tetanic recurvation when drunk.

### III, 17 ἄκανθος, *Acanthus mollis* L., *A. spinosus* L., Bear's-foot

**1.** Bear's-foot: but some call it *melamphyllon* and others *paideros.* It grows in gardens, both on rocky places and watery spots. It has leaves much wider and longer than lettuce, slit like those of rocket, fat, smooth, and dark, and a stem that is two-cubits long, smooth, and thick as a finger; it is surrounded at intervals toward the top by small leaves and by some things that are like elongated little Persian headdresses; they are hyacinth-like; from them grows its flower, which is white.
**2.** The seed is longish and quince-yellow and the head is like a thyrsus. The roots are below ground, sticky, slimy, reddish, and long. They are a suitable plaster for inflammations and spasms; when drunk, they remove the urine, they check diarrhea, and they are useful to tuberculars as well as for spasms and ruptures.
There is also a wild bear's-foot that is similar to the golden thistle, thorny, and smaller than the cultivated one growing in gardens. The root of this one, too, can accomplish all the results that the one before it accomplishes.

### III, 18 ἀνωνίς, *Ononis antiquarum* L., Rest harrow

Rest harrow, but some call it *ononis*. The sprays are a span long or even longer, shrubby, and highly articulated; they have many axils, round heads, thin and small leaves resembling closely the leaves of rue or of the *lotos*[15] that grows in meadows, somewhat hairy, and they are aromatic. It is steeped in brine before it has put out thorns and it is very pleasant. Its branches have sharp thorns, pointed like pales, and strong. It has a warming, white root whose skin is diuretic, shatters stones, and breaks off scabs all around when taken in a drink. Boiled in sour wine, mixed with water, and used as a mouthwash, it assuages toothaches.

---

[15] λωτός refers to various plants and trees providing fodder or fruit.

**III, 19 λευκάκανθα, *Cnicus tuberosus* L. sp. or *Cirstium tuberosum* All., Tuberous thistle**

Tuberous thistle: but some call it *polygonaton,* others *ischias*, others *phyllon,* and others *ladanon.* It has a root that is similar to that of galingale, very bitter, which assuages toothaches when chewed; a quantity of three *cyathoi* of its decoction drunk with wine helps for chronic pleurisy, for hip ailments, ruptures, and spasms. The juice of its root does also the same when drunk.

**III, 20 τραγάκανθα, *Astragallus gummifer* Labill., *A. microcephalus* Willd., Tragacanth**

**1.** Tragacanth has a flat and woody root, visible even above ground, from which grow low, strong branches spreading themselves over a large area. On them grow many delicate little leaves that conceal among them white, strong, and upright thorns. And there is the tragacanth, which is sap that coagulates when the root is severed; the best is translucent, smooth, light, clean, and somewhat sweet.

**2.** It has the same property to stop pores as gum. It is used in eye preparations, for coughs, hoarseness of the trachea, loss of voice, and sniffles in lozenges with honey that one places under the tongue extracting their juice. A quantity of one *drachma,* soaked in grape syrup and combined with burned and washed stag horn or with a small quantity of split alum, is also drunk for kidney pain and for bladder discomfort.

**III, 21 ἠρύγγη, *Eryngium campestre* L., Eryngo**

**1.** The eryngo: but some call it *caryon* and others *eryngion.* It belongs to the group of plants that are thorns; when newly sprouted, its leaves are used as vegetables prepared in brine; they are broad and they have jagged edges and a spicy flavor; as they grow larger they grow prickles at many stem tips, at the top of which there are globular little heads surrounded, in a circle, like a star, by very sharp, stiff thorns of a greenish-yellow or white color; but some times their color is also found to be dark blue.

**2.** The root is long, wide, black on the surface, white in its interior, and thick as a thumb; it, too, is aromatic and spicy in flavor. It grows in plains and in rough terrains.

It has a warming property, it draws down the urine and the menses when drunk, it puts an end to colic and flatulence, and it is suitable to give with wine to people with liver disease and to those bitten by wild animals or who have ingested poisons. For the majority of conditions, a quantity of one *drachma* is drunk with carrot seed. It is reported to disperse growths when hung around a person and when applied as a plaster.

**III, 22 ἀλόη, *Aloe vera* L., Aloe**

**1.** Aloe: it has a leaf nearly resembling the squill's, greasy, somewhat flat, thick where it curves, and curling backward; on each of their edges the leaves have thorns that protrude slightly and that are truncated. It sends up a stem like the flowering stem of asphodel, a white flower, and fruit resembling that of asphodel. However, the entire plant has an oppressive smell and tastes very bitter. It is single-rooted, having its root like a stake.

**2.** A great deal grows in India from where its extracted juice is exported; but it also grows in Arabia, in Asia, along certain coastal areas, and on islands, as for instance on Andros, being not good for extracting juice but suitable for gluing together wounds when plastered on them. The extracted juice is of two kinds: one kind is somewhat sandy, which seems to be sediment of very pure bitter aloe, and the other is liver-like. Choose it oily and free of stones, gleaming, yellowish, brittle and of the texture of liver, liquefying quickly, and intensely bitter; reject that which is dark and hard to break.

**3.** They adulterate it with gum. That which has been adulterated is detected by taste, bitterness, intensity of scent, and by its irreducibility into fine particles when squeezed between the fingers. Some add also shittah.

It has properties that are astringent, desiccative, soporific, and that serve to close the pores; it loosens the bowel and cleanses the stomach when a quantity of two spoonfuls is drunk with cold or tepid water, it controls blood-spitting, and it clears jaundice when a dose of one *triobolon* is taken with water or when one *drachma* is taken in a drink.

**4.** Swallowed with pine resin or taken with water or with boiled honey, it loosens the bowel, but a quantity of three *drachmai* thoroughly purges the bowel, and when mixed with other cathartics it makes them easier on the stomach. Plastered on dry it mends injuries, it cicatrizes and reduces sores, it treats, in particular, ulcerated privy parts, and it attaches severed foreskins. Mixed with sweet wine, it treats both callous lumps and fissures, it stops bleeding from hemorrhoids, and it cicatrizes membranes growing from the inner corner of the eye.

**5.** With honey it removes both livid spots and black eye, it comforts blepharitis and itching at the corners of the eyes, and when rubbed with vinegar and unguent of roses on the forehead and the temples it allays a headache. With wine it stops also the fall of hair, and in combination with honey or wine it is suitable for inflammations of the tonsils, for the gums, and for all conditions associated with the mouth. It is also parched for eye medications on a clean and very hot shell, being stirred with a spoon until it gets evenly hot. It is washed, removing its gritty element because it is useless and keeping its greasiest and smoothest part.

### III, 23 ἀψίνθιον, *Artemisia absinthium* L., Wormwood

**1.** Wormwood: this herb is familiar. The best grows in the Pontic region and in Cappadocia, on the mountain called Taurus.

It has astringent and warming properties and it is capable of purging the bilious elements that pass through the stomach and bowel. It is diuretic, it prevents nausea if drunk before nausea begins, it is suitable for flatulence and for abdominal and stomach pains when drunk with hartwort or Celtic nard, and its infusion or decoction, taken daily in the amount of three *cyathoi*, treats lack of appetite and jaundice.

**2.** It draws down the menses both when drunk and when used topically with honey, it is a suitable drink with vinegar for those choking from poisonous mushrooms, but for pine thistle,[16] hemlock, bites of the shrew mouse, and of the great weever, it is taken with wine; it is used with honey and soda as an unguent for sore throats and with water for pustules that are most painful at night, but for black eye and for dim-sightedness it is used with honey and similarly for purulent ears. The vapor of its decoction is used for earaches, and boiled down with grape syrup it is a poultice for very painful eyes.

[16] See Dsc. Bk. III, 8 and n. 11.

**3.** It is plastered on chronically unwell hypochondria, liver, and stomach, pounded together with Cyprian cerate, but for the stomach it is plastered on with unguent of roses. It is also suitable for people with spleen disease and for those with edemata, being mixed with figs, soda, and meal of darnel.[17]

They also make a wine from it, the so-called *absinthitis,* especially around the Propontis and Thrace, which they use for the conditions mentioned above if the patient does not run a fever. During the summer they drink it as an aperitif believing that it brings about good health.

**4.** It also seems to keep clothing from being eaten by moths when sprinkled into chests of drawers and it keeps mosquitoes away from the body when rubbed with oil. Ink sprinkled with its infusion guards writings from being eaten by mice. It seems that the actions of its juice extract are the same, but we disapprove of using it in drinks because it is bad for the stomach and gives headaches. The juice is adulterated by combining it with the watery substance that runs out when olives are pressed, boiled down.

**5.** Some call even the *seriphon*[18] *absinthion thalassion*; this plant grows abundantly on mount Taurus in Cappadocia and at Taphosiris of Egypt. The priests of Isis use it instead of olive branches. It is a thin-stemmed herb resembling a small wormwood, abounding in seed, somewhat bitter, bad for the stomach, oppressive in scent, and binding with a degree of warmth. Boiled down either by itself or with rice and consumed with honey, it destroys intestinal and round worms, gently purging the bowels.

**6.** It can also accomplish the same results when boiled with lentil gruel and it fattens the sheep that graze on it, especially in Capppadocia.

There is also a third kind of wormwood which grows abundantly in Galatia along the Alps and which they call in the local dialect

---

[17] Modern pharmacopoeias indicate that the dry flowering tops of wormwood are used to make a tea for some of the purposes for which Dioscurides also uses them, viz., to stimulate the appetite, for gastrointestinal complaints, as carminative, to remove bile. See Norman Grainger Bisset, *Herbal Drugs and Phytopharmaceuticals*, p. 46.

[18] "Worm seed."

*Santonicon,* naming it after the land of the Santones[19] that produces it. It resembles wormwood, although it is certainly not as full of seed, it is somewhat bitter, and it can do the same things as *seriphon*.

### III, 24 ἀβρότονον, ~ *Artemisia abrotonum* L., Wormwood

**1.** Wormwood but some call it *Heracleion* and others *glycys angon.* The female of this plant[20] is a tree-like shrub and whitish; its branches teem with leaves that have narrow slits, just like the leaves of wormseed; on top, it has a corymbose flower that is golden, grows in the summer, and is somewhat oppressively aromatic and bitter in taste; it seems that the Sicilian is of this kind. But the other, which is called male, is like vine shoots and its seed is thin like that of wormwood.

**2.** It grows abundantly in Cappadocia, in Asiatic Galatia, and in Syrian Hierapolis.

The seed of these plants, boiled in water or ground raw and drunk, helps for orthopnea, ruptures, spasms, hip ailments, difficult micturition, and for delayed menstruation.

**3.** Drunk with wine, it is also an antidote for deadly poisons and with olive oil an ointment for shiverers. When used as litter or for fumigation, it chases away serpents; it also benefits those whom they have bitten when drunk with wine, and it is especially beneficial for venomous spiders[21] and scorpions. Applied as a plaster with boiled quince or bread, it helps for inflammations of the eyes, and with bruised meal it disperses growths when boiled ground up. It is also mixed into the preparation of oil of iris.

### III, 25 ὕσσωπος, *Satureia graeca* L. = *Micromeria graeca* Benth., Hyssop

**1.** Hyssop: it is a well-known herb, which comes in two kinds; for one grows on mountains and the other in gardens; the best grows in Cilicia.

---

[19] The Santones are people of central western Gaul.

[20] "Lavender cotton."

[21] Especially *Lathrodectus* or *malmignatte*, a highly poisonous, red-spotted spider of southern Europe.

It has a warming property. Boiled with figs, water, honey, and rue, and drunk, it helps inflammations of the lungs, asthmatics, a chronic cough, catarrh, and orthopnea. It also kills intestinal worms and when used as a lozenge with honey it accomplishes the same. Its decoction, drunk with a mixture of vinegar and honey, expels thick masses down the abdomen.

**2.** It is also eaten with brayed green figs for purging the bowel, but it is a more powerful cathartic when mixed with garden cress or with iris or with hedge mustard; it achieves even fresh and healthy looks. It is used as a plaster with fig and soda for the spleen and for edemata and with wine for inflammations; it also disperses black eye when plastered on with hot water. It is an excellent gargle for sore throat with a decoction of figs and it assuages toothaches when cooked with vinegar and employed as a mouthwash. Its vapor stops also inflations around the ears.

### III, 26 στοιχάς, *Lavendula stoechas* L., French lavender

French lavender: it grows on the islands across Gaul, opposite Marseilles, which are called *Stoichades*[22] and after which it was named. It is an herb with delicate seed, having foliage like that of thyme but more elongated, pungent in taste, and somewhat bitter.

Its decoction is effective for chest conditions, just like hyssop; it is also mixed profitably with antidotes.

### III, 27 ὀρίγανος Ἡρακλειωτική, *Origanum heracleoticum vulgare* Rchb. and *O. vulgare* L., Oregano

**1.** Oregano: but some call it *conile.* The leaf is similar to that of hyssop and the flower head is not wheel-like, but as if divided, and at the end of its twigs the seed is not thickly packed.

It does warm, whence its decoction drunk with wine is suitable for people bitten by wild animals, with grape syrup and ash, for hemlock or opium, with vinegar mixed with honey, for those who have drunk chalk or poison that kills on the same day, and for spasms, ruptures, edemata, it is eaten with a fig. Having been dried, an amount of one

---

[22] These islands, east of Marseilles, are now called Iles d'Hyeres. *Stoichas*, French lavender is known in England as cassidony.

*oxybaphon* drunk with hydromel purges the bowel of black elements and sets menstruation in motion; it also assuages coughs when taken as a lozenge with honey.
**2.** Its decoction, used in the bath water, helps for itching, mange, and jaundice. Juice extracted from it when fresh, treats inflamed tonsils, uvulas, and thrush, and it draws blood through the nostrils when instilled with oil of iris. Combined with milk, it also assuages earaches, and there is an emetic made with it, onions, and sumac—the type of sumac that is used in prepared foods—all of these ingredients being placed in a Cyprian copper vessel and set out in the sun for forty days during the burning heat of the Dog Star. Scattered on the ground, this herb chases away reptiles.

**III, 28 ὀνῖτις, *Origanum onitis* L., Oregano *onitis*[23]**

As for the oregano called *onitis*, it has whiter leaves, it is more like hyssop, and it has its seed like clusters set in rows.
It has the same properties as oregano, but it was proven to be not as effective.

**III, 29 ἀγριορίγανος, ~ *Origanum viride* Boiss., Marjoram**

Marjoram. Some people call it *panaces* or *Heracleia* or *conile*. Among these people is also Nicander of Colophon.[24] Its leaves are like those of oregano, the shoots are a span tall and slender, and on top of them rest flower heads like the dill's. The flowers are white and the root is slender and useless.
When drunk with wine, the leaves and flowers are particularly helpful to those bitten by wild animals.

**III, 30 τραγορίγανος, ~ *Thymus graveolens* Sibth. sp., ~ *Th. tragoriganum* L. sp., ~ *Origanum heracleoticum* Richb. sp., Goat's marjoram**

**1.** Goat's marjoram: it is a small shrub the leaves and small stems of which resemble wild tufted thyme. Yet, depending on where it grows,

[23] This is pot marjoram.
[24] *Thrice*, 626 sq.

one plant is rather sturdy, broad-leaved,[25] and quite sticky, and another thin-stemmed and narrow-leaved; some people call the last one *prasion*.[26] The best are the Cilician and those that grow in Cos, Chios, Smyrna, and Crete.

**2.** All of them warm, are diuretic, and ease the bowel when their decoction is drunk, for they do carry downwards the bilious elements. With vinegar they are suitable for people who suffer from spleen disease and with wine for those who drank pine thistle.[27] They also draw down the menses and they are offered in lozenge form with honey for coughs and inflammations of the lungs. Their potion is mild and it is for this reason that it is given to those suffering from nausea, whose stomach is sensitive, who suffer from heartburn, and who are dogged by discomfort, by seasickness, and by a burning sensation in the hypochondria. Applied as a plaster with barley groats, it also disperses growths.

### III, 31 γλήχων, *Mentha pulegium* L., Pennyroyal

**1.** Pennyroyal: it is a familiar herb, warming, thinning, and promoting digestion. When drunk it draws the menses, afterbirth, and embryos/fetuses. It brings up from the lung phlegm when drunk with salt and honey and helps people with spasms, and with sour wine mixed with water it relieves nausea and gnawing pains of the stomach. With wine it drives down the bowel dark matter and helps those bitten by wild animals, and when applied to the nostrils with vinegar it revives those who fainted.

**2.** Ground up dry and burned, it also strengths the gums; plastered on with barley groats, it soothes all inflammations; it is suitable to use all by itself on the gouty until the skin surface becomes irritated, and when used with a cerate it checks facial eruptions; it also helps patients with spleen disease when plastered on with salt. Its decoction used as a wash stops itching and is suitable in a sitz bath for uterine

---

[25] Τραγορίγανος πλατύφυλλος, *Origanum heracleoticum*, "oregano."

[26] Τραγορίγανος λεπτόφυλλος or λεπτόκαρφος," rock savory."

[27] See Dsc. III, 8 and n.11.

inflations, indurations, and twistings. Some people call it *blechon*[28] because sheep that taste it when in bloom bleat continuously.

**III, 32 δίκταμον, *Origanum dictamnus* L., Dittany of Crete**

**1.** Dittany of Crete, which some people call *glechon agria* and others *baition.* It is a Cretan herb, very acrid, similar to pennyroyal, but it has larger and woolly leaves and some sort of woolly ongrowth. It bears neither flower nor fruit.

It accomplishes everything that cultivated pennyroyal accomplishes but much more effectively: for it expels deceased embryos/fetuses not only when drunk but also when used topically and when burned as to produce smoke from below. They say, moreover, that goats in Crete that have been shot with arrows shed the arrows if they should graze on this herb.

**2.** The plant called false dittany grows in many places and while it resembles the above, it is smaller and less acrid. It accomplishes the same results as dittany of Crete but not as efficaciously.

There is another kind of dittany that is also brought from Crete; it has leaves like those of bergamot mint but it has larger stems, on which grows a flower like that of marjoram, dark and soft; the smell of its leaves is between that of bergamot mint and of salvia and very sweet.

It is as good for all the conditions as the above and it is less acrid. It is also mixed with salves for poisonous bites.

**III, 33 ἐλελίσφακον, *Salvia* L. sp., Sage**

**1.** Sage: but some call it *elaphoboscon* and others *sphagnon.* It is a somewhat tall shrub, much branched, having twigs that are quadrangular and whitish, leaves that resemble those of the quince tree, but more elongated, smaller, and imperceptibly rough like the pile of cloth, dense, whitish, highly aromatic, and foul tasting. At the tips of the stems it bears seed like that of uncultivated sage. It grows in rough terrains.

**2.** The decoction of its leaves and branches when drunk has properties that set the urine and menstruation in motion, draw down embryos/fetuses, and help for strokes of the stingray. It also darkens

[28] From βληχάομαι, "bleat."

the hair, it is used for wounds, it staunches the blood, and it cleanses malignant sores. Used as a wash with wine, the decoction of its leaves and branches stops itching around the genitalia.

**III, 34 ὑδύοσμον, *Mentha* L. sp., Green mint**

**1.** Green mint, but some call it *minthe*: it is a well-known little herb having warming, astringent, and drying properties; it is for this reason that its juice, when drunk with vinegar, staunches blood, destroys the round intestinal worm, rouses sexual desire, and when two or three little sprays are drunk with the juice of sour pomegranate, they stop hiccups, vomiting, and cholera. Applied as a plaster with barley groats, it dissipates abscesses, placed on the forehead, it assuages headaches, and it abates distension and swelling of the breasts.

**2.** With salt it is a plaster for people bitten by dogs, and its juice with hydromel is suitable for earaches. Used by women as a pessary before sexual intercourse, it causes barrenness, and if rubbed on a rough tongue it smoothes it; it keeps milk from curdling when little sprays are stirred about in it, and it is through and through wholesome and spicy.

There is also a wild green mint which has thicker leaves, and, all told, it is larger than bergamot mint, rather foul smelling, and less useful for health purposes.

**III, 35 καλαμίνθη, *Calamintha* Lmk. sp., Catmint**

**1.** Catmint: there is a kind that prefers mountains; it has leaves like those of basil and somewhat white, little sprays and twigs that are angular, and purple flowers. And there is another kind that resembles the pennyroyal but bigger, whence some call it wild *glechon*,[29] because it resembles it somewhat even in scent; the Romans call this plant *nepeta*. The third kind resembles wild mint, it has longer leaves, bigger stems and branches than the ones previously mentioned, and it is less effective.

**2.** The leaves of all taste very hot and pungent; the root is useless. It grows in fertile plains as well as in rough terrains and wetlands.

---

[29] One of the names for pennyroyal.

When drunk and when applied as a plaster, it helps people bitten by serpents and its decoction removes the urine when drunk. It helps also for ruptures, spasms, orthopnea, colic, cholera, and chills, and when drunk before hand with wine it is good against deadly poisons and clears up jaundice. Cooked as well as ground up raw, when drunk with salt and honey it kills both worms and ascarids, and it helps people with elephantiasis if they should eat it and wash it down with whey.

**3.** The leaves, ground up and used in a pessary, destroy embryos/fetuses and draw the menses, and, when used for fumigation or when scattered on the ground, they chase away reptiles. Boiled in wine and plastered on, catmint bleaches black scars and removes black eye, and it is applied on people with hip ailments to alter the state of their pores[30] by burning the skin's surface. Its juice also kills worms in the ears[31] when instilled.

**III, 36 θύμος, *Satureia thymbra* L. sp., Cretan thyme**

**1.** Cretan thyme: everybody knows it. It is a small plant belonging to the class of underbrush; it is covered with many narrow leaflets and on top it has very many little heads teeming with purple flowers. It grows mostly on rocky places and in poor soils.

When drunk with salt and vinegar, it is able to drive through the bowel matter full of phlegm.

**2.** Its decoction combined with honey helps those suffering from orthopnea and asthma, expels intestinal worms, and drives out the menses, afterbirth, and embryos/fetuses. It is also diuretic, and, when mixed with honey and sucked, congested matter from the chest is more easily coughed up. Plastered on with vinegar, it disperses fresh swellings, it dissolves blood clots, it removes warty excrescences and warts that have thin necks, it is a suitable plaster with wine and barley groats for people with hip ailments, and when eaten with food it benefits the dim-sighted. It is serviceable also to use as seasoning in the pursuit of good health.

---

[30] The word used is μετασύγκρισις, a term of the Methodic school of medicine.

[31] On earwigs see Dsc. Bk, II, n. 38.

### III, 37 θύμβρα, *Satureia thymbra* L. sp., Savory

Savory: it, too, is well known. It grows in poor soils and rough terrains, it resembles Cretan thyme, but it is smaller and softer, and it bears a greenish spike full of flowers.

It is capable of the same actions as Cretan thyme when similarly used and it is serviceable in the pursuit of good health. There is also a cultivated savory inferior in every respect to the wild but more useful as food, because it is not overly acrid.

### III, 38 ἕρπυλος, *Thymus Sibthorpii*, Tufted thyme

**1.** Tufted thyme: there is a kind that is cultivated, it resembles marjoram in smell, and it is used for making garlands. It was named from its creeping habit[32] and whatever part of it touches the ground strikes root. It has leaves and little stems like those of oregano except they are whiter; it grows faster if it hangs down from dry walls. And there is kind which is wild and which is called also *zygis*; it does not creep but it is erect, sending up delicate little stems, dry like sticks, full of leaves resembling those of rue; they are, however, somewhat narrow, longer, and tougher; the flowers taste acrid, the scent is sweet, and the root is useless.

**2.** It grows on rocks, it is more effective and warms more than the cultivated, and it is more appropriate for medical use: for when drunk it both draws down the menses and it sets micturition going; it helps for colic, spasms, ruptures, inflammations of the liver, and for reptiles when drunk and when plastered on, and when boiled with vinegar and soaked in unguent of roses it assuages a headache. It is especially well suited for lethargic fever and phrenitis. A dose of four *drachmai* drunk with vinegar stops also the vomiting of blood.

### III, 39 σάμψουχον, *Majorana hortensis* Moench, Marjoram

**1.** Marjoram: the best are the Cyzician and the Cyprian; the Egyptian ranks second to them. The people in Sicily and Cyzicos call it *amaracon.* It is an herb with multiple branches, creeping on the ground, with dense and round leaves resembling the leaves of the thin-

---

[32] ἕρπυλος akin to ἕρπειν, "to creep."

leaved catmint. It is highly aromatic, it warms, and it is even braided into garlands.

Its decoction when drunk is good for people with incipient edemata, for difficult micturition, and for the colicky.

**2.** The dry leaves applied as a plaster with honey remove black eye and draw down the menses when used as a pessary; they are plastered on with salt and vinegar for the stroke of the scorpion, for sprains they are applied after being compounded with a cerate, they are similarly compounded with a cerate for swellings, and they are plastered on with very fine meal of barley groats for inflammations of the eyes. They are mixed both with analgesics and with emollients that are used for warming.

**III, 40 μελίλωτος, *Melilotus* Adans., sp., King's clover**

**1.** King's clover: the best grows in Attica, Cyzicus, and Chalcedon;[33] it is saffron-colored and fragrant. It also grows in Campania, around Nola, smelling like fenugreek and being weak in scent.

It has properties that are astringent and that can soften all inflammations, especially those around the eyes, uterus, anus, and testicles when boiled with grape syrup and plastered on; sometimes it is also mixed with a baked egg yolk or flour of fenugreek or linseed or very fine meal or capsules of poppies or chicory.

**2.** Soaked in water, it treats all by itself newly developed impetigo contagiosa and when smeared on with Chian earth and wine or with oak galls it treats scurf; boiled with wine or combined raw with one of the above ingredients, it stops stomach pains; also earaches when its juice is combined raw with grape syrup and instilled into the ears. The plant also assuages headaches when used in compresses with vinegar and unguent of roses.

**III, 41 σισύμβριον, *Mentha silvestris* L., *M. viridis* L., Bergamot mint**

Bergamot mint: but some call it *herpylos agrios megas*. It grows on dry soils, it resembles green mint, although it has broader leaves and it smells sweeter. It is used for making garlands.

---

[33] Chalcedon for Calcedon on the eastern shore of the Propontis opposite Byzantium.

It has a warming property; the seed is suitable for strangury and for diseases of the stone when drunk with wine, and it stops both colic and hiccups. The leaves are plastered on the temples and forehead for headaches; they are also plastered for wasp and bee stings. The seed even stays vomiting when drunk.

**III, 42 μᾶρον ἢ ὑσόβρυον,[34] *Amaracus sipyleus* Rafin., *Maron* or *Hysobryon***

*Maron* or *hysobryon* is a well-known, crackly herb; its flower resembles that of oregano, but its leaves are much whiter and its flower is more aromatic.

It has the same properties as bergamot mint, binding mildly and gently warming; it is for this reason that it stems spreading ulcers when used as a plaster and that it is incorporated into the salves that warm. It grows in abundance in Magnesia and Tralles.

**III, 43 ἄκινος ἢ ἄκονος, ~ *Ocinum pilosum* Willd. or ~ *Thymus acinos* L., Wild basil**

Wild basil: it is a thin-stemmed herb used for making garlands, closely resembling basil, but it is bushier and fragrant. Some even grow it in their gardens.

When drunk it stems diarrhea and the menses, and when plaster on it treats swollen glands and erysipelas.

**III, 44 βάκχαρις, ~ *Helichrysum sanguineum* Boiss. = *Gnaphalium sanguineum* L., Sowbread**

**1.** Sowbread: it is an aromatic herb used for garlands. Its leaves are rough, in size between those of the violet and of the mullein. The stem is angular, one-cubit tall, somewhat rough, and it has offshoots. The flowers are inclining to purple, off-white, and fragrant. The roots are like those of black hellebore, resembling in scent cinnamon. It likes rough and dry terrains.

Boiled in water, its root helps for spasms, bruises, ruptures, dyspnea, chronic coughs, and difficult micturition; it also draws down the

[34] LSJ, "a kind of sage."

menses and it is given with good results to people bitten by wild animals.

**2.** A single of its tender roots, applied as a pessary, draws embryos/fetuses; its decoction is good for sitz baths for women who have just given birth and it is used in scented powders to sprinkle over the body since it is quite aromatic. The leaves, being astringent, are beneficial for headaches, inflammations of the eyes, incipient lachrymal fistulas, breasts that are inflamed as a result of childbirth, and erysipelas when plastered on. Their scent is even soporific.

### III, 45 πήγανον, *Ruta graveolens* L., Rue

**1.** Rue that grows on mountains and that is wild is harsher than the cultivated and it is unfit to eat, and of the cultivated rue the one that grows near fig trees is more edible.

Both, however, warm, burn, ulcerate, are diuretic and emmenagogic; when eaten as well as when drunk, they end diarrhea and they are an antidote to deadly poisons when a quantity of one *oxybaphon* of the seed is drunk with wine. The leaves, if eaten in advance all by themselves or with walnuts and dry figs, render deadly poisons ineffectual; similarly taken, they are suitable for reptile poisons and the seed quells the organ of generation when eaten and when drank.

**2.** Boiled with dry dill and drunk, it stops colic; it is also good for pains on the side and chest, dyspnea, coughs, inflammation of the lungs, pains of the hip joints, of joints, and for periodic shiverings when drunk as indicated above; boiled with olive oil and infused, it is good for inflations of the colon, of the uterus, of the intestinum rectum, and when applied ground up with honey from the genitalia to the anus it relieves uterine suffocation.

**3.** Boiled with olive oil and drunk, it expels intestinal worms; it is also plastered on with honey for pains of the joints and with fig for internal edemata; it also helps these conditions when drunk, having first been boiled in wine until the wine is reduced by half. Eaten either raw or preserved, it sharpens the vision, it assuages severe eye pains when applied as a plaster with barley groats, in combination with unguent of roses and vinegar it helps for headaches, and when ground and inserted it stops nosebleeds. Plastered on with leaves of sweet bay, it is good for inflammations of the testicles and with cerate of myrtle for their pustules.

**4.** Rubbed on with soda and pepper, it treats dull-white leprosy; plastered on with the same ingredients, it lifts warty excrescences and warts that spread under the skin, and when applied with honey and alum it is good for lichen-like eruptions of the skin. Its juice, heated in the shell of a pomegranate and instilled, is good for earaches; smeared on with fennel juice and honey, it helps for dim-sightedness; coated on with vinegar, white lead, and unguent of roses, it treats erysipelas, shingles, and scurf, and when chewed it stops the smell and pungent taste of garlic and onion.

**5.** But eating much wild rue is fatal; gathered for pickling when in bloom, it does redden and puff up the skin with itching and with a violent rash. People must thus harvest it after they have anointed their face and hands. They say that its juice keeps cats at bay when sprinkled on fowl and that the rue that grows in Macedonia by the river Haliacmon is fatal when eaten; this place is mountainous and full of vipers. Its seed is good for internal ailments when drunk and it is mixed beneficially with antidotes.

### III, 46 πήγανον ἄγριον, *Peganum harmala* L., Wild rue

**1.** Wild rue: some people call wild rue the plant that both in Cappadocia and in Asiatic Galatia is called *moly*. It is a shrub that sends up many shoots from one root, having much longer and more tender leaves than the other rue, an oppressive scent, a white flower, and on top little heads slightly larger than the heads of cultivated rue, composed of about three sections wherein lie yellowish, triangular seed, rather bitter in taste, of which there is also use.

**2.** The seed ripens in the fall. Triturated with honey, wine, bile of hens, saffron, and fennel juice, it is suitable for dim-sightedness. Some call this plant *harmala*, the Syrians *bessasa*, and the Cappadocians *moly* because to some extent it preserves a likeness to *moly*, having a black root and white flower. It grows on hillocks and fertile places.

### III, 47 μῶλυ, *Alium nigrum* L., Garlic

Garlic: it has leaves similar to the leaves of dog's-tooth grass, but wider and bending toward the ground, blossoms closely resembling

gillyflowers, milk-colored, but smaller as compared with those of gillyflower, and a slender stem, four-cubits tall. At the top there is something that is like garlic. The root is small and bulb-shaped.
The root, triturated and inserted as a pessary with darnel flour, is very good for opening the uterus.

### III, 48 πάνακες Ἡράκλειον, *Opoponax hispidus* Grisb., Hercules' woundwort

**1.** Hercules' woundwort, from which opopanax is collected, grows so well in Boeotia and in Psophis of Arcadia that it is cultivated on purpose in gardens for the revenue derived from its gum. It has rough leaves, lying on the ground, light green, nearly resembling the leaves of the fig tree and split at the periphery into five sections; it has a stalk like that of giant fennel, very tall, having delicate white down and tiny leaves all around it; and it has an umbel at the top, like that of dill, a quince-yellow flower, seed that is aromatic and burns, and many roots from one beginning, which are white and oppressive in scent and which have a thick skin that is somewhat bitter in taste. It grows also in Cyrene of Libya and in Macedonia.
**2.** Juice is extracted from the root, which is cut when the stalks are newly sprouting; it releases a white juice, which is saffron-yellow on the surface when it has dried. The run-off is received on leaves previously placed on hollowed ground below and collected after they have dried. They also extract juice from the stalk, around wheat-harvest time, and collect the run-off in a similar manner.
**3.** The best roots are white and dry, smooth and not worm-eaten, burning in taste and aromatic. The fruit is useful if it comes from the middle stalk, because that from the suckers is less nutritious. The juice is superior if it is rather bitter in taste, white in its interior, saffron-colored on the outside, smooth, greasy, friable, easily dissolved, and heavy in scent. But the black is inferior, so is that which is soft. For they do adulterate it with gum ammoniac and wax. They test it with water, rubbing it with their fingers; for the unadulterated dissolves and becomes milky.
**4.** It has warming, thinning, and softening properties; it is for this reason that it is good for shiverings, for fits of intermittent fever, spasms, ruptures, pains on the side, coughs, colic, strangury, and

itching of the bladder when offered to drink with hydromel or with wine; and it draws down the menses, it destroys embryos/fetuses, and it dissipates uterine inflations and indurations when laid on with honey. It is also an ointment for hip ailments, it is mixed both with analgesics and with medications for headaches, it breaks all around carbuncles, and it is good to plaster with cultivated raisins on the gouty.
**5.** Placed into cavities of teeth, it relieves toothaches, it is rubbed on the eyes for sharp-sightedness, and it is an outstanding salve for people bitten by a rabid dog when mixed with pitch. The root, too, grated and applied as a pessary to the uterus draws embryos/fetuses, it is good for old sores, and when plastered on ground up or smeared on with honey, it fleshes bones that were stripped bare. Its fruit, taken with wormwood *Artemisia absinthium,* draws down the menses, with birthwort, it is good for venomous animals, and it is drunk with wine for uterine suffocation.

### III, 49 πάνακες Ἀσκληπί‹ει›ον, ~ *Ferula nodosa* L. or ~ *Echinophora tenuifolia* L., Aesculapius' allheal

Aesculapius' allheal: it sends from the ground up a slender stalk, one-cubit tall, marked at intervals by knots, and surrounded by leaves similar to those of fennel; but they are larger, denser, and aromatic. At the top it has an umbel on which there are flowers that are golden, pungent, sharp, and aromatic. The root is small and slender.
Its flower and seed ground and laid on with honey have a property that is well-suited for sores, growths, and cankers, and, when drunk with wine or rubbed on with olive oil, for bites of reptiles. Some call even the marjoram allheal and others *conile*, about which I spoke in the section on marjoram (III, 29.)

### III, 50 πάνακες Χειρώνιον, *Panaces olympicum* Chiron's allheal

Chiron's allheal: it grows mostly on mount Pelion. It has leaves like those of marjoram, golden flowers, and a slender and shallow root that tastes pungent.
The root is effective for venoms of reptiles when drunk, as is also its foliage when plastered on.

**III, 51 λιγύστικον, *Levisticum officinale* Koch, Lovage**

**1.** Lovage: it grows abundantly in Liguria, from where it was named, on the so-called Apennines, a mountain range adjacent to the Alps. The natives call it, not unreasonably, *panaces* since its root is similar to that of the Hercules'woundwort and its efficacy has been proven to be the same. It grows on very high, rather rough, and thickly shaded mountains, especially along rushing streams.

**2.** It bears a slender little stalk similar to that of dill, knotty, surrounded by leaves resembling the leaves of king's clover, but they are more tender and aromatic, and the ones toward the top of the stalk are thinner and more incised; on top there is an umbel whereon is also the seed, black, firm, longish, somewhat like that of fennel, and tasting pungent and aromatic; the root is white, similar to the root of Hercules' woundwort and aromatic.

**3.** The seed and root have warming and digestive properties that are well suited for internal pains, for swellings, for gas, especially in the area of the stomach, and for strokes of wild animals. They set micturition and the menses going when drunk, and the root does the same when applied. The seed is also quite tasty so that the locals use it instead of pepper, mixing it in their side dishes. It is adulterated with some kind of seed that resembles it. You can discern it from its taste, for it is bitter. Some people, moreover, adulterate it by mixing it with seed of fennel or of hartwood.

**III, 52 σταφυλῖνος ἄγριος, *Daucus guttatus*, Wild carrot**

**1.** Wild carrot: but some call it *ceras*. It has leaves like those of the carrot but wider and somewhat bitter, an upright stem that is rough and that has an umbel like that of dill on which there are white flowers, and in the middle there is something small and purplish, as if it were nap on woolen cloth; the root is as thick as a finger, a span long, aromatic, and edible when boiled.

**2.** When drunk or even when applied, its seed sets the menses going, it is suitable for those that pass water painfully and with difficulty, for those with edemata, for pleurisy in potions, and for bites and strokes of wild animals. They say that reptiles do not harm people who have taken it in advance; it also aids conception. As for the root, it, too, is diuretic, aphrodisiac, and expels embryos/fetuses when used as a

pessary. The leaves ground and applied with honey clear cancerous sores completely.
The cultivated carrot, which is more edible, is suitable for the same purposes but it acts more weakly.

**III, 53 σέσελι, *Seseli tortuosum* L., Massilian hartwort**

**1.** The Massilian hartwort has leaves like those of fennel but they are thicker, and its stalk sprouts better; it has an umbel similar to that of dill, on which lies seed that is longish, angular, pungent, and pleasant to eat; the root is long and aromatic.
The fruit and root have warming properties. When drunk, they treat strangury and orthopnea, they help for uterine suffocation and epileptics, they draw the menstrual period and embryos/fetuses, they are good for all internal ailments, they cure old coughs, and when the fruit is drunk with wine it aids digestion, it counteracts colic, and it is useful for high fevers; it is also drunk with pepper and wine for chills incurred on the road. It is given as a drink to she-goats and to the other animals to ease their deliveries.
**2.** The so-called Ethiopian hartwort (hare's ear) has leaves like those of ivy but they are smaller and oblong, tending toward the honeysuckle's; it is a large shrub with vine-twigs about two-cubits long from which grow branches a span's length; the flower heads are like those of dill, the seed is black, dense like that of wheat but more pungent and more aromatic than the seed of the Massilian hartwort, and it is very sweet. It can do the same things.
**3.** As for the hartwort that grows on Peloponnesos (golden cow-parsnip), it has leaves nearly resembling those of hemlock but rougher and fatter, a stalk that is longer than the stalk of the Massilian hartwort, resembling the stock of giant fennel, and at the top it has a wide umbel; on this one the seed is broader, fleshier, and more aromatic. It has the same properties. It grows in rough, moist, and hilly terrains; it also grows on Ida.

**III, 54 τόρδιλον, *Tordylium officinale* L., Cretan hartwort**
Some call this one, too, *seseli* (see III, 53, above.) It grows on Amanos[35] in Cilicia. It is a shrubby little herb. It has a small, round, double seed, resembling little shields, which is somewhat pungent and aromatic and which is drunk for difficult micturition and to induce menstruation. But the juice of its stem and seed extracted while still green, when drunk in the amount of one *triobolon* with grape syrup for 10 days cures patients with kidney disease. The root, too, is effective in bringing up substances from the chest when licked like a lozenge with honey.

**III, 55 σίνων, *Sison amomum* L., Stone parsley**
Stone parsley is a seedlet growing in Syria, resembling celery, longish, black, and warming; it is drunk for the spleen, for difficult micturition, and to suppress the menses. The locals use it as condiment with boiled bottle gourd, taking it with vinegar.

**III, 56 ἄνησσον, *Pimpinella anisum* L., Anise**
Anise: in general, it has properties that warm, sweeten the breath, allay pain, disperse substances, promote micturition, further perspiration, relax, and quench thirst when drunk. It is suitable both for animal venoms and for inflations. It stems diarrhea and leucorrhea, it draws forth the milk, and it is aphrodisiac. Burned below the nostrils as to produce thick smoke, it stops headaches; it also treats discharges from the ears ground up and instilled with unguent of roses. The best of it is that which is new, full, not bran-like, and vigorous in scent. The Cretan ranks first, the Egyptian second.

**III, 57 καρώ, *Carum carvi L.*, Caraway**
Caraway: it is a well-known seedlet, diuretic, tasty, warming, wholesome, and it promotes digestion; it is combined beneficially with antidotes and fast acting medicines and it is comparable to anise seed. Boiled, the root is edible just like the carrot.

---

[35] A mountain between Cilicia and Syria.

**III, 58 ἄνηθον, *Anethum graveolens* L., Dill**

Dill; the decoction of the dry foliage and seed of dill when drunk draws down the milk, stops colic and inflations, ends diarrhea and mild vomiting, sets micturition in motion, assuages hiccups, dulls the sight, and when drunk continuously quells the organ of generation.[36] Its decoction is also useful for sitz baths of women with uterine ailments. The seed removes callous lumps when burned then plastered on.

**III, 59 κύμινον ἥμερον, *Cuminum cyminum,* L., Cultivated cumin**

**1.** Cultivated cumin: it is wholesome, especially the Ethiopian, which Hippocrates (V 490 L) named "royal"; the Egyptian ranks second, then the rest. It grows in Galatia, in Spain, in Cilicia, and in very many other places.

It has warming, drying, and astringent properties that are good for colic and inflations when it is used boiled with olive oil as a clyster and as a plaster with bruised meal of raw corn.

**2.** It is also given to people who suffer from orthopnea with sour wine and water, but to those bitten by wild animals it is given with wine; plastered on with raisins and with flour made of bruised beans or with cerate, it is good for testicular inflammations; ground fine and applied with vinegar, it keeps in check the female flux and nosebleeds; it also changes skin to a paler color when drunk and when smeared on.

**III, 60 κύμινον ἄγριον, *Lagoecia cuminoides* L., Wild cumin**

**1.** Wild cumin: it grows in very large quantities and quite vigorously in Carthage of Spain. It has a delicate little stalk that is a span tall and four or five delicate little leaves, as if slit by a saw, the way the leaves of *gingidion* are slit. At the top it has five or six round soft heads in which is the fruit, chaffy and more pungent in taste than the fruit of cultivated cumin; it grows on hillocks.

**2.** The seed is drunk with water for colic and flatulence, with vinegar it stops hiccups, and for venoms and excessive accumulation of stomach fluids it is drunk with wine. Chewed and plastered on with

---

[36] See Dsc. Bk. I, n. 130.

honey and raisins, it removes black eye and it treats testicular inflammations when plastered on with the same.

**III, 61 ἕτερον γένος ἀγρίου κυμίνου, *Nigella arvensis* L., Another kind of wild cumin**

There is also another kind of wild cumin that resembles the cultivated. It sends out from each flower little horns that float in the air and that contain seed like black cumin.

When drunk, this is an excellent defense against bites of reptiles. It helps those who suffer from strangury, from stones, and those who pass clots of blood with their urine. But they should drink afterwards celery seed.

**III, 62 ἄμι, *Carum copticum* B. and H., Ajowan**

**1.** Ajowan: some call this one also Ethiopian cumin and others call it royal cumin, but some said that Ethiopian cumin is of one nature and ajowan of another. Its seedlet is well known, being a great deal smaller than the seed of cumin and tasting like oregano. Choose that which is clean and not chaffy.

This one also has warming, heating, and drying properties, operating on colic, difficult micturition, and on animal bites when drunk with wine.

**2.** It also draws down the menses; it is mixed with exfoliating medications made from blister beetles to counteract the ensuing dysurias and it removes black eye when smeared on with honey. When drunk and when anointed, it also changes skin to a paler color, and when burned from below with raisins and pine resin as to make a thick smoke it cleanses the uterus.

**III, 63 κόριον, *Coriandrum sativum* L., Coriander**

Coriander: it has a cooling property, wherefore, when plastered on with bread or barley groats, it cures erysipelas and shingles; with honey and raisins, it treats pustules that are most painful at night, testicular inflammations, and carbuncles, and with bruised corn it dissolves scrofulous swellings of the glands and tumors. A small quantity of its seed drunk with grape-syrup expels intestinal worms and furthers the production of semen, but if too much is taken, it dangerously disturbs the thinking process; this is why one must guard against drinking it to excess and continuously. Anointed with white lead[37] or with litharge, and with vinegar and unguent of roses, the juice benefits surface tumors that are inflamed.

**III, 64 σέλινον κηπαῖον, *Apium graveolens* L., Garden celery**

**1.** Garden celery: this herb is suitable for all the things for which coriander is also suitable, as well as for inflammations of the eyes when applied with bread or with very fine barley groats; it allays heartburn, it relaxes breasts swollen with clots of milk, and when eaten either raw or cooked it is diuretic. Both its decoction and the decoction of its roots when drunk counteract deadly poisons, are emetic, and antidiarrheic.

**2.** The seed is more diuretic, helping those bitten by wild animals and those who have drunk litharge; it is also dissolvent of flatulence. It is profitably mixed with analgesics, with antidotes for poisonous bites, and with cough medications.

The marsh celery, which grows in moist places and which is larger than garden celery, can also accomplish the same cures as garden celery.

**III, 65 ὀρεοσέλινον, *Athamanta macedonica* L. sp., Mountain parsley**

Mountain parsley: it is a stalk, one-span tall, growing from a slender root, surrounded by little sprays and tiny heads like those of hemlock, but much more delicate, whereon lies the seed which is longish, pungent, sweet-smelling, and resembling cumin. It grows on rocks and on mountainous places.

The seed and root drunk in wine have a diuretic property; they also bring on the menstrual period; they are mixed both with antidotes and with heating medicines. One must not confuse the mountain parsley that grows on rocks with parsley.

[37] Used as a pigment especially to whiten facial skin, also hair, and in salves.

**III, 66 πετροσέλινον, *Petroselinon hortense* Hoffm., Parsley**

Parsley: it grows in Macedonia on precipitous spots. The seed is like that of ajowan, but more fragrant, more pungent, spicy, diuretic, drawing forth the menses, suitable for stomach and colon gases, for colic, for pains on the side, kidneys, and bladder when taken in a drink. It is mixed both with diuretics and with antidotes.

**III, 67 ἱπποσέλινον, *Smyrnium olusatrum* L., Alexanders**

**1.** Alexanders: but some call it *agriolon*, others *agrioselinon*, others *smyrnion*, and the Romans *olesathrum*. It is different from the plant properly called *smyrnion,* as I shall discuss in a moment. It is larger and whiter than garden celery and the stalk is hollow, tall, tender, having lines, as it were; the leaves are wider and somewhat purple, among which, just like among the foliage of rosemary frankincense, there are many flowers that combine into clusters before withering. The seed is black, oblong, firm, pungent, and spicy. The root is white, aromatic, tasty, and not thick.

**2.** It grows in shady <spots> and near marshlands. It is used as a vegetable like celery. The root is eaten both boiled and raw, the leaves and stalks are eaten boiled; they are prepared by themselves as well as with fish. They are also preserved raw in brine.

When drunk with honey and wine, the seed can bring on the menstrual period, it warms shiverers when drunk and when anointed and it helps for strangury. The root, too, does the same.

**III, 68 σμύρνιον, *Smyrnium perfoliatum* Mill., Cretan alexanders**

**1.** Cretan alexanders, which in Cilicia they call *petroselinon*, grows abundantly on the mountain called Amanos. It, too, has a stem like that of celery, having many side-growths, but the leaves are broader — the ones near the ground even bend around a little — somewhat fat, sturdy, pungently fragrant, with a medicinal smell and of yellowish color. It has a dill-like umbel on the stem. The seed is round, similar to that of cabbage, black, pungent in taste, <smelling of> frankincense, and most efficacious. The root is pungent, fragrant, soft, and juicy; it bites the throat; its skin is black on the outside but pale yellow or whitish on the inside. It grows in rocky places and on hillocks.

**2.** The root, herb, and seed have a warming property. The leaves are used as vegetables preserved in brine and they stop diarrhea. The root is suitable for those bitten by reptiles when drunk; it calms coughs and it treats both orthopnea and difficult micturition; plastered on, it disperses recent swellings, inflammations, and indurations; it brings wounds to the point of cicatrisation and when grated and used as a pessary, it induces miscarriage. Its seed, too, is good for the kidneys, spleen, and bladder; it draws both the afterbirth and the menstrual period, it is suitable for hip ailments when drunk with wine, and it soothes inflations of the stomach. It also promotes perspiration and eructation and it is especially drunk for edemata and for fits of intermittent fevers.

**III, 69 ἐλαφοβόσκον, *Pastinaca sativa* L., Parsnip**

Parsnip: it is a stalk that resembles the rosemary frankincense or the fennel, jointed, having leaves that are two fingers wide, quite long like the leaves of the terebinth, arching and incised, and somewhat rough. The stalk has quite a few offshoots that have umbels similar to the dill's, flowers that are yellowish, and the seed is like the dill's. The root is about three-fingers long and one-finger thick. It is white, sweet, and edible. The stalk is also used as a vegetable when fresh.

They say that deer that graze on this herb develop a resistance to the bites of reptiles; wherefore the seed is given with wine to those bitten by reptiles.

**III, 70 μάραθον, *Foeniculum vulgare* Gaertn., Fennel**

**1.** Fennel: this herb can draw down milk when eaten, as can also its seed when drunk or when cooked together with barley gruel. The decoction of its foliage, being diuretic, is suitable for kidney and bladder <diseases>; it is given with wine to people bitten by reptiles, it brings on the menstrual period, and it relieves the nausea and heartburn of people who have a fever when drunk with cold water. The roots, smeared on ground up with honey, treat those bitten by dogs.

**2.** The juice, expressed from the stalks and leaves and dried in the sun, is prepared advantageously for such eye medications as are made for sharpening the vision. For the same purposes juice is extracted from its seed, while <it is> still green, together with the leaves and branches, and from the root when it first grows. In Spain to the west, it releases also a juice that is similar to gum. The locals cut the stem in the middle at the time the plant is in bloom and place it near the fire so that by sweating, as it were, from the heat it may release the gum. This is more active for eye preparations than the juice.

**III, 71 ἱππομάραθον, ~ *Prangos ferulacea* L., Horse fennel**

Horse fennel: it is a large wild fennel; its seed is like that of rosemary frankincense and the root, which is below ground and fragrant, when drunk treats strangury <and> it brings on the menstrual period when used as a pessary. The seed and root stem diarrhea, help those bitten by wild animals, break up stones, and clear away jaundice when drunk. The decoction of its leaves when drunk activates lactation and cleanses women after they have given birth.

There is also another plant called horse fennel that has small, narrow, and elongated leaves and round seed tending toward that of coriander, pungent, fragrant, and warming. Its properties correspond to those of the above but they are weaker.

**III, 72 δαῦκος,[38] ~ *Athamanta cretensis* L., *Daucos***

**1.** *Daucos:* there is one kind called Cretan, having leaves like those of fennel but smaller and finer, a stem that is one-span tall, an umbel like that of coriander, and white flowers; they contain seed that is white, rough, pungent when chewed, and fragrant; the root is a finger thick and one-span long. It grows in rocky and sunny places. And there is another kind that nearly resembles wild celery; it is spicy and fragrant, and it tastes pungent and hot. The Cretan is superior.

**2.** The third kind resembles coriander in foliage and it has white flowers. Its top and fruit are similar to the dill's, the umbel is like that of carrot, it is full of longish seed like cumin and it is pungent.

The seed of all of them warms; when drunk, it draws out the menstrual period, embryos/fetuses, and urine, it relieves colic, and it allays chronic coughs; it comes to the aid of people bitten by poisonous

---

[38] According to LSJ *s.v.* δαῦκος, the three species discussed in this chapter are Athamanta *cretensis*, *Peucedanum cervaria* and *Psychotis amnis.*

spiders when drunk with wine, and it disperses swellings when plastered on. All of them are used for their seed, but the Cretan is also used for its root, which is mostly drunk with wine as an antidote to poisonous animals.

**III, 73 πύρεθρος, *Anacyclus pyrethrum* DC = *Anthemis pyrethrum* L., Pellitory**

Pellitory: it is an herb that sends out a stalk and leaves like those of the wild carrot or fennel. The umbel is wheel-like, resembling the dill's. The root is thick as a thumb, long, extremely hot if one were to taste it, and it draws phlegm. Therefore, when boiled with vinegar and used as a mouthwash it helps for toothaches. It also draws out phlegm when chewed, and it causes perspiration when smeared on with olive oil, helping for chronic shiverings. It is also highly suitable for chilled or weakened body parts.

**III, 74 λιβανωτίς, ~*Cachris libanotis* Koch, ~*Lecokia graeca* (Andrews), ~*Prangos ferula*, Rosemary frankincense**

**1.** Rosemary frankincense: it is of two kinds. One kind bears fruit. Some call this kind *zea* or *campsanema*; its fruit is called *cachry*. It has leaves like those of fennel, but they are wider and thicker. They lie on the ground in a circle and they are fragrant. It has a stem that is one-cubit tall or even taller, having many branches and at the tip umbels, whereon there is a great deal of white fruit resembling vertebrae, round, having many nooks, pungent, smelling like pine resin, and burning the taste buds when chewed.

**2.** Its root is white, sizable, and smells of frankincense. The other kind is similar to the above in every respect; it has a broad seed, which is dark like the seed of cow parsnip, fragrant, it does not burn, and a root which is black on the outside but white when broken. The rosemary frankincense called fruitless is in all respects similar to the above; it grows no stem, nor flower, nor seed. It grows on rocky and rough terrains.

In general, the foliage of all three ground and applied as a plaster shrink hemorrhoids, allay anal inflammations, and bring to a head callous lumps, scrofulous swellings of the glands, and those elements of abscesses that refuse to be assimilated.

**3.** Combined with honey, the dried roots cleanse sores, treat colic and are suitable for people bitten by wild animals when drunk with wine, draw the menstrual period and urine, and disperse old swellings when plastered on. The juice of the root and of the herb, combined with honey and smeared on, promotes sharp-sightedness. The fruit accomplishes the same results when drunk; it helps for epilepsy, for chest conditions of old standing, and for jaundice when given with wine and pepper. Rubbed on with olive oil, it causes one to perspire, it is suitable for spasms, ruptures, and gout when plastered on ground with meal of darnel and vinegar, and it clears off dull-white leprosies when mixed with very sharp vinegar.
**4.** One must use for drinks the seed of rosemary frankincense that does not bear *cachry,* because *cachry* is sharp and roughens the throat. Theophrastus[39] reports that there is a rosemary frankincense that grows among heath, having leaves like those of wild lettuce, the kind of lettuce that is bitter, and a short root that purges upward and downward when drunk, but that the leaves are whiter and more prickly than those of lettuce. *Cachry* has warming and extremely drying properties, therefore, when mixed with unguents it is suitable for rheumy eyes, being plastered on the head and wiped off after three days.

**III, 75 λιβανωτίς, *Rosmarinus officinalis* L., Rosemary**

Rosemary which the Romans call *rosmarinum* and which wreath-makers use: it has slender shoots surrounded by leaves that are delicate, dense, somewhat long, thin, white on the inside, pale green on the outside, and oppressive in smell.
It has properties that warm and that cure jaundice if one after boiling it in water gave it to drink prior to exercise and after exercising the person bathed and drank wine. It is also mixed with analgesics and with ointment of sweet new wine.

---

[39] Theophrastus, *H. P.* IX, 11, 11. This seems to be a kind of lettuce. See LSJ *s.v.* λιβανωτίς.

**III, 76 σφονδύλιον, *Heracleum sphondylium* L., Cow-parsnip**

**1.** Cow parsnip: its has leaves that resemble somewhat those of the plane, tending toward the leaves of allheal, stalks one-cubit tall or even taller, similar to those of the fennel, and at their tip there is seed like that of hartwort, double but wider, whiter, more chaffy, and oppressive in scent; it has white flowers and a white root that resembles the cabbage's. It grows in marshlands and wet places.

**2.** When its fruit is drunk, it expels through the bowels matter full of phlegm. It treats people with liver disease, jaundice, orthopnea, epilepsy, and uterine suffocation when drunk; burned to produce smoke from below, it revives people who faint, and in combination with olive oil it is used to moisten the head of those suffering from phrenitis, lethargic fever, and headaches; it also keeps shingles in check when plastered on with rue. The root, too, is given to those with jaundice and liver disease, and it does melt away the hardness of fistulous sores when scraped all around and inserted into them. Juice extracted from its fresh flowers is suitable for lacerated and purulent ears. Having been baked in the sun, it is stored like the other juice extracts.

**III, 77 νάρθηξ, *Ferula communis* L., Giant fennel**

Giant fennel: the pith of fresh giant fennel benefits people who spit blood and those suffering in the bowel when drunk. It is also given with wine to those bitten by vipers and it stops nosebleeds when placed into the nostrils ground up. The seed benefits the colicky when drunk and it promotes perspiration when smeared on with olive oil. The stalks, however, cause headaches when eaten. It is preserved in brine.

**III, 78 πευκέδανον, *Peucedanum officinale* L., Sulphurwort**

**1.** Sulphurwort: it sends up a thin stalk like the fennel; it has ample and dense foliage around the root, quince-yellow flower, and a root that is black, oppressive in scent, strong, and full of juice. It grows on thickly shaded mountains.

The root is tapped when tender by cutting it with a knife and immediately putting the run-off in the shade. For the sun weakens it. But while it is collected, it causes headaches and dizziness unless one first smeared his nostrils with unguent of roses and wetted his head. Once tapped, the root becomes useless.

**2.** The stalks are also squeezed to express their juice and the root is tapped like the mandrake. But the expressed juice is weaker than the tapped and it swiftly looses its power. At times one finds formed on the stalks and roots resin, which is similar to frankincense. The best tapped juice is that produced in Sardinia and in Samothrace; it is oppressive in scent, pale-yellow, and warming in taste.

Smeared on with vinegar and unguent of roses, it is suitable for people suffering from lethargic fever, phrenitis, dizziness, epilepsy, chronic headaches, paralysis, hip ailments, spasms, and, in general, it is rubbed on with olive oil and vinegar for diseases relating to the nerves.

**3.** It is also smelled for uterine suffocation and it revives those who faint. When used for fumigation, it chases away wild animals, dribbled with unguent of roses, it is suitable for earaches, also for toothaches when placed into the decayed teeth. Taken with an egg, it is good for coughs, it is fitting for dyspnea, colic, and for afflictions where distention is involved, it gently softens the stool, it reduces the spleen, it helps beyond measure difficult deliveries, and it is beneficial to drink for pains and obstructions in the bladder and kidneys. It even opens the womb.

**4.** The root, too, is useful for the same purposes, although its activity is less strong; it is its decoction that one drinks. Ground up dry, it cleanses sordid sores, it removes spurs from bones, and it cicatrizes old sores. It is mixed both with cerates and with warming emollients. Choose that which is fresh, not worm-eaten, solid, and full of scent. The expressed juice is dissolved into drinks with bitter almonds or rue or dill or warm bread.

### III, 79 μελάνθιον, *Nigella sativa* L., Black cumin

**1.** Black cumin: it is a small shrub, thin-stemmed, two-spans tall or even taller, [having] small leaves like those of groundsel but a great deal thinner, and at the top a delicate little head, small as a poppy's, longish, having internal partitions within which lies its seed. It is black, sharp, and fragrant and it sprinkled on breads.

It is suitable for people who have headaches, their forehead being plastered with it, and for incipient cataracts when poured <ground up> into the nostrils with unguent of iris.

**2.** Plastered on with vinegar, it removes birthmarks, leprosies, old swellings, and indurations, and when applied with old urine it sheds warts demarcated with a circular incision; it is beneficial for toothaches boiled with a fragment of pinewood and vinegar and used as a mouthwash, and it expels round intestinal worms when plastered on the navel with water. Triturated, tied in a bag, and smelled, it helps those who have catarrhs; when drunk for many days, it brings on the menstrual period, urine, and milk; it stops dyspnea when drunk with soda, and an amount of one *drachma* drank with water helps people bitten by poisonous spiders. Burned for fumigation, it also chases away reptiles. But they say that it is also fatal if one drank too much of it.

**III, 80 σίλφιον, ~ *Ferula tingitana* L., Laserwort**

**1.** Laserwort: it grows in places around Syria, Armenia, Media, and Libya. Its stem is called *maspeton*; it resembles that of giant fennel. It has leaves similar to celery and seed that is wide and leaf-like, which is called *magydaris*.

The root warms, <causes flatulence, eructation, and drying up>, is hard to digest, and is bad for the bladder. Compounded with cerate, it treats scrofulous swellings of the glands and tumors and when applied with olive oil it treats black eye; with cerate of iris or of henna, it is suitable for those with hip ailments, and, when boiled with vinegar in the shell of a pomegranate and plastered on, it removes excrescences around the anus; it is also an antidote for deadly poisons when drunk and it is tasty when mixed into sauces and salts.

**2.** Juice is extracted from the root and stalk by incision. The best juice[40] is reddish and translucent, myrrh-like and lively in scent, not greenish nor unpleasant in taste and passing quickly into white color. One should know that the Cyrenaic, even if one tasted a tiny amount of it, causes the entire body to break out immediately in a sweat and that it has a very mild scent so that the taster's mouth smells only

[40] See Dsc. Bk. I, n. 17.

briefly. The Median and Syrian are decidedly weaker and their smell is rather foul.

**3.** All the juices are adulterated before they are dried by mixing them with *sagapenon*[41] or with flour made from bruised beans. Taste, smell, appearance, and viscosity determine whether they have been adulterated. Some called the stalk *silphion,* the root *magydaris*, and the leaves *maspeta*. The juice is the most effective, then the leaves, then the stalk.

It causes inflation and it is pungent; smeared on with wine, pepper, and vinegar, it treats bald spots; it effects sharp-sightedness, it can disperse incipient cataracts when coated on with honey, and it is placed into cavities or it is smeared on a linen cloth with rosemary frankincense and wrapped around the tooth for toothaches.

**4.** It is used as a mouthwash with hyssop and figs boiled in sour wine and water; it is a beneficial application both for the injuries of those bitten by a mad dog and for the injuries caused by all poisonous animals and poisoned arrows when anointed and when drunk; diluted in olive oil, it is smeared all around scorpion bites; it is injected into gangrenous sores before they have scarified; it is used with rue, soda, and honey or by itself for carbuncles, and when softened with cerate or with the inner part of dry figs it removes warts and calluses that have been demarcated with a circular incision. It treats with vinegar fresh lichen-like eruptions of the skin, but for fleshy excrescences and polyps it is anointed for a few days with a solution of blue vitriol or verdigris. But do pull the excrescences with forceps.

**5.** Diluted in water and gulped down, it helps also for chronic harshness of the throat and it immediately clears the voice should it suddenly become hoarse; anointed with honey, it shrinks the uvulas, it is a useful gargle with hydromel for sore throats, it gives a rather nice complexion when taken in the diet, it is suitable for a cough when given with a soft-boiled egg, it is given in thick gruel for pleurisy, and it is given successfully with dry figs to the jaundiced and to those with edemata. Drunk with pepper, rue, and wine, it stops shiverings; give to those with tetanus and with tetanic recurvation to swallow an amount of one *obolos* kneaded with cerate. Used as a gargle with vinegar, it

---

[41] The juice of *Ferula persica.*

expels leeches that cling to the throat, and when taken with oxymel it helps those whose milk curdles inside them and epileptics.

**6.** Drunk with pepper and myrrh, it brings on the menstrual period and when taken enclosed in a grape it benefits those with bowel ailments; drunk with ash it is good for sudden spasms and ruptures. It is dissolved in potions with bitter almonds or rue or dill or warm bread. Its seed does the same but much less effectively; it is eaten with oxymel, being suitable for conditions associated with the trachea and especially for loss of voice. They also use it with lettuces, eating it instead of rocket.

There is also another plant called *magydaris* that grows in Libya. Its root is similar to that of the laserwort but it is less thick, pungent, and porous; it has no juice but it accomplishes the same as laserwort.

### III, 81 σαγάπηνον, *Ferula persica* Willd., *Sagapenon*

**1.** *Sagapenon*[42] is the juice[43]of an herb that resembles the giant fennel and that grows in Media. The best is clear, outwardly yellow but internally white, smelling between the juice of laserwort and *galbanum*, and it is pungent in taste.

It is effective for chest pain and for pains on the side, for ruptures, spasms, chronic coughs, and it clears thick matter from the lungs. It is given in a drink to people with epilepsy, tetanic recurvation, spleen disease, paralysis, to those who are chilled, and for intermittent fevers; it is also added profitably to ointments.

**2.** Drunk with hydromel, it brings on the menstrual period and destroys embryos/fetuses; taken with wine, it helps those bitten by wild animals; smelled with vinegar, it revives those suffering from uterine suffocation, and it clears scars in the eyes, dim-sightedness, the elements that cast a shadow over the pupils of the eyes, and cataracts. It is dissolved with rue and water or with bitter almonds or with honey or with warm bread, just like the juice [of laserwort.][44]

---

[42] Both the plant and the juice are called *sagapenon.*

[43] J. Innes Miller, *The Spice Trade of the Roman Empire, 29 B.C. to A.D. 641*, p. 100, describes the juice as gum-like.

[44] See Dsc. Bk. III, 80.6 above, where the prescription is similar to that in this passage. The Latin Dioscorides, "*…si* [*sacopenium=segapenon*] *suco rutae aut amigdale aut melli fuerit unctus,*" is clearer, …if [*sagapenon*] is smeared on with

**III, 82 εὐφόρβιον, *Euphorbia resinifera* Berg., Spurge**

**1.** Spurge: it is a Libyan plant that resembles the giant fennel, growing in Autololia[45] next to Mauretania, full of very pungent juice, which the inhabitants there collect with much trepidation because of the intensity of its heat. Therefore, after tying on the plant washed sheep's stomachs, they sever the stalk with javelins from a distance; right away a great deal of juice pours into the stomachs, as if from some sort of a vessel; as it darts forth, it also gushes on the ground.

**2.** There are two kinds of this juice: one is clear like *sarcocolla*,[46] about the size of bitter vetches,[47] and the other which is in the stomachs is full of particles and firm. It is adulterated with a mixture of *sarcocolla* and gum. Choose that which is clear and pungent. It is hard to test it by taste, because once it has stung the tongue its burning sensation lasts for a long time so that everything that is put to the tongue seems to be spurge. It was discovered when Juba was king of Libya.[48]

**3.** The juice has the property of dispersing cataracts when smeared on, but it surely burns all day long. It is for this reason that it is mixed with honey and with eye salves in proportion to its sharpness. It is suitable for diseases of the hips when mixed with an aromatic potion and drunk. It also quickly removes spurs. Users must secure, however, the flesh that surrounds the bones with lint pledgets or with cerate. Some say that no harm will befall those whom serpents bite if one, cutting the skin of their head to the bone, inserted the smooth juice and sowed up the wound.

---

juice of rue or almond or honey.

[45] In Northwest Africa.

[46] A Persian gum, *Astragallus fasiculifolius.*

[47] This is the one that spills on the ground and condenses into small, solid masses, of the size of bitter vetch seeds.

[48] Juba, ca. 50 B.C. to ca. 23 A.D. Actually it was Juba who discovered it, named it in honor of his personal physician, Euphorbos, and wrote a treatise about it, which is lost as are all of Juba's writings. See F. Jacoby, *DieFragmente der griechischen Historiker*, III A (1940), pp. 127 ff.

## III, 83 χαλβάνη, Galbanum

**1.** Galbanum: it is the juice of a giant fennel (*Ferula galbaniflua* Boiss. and Buhse) growing in Syria; some call this juice *metopon.* The best is like frankincense, granular, clean, greasy, free of wood particles, having some seed and some giant fennel mixed with it, heavy in scent, and neither too moist nor too dry. They adulterate it by mixing it with pine resin, bruised corn, and gum ammoniac.

It has warming, burning, drawing, and dispersive properties. When applied as a pessary and when burned to produce smoke from below, it draws the menstrual period and embryos/fetuses, and when plastered on with vinegar and soda it removes birthmarks. It is also drunk for a persistent cough, dyspnea, asthma, ruptures, and spasms.

**2.** Drunk with wine and myrrh, it counteracts arrow poisoning; taken similarly, it expels dead embryos/fetuses; it is applied both for pains on the side and for abscesses; when smelled, it revives epileptics, those having an attack of uterine suffocation, and those suffering from dizziness; burned for fumigation, it chases away wild beasts, and when smeared on it keeps people free from bites. Set out with cow parsnip and olive oil, it kills reptiles and, when kneaded and inserted into a decayed tooth, it stops the toothache. But it is thought to cause difficult micturition.

**3.** It is dissolved into drinks with bitter almonds and water or with rue or with hydromel or with warm bread or, as alternatives, with *meconion*,[49] burned copper,[50] liquid bile.

But if you wish to purify it, place it into hot water, because when it has melted, the filthy part will come to the surface; you will separate the valuable part as follows: after tying it in a clean and loosely woven linen cloth, hang it over a copper box or a clay vessel so that the bundle does not touch the bottom of the vessel then covering it with a lid let it down into boiling water; for this way the valuable part will dissolve in the vessel as through a strainer, but its woody part will remain in the linen cloth.

---

[49] Which can mean a number of things: poppy, opium, spurge, etc.

[50] On burned copper, see Dsc. Bk. V, 76.

**III, 84 ἀμμωνιακόν, *Ferula marmarica* L., Gum ammoniac**

**1.** Gum ammoniac: it, too, is the juice of a giant fennel growing in that part of Libya that is near Cyrene. The entire shrub from which it comes together with the root is called *agasylis.* One must choose it nicely colored, free of stones, free of wood, with granules that are like frankincense, clean, dense, devoid of all filth, smelling like castor, and bitter in taste. Such as this is called *thrausma,* but that which is earthy and stony is called *phyrama.* It is produced in that area of Libya where Ammon is,[51] being the juice of a tree resembling a giant fennel.

**2.** It has properties that warm, soften, draw, and dissolve indurations and growths, and it purges the bowels when drunk; one *drachma,* when drunk with vinegar pulls down embryos/fetuses, reduces the spleen, and relieves ailments of the joints and of the hips. Used as a lozenge with honey or gulped down with barley-water, it helps asthmatics, those suffering from orthopnea, epileptics, and people who have liquids in the chest; it also drives out bloody urine.

**3.** It washes away leucomas and it reduces roughness of the eyelids. Dissolved in vinegar and plastered on, it stops indurations around the spleen and liver. Plastered on with honey or mixed with pitch, it dissolves the chalkstones that are formed around the joints. It is also good, instead of an analgesic, both for exertion and for hip ailments when anointed after being mixed with vinegar, soda, and oil of henna.

**III, 85 σαρκοκόλλα,[52] *Astragalus fasiculifolius* Boiss. sp., Sarcocolla**

Sarcocolla is the resin of a tree that grows in Persia. It resembles fine frankincense, it is yellowish, and it is bitter in taste.

It has properties that close wounds and stop running eyes; it is also compounded with salves. But they do adulterate it by mixing it with gum.

---

[51] I.e. where the temple of Ammon is.

[52] The property of this substance to glue together flesh and therefore to close wounds is embedded in the component parts of the word, σαρκοκόλλα, viz. σάρξ, "flesh" and κόλλα, "glue." See Miller, *The Spice Trade of the Roman Empire,* 29 B.C. to A.D. 641, p. 100.

**III, 86 γλαύκιον, *Glaucium corniculatum* Curtis, *Glaucion***

*Glaucion* is the juice of an herb growing in Hierapolis of Syria. Its leaves resemble the leaves of horned poppy but they are thicker and low growing, oppressive in scent, and bitter in taste. They contain much saffron-colored juice. The locals place its leaves in a small pot, warm them in lukewarm ovens until they wither, then after chopping them squeeze out the juice.

It is used for incipient eye problems because it cools.

**III, 87 κόλλα, Glue**

Glue, which some call wood glue or bull's hide glue: the best is the Rhodian made from hides of bulls. This type is white and translucent but the black is inferior.

Dissolved in vinegar, it has a property that removes lichen-like eruptions and superficial leprosies and it does not allow burns to blister when smeared on them diluted with warm water. Diluted with honey and vinegar, it is also used for wounds.

**III, 88 ἰχθυοκόλλα, Fish glue**

Fish glue: but what is called fish glue is the belly of a whale-type fish. The best is made in the Pontic region; it is white, somewhat thick, not scabby, and it dissolves very quickly.

It is suitable for head salves, for medications for leprosies, and for facial lotions.

**III, 89 ἰξός, *Hozanthus europaeus* L. Birdlime, Oak-mistletoe**

**1.** Birdlime: it is of good quality when smooth, greenish internally, somewhat yellow on the outside, and devoid of anything rough or bran-like. It is collected from a certain round fruit that grows on the oak-mistletoe, the kind of mistletoe that has leaves like those of box. The fruit is chopped, then washed, and then boiled in water. But some make it by chewing the fruit. It is also collected from apple, pear, and other trees; it is found also near the roots of certain shrubs.

**2.** It can disperse, soften, draw, and contract growths, tumors of the parotid gland and the other suppurating inflammations when mixed in equal amounts with pine resin and cerate, and it treats pustules that are most painful at night when plastered with a linen compress. In combination with frankincense, it softens old sores and malignant suppurative inflammations, and, when boiled together with unslaked lime and jet or Asian stone then applied, it softens the spleen. Plastered on with yellow orpiment or with red sulfide of arsenic, it draws off nails, but when mixed with unslaked lime and new wine it increases their strength.

**III, 90 ἀπαρίνη, *Galium aparine* L., Cleavers**

Cleavers: but some call it *ambelocarpon*, others *omphalocarpon*, and others *philanthropon.* It has many, long, quadrangular, rough sprays, leaves at a distance from each other lying whorled like those of madder, white flowers, and seed that is hard, round, somewhat indented in the middle like a navel. The herb clings onto clothing. Shepherds use it as a strainer for milk to remove the hair in it.

Juice extracted from its seed, twigs, and leaves helps those bitten by poisonous spiders and snakes when drunk with wine and it also treats earaches when instilled. Compounded with lard, the herb disperses scrofulous swellings of the glands.

**III, 91 ἄλυσσον, *Biscutella* L. sp., Madwort**

Madwort: it is a small undershrub, somewhat rough, single-stalked, having round leaves. Adjacent to them is the fruit, resembling small double shields and containing somewhat wide seed. It grows in mountainous and rough places.

When drunk, its decoction stops feverless retchings; it does the same also when held in the mouth or when smelled. Ground up with honey, this undershrub removes birthmarks and freckles. It is thought that it also treats rabies[53] when chopped together with food and served. They say that it is good for the health of humans and beasts when hung in the home. Suspended with a purple strip of cloth, it cures young domesticated animals.

---

[53] The connection of this plant to rabies is evident not only from its English name, madwort, but also from its Greek, ἄλυσσον, the components of which are from alpha privative and λύσσα, "rabies."

**III, 92 ἀσκληπιάς, *Vincetoxicum officinale*, Moench, Swallowwort**
Swallowwort: it sends out small sprays on which the leaves are like those of ivy; it has many slender and fragrant roots, a flower that has a heavy smell, and seed like the axeweed's. It grows on mountains.
Drunk with wine, the roots help the colicky and those bitten by wild animals, as do also the leaves when plastered on. They are also suitable for breast and uterine malignancies.

**III, 93 ἀτρακτυλίς, *Cartharmus lanatus* L., Spindle thistle**
Spindle thistle: but some call it *cnecos agrios*. It is a thorny plant that resembles the safflower, although it has much smaller leaves at the end of its shoot; yet, by and large, it is bare and this is why women use it as spindle. It also has on top hair that is thorny and a pale flower; the root is delicate and useless.
Its leaves, hair, and fruit ground and drunk with pepper and wine benefit those stung by a scorpion. Some report, moreover, that people who have been stung remain free of pain as long as they hold onto this herb but that they hurt when they let go of it.

**III, 94 πολύκνημον, *Zizyphora capitata* L., Field basil**
Field basil: it is a little bush that belongs to the class of undershrubs, having leaves like those of oregano and a stem that has many joints like the pennyroyal. It does not have a flower head but small clusters on top that smell of something pungent and sweet at the same time.
Plastered on with water either fresh or after it was dried, it is good for wounds, gluing them together. But one must remove the plaster every fifth day. It is drunk with wine both for strangury and for ruptures.

**III, 95 κλινοπόδιον, *Calamintha clinopodium* Moris = *Clinopodium vulgare* L., Horse thyme**
Horse thyme: but some call it *cleonicon*, others *ocimoides*, and others *Zopyrion*. It, too, is a small shrub belonging to the class of undershrubs, two-spans tall, growing on rocks, having leaves very nearly resembling those of tufted thyme and, at intervals, flowers that are like bed-feet[54] and that resemble those of horehound.

---

[54] Hence its name κλινοπόδιον, composed of the elements κλίνη, "bed" and πόδιον,

The herb and its decoction is drunk for animal bites, spasms, ruptures, and strangury. It also draws the menstrual period and embryos/fetuses, and if drunk for several days it sheds warts that have a thin neck; it also stops diarrhea when boiled down to one-third and drunk with wine by patients who are fever-free and with water, if they have a fever.

**III, 96 λεοντοπέταλον, *Leontice leontopetalum* L., *Leontopetalon***

*Leontopetalon*: but some call it *leontopodion*, others *pardalion*, others *thorybethron*, and others *leucethron*. It sends up a stem as tall as a span that has several branches and on top there are pods like chick-peas containing two or three small seeds. It has leaves like those of cabbage, a root that is black like that of the turnip, having protuberances as if they were some knobs; it grows in fields and among the grain.

When drunk with wine, its root helps people that have been bitten by reptiles, rendering them quickly free of pain. It is also mixed into rinses that are good for hip ailments.

**III, 97 Τεύκριον, *Teucrium flavum* L., Tree germander**

Tree germander: it is a rod-like herb, somewhat similar to germander; the leaves are thin, resembling the chick-pea's. It grows extensively in Cilicia around that part which is near what is called Selentis and Cetis. When drunk fresh with sour wine mixed with water or when boiled dried and drunk it can substantially reduce the spleen. It is also plastered with fig and vinegar on people with spleen disease but it is applied only with vinegar, without the fig, on people bitten by wild animals.

**III, 98 χαμαίρωψ, *Teucrium chamaedrys* L. and *T. lucidum* L., Wall germander**

**1.** Wall germander or *chamaidrys* or *linodrys*: but some call this plant, too, *Teucrion* because it maintains a degree of likeness to tree germander. It grows in rough and stony terrains. It is a small shrub, one-span tall, which has small bitter leaves shaped and lobbed like the

---

"small foot."

leaves of the oak and a small reddish flower. One must harvest the plant when big with seed.
Fresh as well as dried, when boiled with water and given to drink, it has properties that help for spasms, coughs, an indurated spleen, difficult micturition, and people with incipient edemata.
**2.** It does draw both the menstrual periods and embryos/fetuses, and it reduces the spleen when drunk with vinegar. Drunk with wine or applied as a plaster, it is efficacious for venoms of animals. For the above conditions, it can also be ground up and molded into capsules, and with honey it cleanses old sores. Ground up and anointed with oil, it eliminates misting of the eyes and it warms when rubbed on.

**III, 99 λευκάς, ~ *Lamium album* L., Dead nettle**
Dead nettle: the one growing on mountains has wider leaves than the cultivated and is <more pungent>. It has a more pungent, bitter, and less tasty fruit. It is certainly more potent than the cultivated.
Both are suitable for venoms of animals and especially of sea-animals when plastered on and when drunk with wine.

**III, 100 λυχνὶς στεφανωματική, *Lychnis coronaria* L., Rose campion**
Rose campion: it is a flower like the gillyflower, somewhat purple, which is plaited into the garlands. Its seed helps those stung by scorpions when drunk with wine.

**III, 101 λυχνὶς ἀγρία, *Agrostemma githago* L., Corn cockle**
Wild corn cockle resembles the cultivated in every respect. Two *drachmai* of its seed drunk with wine draw bilious matter down the bowel. They say also that scorpions become lethargic and inactive when the herb is set next to them.

**III, 102 κρίνον, *Lilium candidum* L., Lily**
**1.** The lily,[55] whose flower is used for making garlands, which some call *leirion* and from which the unguent that some call *leirinon* and others *sousinon* is made, softens tendons and especially indurations around the uterus.

---

[55] This is the white lily.

Plastered on, the leaves of this plant have the capacity to help those bitten by reptiles. They are also good boiled for burns, and preserved in vinegar they are a remedy for wounds.

**2.** Their juice, mixed with vinegar and honey and boiled in a copper cauldron, becomes a liquid medication for old sores and for fresh injuries. The root, ground up and boiled with unguent of roses, treats burns, softens the uterus, draws the menstrual period, and cicatrizes sores. Triturated with honey, it treats ruptured tendons and sprains, it clears dull-white leprosies, and it washes off leprosies, dandruff, and scurf.

**3.** It also cleans the face and makes it wrinkle-free and, when triturated with vinegar or with leaves of henbane and wheat meal, it relieves testicular inflammations. The seed is an antidotal potion for bites of reptiles and both the seed and the leaves triturated with wine are a plaster for erysipelas. Some say that lilies are also purple.[56] The most potent flowers for making the unguent grow in Syria, Pisidia, and Pamphylia.

### III, 103 βαλλωτή, *Ballota nigra* L., Black horehound

Black horehound: but some call it *melamprasion.* It sends out from one root many quadrangular stems that are black and somewhat hairy; its leaves are like the horehound's, except bigger, rounder, dark, and downy, growing on the stem at intervals, very nearly resembling the leaves of balm, and ill-smelling; it is for this reason that some people have called this plant also balm. Its flowers lie around the stems like a circle.

Its leaves, plastered on with salt, are good for dog bites, wilted on hot ashes, they reduce knobs, and with honey they cleanse thoroughly filthy sores.

### III, 104 μελισσόφυλλον, *Melissa officinalis* L., *M. altissima* Sibth. and Sm., Balm

**1.** Balm: some people call the balm *melittaina*[57] because bees take a great deal of pleasure in this plant. Its leaves and stems resemble the

[56] The reference is to Turk's cap lily, *Lilium chalcedonicum* L.

[57] The meaning is made clear by the etymology of μελίτταινα, a compound word from

horehound's mentioned above, but the balm's are larger and thinner, they are not as downy, and they smell of citrons.
Drunk with wine or plastered on, the leaves are suitable for people bitten by scorpions, spiders, and dogs.
**2.** Their decoction also accomplishes the same when used as rinse, it is suitable in sitz baths for bringing on the menstrual period, it is a mouthwash for toothaches, and it is a clyster for dysenteries. When drunk with soda, the leaves help those choking from mushrooms and the colicky, and they are made into lozenges for people with orthopnea. Plastered on with salt, they disperse scrofulous swellings of the glands and cleanse sores; they also relieve arthritic pains when plastered on.

### III, 105 πράσιον, *Marrubium vulgare* L., *M. creticum* Miller, Horehound

**1.** Horehound, but some call it *philophares*: it is a shrub that has many branches growing from a single root. It is somewhat hairy and white and it has quadrangular stems. The leaf is as big as the thumb, somewhat round, thick, somewhat wrinkled, and bitter in taste. Spaced on the stem at intervals are the seeds and the flowers, as if they were vertebrae. They are rough. It grows around building lots and ruins.
Its dry leaves are boiled in water with its seed or are converted into juice when green and the liquid is given with honey to tuberculars, asthmatics, and to people who cough. It also brings up congestive matter from the chest when mixed with dry iris.
**2.** It is given to women that have not been cleansed to bring on the menstrual period and afterbirth, to those having difficult deliveries, to people bitten by wild animals, and to those who drank deadly poisons. But you should know that it is not suitable for the bladder and kidneys. The leaves, plastered on with honey, cleanse filthy sores, remove fleshy excrescences and spreading ulcers, and relieve pain on the sides. Also their juice, made by squeezing the leaves and condensing the liquid in the sun, is good for the same purposes. It sharpens the sight when anointed with honey, it purges jaundice

---

μέλιττα, "bee" and αἴνυμαι, "enjoy," "feed on."

through the nostrils, and it is suitable for earaches when instilled either by itself or with unguent of roses.

**III, 106 στάχυς, *Stachys* L. sp., Base horehound**

Base horehound: it is a shrub resembling the horehound, but it has very many little leaves, more elongated, somewhat hairy, tough, fragrant, and white. It has many little shoots from the same root; they are whiter than the shoots of horehound. It grows on mountainous and in rough terrains.

It has warming and sharp properties; it is for this reason that the decoction of its leaves draws the menstrual period and afterbirth when drunk.

**III, 107 φυλλῖτις, *Scolopendrium officinale* L. sp., Hart's tongue**

Hart's tongue: it sends out leaves that are similar to the leaves of monk rhubarb, but they are longer and more luxuriant, six or seven, upright, smooth in front, and on the back side they have, as it were, fine worms hanging. It grows in thickly shaded places and gardens, and it tastes sour; it bears neither flower, nor stem, nor fruit.

Its leaves when drunk with wine benefit people bitten by reptiles. Its infusion, introduced orally, helps quadrupeds. It is drunk both for dysentery and for diarrhea.

**III, 108 φαλλάγγιον, *Lloydia graeca* L., Spiderwort**

Spiderwort: but some people call it *phalangitis* and others call this one also *leucacanthon.* It has two or three or more slips at a distance from each other, white flowers nearly resembling white lilies, having many slits, seed that is broad, dark, like half a lentil but a great deal thinner, and a rootlet that is small, delicate, and lively when first pulled from the ground; for afterwards it contracts. It grows on hillocks.

Drunk with wine, its leaves, seed, and flower help those bitten by scorpions and by poisonous spiders; they also stop colic.

**III, 109 τρίφυλλον, *Psorolea bituminosa* L., Treacle clover**

**1.** Treacle clover: but some call it *minyanthes*, others *asphaltion*, others *cnecion,* and others *oxyphyllon*. It is a shrub, one-cubit tall or taller, having slender, black, stringy shoots that have many offshoots.

On them grow leaves that resemble those of the nettle tree. There are three at each budding. When newly sprouted, they smell of rue but after they have grown bigger, of asphalt. It sends out a purple flower and seed that is somewhat broad, somewhat hairy, and at one end it has a projection so to speak. The root is slender, long, and solid.
**2.** When drunk with water, the seed and leaves are good for people suffering from pleurisy, from difficult micturition, epileptics, for those with incipient edemata, and for women suffering in the womb; it also brings on the monthly period. One must give of the seed three *drachmai* and of the leaves four. Drunk with oxymel, the leaves help people bitten by wild animals. Some reported that the decoction of the entire shrub and of both the root and leaves, used as a fomentation on those bitten by reptiles, relieves their pains. But if the fomentation that was used to cure somebody is poured over the sore of another person, that person will suffer as the bitten. Some give three leaves or three seeds in wine for tertian fever and four for quartan fever, on the assumption that they stop the periodic fever. Its root is also mixed with antidotes.

### III, 110 πόλιον, *Teucrium polium* L., Hulwort

Hulwort: there is a kind that grows in mountains; it is also called *teuthrion* and it is useful. It is a tiny shrub that is white, with delicate leaves, one-span tall, full of seed, having small corymboid heads on top, as if they were grey hair, oppressive in scent with a degree of sweetness. The other kind is a smaller shrub, neither quite as vigorous in scent nor as efficacious in strength.
When drunk, their decoction helps those bitten by wild animals, those with edemata, and those who have jaundice, and with vinegar it helps those suffering from spleen disease. It does, however, give headaches, it is bad for the stomach, and it moves both the bowels and the menstrual period. Strewn around and burned for fumigation, it chases away wild animals and when plastered on it closes wounds.

### III, 111 σκόρδιον, *Teucrium scordium* L., Garlic germander

**1.** Garlic germander: it grows in mountainous and marshy areas, having leaves like the germander's but bigger and not as incised at the periphery, smelling somewhat like garlic, astringent and bitter in taste. The little stems are quadrangular; there is a reddish flower on them. The plant has warming and diuretic properties when given to drink fresh, ground up. It is also given dry, boiled with wine, for snakebites and for deadly poisons, and for gnawing pains in the stomach, for dysentery, and for difficult micturition a weight of two *drachmai* is offered with hydromel.

**2.** It also purges pussy matter from the chest, it is mixed with garden cress, honey, and dry pine resin into lozenges, it is good for an old cough, ruptures, and spasms, and it comforts a chronically inflamed hypochondrium when made up with cerate. It is also good for gout when smeared on with sharp vinegar or plastered on with water; inserted as a pessary, it draws the menstrual period; with honey, it glues injuries <and> it cleanses and cicatrizes old sores. When dry, it reduces overgrown flesh. Its juice, too, is drunk for the ailments that have been mentioned. Most effective are the Pontic and Cretan.

### III, 112 βήχιον, *Tussilago farfara* L., Colt's foot

**1.** Colt's foot: but some call it *pithion*, others *pechion*, and others *petronion*. It has leaves like those of ivy but bigger, six or seven from the same root; they are quite white on the underside, green on the upper side, and polygonal; it has a stem that is a span tall, and in the spring a pallid flower; but it quickly looses both its flower and small stem. It is for this reason that some people supposed that this herb is stemless and flowerless. The root is slender and useless. It grows near springs and wetlands.

**2.** Its leaves, ground up and applied with honey, treat erysipelas and all inflammations; burned when they are dry so as to create fumes, they treat those troubled by a dry cough and orthopnea if opening their mouth wide they should catch the smoke in it and swallow it. It also breaks abscesses in the chest. The root, too, accomplishes the same[58]

[58] Note that in the first paragraph of this chapter the root of colt's foot is said to be useless, ἄχρηστος. It has been suggested that "useless" be read as useful, εὔχρηστος, see Max Wellmann, *Pedanii Dioscuridis Anazarbei De Materia Medica,* Bk. III, p. 124.

when burned as to produce smoke and it expels a dead embryo/fetus when drunk boiled in hydromel.

### III, 113 ἀρτεμισία, *Artemisia arborescens* L., *A. campestris*, *A. genipi* Weber, Wormwood

**1.** Wormwood: by and large, it grows on coastal lands. It is a shrubby herb, very much like *artemisia absinthium*, but having larger and shinier leaves. And one kind of this plant sprouts well, having leaves and shoots that are rather broad, but the other is more delicate, having small and delicate white flowers that are oppressive in scent; it blooms in summer. Some, however, call wormwood the small herb of midlands, which is more slender-stemmed, has a single stalk, is quite small, and is full of flowers of a delicate wax-color. It is more fragrant than the previous one.

**2.** Both warm and thin; when boiled they are suitable to use in sitz baths for drawing the menstrual period, afterbirths, embryos/fetuses, for uterine closing and uterine inflammation, for breaking stones, and for retention of urine. The herb when liberally plastered against the lower part of the abdomen sets the menstrual period in motion. Its juice, triturated with myrrh and applied, draws from the uterus as many things as the sitz bath; the foliage is also given to drink in the amount of three *drachmai* to draw out the same.

### III, 114 ἀμβροσία, *Artemisia maritima* L., Ambrose

Ambrose, which some call *botrys* and others *artemisia.* It is a small shrub with many branches, about three-spans tall, having leaves all around where the stem grows that are small like those of rue; its small twigs are full of seedlets resembling grape clusters that never bloom; it smells like wine. Its root is slender, two-spans long. In Cappadocia, it is weaved in garlands.

It has properties that bind, staunch, and dissipate the accumulations of humors when applied as a plaster.

### III, 115 βότρυς, *Chenopodium botrys* L., Oak of Jerusalem

Oak of Jerusalem: it is a plant entirely quince-yellow, shrubby, not compact, and having many branches; its seed grows all around on all the sprays, the leaves resemble chicory, and the whole plant is quite

fragrant. It is for this reason that it is placed between clothing. It grows mostly near mountain streams and torrents.
When drunk with wine, it is able to relieve orthopnea. The Cappadocians call this plant also *ambrosia* but some call it *artemisia*.

**III, 116 γεράνιον, *Geranium tuberosum* L., Cranesbill**

Cranesbill: its leaf is like that of anemone, split <but> longer. It has a round, sweet, and edible root; an amount of one *drachma* of it drunk with wine stops uterine inflations.
Some call another plant also cranesbill; it has delicate and fuzzy stems that are two-spans tall, leaves resembling those of the mallow, and at the end of the branches they have some upright growths, like heads of cranes or dogs' teeth. It is not used at all in medicine.

**III, 117 γναφάλλιον, *Gnaphalium* L. sp. and *Filago* L. sp., Cottonweed**

Cottonweed: the leaves of which are used as flock of wool because they are white and soft. Its leaves are good for dysentery when given to drink with harsh wine.

**III, 118 τύφη, *Typha* L. sp., Reed mace**

Reed mace: it sends out a leaf like that of galingale and a smooth and uniform stem, surrounded by a dense flower at the top which becomes plumose and which some call *anthele*.
Its flower, compounded with washed and aged pork fat, treats burns. It grows in marshes and in places with stagnant water.

**III, 119 κιρκαία, *Vincetoxicum nigrum* Moench., Black swallow-wort**

Black swallowwort: but some call it *dircaia*. It has leaves like those of hound berry, many offshoots, many small dark flowers, fruit that is like grains of millet, as if in some tiny horns, and roots that are a span long, three or four of them, white, fragrant, and warming; it grows mostly on stony and [breezy,] sunny places.
A quarter of one *mna* of its root, bruised and soaked for a day and a night in six *cotylai* of sweet wine, when drunk for three days, cleanses the uterus; the fruit draws down milk when taken in porridge.

**III, 120 οἰνάνθη *Spiraea filipendula* L., Dropwort**

Dropwort: it has leaves just like the carrot, white flowers, and a thick stem one-span tall; it has fruit just like the orach's and a large root that has many round heads. It grows on rocks.

Its fruit, stem, and leaves are given to drink with honey mixed with wine to drive out the afterbirth, and the root is given with wine for strangury.

**III, 121 κόνυζα, *Inula graveolens* Desf., *I. viscosa* Aiton, *I. Britannic*a L., Fleabane**

**1.** Fleabane: one is called small and smells rather sweet; the other is called bigger, being more sizable as a bush and in foliage; it is broader and oppressive in scent. Both have leaves that resemble the leaves of the olive tree although these are rough and shiny. The stem of the bigger is two-cubits tall and of the smaller one-foot. The flower is airy, quince-yellow, somewhat bitter, and becoming plumose. The roots are useless.

**2.** The shrub with its leaves strewn around and burned as to produce smoke, can chase away wild animals and drive away mosquitoes. It also kills fleas. The leaves are plastered to good avail on those bitten by reptiles, on growths, and on wounds. The flower and leaves are drunk with wine to bring about the menstrual period, to expel embryos/fetuses, for strangury, colic, and jaundice, and they benefit epileptics when drunk with vinegar. Also their decoction treats uterine ailments when used in a sitz bath.

**3.** Used topically, the juice causes abortions. The herb is good also for shiverings when smeared on with olive oil. The small one treats also headaches when plastered on.

There is even a third kind of fleabane; its stem is thicker and softer and its foliage is larger than the small one's but smaller than the bigger one's. It is not shiny, it smells much more oppressive and unpleasant, and it is less efficacious. It grows in wetlands.

**III, 122 ἡμεροκαλλές, *Lilium martagon* L., Martagon lily**

Martagon lily: but some call it *hemerocatallacton.* Its leaves and stem are similar to those of the white lily and green like leeks. On the stem grow three or four flowers, resembling white lilies in the way they are sectioned when they begin to open up; they are of a deep yellow color. It has root like a bulb and it is sizable; reduced into powder and drunk or inserted in a woolen wad, it draws out water and blood. The leaves, ground up and plastered on, assuage breast inflammations that are the result of childbirth and inflammations of the eyes. The root and leaves are beneficially plastered on burns.

**III, 123 λευκόϊον, *Matthiola incana* L., Gillyflower**

The gillyflower is well known. Its flower comes in different colors: for it is found either in white or quince-yellow or purple. Highly useful for medical purposes is the quince-yellow. Boiled when dry, the flowers are good in sitz baths for inflammations in the area of the uterus and for driving out the menstrual period; made up with cerate, they treat anal fissures and with honey the thrush. Its fruit, when drunk in wine in the amount of two *drachmai* or when used as a pessary with honey, draws the menstrual period and embryos/fetuses. The roots reduce the spleen and help the gouty when plastered on with vinegar.

**III, 124 κραταιόγονον, *Polygonum persicaria* L., Willow weed**

Willow weed: it has leaves like those of wheat—very many knotty shoots grow from one root—and seed like millet. By and large, it grows on shady and shrubby places and it is very pungent.

It is reported by some that drinking its seed makes a woman give birth to a boy, if after having had her menstrual period and before intercourse she drank, on an empty stomach, three times a day for 40 days, one *triobolon* of seed with two *cyathoi* of water; but her man, too, must drink it similarly for the same number of days and then he must have sexual intercourse with her.

**III, 125 φύλλον, Mercurialis *perennis* L., Dog mercury**

Dog mercury: it grows on rocks. The kind called *thelygonon* is just like moss, having foliage of a paler color than that of the olive, a delicate and short stem, a delicate root, white flower, and small seed just like the seed of poppy. But the kind called *arregonon*, while it resembles the previous one in all other respects, differs in seed; for it is somewhat similar to an olive that freshly burst into bloom and it is cluster-like.

It is said that the *arregonon* produces males when drunk and that the *thelygonon* females. It is Crateuas who recounts these things, but it seems to me that he says such things from hearsay.

**III, 126 ὄρχις, ~ *Orchis papilionacea* L., ~ *O. longicruris* L., Orchid**

**1.** Orchid: but some people call it *cynos orchis*. It has leaves that are spread on the ground around its stem and base; they are similar to the leaves of the olive but softer, narrower, and longer.[59] The stem is one-span long, bearing purplish flowers. It has a bulbous root that is somewhat long, it has two parts, and it is narrow like an olive. One part is high up, the other lower down, one is full the other soft and shriveled. The root is eaten boiled like a bulb.[60]

**2.** About this plant, too, it is said that men who eat the larger root sire males, and that women eating the smaller give birth to females. And they say that women in Thessaly drink its soft growth with goat's milk to arouse sexual desires, and the dry one to check and abate them, and that the activity of the one is cancelled by the activity of that which is drunk afterwards. It grows on stony and sandy places.

**III, 127 ὄρχις ἕτερος, *Orchis morio* L., Another orchid**

Another orchid which some people call *serapias,*[61] as does Andreas, because its root is highly useful. It has leaves like those of the leek, longish but wider and shiny, a stem that is one-span long, and purplish flowers. The root is below ground, resembling small testicles. It has properties that disperse swellings, cleanse sores, and control shingles when plastered on; it also removes fistulas and it soothes festering sores when plastered on them. Dry, it halts spreading ulcers and it treats both putrid humors and malignancies in the mouth. It also stops diarrhea when drunk in wine. About this orchid there are as many stories told as of the former.

---

[59] The text, ἐλαίᾳ μαλακῇ ὅμοια is corrupt and several codices have different readings. The Latin Dioscorides, has *similia sunt olivae folia ipsa, sed molliora et angusta et longiora.*

[60] The dried roots of many species of orchids are referred to as salep. It contains gum and starch and it is used for food like tapioca and as a demulcent.

[61] *Serapias* derives from the Egyptian god Serapis whose attributes include healing.

**III, 128 σατύριον, *Fritillaria graeca* L., Man orchis**

**1.** Man orchis: but some call it *triphyllon*, because it commonly bears no more than three leaves that bend toward the ground; they resemble the leaves of the monk's rhubarb or of the white lily, but they are smaller and somewhat red; and it has a tall soft stem, about a cubit tall, a lily-like flower that is white, and a bulbous root, as big as an apple and red; internally, however, it is white like an egg; it is tasty and sweet.

One must drink this one in black harsh wine for tetanic recurvation and they say that it is aphrodisiac.

**2.** There is also one called *erythraicon*. Its seed resembles linseed but it is larger, shiny, smooth, and strong; it, too, is reported to be aphrodisiac just like the skink.[62] The rind of its root is somewhat thin and tawny but the root's inner part is white, tasty, and sweet. It grows in sunny and mountainous places. The root is said to be aphrodisiac even when held in the hand but more so when drunk with wine.

**III, 129 ὅρμινον, *Salvia horminum* L., Clary**

Clary: it is an herb that resembles the horehound in foliage; the stem is quadrangular, one-half-cubit tall, surrounded by pod-like excrescences that float over the root, as it were, containing seed that varies: for on the uncultivated clary the seed is round and of a drab color, but on the other, which is the one that is used, it is elongated and black.

When drunk with wine this one, too, is believed to be aphrodisiac. With honey it clears albugo and leucomas, and when plastered on with water it disperses swellings and draws out splinters. The herb does also the same when plastered on. But the uncultivated has greater strength; it is for this reason that it is compounded with ointments, especially with ointment of sweet new wine.

**III, 130 ἡδύσαρον, *Securigera securidaca* L., Axweed**

The axweed which unguent makers call *pelecinos*:[63] it is a shrub having little leaves like the leaves of the chick-pea and pods resembling little horns, wherein lies red seed similar to a two-edged

---

[62] On the skink, see Dsc. Bk. II, 66.

[63] From πέλεκυς, "battle-axe."

battleaxe, whence it was named. It tastes bitter and it is wholesome when drunk. They mix it with antidotes. Applied as a pessary prior to intercourse, it is believed to cause barrenness. It grows among barley and wheat.

**III, 131 ὄνοσμα, *Onosma echinoids* L., Stone bugloss**

Stone bugloss: but some call it *osmada*, others *phlonitis* and others *ononis*. It has leaves similar to those of alkanet, longish, soft, about four-fingers long and one-finger wide, spread on the ground very much like the leaves of alkanet. The plant has neither stem, nor seed, nor thorn; a longish little root is below ground, weak, delicate, and slightly red. It grows in rough terrains

Drunk with wine, its leaves draw embryos/fetuses. They say that a pregnant woman miscarries even if she steps over this plant.

**III, 132 νυμφαία, *Nymphaea alba* L., White water lily**

**1.** White water lily: it grows in marshlands and stagnant waters. It has many leaves from the same root. They are similar to the Egyptian bean but smaller and longer, rising somewhat above water, although some are even in the water itself. The flower is white, like the white lily, with a saffron-colored center. Once it has finished blooming, it becomes round, nearly resembling an apple in its roundness or a poppy head. It contains seed that is broad, firm; it feels sticky to the taster. The stem is smooth, not thick, black, similar to the stem of the Egyptian bean. The root is black, rugged, and club-like. It is harvested in the fall.

**2.** Drunk dry with wine, it benefits the colicky and dysenteric, and it reduces the spleen. The root is plastered on for stomach and bladder pains, it clears dull-white leprosies with water, and it treats bald spots when applied with pitch. The root is also drunk to combat ejaculations during sleep; for it does allay them and it effects a slackness of the genitalia for a few days if one kept on drinking it. The seed, too, accomplishes the same when drunk.

**3.** It seems that it was named from the nymphs because it likes watery places. Much is found at Elis on the river Anigros and at Haliartos of Boeotia.

There is also another water lily that has leaves similar to the leaves of the above, but a root that is white and rugged and a quince-yellow flower that shines and that resembles a rose. Its root and seed drunk in red wine[64] are good for leucorrhea. It grows in areas around Thessaly, by the river Peneios.

**III, 133 ἀνδρόσακες, *Acetabularia mediterranea* L., Sea navel**
Sea navel: it grows in Syria, along the shore. It is a white plant, thin-stemmed, bitter, leafless, having a sack on top that contains seed.
It has properties that draw out much urine from those with edemata when an amount of two *drachmai* is drunk with wine; both the decoction of the plant and the seed do the same when drunk. It is also beneficially plastered on the gouty.

**III, 134 ἄσπληνος, *Ceterach officinarum* Willd., Miltwaste**
**1.** Miltwaste:[65] but some call it *scolopendrion*, others *hemionion*, others *splenion*, and others *pteryga*. It has leaves resembling the creature scolopendra, many growing from one root on rocks and on thick-shaded walls that are made from pebbles; they are stemless, flowerless, fruitless, slit like the leaves of polypody, yellowish and rough on the underside, and greenish on top.
**2.** The leaves, boiled with vinegar and drunk for 40 days, can reduce the spleen; but one must also plaster the spleen with leaves ground up with wine. They can also help for strangury, hiccups, and jaundice, and they break stones in the bladder. When hung about a person by itself or with the hoof of a mule, the plant is thought to cause barrenness. And they say that in order to cause barrenness it must be dug up when the night is moonless.

**III, 135 ἡμιονῖτις, *Scolopendrium hemionitis* Lag., Mule fern**
Mule fern, but some call it *splenion*. It sends out a leaf like that of edderwort, crescent-shaped. It has many delicate roots below the

---

[64] See Dsc. Bk. V, n. 2.
[65] Miltwaste refers to the alleged ability of this plant to reduce the spleen, milt being a synonym for spleen. This plant is also known as spleenwort. Its etymology is also imbedded in its Greek name from alpha privative and σπλήν, "spleen."

ground. It bears neither stem, nor fruit, nor flower. It grows on rocky places. The plant tastes astringent and it reduces the spleen when drunk with vinegar.

**III, 136 ἀνθυλλίς, *Cressa cretica* L., *Ajuga iva* Schreb., *Anthyllis***

**1.** *Anthyllis* is of two kinds: for one kind has leaves very much like those of lentil and twigs that are one-span tall and upright, and its leaves are soft. The root is thin and small. It grows on sandy and sunny places, tasting somewhat salty. The leaves and twigs of the other resemble those of the ground pine although they are rougher and shorter. Its flower is purple, very oppressive in scent, and the root is just like the chicory's.

**2.** An amount of four *drachmai* of root can help those greatly distressed by difficult micturition and kidney disease. Ground up and inserted as a pessary with unguent of roses and milk, the roots soften uterine inflammations. They treat also injuries. The one that resembles ground pine, in addition to its other benefits, also helps epileptics when drunk with oxymel.

**III, 137 ἀνθεμίς, *Chamomilla* sp., Camomile**

**1.** Camomile: but some call it *leucanthemon*, others *eranthemon*, because it blossoms in spring,[66] others *chamaemelon*, because of the similarity of its scent to apples,[67] others *melanthemon,* others *chrysocallia*, and others *callia.* There are three kinds of this plant differing only in flowers; the sprays are one-span tall, shrubby, they have many axils, tiny little leaves, delicate, round little flower heads that have a small, whitish brilliancy in the center, but at the periphery, disposed in a circle are <little petals> the size of rue, that are white or yellow or purple. It grows in rough terrains and by the roadside, and it is collected in the spring.

**2.** The roots, flowers, and greens have warming and thinning properties. When drunk and when used in sitz baths, they draw the menstrual period, embryos/fetuses, stones, and urine. They are given to drink for inflations and for intestinal obstructions, they cleanse

---

[66] From ἔαρ, "spring" and ἄνθεμον, "flower."

[67] From χαμαί, "on the ground" and μῆλον, "apple."

away jaundice, and they treat people with liver disease. Their decoction is also used in vapor baths for the bladder. But for people with stone disease the one that is purple-flowered, which is bigger in every respect and which is properly called *eranthemon*, is more effective; the one called *leucanthemon* is more diuretic as is also the *chrysanthemon.* When plastered on they cure lachrymal fistulas and when chewed they treat the thrush.

**3.** Some, triturating them with oil, use them also as a salve to cure intermittent fevers. You must store them, after chopping the leaves and flowers separately and forming them <into> little lozenges, and you must store the root after you have dried it. When the need arises, you must give sometimes two parts flowers and one part greens or root, and at other times the opposite, <one> part flowers and two parts greens, doubling the amount alternately every other day. It must be drunk in diluted mead.

**III, 138 παρθένιον, *Chrysanthemum parthenium* Bernh., Feverfew**

Feverfew: but some call it *amaracon* and some call this plant, too, *leucanthemon.* It has leaves like those of coriander and flowers that are white around the periphery, but their center is quince-yellow, slightly malodorous, and bitter in taste.

Dried and drunk with vinegar mixed with hydromel or with salt, it is capable of driving phlegm and bile downward just like *epithymon*,[68] and it is beneficial to asthmatics and melancholiacs. The plant without the flower is given to drink with good results to people suffering from stones and asthma and its decoction is a sitz bath for an indurated and inflamed uterus. It is also plastered on with the flowers for erysipelas and inflammations.

**III, 139 βούφθαλμον, *Chrysanthemum coronarium* L., Oxeye**

Oxeye: but some people call it *cachla.* It puts out a tender stem and leaves like those of fennel, quince-yellow flowers, larger than the flowers of chamomile, shaped like eyes, whence it was named. It grows around cities.

---

[68] A parasitic plant that grows on thyme, *Cuscuta epithymum,* See also Dsc. Bk. IV, 177, where its activity is fully discussed.

Its flowers ground with cerate disperse swellings and indurations. And they say that it gives people with jaundice a healthy complexion for a while if they drank it in the bathroom, right after getting out of the tub.

### III, 140 γλυκισίδη, *Paeonia* L. sp., Peony

**1.** Peony: but some call it *pentorobos* and others *Idaioi dactyloi*, and they call its root *paionia*, but others call it *aglaophotis.*
The stem grows two-spans tall, having many offshoots. The male has leaves like those of the walnut, but the leaves of the female are split like those of Cretan alexanders. It also sends out some pods on top of the stem resembling almonds. After they have opened, one finds many small red seeds resembling those of pomegranate, and in the middle they are black tending to purple, five or six.
**2.** The root of the male is about a finger thick, one-span long, binding in taste, and white; but on the female, the roots have seven or eight side-growths like acorns, as the asphodel.
The root is given to women who are not cleansed after giving birth, it draws down the menses when a quantity the size of an almond is drunk, and it helps for belly aches, the jaundiced, people with kidney disease, and those smarting in the bladder when drunk with wine. Boiled down in wine and drunk it stops diarrhea.
**3.** Ten or twelve red seeds of its fruit drunk in harsh red wine[69] stem the red flux, they help people who have stomach problems and gnawing of the stomach when eaten, and they avert the starting of stones when children drink them and eat them. A quantity of 15 black seeds, drunk with a mixture of hydromel or with wine, is good for those who gasp from nightmares,[70] for uterine suffocation, and for uterine pains.

### III, 141 λιθόσπερμον, *Lithospermum officinale* L., Groomwell

Groomwell: but some call it *aetonychon,* others *exonychon,* others *Dios pyros*, and others *Heracleia* on account of the toughness associated with its seed.[71] It has leaves like those of the olive but

---

[69] See Dsc. Bk. V, n. 2.
[70] The nightmare was conceived as a throttling demon.
[71] The reference here is to Hercules.

longer, wider, softer, and the ones near the base lie on the ground; the sprays are erect, slender, having the thickness of the great sea-rush, solid, and woody; at the tips there is a two-pronged growth, resembling a stem, having small leaves, between which there is seed that is stone-like, round, white, and like a small bitter vetch in size. It grows in rough terrains and high elevations.
When drunk with white wine, the seed has properties that break stones and draw out the urine.

**III, 142 φαληρίς, *Phalaris canariensis* L., Canary grass**
Canary grass: it sends up many little stems from thin and useless roots, two-palms tall, knobby, reed-like, resembling the stems of *zea*[72] but thinner and sweet in taste; the leaves also resemble the leaves of *zea*, but the seed it bears is of the size of millet, white, and longish.
This plant when chopped up, converted into juice by means of water or wine, and drunk has properties that help for pains of the bladder. A spoonful of the seed also is good for the same purposes when drunk with water.

**III, 143 ἐρυθρόδανον ἢ ἐρευθέδανον, *Rubia tinctorum* L., *R. peregrina* L., Madder**
**1.** Madder, but some call it *teuthrion*. The root is red and suitable for dyeing. One kind is wild and the other cultivated, as in Ravenna of Italy where it is profitably sown in the middle of marshes because of the large revenues derived from it. Its stems are quadrangular, long, resembling in every respect the stems of cleavers, although they are larger and more vigorous, having the leaves spaced at each joint in a circle like stars. It has round fruit, greenish at first, then red, then as it ripens turning black.
**2.** The root is slender, long, red, and diuretic; it is for this reason that when drunk with hydromel it helps the jaundiced, also those suffering from hip ailments and paralytics; it also drives out much thick urine and at times even blood. But the people who drink it must bathe daily. The stem with the leaves when drunk helps those bitten by wild animals, and the fruit when drunk with oxymel reduces the spleen.

---

[72] On *zea*, see Dsc. Bk. II, 89.

Applied as a pessary, the root draws the menstrual period and embryos/fetuses and treats dull-white leprosies when anointed with vinegar.

**III, 144 λογχῖτις, *Serapias lingua* L., *Lonchitis***

*Lonchitis* has leaves like sliced leek but wider and reddish; very many of them are near the root, bending on the ground, as it were; it also has a few around the stem upon which there are flowers resembling little felt hats, shaped like gaping comic masks; they are black, and there is something white that protrudes from their opening toward the lower lip, as if it were a little tongue. The seed is like a spearhead, triangular and encapsulated, whence it earned its name.[73] The root is like that of *daucos.*[74] It grows in rough and arid lands.
Its root is diuretic when drunk with wine.

**III, 145 λογχῖτις ἑτέρα, *Aspidium lonchitis* L., Holy fern**

Holy fern: it sends out leaves resembling the leaves of miltwaste except rougher, larger, and more incised.
The leaves have the property of healing injuries and of countering inflammations. They also reduce the spleen when drunk with vinegar.

**III, 146 ἀλθαία, *Althaia officinalis* L., Marsh mallow**

**1.** Marsh mallow, which some call *ebiscos*, is a kind of wild mallow; it has rounded leaves like the cyclamen and they are downy; the flower is rose-like, the stem is a cubit tall, and the root sticky and white inside. It was named *althaia*[75] because it can cure many diseases and because it is very useful: for boiled in hydromel or in wine or chopped all by itself, it is good for injuries, tumors of the parotid gland, scrofulous swellings of the glands, abscesses, inflamed breasts, anal <inflammations>, bruises, inflations, and tension in the tendons; for it disperses, it brings to a head, it breaks loose, and it cicatrizes.
**2.** Softened with pork or goose fat and turpentine, after it has been boiled, as indicated, it is good in pessaries for uterine inflammations

---

[73] From λόγχη, "spear-head."
[74] On *daucos, s*ee Dsc. Bk. III, 72.
[75] ἀλθαία from ἀλθαίειν, "to heal."

and closings. Its decoction, too, accomplishes the same, removing the so-called discharges of childbirth. Drunk with wine, the decoction of its root benefits those having difficult micturition, stones, hip ailments, dysenterics, quiverers, people with ruptures, and it assuages toothaches when boiled with vinegar and used as a rinse.

**3.** The seed both fresh and dry, ground and smeared on with vinegar in the sun, clears dull-white leprosies, and with vinegar and oil it is a prophylactic ointment against animal poisons; it is also good for dysentery, for coughing up blood, and for diarrhea. The decoction of its seed is a good drink for bee-stings also for the strokes of all small animals when drunk with sour wine mixed with water or wine. The leaves, too, are plastered with a little olive oil on bites and burns. The root thickens even water when mixed with it ground up and set outdoors.[76]

**III, 147 ἀλκαία, *Malope malacoides* L., Vervain mallow**

Vervain mallow: it, too, is a kind of wild mallow. It has leaves that are cut like those of the vervain, three or four stems that have bark closely resembling the hemp's, a small flower, resembling a rose, and five or six white roots growing sideways, about one-cubit long, which treat dysentery and ruptures when drunk in wine or water.

**III, 148 κάνναβις, *Cannabis sativa* L., Hemp**

Hemp: it is a useful plant in daily life for braiding very strong ropes. It has leaves that nearly resemble those of manna ash, malodorous, long and hollow stems, and round, edible fruit that quells the organ of generation when eaten in large quantities. The juice extracted from it when green and instilled is appropriate for earaches.

**III, 149 ἀγρία κάνναβις, *Althaea cannabina* L., Hemp mallow**

Hemp mallow: it has little shoots resembling those of elm, although they are darker, smaller, and one-cubit tall. Its leaves are like those of the cultivated hemp, but tougher and darker. The flowers are reddish,

---

[76] Marsh mallow is now used as antitussive and to allay inflammations of the gastrointestinal tract. Freshly bruised leaves are used in folk remedies to cover insect bites, see Norman Grainger Bisset, *Herbal Drugs and Phytopharmaceuticals,* p. 64.

resembling those of rose campion. The seed and root are similar to those of the marsh mallow.
The root can soothe inflammations and disperse chalkstones in the joints when plastered on boiled. Its bark, too, is useful for braiding ropes.

### III, 150 ἀνάγυρος, *Anagyris foetida* L., Stinking bean trefoil

**1.** Stinking bean trefoil: but some call it *anagyris* and others *acopon.* It is a shrub, which in foliage and shoots resembles the chaste tree; it is tree-like and it has a very oppressive smell. The flower is like a cabbage; the fruit is in long little horns, kidney-shaped, mottled, and firm. It becomes hard around the time grapes ripen.
**2.** Its leaves, ground up when tender and plastered on, reduce swellings; an amount of one *drachma* is given to drink in grape syrup for asthma and for getting out the afterbirth, embryo/fetus, and the menstrual period; but for strokes of poisonous spiders, it is given with wine. It is also an amulet for women whose labor is difficult. Immediately after giving birth, however, the amulet must be removed and thrown away. The bark of the root disperses and digests. The fruit is a violent emetic when eaten.

### III, 151 κηπαία, *Sedum cepaia* L., *Cepaia*

*Cepaia* resembles purslane, but it has darker leaves and a delicate root. The leaves help those with difficult micturition and those itching in the bladder when drunk with wine; but it is <the root in grape syrup> that is most effective when drunk with the decoction of the roots of the asparagus called *myacanthos.*

### III, 152 ἄλισμα, *Alisma plantago* L., *A. arcuatum* Mich., Water plantain

**1.** Water plantain: but some call it *damasonion* and others *lyron.* It has leaves like those of plantain but narrower and bent back toward the ground; the stem is slender, single, over a cubit tall, having a thyrsus-like little head; the flowers are delicate and pale-yellow, and the roots are like the black hellebore's, thin, fragrant, sharp, and somewhat greasy. It likes moist places.

**2.** A weight of one or two *drachmai* of the root drunk with wine is a suitable antidote for sea hare, toad, and opium; it stops colic and dysentery when drunk by itself or with an equal amount of *daucos*,[77] and it is suitable for spasms and for uterine ailments. The plant stops diarrhea, sets the menstrual period going, and assuages swellings when plastered on.

**III, 153 ὀνοβρυχίς, *Onobrychis caput galli* Link. and *O. viciaefolia* Scop., Cock's head**

Cock's head: the leaves are like those of the lentil but slightly longer, the stem is one-span tall. It has a red flower and a small root. It grows on wet and fallow lands.

Ground up and plastered on, the plant can disperse swellings; drunk with wine, it treats difficult micturition, and it causes sweating when daubed with olive oil.

**III, 154 ὑπερικόν, *Hypericum crispum* L., St. John's wort**

**1.** St. John's wort: but some call it *androsaimon,* others *corion,* and others *chamaipitys* because the smell of its seed resembles that of pine resin.[78] It has leaves similar to those of the rue. It is a bush that belongs to the class of undershrubs, about one-span tall, reddish, bearing a flower that is like a gillyflower, and a capsule that is somewhat hairy, longish in circumference, of the size of barley; it contains black seed smelling of resin. It grows on cultivated lands and on rough terrains.

**2.** It has properties that are diuretic and emmenagogic when it is used as a pessary and it gets rid of quartan fevers when drunk with wine. The seed, drunk for 40 days, treats hip ailments, and the leaves with the seed treat burns when plastered on.

**III, 155 ἄσκυρον, *Hypericum perforatum* L., St. John's wort**

St. John's wort: but some call it *ascyroeides* and others *androsaimon.* This plant, too, is a kind of *hypericon*, differing in size, having bigger

---

[77] *Daucos* seed probably, because it is the seeds of *daucos* that are mostly useful. See Dsc. Bk. III, 72.

[78] The πίτυς element of χαμαιπίτυς means pine.

branches, but they are more twiggy and redder; it bears quince-yellow flowers, fruit like the fruit of *hypericon*, smelling of pine resin, and when crushed staining the fingers as if they were bloody. It is for this reason that it is called *androsaimon.*[79] When drunk with two *cotylai* of hydromel, the fruit of this plant, too, is good for hip ailments. It also draws out much bilious matter and excrement. But it must be given continuously until the patients are cured. It is also good for burns when plastered on.

**III, 156 ἀνδρόσαιμον, *Hypericum perfoliatum* L., St. John's wort**

**1.** St. John's wort: but others call it *Dionysias* and others call this plant, too, *ascyron*. It is different from *hypericon* and *ascyron* in that it is a thin-stemmed and twiggy bush; its little stems are red. The leaves are three times the size of rue releasing a wine colored juice when brayed. It has many branches that have many pinnatifid leaves at the end and that are surrounded by small quince-yellow flowers.

**2.** The seed, in capsules, is like that of corn poppy, striped as it were; the foliage releases a resinous smell when rubbed.

The seed of this plant also drives out bilious matter and excrement when an amount of two *drachmai* is drank ground up. But above all, it treats hip ailments. One must drink <a little> water after the purging. The plant also treats burns and stays bleeding when plastered on.

**III, 157 κόρις, *Hypericum empetrifolium* and ~ *H. coris* L., St. John's wort**

St. John's wort: but some call this plant also *hypericon.* It has a leaf nearly resembling that of heath, except it is smaller and shinier. It is a shrub a span tall, tasty, pungent, and fragrant.

Its seed sets in motion micturition and the menstrual period when drunk. It helps those bitten by venomous spiders, those with hip ailments, and for tetanic recurvation when drunk with wine, but for shivering fits it is drunk with pepper; it is also a suitable ointment with olive oil for tetanic recurvation.

---

[79] *Androsaimon* from ἀνήρ, genitive ἀνδρός, "man" and αἷμα, "blood."

**III, 158 χαμαίπιτυς, *Ajuga hamaepitys Schreb.* L., Ground pine**

**1.** The ground pine, which some people in Pontus call *holocyros*, in Euboea *sideritis*, and in Athens *Ionia*: it is an herb that creeps on the ground and that is humped; it has leaves similar to the houseleek, but thinner, shinier, rough, closely packed around the branches, and smelling like pine, flowers that are delicate and quince-yellow, and a root like that of chicory.

Its leaves treat jaundice when drunk with wine for seven days and they cure hip ailments when drunk for 40 days with hydromel. They are given to liver patients, to people having difficult micturition, and to kidney patients; they are especially well suited also for the colicky.

**2.** The people in Pontic Heracleia use it as antidote and give its decoction to drink for hemlock. It is also plastered for the above conditions with groats soaked in the decoction of the plant. Triturated with figs and given as a little pill, it softens the stool and when combined with roughage and pine resin it purges. Applied in a pessary with honey, it draws matter from the uterus, it disperses indurations of the breasts, it closes wounds, and it keeps shingles in check when daubed with homey.

**3.** There is also another ground pine (mountain germander) which has branches a cubit long, anchor-shaped and thin, foliage and flower like the one before it, and black seed; it, too, smells of pine. There is even a third kind (herb ivy) which is called male. It is a tiny herb having very small, delicate, white, and closely packed little leaves, a rough white stem, little quince-colored flowers, and small seeds near the axils. It, too, smells of pine.

These, too, have the same properties as the above, but not quite as strong.

# BOOK IV

Dear Areios,
In the previous three books we discussed aromatics, oils, unguents, trees, animals, cereals, garden vegetables, roots, plant extracts, herbs, and seeds. In this fourth book we shall talk about the balance of herbs and roots.

### IV, 1 κέστρον, *Stachys officinalis* L., Betony

**1.** The betony, which is called *psychrotrophon*[1] because it is found in very cold places and which the Romans call *bettonica* or *rosmarina.* It is a plant having a slender, quadrangular stock, a cubit tall or even taller, long and soft leaves resembling the leaves of oak, slit in the periphery, and fragrant; the ones near the root are larger. At the top of the stock, lies the seed growing in a spike just like that of savory. Its leaves must be dried after they have been collected. It is the leaves that are mostly used.

**2.** The roots are below ground and they are delicate like the hellebore's; when drunk with hydromel they provoke vomiting that is full of phlegm. One *drachma* of the leaves is given with either hydromel or water for spasms, ruptures, uterine problems, and uterine suffocations; but to people bitten by wild animals three *drachmai* with two *cotylai* of wine are given. When plastered on, the plant benefits those bitten by wild beasts and it is suitable for deadly poisons when one *holce* is drunk with wine. And should one drink it before hand he will not in the least be harmed on ingesting a deadly poison.

**3.** It is both diuretic and it purges the bowels; it treats epileptics, the insane, and people with liver disease when drunk with water, and a weight of one *drachma* drunk with vinegar and honey, treats those with spleen ailments. It even aids digestion if one drank after dinner a dose the size of a bean with boiled honey; it is similarly given also for heartburn and to those with stomach problems to chew and swallow, then they are given diluted wine to gulp down.

---

[1] ψυχρός, "cold" and τροφή, "nourishment".

**4.** A weight of three *obols* is given with one *cyathos* of diluted tepid wine to those spitting blood; to those with hip ailments, with kidney problems, and to those hurting in the bladder it is given with water, and to those with edemata, if they have fever, <a weight of> two *drachmai* is given with hydromel, but if they are fever-free, it is given with honey mixed with wine. When one *drachma* is drunk with wine, it cures the jaundiced and it draws down the menses. Four *drachmai* drunk with ten *cyathoi* of hydromel purge the bowels; it is also good for tuberculars and for those with internal abscesses with honey. The leaves, dried and ground up, must be stored in a clay vessel.

**IV, 2 βρεττανική, *Rumex aquaticus* L., Water dock**

Water dock: it is a plant that has leaves like those of dock but darker, more downy, and astringent in taste; it sends out a stem that is not large and a root that is delicate and short. Juice is extracted from its leaves and the juice is concentrated either in the sun or with fire. It has an astringent property singularly suitable for spreading ulcers in the mouth and in the tonsils.

It is also good for all other conditions that require astringency.

**IV, 3 λυσιμάχειος, *Lysimachia vulgaris*, L., Loosestrife**

Loosestrife: it sends out stems a cubit tall or even taller, slender, and shrubby; at their joints there are outgrowths of delicate leaves that closely resemble the leaves of the willow and that are astringent in taste. It has a purple or a golden flower. It grows in marshlands and near waters.

Because its leaves are astringent, their juice is suitable as a draught and as a clyster for coughing up blood and for dysentery; the plant stops leucorrhea when used in a pessary and is suitable for plugging nosebleeds. It is good both for wounds and for staunching blood. Burned for fumigation, it releases smoke so acrid that it routs reptiles and kills rodents.

**IV, 4 πολύγονον ἄρρεν, *Polygonon aviculare* L., Knotgrass**

**1.** Knotgrass: but some call it *carcinothron*, others *teuthalis*, others *clema*, others *myrtopetalon*, and others *polycarpon.* It is a plant that has many thin, tender sprays covered with joints, creeping on the ground like dog's-tooth grass, and leaves that are like those of rue <but> somewhat longer and softer. It has fruit right next to every leaf, whence it is even called *arren*,[2] and a flower that is either white or purple.

It has astringent and cooling properties. When drunk its juice is suitable for people who spit blood, for diarrhea, for those suffering from cholera, and for patients with strangury. For it does vigorously flush out the urine.

**2.** When drunk with wine it does help both people bitten by wild animals and for intermittent fevers if taken an hour before their access. Applied as a pessary it quells leucorrhea, dispensed drop-by-drop it is suitable for earaches and for suppurating matter, and when boiled in wine and taken with honey, there is nothing like it for genital sores. The leaves are plastered on for heartburn, for spitting blood, for shingles, erysipelas, inflammations, swellings, and for fresh wounds.

### IV, 5 πολύγονον θῆλυ, *Hippuris vulgaris* L., Mare's tail

Mare's tail is a small shrub, single-stemmed, tender, and reed-like, having continuous joints disposed one after the other, as are those of a trumpet,[3] and, in a circle all around the joints, it has prominences resembling small pine needles; the root is useless. It grows near water. It has astringent and cooling properties that are effective for the same conditions as the one before it, except more weakly.

### IV, 6 πολυγόνατον, *Polygonatum verticillatum* All., *P. officinale* All., *P. multiflorum* L., Solomon's seal

Solomon's seal: it grows on mountains. The shrub is taller than a cubit. It has leaves like those of sweet bay but wider and smoother, releasing something tasting like quince or pomegranate with astringency. Next to each outgrowth of leaves, it has white flowers that surpass the number of leaves, joined together at the base. It has a root that is white, soft, long, highly articulated, thick, oppressive in

---

[2] ἄρρεν, "male."

[3] The word used is σάλπιγξ, "trumpet," the musical instrument, which has a smooth surface, instead of σύριγξ, "shepherd's pipe," which has knots or joints.

smell, thick as a finger, and effective for wounds when plastered on. It also removes facial blemishes.

### IV, 7 κληματίς, *Vinca minor* L., Periwinkle

Periwinkle: but some call it *daphnoeides*, others *myrsinoeides*, and others *polygonoeides*. It is a ground cover having long twigs about as thick as those of the club rush and a small leaf resembling sweet bay both in shape and color but a great deal smaller.

Its leaves and stems stop diarrhea and dysentery when drunk with wine. Applied as a pessary with milk and with either unguent of roses or unguent of henna, periwinkle treats uterine pains, stops toothaches when chewed, and helps those bitten by wild animals when used topically. It is reported to help also people bitten by asps when drunk with vinegar. It grows on arid soils.

### IV, 8 πολεμώνιον,[4] ~ *Polemonium caeruleum* L., ~ *Hypericum olympicum* L., Jacob's ladder

**1.** Jacob's ladder: but some call it *Philetairion*[5] and the Cappadocians *chiliodynamon*. It has slender sprays, pinnatifid leaves, a little larger than those of rue and somewhat longer than the leaves of knotgrass or of catmint, and at their tips there are clusters, so to speak, containing the seed, which is black. Its root is thick, whitish, and resembling that of the soapwort. It grows on mountainous and rough terrains.

**2.** Its root is drunk with wine for malignant ulcers and dysentery and with water for difficult micturition and hip disease; a quantity of one *drachma* is given with vinegar for spleen disease.

The root is also worn against the stroke of the scorpion. They say that those who wear it are not struck by scorpions and that they would suffer no harm even if they were struck. It also stops toothaches when chewed.

---

[4] So named from Polemon, King of Pontus, first century B.C. See Pliny, *N. H,* XXV, 64.

[5] From Philetaerus, king of Pergamum, 343-263 B.C. who allegedly discovered it. See Pliny, *N. H.*, 64, XXV.

**IV, 9 σύμφυτον πετραῖον, *Symphytum tuberosum* L., Low pine**
**1.** Low pine: it grows on rocks. It has little sprays resembling those of oregano, delicate leaves, and little heads like those of thyme. The entire plant is woody and fragrant, tastes sweet, and stimulates salivation. It has a long, reddish root, about one-finger thick.
Boiled with hydromel and drunk, this plant thoroughly cleanses impurities from the lung, and it is given with water to those spitting blood and to kidney disease patients.
**2.** It is drunk boiled in wine for dysentery and for the red female discharge, and with vinegar and honey for spasms and ruptures. When chewed it also quenches thirst and it is suitable for roughnesses in the area of the throat. Applied as a plaster it closes fresh wounds, it controls intestinal hernias, and it compacts the meats when boiled with them.

**IV, 10 σύμφυτον ἄλλο, *Symphytum bulbosum*, Comfrey**
**1.** Comfrey, but some call it *pecte*: it sends up a thick stem, two cubits tall or even taller, angular, hollow like that of sow-thistle, around which grow at small intervals downy, narrow, and longish leaves resembling those of the bugloss. But the stem has also at the corners some protuberances, stretching out from leaves, which lie flat at each axil. The flowers are quince yellow and the fruit around the stem is just like that of mullein.
**2.** The entire stem and leaves have a somewhat rough down, causing itching on contact. The roots are below ground, black on the surface but white and slimy inside. It is the roots that are used.
Ground and drunk, they are good for people who spit blood and who have raptures, and they are plastered on for inflammations, being especially beneficial with leaves of groundsel for anal inflammations. Plastered on, they close fresh wounds and they compact meats when boiled with them.

**IV, 11 ὁλόστεον, ~ *Plantago Bellardii* All., ~ *P. albicans* L., Allbone**
Allbone: it is a small herb, about three or four fingers above ground. It has leaves and tendrils that nearly resemble those of hartshorn or dogs-tooth grass and that are astringent, and a root that is as fine as

hair, white, smelling of wine, and four-fingers long. It grows on hillocks.
It, too, when boiled with meats can contract them and it is given to drink with wine for ruptures.

**IV, 12 στοιβή, *Poterium spinosum* L., Thorny burnet**
Thorny burnet: its fruit and leaves are astringent. This is why their decoction is used in clysters for dysenterics; it is also instilled into purulent ears. Plastered on, the leaves benefit eye injuries caused by a blow and stop hemorrhages.

**IV, 13 κλύμενον, *Scorpiurus vermiculatus* L., Bearbind**
Bearbind: it sends out a quadrangular stem like the stem of the bean, leaves somewhat like the plantain's, and little bags on the stem nodding to one another, resembling an iris and tentacles of octopus. The one growing on mountains is best. Juice is extracted from the whole plant together with the root.
When drunk the juice is good for blood spitting, for the colicky, and for the red flow, cooling and binding. It also stops nosebleeds. The little bags, ground up, are efficacious for fresh sores when applied on them until they develop a scar.

**IV, 14 περικλύμενον, *Lonicera etrusca* L., Honeysuckle**
**1.** Honeysuckle: but some call it *splenion* and others call this plant also *clymenon.* It is a plain little shrub, surrounded at intervals by small, whitish, ivy-like leaves, and next to the leaves it has buddings on which there is fruit closely resembling that of ivy, lying recumbent, so to speak, upon the leaf, hard, and difficult to tear off. The root is thick. It grows in tilled lands and hedges and it winds itself around the adjacent shrubs.
**2.** Harvested when ripe and dried in the shade, its fruit is drunk in the amount of one *drachma* with wine for 40 days; it reduces the spleen, it abates fatigue, it is good for orthopnea and hiccups, but from the sixth day, it makes the urine bloody. It also induces a quick delivery. The leaves, too, have the same property, but it is reported that they make people sterile when drunk for 37 days, and they allay shiverings when rubbed on with olive oil during intermittent fevers.

### IV, 15 τρίβολος χερσαῖος, *Tribulus terrestris* L., Caltrops

**1.** Caltrops: it has leaves that are like the leaves of purslane except thinner, its twigs are long, spread along the ground, and on them there are thorns that are stiff and hard. It grows near rivers and on building lots. There is also a kind that is a water plant,[6] growing in rivers, having its foliage above water but hiding its thorn; the leaves are broad, having a long petiole, and the stem is thicker at the top than at the bottom. It has also some hairy growth that is like a spike of wheat; the fruit is tough just like the fruit of the other kind.

**2.** Both cool and are astringent. They are plasters for all kinds of inflammations, and with honey they treat the thrush, putrid humors in the mouth, inflammations of the tonsils, and the gums. Their juice is extracted also for eye medicines. When taken in a drink their unripe fruit benefits also those who have stones. About one *drachma* of the fruit of the land caltrops when drunk and when used as a plaster restores those bitten by vipers and it is suitable to drink with wine for deadly poisons. Its decoction kills even fleas when sprinkled around. The Thracians who live around the Strymon River feed the herb when green to horses and they prepare the fruit, which is sweet and edible, for food, using it instead of bread.

### IV, 16 λειμώνιον, *Beta maritima* L., Sea lavender

Sea lavender: but others call it *neuroeides*. It has leaves like the beet's but slenderer and smaller, ten or more, and a slender stem, upright just like the white lily's, full of red fruit that is astringent in taste. A quantity of one *oxybaphon* of fruit ground up and drunk with wine can benefit those with dysentery and colic and it stems the red discharge. It grows in meadows and marshlands.

### IV, 17 λαγώπουν, *Trifolium arvense* L., Hare's foot trefoil

Hare's foot trefoil: when drunk with wine its property stops diarrhea, but people who run a fever should drink it with water. It is also worn suspended for inflammation of the groin. It grows in garden plots.

---

[6] Water chestnut.

**IV, 18 μήδιον, ~ *Campanula lingulata* L., *Medion***

*Medion* grows in thickly shaded and rocky places. The leaves are like the endive's, the stem is three-cubits tall, the flowers are purplish, large, and round, the seed is small, resembling safflower, and the root is a span long, thick as a cane and astringent in taste. The dried root, ground up and taken as a lozenge with honey for several days, stops the red discharge. But the seed when drunk with wine brings on the menstrual period.

**IV, 19 ἐπιμήδιον, *Epimedion***

*Epimedion* is a stem, not a large one, having leaves that resemble ivy, about ten or twelve; it bears neither fruit nor flower. The roots are thin, black, oppressive in scent, and insipid in taste. It grows in moist places.

Its leaves ground up with olive oil are a plaster for breasts to prevent them from growing, the root causes barrenness, and the leaves, ground up and drunk with wine in the amount of five *drachmai* for five days after the menstrual period, guard against conception.

**IV, 20 ξίφιον, *Gladiolus segetum* Gawler, Corn flag**

**1.** Corn flag: but some call it *phasganion* and others *machairion*,[7] on account of the shape of its leaf; for it does resemble the iris's, although it is smaller and narrower, tapering like a dagger, and fibrous. The plant sends out a stem that is a cubit tall, on which there are purple flowers that are in a row, at a distance from each; it has round seed, two roots, the one pressing upon the other like little bulbs: the lower of these is weak, the upper stronger. It grows mostly on tilled lands.

**2.** The upper root when plastered on with wine and frankincense can draw splinters and thorns and with meal of darnel and hydromel it can disperse swellings of the glands.[8] It is for this reason that it is also mixed with such plasters as disperse swellings. Applied as a pessary, it also brings about the menstrual period. They say that the upper root when drunk with wine rouses sexual appetite, that the lower makes

---

[7] From φασγάνιον, "little sword" and μάχαιρα, "short sword" or "dagger."

[8] See Dsc. Bk. I, n.100.

people sterile, and that the upper is beneficially given in a drink of water to children suffering from intestinal hernias.

**IV, 21 σπαργάνιον, *Sparganium ramosum* Curtis, and *S. simplex* Huds., Bur reed**

Bur reed: it has leaves like those of the corn flag but narrower, more bent, and longer, and at the top of the stem there are little balls, as it were, wherein is the fruit. The root and fruit are given with wine to people bitten by wild animals.

**IV, 22 ξυρίς, *Iris* L. sp., Gladwyn**

**1.** Gladwyn: but others call it *xiris*, others *iris agria*, and the Romans call it *gladiolus*. Its leaf is similar to that of the iris but wider and sharp at the tip; and it has a stem, rising from the middle of the leaves that is a cubit tall and quite thick; on it are triangular pods and on them there is a purple flower, but the part in the middle is red; the fruit, which is in little fig-like sacks, is round, black, and sharp; the root has many joints; it is long, red, and good for injuries and fractures on the head.

**2.** It restores bones and it draws out thorns and all kinds of missiles painlessly when mixed with one-third solution of copper sulfate, one-fifth root of centaury, and enough honey. Plastered on with vinegar it treats both swellings and inflammations. The root is also drunk with grape syrup mixed with seawater for spasms, ruptures, hip ailments, strangury, and diarrhea. The fruit is very diuretic when about a *triobolon* is drunk with wine; it also reduces the spleen when drunk with vinegar.

**IV, 23 ἄγχουσα, *Anchusa tinctoria* L., Alkanet**

**1.** Alkanet, which some call *calyx* and others *onocleia*: it has leaves that nearly resemble the leaves of the lettuce that has pointed leaves. They are thick, rough, dark, and many, growing on the ground from all around the root. They are thorny. The root is thick as a finger becoming red in the summer and staining the hands. It grows in fertile lands.

**2.** The root is astringent; boiled down with wax and olive oil, it is good for burns and old sores. Plastered on with barley groats it treats erysipelas; applied with vinegar it treats both dull-white leprosies and leprosies, and when applied as a pessary it draws down embryos/fetuses. Its decoction is given with honey and water to people with jaundice, kidney disease, and spleen disease if they have fever, <but if they have no fever> it is given to them with wine. The leaves stop diarrhea when drunk with wine. Unguent makers also use the root for thickening perfumes.

**IV, 24 ἄγχουσα ἑτέρα, *Echium diffusum* Sibth., Another alkanet**

Another kind of alkanet, which some called *Alcibiadeion* or *onocheiles*. This one differs from the first in that it has smaller leaves, but they are equally rough and its sprays are slender; on them there is a purplish, somewhat red flower. It has red roots, of a good length, which at the time of the wheat-harvest contain something that looks like blood. It grows in sandy places.

When eaten or taken in drink or plastered on, this plant and its leaves can help people bitten by wild animals, especially by reptiles; and if someone after chewing it spat it out into the mouth of the animal, it kills it.

**IV, 25 ἄγχουσα ἄλλη, *Lithospermum fruticosum* L., Another alkanet**

There is yet another kind of alkanet that resembles the latter except it is smaller and it has a red fruit; if one after chewing the fruit spat it out into the mouth of a reptile, he will kill it. An amount of one *oxybaphon* of the root drunk with hyssop and garden cress expels the flat intestinal worm.

**IV, 26 λυκαψός, *Echium italicum* L. sp., Viper's herb**

Viper's herb: But some called this plant also *anchousa*. It has leaves like those of lettuce, except they are longer, thicker, rougher, and lying down all around the head of the root. It sends up a stalk that is long, rough, and straight that has many offshoots about a cubit long; they, too, are rough. The flowers are small and purple and the root is red and astringent. It grows in plains.

Plastered on with barley groats, the root treats erysipelas and it is sudorific if it is rubbed on ground up with olive oil.

**IV, 27 ἔχιον, Echium *plantagineum* L., *E. rubrum* L., *Echion***

*Echion*: but some call it *Doris* and others call this plant also *Alcibiadeion*. It has leaves that are longish, rough, somewhat thin, resembling the leaves of alkanet but smaller and shiny. The small thorns that are on the leaves make them rough. It has many thin little stems. On either side they have many thin, pinnatifid little leaves, proportionately smaller at the end of the stem. The flowers next to the leaves are purplish; they contain the fruit, which is like the head of a viper; the root is thinner than a finger and somewhat black; when drunk with wine not only it helps those bitten by vipers but it also keeps those who drink it beforehand from being bitten; the same is true of both the leaves and fruit. Taken with wine or porridge, it stops pain of the lower back and it draws down milk.

**IV, 28 ὠκιμοειδές, *Silene gallica* L., Catchfly**

Catchfly: but some people call this one also *echion* or *Philetairion*. It has leaves similar to basil, twigs that are a span long and rough, and pods that nearly resemble the pods of henbane, full of black seed resembling black cumin.

Drunk with wine the seed has the property to treat those bitten by vipers and the other bites of reptiles.[9] It is also given with myrrh and pepper to those suffering from hip ailments. The root is below ground, thin, and useless.

**IV, 29 ἄγρωστις, *Cynodon dactylon* Pers., Dogs-tooth grass**

Dog's-tooth grass: it is a familiar plant; it has small, articulated runners that creep on the ground and that sprout from the stalks, roots that are articulated and sweet, pointed and hard leaves that are as wide as of a small reed and that are fodder for cattle and herds.

Its root, ground up and plastered on, closes wounds; its decoction when drunk is good for colic, difficult micturition, sores in the area of the bladder, and it breaks up stones.

[9] The text reads: καὶ τὰ ἄλλα τῶν ἑρπετῶν δήγματα θεραπεύειν instead of καὶ τά τῶν ἄλλων ἑρπετῶν δήγματα θεραπεύειν.

**IV, 30 καλαμάγρωστις,[10] ~ *Calamagrostis epigeios* Roth, ~ *Sorgum halepense* L., ~ *Dactyloctenium aegyptiacum* Willd. = *Cynosurus aegiptius* L., *Calamagrostis***

*Calamagrostis* is larger than dog's-tooth grass in every respect. It is poisonous to animals that eat it, and that is especially true of the kind of *calamagrostis* that grows in Babylon by the roadsides.

**IV, 31 ἡ δέ ἐν τῷ Παρνασσῷ ἄγρωστις, *Parnassia palustris* L., Grass of Parnassus**

Grass of Parnassus is more branched. It has leaves similar to those of ivy, a white fragrant flower, small seed which is not useless, and five or six roots that are a finger thick, white, soft, and quite sweet. Their juice, boiled with wine and with an equal amount of honey, with half as much myrrh, and with one-third of pepper and frankincense, is an excellent medication for the eyes; it is stored in a brazen box. The decoction of the roots is good for the same conditions as the plant itself. Its seed is highly diuretic and it stops vomiting and diarrhea.

**IV, 32 ἡ δέ ἐν Κιλικίᾳ γεννωμένη [ἄγρωστις], *Hordeum marinum* L., Wall barley**

Wall barley, which they call locally *cinna,* if eaten damp often distends cattle.

**IV, 33 σιδηρῖτις, *Sideritis romana* L., Ironwort**

Ironwort, but some call it *Heracleia.* It is an herb having leaves like those of horehound, but more elongated compared with the leaves of salvia or oak, yet smaller and rough. It sends out quadrangular stalks, a span tall or even taller, not disagreeable in taste and somewhat astringent, on which at intervals are round vertebrae, just like those of horehound, containing black seed. It grows in rocky places.

When plastered on, the leaves have properties that close wounds and control inflammations.

---

[10] See Jacques André, *Les noms des plantes dans la Rome antique*, p. 44, who says that the last of the three possible candidates for this plant, ~ *Dactyloctenium aegyptiacum* Willd. = *Cynosurus aegiptius* L., contains cyanogenetic glucosides that can be, in some cases, toxique to animals.

**IV, 34 ἄλλη σιδηρῖτις, *Sanguisorba minor* Scop. = *Poterium sanguisorba* L., [Another *sideritis*], Burnet**

Burnet: it has sprays that are two-cubits long and delicate, and leaves on long petioles resembling the leaves of the male fern, cloven repeatedly at the end on either side. From the upper axils it has long delicate side-shoots that have at the end a rough and globular head containing seed like that of the beet, but it is rounder and harder.

The property of the leaves of this plant, too, is good for wounds.

**IV, 35 σιδηρῖτις ἑτέρα, *Scrofularia lucida* L., (Another *sideritis)*, Figwort**

Figwort. There is yet another *siderit*is, which Crateuas calls also *Heracleia.* It grows on walls and vineyard; it has from one root many small leaves, similar to coriander, which surround stems that are one-span long, smooth, soft, and whitish with a touch of red. The flowers are red, small, bitter in taste, and slimy.

This plant, too, can close bleeding and fresh wounds when plastered on.

**IV, 36 Ἀχίλλειος, *Achillea millefolium* L., Achilles woundwort**

Achilles woundwort. Some people call even Achilles woundwort *sideritis*. It bears shoots that are a span long or even longer, spindle-shaped, and surrounded by thin little leaves that have frequent slits at the sides; they resemble the leaves of coriander, they are somewhat bitter, slimy, strong-smelling, not unpleasant but medicinal in scent. On top, it has a rounded flower head. The flowers are white, later becoming golden. It grows on fertile lands.

The foliage of this plant, too, when ground up closes bleeding wounds, it relieves inflammations, and it can quell bleeding, including uterine bleeding when applied as a pessary; its decoction is a sitz bath for women suffering from discharges and it is drunk for dysentery.

**IV, 37 βάτος, *Rubus ulmifolius* Schott, Bramble**

The bramble is a familiar plant. The decoction of its branches contracts, desiccates, dyes hair, and stops diarrhea when drunk, keeps in check leucorrhea, and is suitable for the bite of the *plester*.[11] When chewed, the leaves strengthen the gums and heal the thrush; plastered on they keep in check shingles, treat head scurf, prolapses of the eyes, callous lumps, and hemorrhoids, and they are suitable to apply ground up on those with stomach and heart ailments. But its juice, extracted from the stems and leaves and condensed in the sun, will accomplish everything better. The juice of its fully ripened fruit is suitable for mouth ailments, its half-ripe fruit stops diarrhea when eaten, and its flower checks diarrhea when drunk with wine.

### IV, 38 βάτος Ἰδαία, *Rubus idaeus* L., Raspberry

Raspberry: it was named so because a great deal of it grows on Ida. It is much softer than the previous one, having small thorns. But it is also found without thorns.
It can treat the same conditions as the one before it, but its flower, triturated with honey and smeared on eye inflammations, is extremely effective; it also cools erysipelas and it is given in a drink with water to those with stomach problems.

### IV, 39 ἐλξίνη, *Convolvulus arvensis* L., Bindweed

Bindweed: but some people call it *amersine* and others *cissambelon*. It has leaves similar to ivy but smaller, and small sprays wrapping themselves around whatever they can. It grows on fences, vineyards, and in grain fields.
When drunk the juice of its leaves is diarrheic.

### IV, 40 ἐλατίνη, *Linaria spuria* Miller, Cankerwort

Cankerwort: it has leaves similar to the bindweed but smaller, rounder, and downy, and delicate sprays, a span long, five or six from the same root, full of sour tasting leaves. It grows among grains and on cultivated lands.
The leaves when plastered on with barley groats can help inflamed and running eyes. The plant stays dysenteries when boiled and sipped.

[11] A kind of serpent whose bite is poisonous.

**IV, 41 Εὐπατόριος, *Agrimonia eupatoria* L., Agrimony**

**1.** Agrimony: it is a plant that belongs to the class of undershrubs, putting out a single upright shoot that is woody, slender, dark, somewhat rough, and a cubit tall or even taller. Its leaves are at intervals, deeply slit in about five sections or even more, resembling the leaves of cinquefoil or rather of hemp, and they, too, are somewhat dark, serrated at the periphery like a saw.

**2.** The seed grows from around the middle of the stem; it is somewhat hairy and flops downwards so that it clings to clothing when dry.

Its leaves, ground up and plastered on with aged pork fat, treat sores that are hard to cicatrize, and the seed and plant when drunk with wine benefit dysenterics, people suffering from liver disease, and those bitten by reptiles.[12] Some have mistakenly called it *argemonion*; and we say mistakenly because agrimony is different, as we have demonstrated (II 207.)[13]

**IV, 42 πεντέφυλλον, *Potentilla reptans*, L., Cinquefoil**

**1.** Cinquefoil: but some call it *pentapetes*, others *pentatomon*, others *pentadactylon*, others *pseudoselinon*, others *callipetalon*, others *xylolotos*, and others *xylopetalon.* It has sprays that are like dry sticks, slender, a span long, whereon is the fruit. It has leaves resembling the leaves of mint, five on each petiole, rarely more, if ever, split all around in a saw-like manner, and the flower is pale white. It grows on moist places and next to water conduits. It has a reddish root, somewhat longish, thicker than that of black hellebore. It is very useful.

**2.** The decoction of its root reduced to one-third and held in the mouth can stop toothaches, it controls putrid humors in the mouth when used as a rinse, it assuages hoarseness of the trachea when used as a gargle, and it helps for diarrhea, dysentery, and those suffering in the joints and from hip ailments when drunk. Boiled ground up in vinegar and

---

[12] Tea made from its leaves is now used to combat inflammations of the throat, gastroenteritis, and intestinal catarrh. It is also used in small amounts to compound teas for the liver, bile, stomach and kidneys, Norman Grainger Bisset, *Herbal Drugs and Phytopharmaceuticals* p. 50.

[13] This reference in Max Wellmann, *Pedanii Dioscuridis Anazarbei De Materia Medica* Bk. IV, p. 199, is incorrect. The correct reference is II, 176.

plastered, it keeps shingles in check; it disperses scrofulous swellings in the glands,[14] indurations, swellings, aneurisms, abscesses, and erysipelas, and it treats fleshy excrescences in the fingers, callous lumps, and mange. The juice, extracted when the root is soft, is good for ills of the liver and lung and for deadly poisons.

**3.** The leaves are drunk with hydromel or with diluted wine and a little pepper for fits of intermittent fevers: for quartan fevers the leaves of four sprays, for tertian, the leaves of three sprays, and for the quotidian, the leaves of one spray. About 30 leaves when drunk for 30 days help for epilepsy; the juice of the leaves, when drunk for a few days in the amount of three *cyathoi*, quickly cures also jaundice, and the leaves treat fistulas and membranes that grow over the eyes from the inner corner when plastered on with salt. When drunk as well as when applied as a plaster, the plant also helps those suffering from intestinal hernias and it stems bleeding. It is cut for expiations, religious services, and purifications.

### IV, 43 φοῖνιξ, *Lollium perenne* L., Rye grass

Rye grass: but some call it *rhous* and others *anchynops*. Its leaves are like those of barley but shorter and narrower, the ear resembles darnel, the stalks are six-fingers tall in a circle from the root, and it has seven or eight ears. It grows on tilled lands and on newly caulked roofs.

When drunk with harsh wine, it can stay diarrhea, bleeding from the uterus, and excessive flow of urine. Some say that it also stops bleeding when wrapped in red wool and hung around the patient.

### IV, 44 Ἰδαία ῥίζα, *Ruscus hypoglossum*, *Idaia rhiza*

*Idaia rhiza* has leaves like those of butcher's broom and next to them grow, as it were, long tendrils from which grows the flower.

The root of this plant is highly astringent and suitable for such conditions as need astringency. It is drunk both for diarrhea and leucorrhea and it stems all hemorrhaging.

---

[14] See Dsc. Bk. I, n. 100.

**IV, 45 Ῥοδία ῥίζα, *Sedum roseum* Scip., *Rhodia rhiza***

*Rhodia riza* grows in Macedonia; it resembles costusroot, but it is lighter and more uneven, and when reduced into fine particles it releases a scent of roses. Wetted with plain oil of spikenard and placed on the forehead and temples, it is useful to people who have headaches.

**IV, 46 ἵππουρις, *Equisetum silvaticum* L., Horsetail**

**1.** Horsetail: but some call it *anabasion* and others *hephedron.* It grows in moist places and in ditches. It has hollow little stalks, reddish, somewhat rough, solid, divided by joints that grow into each other, and around the stalks there are many stringy and thin leaves. It grows tall, climbing on nearby tree trunks and it hangs from them, spreading itself all around with much black hair like a horse's tail. The root is woody and tough.

**2.** The plant is astringent, wherefore its juice stops nosebleeds and is beneficial for dysentery when drunk with wine; it is also diuretic. Ground up and plastered on, its leaves close bleeding wounds and the root and plant help those who cough, those with orthopnea, and those with ruptures. It is reported that the leaves mend breaks of the intestine, ruptured bladders, and intestinal hernias when drunk with water.

**IV, 47 ἑτέρα ἵππουρις, *Equisetum maximum* Link. = *E. telmateia* Ehr., Another horse tail**

There is also another horsetail, having shorter, whiter, and softer foliage; this one, too, ground up with vinegar, treats wounds.

**IV, 48 κόκκος βαφική, *Quercus coccifera* L., Kermes oak**

Kermes oak: it is a bush belonging to the class of undershrubs to which cling galls, as if they were lentils; these galls are collected and stored. The best gall is the Galatian and the Armenian, then the Asian and the Cilician, and worst of all is the Spanish.

It has an astringent property, suitable for wounds and injuries of tendons when ground up and plastered on with vinegar. In Cilicia, one finds on the oaks <something> like a little snail, which the women there, harvesting with a steel blade, call gall.

**IV, 49 τράγιον, *Pistacia palestina* Boiss., Stinking tutsan**

Stinking tutsan: it grows only on Crete. Its leaves are like those of mastic as are also its shoots and fruit, except they all are smaller. It produces also a sap that closely resembles gum. Its leaves, fruit, and sap when plastered on with wine draw splinters and all imbedded materials, and when drunk treat strangury, break stones in the bladder, and bring on the menstrual period. The amount to take is one *drachma*. And they say that even wild goats that have been shot by arrows when grazing on this herb shed their arrows.

**IV, 50 τράγιον ἄλλο, *Pimpinella tragion* Vill., Pimpinell**

Pimpinell: it has leaves similar to miltwaste and a white, thin root that closely resembles that of the tuberous spurge and that helps dysenterics when eaten either raw or boiled. In the fall, the leaves throw off a smell of he-goat on account of which it was named *tragion*.[15]

**IV, 51 τράγος, *Ephedra distachya* L., *Tragos***

*Tragos*: but some call it *scorpion* and others *targanon*. It grows mostly by the sea. It is a small shrub, not much above ground, a span or more tall, and it has no leaves. On the branches cling small berries, so to speak, that are red, in size like wheat, pointed at one end, and very astringent in taste.

The fruit of this plant, about ten berries, when drunk with wine benefits those suffering in the bowels and women suffering from discharges. After braying it, some mold it into troches for storage and use it this way.

**IV, 52 σχοῖνος ἐλείας, *Scirpus* L. sp., *Juncus* L. sp., Rush**

**1.** There is a rush called *oxyschoinos* that tapers at the end. This plant, too, is of two kinds. For one has no fruit and the other has round, black fruit, and its reeds are thicker and fleshier. There is even a third kind much more fleshy and much more thick than these two, called *holoschoinos*. At the tip, it, too, has fruit resembling the fruit of the previous one.

---

[15] τράγιον akin to τράγος, "he-goat."

**2.** The fruit of both plants roasted and drunk with diluted wine checks diarrhea and the red discharge and promotes micturition; it does, however, give headaches. Plastered on, the tender leaves that grow near the root are suitable for people bitten by poisonous spiders. But the Euripic[16] rush has soporific fruit. One must guard against drinking too much of it for it is a powerful somnifacient.

**IV, 53 λειχήν ὁ ἐπί τῶν πετρῶν, The lichen growing on stones**[17]

The lichen growing on stones: it is a growth attaching itself to dewy stones. When plastered on, it stops bleeding, it assuages inflammations, and it treats the lichen like-eruptions on the skin. It also benefits people with jaundice when smeared with honey on the mouth and tongue and it relieves rheums.

**IV, 54 παρωνυχία, Paronychia Mill. sp., *Paronychia***[18]

*Paronychia* grows on rocks. It is a little shrub similar to wartweed, not as long, but with bigger leaves. It treats whitlow and impetigo contagiosa when the entire plant is plastered on them.

**IV, 55 χρυσοκόμη, *Aster linosyris* Bernh., Immortelle**

Immortelle: but some call it *chrysitis*. It is a little shoot the size of a span, having foliage in clusters, resembling that of hyssop, a shaggy and thin root like the root of black hellebore, tasting not unpleasant, reminiscent of cypress, and somewhat sweetly sour. It grows in shady and stony places.

The root has warming and astringent properties suitable for people with liver disease and for those affected with inflammations of the lungs. It is also taken boiled with hydromel to clean the uterus.

---

[16] The adjective derives from εὔριπος, "any straight or narrow sea, where the flux and reflux is violent, especially the straight that separates Euboea from Boeotia." It also means canal or ditch, LSJ.

[17] In general, the ancients did not identify the various kinds of lichens that attach themselves on rocks, Jacques André, *Les noms des plantes dans la Rome antique,* p. 144.

[18] The name of this plant, *paronychia*, is the same as *paronychia*, "whitlow," one of the aflictions it was reputed to treat.

**IV, 56 χρυσόγονον, *Leontice chrysogonon* L. sp., Black turrnip**
The black turnip: but some call it *iaspis* and others *linon.* It has leaves like those of oak — but the shrub is compact — a flower that nearly resembles the flower of the mullein that is used for making garlands, and a root like a turnip, inside very red but outside black. The root triturated with vinegar and plastered on helps for bites of the shrewmouse.

**IV, 57 ἑλίχρυσον ἢ χρυσάνθεμον, *Helichrysum orientale* L., *H. Stoechas* L., *H. sicelum* L., Gold flower**
Gold flower or *chrysanthemon* or *amaranton* and with which they crown the gods' images. It is a small, <upright>, white shoot, having at intervals narrow leaves like those of wormwood, foliage in a circle, umbels shining like gold, round, as if they were dry clusters, and a thin root. It grows in rough terrains and in places abounding in gullies. The foliage when drunk with wine helps for difficult micturition, bites of reptiles, hip ailments, and ruptures; drunk with wine or with honey mixed with wine, it brings on the menstruation and dissolves blood clots in the bladder or abdomen. It also controls catarrhs when about one *triobolon* is given to drink on an empty stomach with diluted white wine. It is placed even between clothes because it guards them from being eaten by moths.

**IV, 58 ἀγήρατον, *Achillea ageratum* L., Pot marjoram**
Pot marjoram: it is a bush that belongs to the class of undershrubs, measuring two-spans; it is low, plain, resembling a great deal the oregano, having an umbel on which grows a golden, bubble-like flower, smaller than the gold flower. It was named *ageraton*[19] because, by and large, the flower stays unaltered.
Its decoction has a burning property and the herb itself, burned as to produce smoke, is able to draw down the urine and to soften the areas around the uterus.

---

[19] ἀγέρατον, "ageless."

**IV, 59 περιστέριον, *Lycopus europaeus* L., Vervain**

Vervain: it grows in moist places and it seems that it was so named because doves[20] like to spend time near it. It is a plant that has a height of a span or even greater, and leaves that are split and whitish, growing from the stem. It is generally found with a single stem and a single root.

It seems that its leaves, applied as a pessary with either unguent of roses or with fresh pork fat, stop uterine pains. Applied as a cataplasm with vinegar, the plant checks erysipelas, and with honey it controls putrid humors, closes wounds, and cicatrizes wounds that are old.

**IV, 60 ἱερὰ βοτάνη, *Verbena officinalis* L., Holy vervain**

**1.** Holy vervain: some called it *peristereon.* It sends out shoots that are one-cubit tall or even taller, angular and knobby, surrounded at intervals by leaves resembling oak leaves, except they are narrower, less indented at the periphery, and grayish; it has a somewhat long and slender root.

Its leaves and root, when drunk with wine and when applied as a plaster, are good for bites of reptiles. For jaundice, about one *drachma* of the leaves is drunk on an empty stomach with one *triobolon* of frankincense and one *cotyle* of aged warm wine for four days. The leaves assuage both chronic swellings and inflammations, and they cleanse filthy sores.

**2.** The entire plant, boiled in wine, breaks off tonsillar scabs, stops spreading ulcers of the mouth when used as a gargle, and its infusion sprinkled around at a drinking party is said to make the guests merrier. The third joint from the ground with the surrounding leaves is given to people who have tertian fever and the fourth to those who have quartan. It is called sacred herb[21] because it is used in amulets during purificatory offerings.

**IV, 61 ἀστράγαλος, *Astragalos* L. sp., Milk vetch**

Milk vetch: it is a small shrub, a ground cover, resembling the chick-pea in foliage and sprigs. The flowers are purple and small. The root is

---

[20] The name of this plant, περιστέριον, is from περιστέρα, "pigeon" or "dove."

[21] This is the literal translation of ἱερὰ βοτάνη.

below ground, round just like a good-sized radish, having firm offshoots that are black, hard as horns, entwined with each other, and astringent in taste. It grows in places sheltered from the wind, shady, and snowy; a great deal of it grows at Pheneos of Arcadia.
When drunk in wine, the root stems diarrhea and moves the urine; sprinkled dry, it is good for old sores and checks bleeding. But it is brayed with difficulty because of its toughness.

**IV, 62 ὑάκινθος, *Scilla bifolia* L., Wild hyacinth**

Wild hyacinth:[22] it has leaves like those of purse-tassels, a stem that is a span tall, smooth, thinner than the little finger, pale-green, and a curled, overhanging top full of purplish flowers. The root, too, is like the root of purse-tassels; when plastered with white wine on young boys, it is believed to keep them from coming to manhood and when drunk it stems diarrhea, it is diuretic, and it benefits those bitten by poisonous spiders. Since the fruit is rather astringent, it, too, helps those suffering in the bowels and it clears away jaundice when drunk with wine.

**IV, 63 μήκων ῥοιάς, *Papaver rhoeas* L., Corn poppy**

**1.** Corn poppy: it has been so named because it quickly loses its flower.[23] It grows on tilled fields in the spring, at which time it is also collected. Its leaves are similar to those of chicory or of Cretan thyme, incised, but longer and rougher. It has a stringy stem, erect, rough, about a cubit tall, and a red flower, but sometimes it is white, resembling the scarlet windflower. The head is elongated, yet less so than the head of the poppy, the fruit is red, and the root is longish, whitish, having the thickness of the small finger, and bitter.
**2.** After boiling five or six of its heads in three *cyathoi* of wine until reduced to two, give it to those you wish to fall asleep. An amount of one *oxybaphon* of its seed, drunk with hydromel, gently softens the bowel and it is mixed both with honey-cakes and tortes for the same purpose. The leaves together with the heads treat inflammations when

---

[22] Also known as bluebell.

[23] Μήκων, generic name for poppy; ῥοιάς is cognate with ῥέω, "flow or drop off."

plastered on. Their decoction, too, is soporific when poured on a patient.

### IV, 64 μήκων, *Papaver somniferum* L., Opium poppy

**1.** Opium poppy: there is one kind that is cultivated and that is grown in gardens; its seed is used roasted for a health-promoting diet; they also use it with honey instead of sesame; it is called *thylacitis,* having an oblong little head and its seed is white. And there is another kind that is wild, having a capsule that hangs down, and black seed; this one is also called *pithitis,* but some call even this one *rhoias*, because of the juice that flows from it.[24] A third kind is wilder, smaller, and more medicinal than these, having the capsule oblong.

**2.** Their common property is cooling; it is for this reason that the leaves and capsules, boiled in water and fomented, are soporific; the decoction is also drunk for insomnia and the capsules, ground up and mixed with barley groats, are suitable for inflammations and erysipelas. Brayed when green, they must be molded into little troches, and after they have dried, they must be stored and so used. The capsules, boiled in water until they are half-cooked, then boiled again with honey until the liquid condenses, make anodyne lozenges for coughs, rheums of the trachea, and for conditions relating to the abdomen.

**3.** And it does become more effective if one mixed with it juice of hypocist and of shittah tree. The seed of the black poppy, ground up, is given to drink with wine for diarrhea and leucorrhea, and it is plastered on with water on the forehead and temples of insomniacs. And the juice, since it, too, cools a great deal, befuddles, and dries, taken in an amount as small as a bitter vetch is analgesic, soporific, helpful for digestion, and comes to the aid of coughs and abdominal conditions; but when too much of it is drunk, it plunges into a coma and it is deadly.

**4.** Soaked with unguent of roses, it is good also for headaches, but for earaches it is good when instilled with unguent of almonds, saffron, and myrrh; it is good for eye inflammations with a boiled egg yolk and saffron, for erysipelas and wounds with vinegar, and for gout with

---

[24] See Dsc. Bk. IV, n. 23.

a woman's milk and saffron. Inserted into the anus as a suppository, it is soporific.

**5.** The best juice is thick and heavy, it induces sleep when smelled, it is bitter in taste, it easily dissolves in water, it is smooth, white, not rough nor lumpy, nor hardens when soaked as does wax. Additionally, it flows easily when exposed to the sun, when dripped on a lamp the flame is not dark-colored, and it preserves the intensity of its scent after it has been quenched. Some, however, adulterate it by mixing it with juice of horned poppy or with gum or with juice of wild lettuce. But the juice that is mixed with juice of horned poppy is yellow, the one made with juice of wild lettuce is faint in scent and rather rough, and the one with gum is weak and translucent.

**6.** Some reach such madness as to mix even suet with it. It is roasted for eye medication in a new clay vessel until it becomes soft and appears to be of a more orange-tawny color. You should know, however, that Diagoras says that Erasistratos rejects its use for earaches and ophthalmia because it weakens the sight and it is soporific. Andreas says that if it were not adulterated those anointed with it would be blinded, and Mnesidamos that the only suitable use of it is for sleep through smell, otherwise it is harmful; these assertions are decidedly false, being refuted by experience, because the efficacy of a drug is confirmed by its performance.

**7.** Nor is it inappropriate to describe also how they collect the juice: and so, some people after braying the capsules together with the leaves squeeze them through a press and after pounding them in a mortar they shape them into troches. Such a product is called *meconion*; it is less efficacious than the juice. In extracting the juice after the dew dried off, it is necessary to scratch all around the capsule with a knife in a way as not to pierce through its inner part and to make superficially straight cuts at the side of the capsule, then wipe up the tear that flows with the finger into a spoon and repeat the process shortly thereafter; for a tear is found formed, and it is found also on the following day. This, too, must be pounded in a mortar, shaped, and stored. But, as the cuts are made, one must stand back so that the juice does not come in contact with the clothing.

**IV, 65 μήκων κερατῖτις, *Glaucium flavum* L., Horned poppy**

**1.** The horned poppy which some call *paralios* and others *agria mecon*: it has pale leaves, rough, they are like the leaves of mullein, swollen at the periphery just like the leaves of wild poppy and similar in stem. The flower is pale-yellow; it has a small fruit, curved like a horn, similar to the fruit of fenugreek from which it was named.[25] It has small black seed, like that of opium poppy, and a root that grows close to the surface and that is black thick. It grows in coastal and rugged places.

**2.** The root, boiled in water until the water is reduced by half and drunk,[26] has properties that treat hip ailments and liver diseases and that benefit those passing thick or filamentary water. A quantity of one *oxybaphon* of seed drunk with hydromel mildly purges the bowel. The leaves and flowers plastered on with olive oil break off all around scabs, and when smeared on wipe off albugo and cloud-like opacities on the eyes of animals. Some have been mistaken in thinking that *glaucion*[27] is made from it on account of the similarity of their leaves.

**IV, 66 μήκων ἀφρώδης, *Silene inflata* Sm. and *S. muscipula* L., Frothy poppy**

The frothy poppy, called by some *Heracleia*, has a stem a span tall, very small leaves like those of soapwort and next to them white fruit — the entire little plant is white and frothy — and it has a thin root close to the surface. Its fruit is collected in the summer, when fully ripe, and it is stored after it has dried.

A quantity of one *oxybaphon* taken with hydromel purges through vomiting; this type of purging is especially suitable for epileptics.

**IV, 67 ὑπήκοον, *Hypecoum procumbens* L., Horned cumin**

Horned cumin: it grows among grains and on tilled lands. The leaf is like that of rue and the sprigs are small.

It has properties comparable to those of the juice of opium poppy.

---

[25] κερατῖτις, "horned."

[26] "drunk" refers to the root and it is the water in which the root was boiled that is drunk.

[27] See Dsc. Bk. III, 86.

**IV, 68 ὑοσκύαμος, *Hyoscyamus* sp., L., Henbane**

**1.** Henbane: but some call it *adamanta*. It is a shrub that sends out thick stems and its leaves are wide, oblong, split, dark, and rough. The flowers, which are fenced in with little disks, grow on the stem in a row, just like the flowers of the pomegranate; they are full of seed like the flower of opium poppy. There are three kinds of this plant: for one kind has somewhat purple flowers, leaves like bindweed, black seed, and the calyces are hard and thorny; another has quince-yellow flowers, softer leaves and capsules, and yellowish seed like hedge-mustard.

**2.** Both these plants cause madness and are soporific; they are difficult to use. But the third one is highly useful for treatments, being very mild, fatty, soft, and downy, having white flowers and the seed is white; it grows by the sea and among ruins.

Therefore, it is the one with the white seed that must be used; if this kind is unavailable, then the kind with the yellow seed must be used, but the henbane with black seed must be rejected as being the worst. Juice is extracted from fruit that is soft, from the leaves, and from the stems after braying and pressing them, and the liquid is dried in the sun. It is good for one year because it spoils easily.

**3.** But juice is also extracted separately from the seed, which is brayed when dry, doused with hot water, and squeezed. The juice is better than poppy juice and a more powerful analgesic. The first green shoots pounded and mixed with this year's flour are shaped into little pastilles and stored.

The juice and the juice from the dry seed are primarily suitable for analgesic pessaries, for severe and fevered rheums, for earaches, for ailments associated with the uterus, and with meal or with barley groats for inflammations of the eyes, of the feet, and for the other <inflammations>.

**4.** The seed also offers the same cures, being good for coughs, catarrh, running eyes, and for severe pain; also for the female flow and for the other bleedings when an amount of one *obol* is drunk with poppy seed and hydromel. It is also suitable for gout, for swollen testicles, and for swollen breasts during pregnancy when applied as a plaster ground up with wine, and it is mixed beneficially into the other pain allaying plasters. The molded leaves are useful for all the other anodyne plasters when mixed with barley groats or when plastered on by themselves; but the fresh leaves applied as a plaster are most effective analgesics for all pains.

**5.** Three or four taken in a drink with wine, treat shivering fits of fevers, but if a bowlful of them is eaten boiled like vegetables, they cause delirium. And they say that if one uses them in a clyster on a person with a colon ulcer, they cause the same. The root boiled with vinegar is a mouthwash for toothaches.

### IV, 69 ψύλλιον, *Plantago psyllium* L., and *P. cynops* L., Fleawort

**1.** The fleawort: but some call it *cynocephalon*, the Sicilians *crystallion*, and others *cynomyia*. It has a leaf isimilar to that of the hartshorn, it is rough, and it has branches that are a span long. Also, it is an entirely grass-like little herb. Its foliage starts from the middle of the stem. On top there are two or three compact little heads which contain the seed and which is like fleas, black, and hard. It grows on tilled lands.

**2.** It has a cooling property. Applied as a plaster with unguent of roses, vinegar, and water, it is beneficial for joint diseases, tumors of the parotid glands, growths, swellings, sprains, and headaches, and when plastered on it cures children's hernias and protruding navels. After triturating a quantity of one *oxybaphon,* one must soak it in two *cotylai* of water and when the water has thickened one must plaster it on; it chills considerably.

### IV, 70 στρύχνον κηπαῖον, *Solanum nigrum* L., Hound's berry

**1.** Hound's berry: it is edible. It is a little shrub, having many branches, dark leaves, larger and wider than those of basil, and round fruit, either pale-green or black; it becomes pale-yellow after it has ripened. The herb is inoffensive in taste.

It has a cooling property, whence the leaves are a suitable plaster with very fine meal of barley for erysipelas and shingles; ground up and applied by themselves, they treat lachrymal fistulas, they help for headaches and heartburn, and they dissipate tumors of the parotid glands when plastered on ground with salt.

**2.** Its juice, too, is good for erysipelas and shingles with white lead, litharge, and unguent of roses; but for lachrymal fistulas it is used with bread. It is also good for children suffering from heatstroke, being sprinkled on with unguent of roses. It is mixed also, instead of water or egg, with eye-salves that are used in ointments for severe fluxes and it is good for earaches when instilled. It also stems leucorrhea.

**IV, 71 ἕτερον στρύχνον, *Physalis alkekengi* L., Another hound's berry = Winter cherry**

Winter cherry: there is also another hound's berry, which they call idiomatically *halicaccabon.* It has leaves similar to those of the above but wider. Its stems bend toward the ground when they have grown big. It has fruit in small round capsules that resemble bladders; it is yellowish-red, round, and smooth like a grape. Wreath makers use it in plaiting their wreaths.

Its properties and uses are the same as of the hound's berry mentioned above but it is not edible. Being diuretic, its fruit can clear jaundice when drunk. Juice is extracted from both plants and it is dried in the shade for storage. It is good for the same purposes.

**IV, 72 στρύχνον ὑπνωτικόν, *Withania somnifera* Dun., Sleepy nightshade**

**1.** Sleepy nightshade: but some call it *halicaccabon* and others *caccalia.* It is a shrub that has many branches, thick, trunk-like, hard to break, full of fatty leaves resembling the leaves of quince, a red flower that is sizable, saffron-colored fruit that is in pods, and a sizable root that has a reddish peel. It grows in stony places.

**2.** An amount of one *drachma* of its root's peel drunk in wine has a soporific property that is milder than that of the juice of opium poppy, and its fruit is very diuretic. A cluster of about 12 fruits is given to those with edemata, but when more are drunk they cause severe mental distress. Drinking large quantities of hydromel helps. Its peel is mixed also with analgesics and lozenges and it helps for toothaches when boiled down in wine and held in the mouth. The juice of the root anointed with honey allays dim-sightedness.

**IV, 73 στρύχνον μανικόν, *Datura stramonium* L., Thorn apple**

**1.** Thorn apple which some called *perseion,* others *perisson*, others *anydron*, others *pentodryon*, others *enory*, others *thryon*, and others *orthogyion*. Its leaf closely resembles that of the rocket, but it is bigger, more like the leaf of the thorn called *paideros*.[28] It sends out very tall stalks from the <same> root, 10 or 12 of them, about six-feet tall, a head that lies on top just like an olive, but rougher, as if it were the globular catkin of the plane tree, but bigger and broader, and a black flower.

**2.** This is followed by clusters of fruit, round, black — 10 or 12 berries like the corymbs of ivy — and soft like a grape. The root is below, white, thick, hollow, about a cubit long; it grows in areas that are mountainous, exposed to the wind, and among groves of plane trees.

The root has a property that causes not unpleasant fantasies when a quantity of one *drachma* is drunk with wine, but when a quantity of two *drachmai* is drunk, it drives a person out of his senses for up to three days; and if a quantity of four *drachmai* is drunk, it kills; drinking and vomiting large quantities of hydromel is its antidote.

### IV, 74 δορύκνιον, *Convulvulus oleaefolius* Desr. *Dorycnion*

*Dorycnion,* which Crateuas calls *hallicaccabon* or *calleas*. It is a shrub similar to a newly sprouting olive tree, having branches shorter than a cubit, leaves nearly resembling the olive's in color, but smaller, narrower, and very rough, and a white flower; at the top it has little seed-capsules, firm like chick-peas, enclosing round seedlets, five or six, in size like small bitter vetch seeds, smooth, strong, and pied. It has a root a finger thick and a cubit long. It grows on rocks not far from the sea.

This, too, seems to be soporific and to kill if taken in excess. Some say also that its seed is taken for love-potions.

### IV, 75 μανδραγόρας, *Mandragora* L. sp., Mandrake

**1.** Mandrake: but some call it *antimimon*, others *bombochylon,* and others *Circaia* because its root seems to be good for making love-potions. One kind of this plant is female, the black one, called *thridacias*, having leaves narrower and smaller than the leaves of lettuce, fetid and heavy in scent, streaming on the ground, and among

---

[28] Described in Dsc. Bk. III, 17. n

them fruit resembling sorb apples, pale-green in color, sweet-smelling, containing seed like the seed of the pear. The roots are sizable, two or three entwined with each other, black on the surface but white inside, having thick skin. It has no stem.

**2.** The leaves of the male and the on that is white, which some called *morion*, are white, large, broad, and smooth like the leaves of beet; its fruit is twice as large, saffron in color, and somewhat oppressively fragrant; shepherds eat it and are reduced to a state of stupor; the root is like that of the former, but bigger and whiter. It, too, is stemless.

**3.** Juice is extracted from the skin of the root when fresh, by chopping it and putting it under a press. After it has been condensed, it must be stored in a clay vessel. Juice is extracted also from the fruit in a similar fashion, but the juice from the fruit becomes weak. The skin is also peeled from the root, threaded with a linen thread, and hung for later use. But some boil down the roots with wine until reduced to one-third, strain, and store, administering about one *cyathos* to insomniacs, to those in much pain, and to those they wish to anesthetize either for surgery or cauterization.

A quantity of two *obols* of its juice drunk with hydromel brings up phlegm and bile as hellebore does; but when too much of it is drunk, it is lethal.

**4.** It is compounded with ophthalmic and analgesic medications and with emollient pessaries; about one *hemiobolon* inserted by itself as a pessary, draws the menstrual period and embryos/fetuses; and when placed in the anus as a suppository it is soporific. The root boiled with ivory for six hours is said to soften the ivory and to make it malleable enough for molding into whatever shape one may wish. When new, the leaves are suitable plasters with barley groats both for inflammations of the eyes and for inflammations of sores; they dissipate all indurations and abscesses, scrofulous swellings of the glands, growths, and when gently rubbed on for five or six days they erase blemishes without ulceration; the leaves are also put up cured for the same uses.

**5.** The root, ground up with vinegar, cures erysipelas, it is good with either honey or oil for strokes of reptiles. With water it disperses scrofulous growths and tumors and with barley groats it puts an end to pains of the joints. From the skin of the root they also make, without boiling, a wine: one must cast three *mnai* of root skin into one *metretes of* sweet wine and give three *cyathoi* of it to those about to undergo surgery or cautery, as indicated above. For they become unaware of the pain because they sink into deep sleep.

**6.** Its fruit is soporific when eaten as well as when smelled, as is also its juice, but eaten to excess it even makes people unable to speak. The seed of the fruit cleanses the uterus when drunk and it stops the red discharge when inserted with native sulfur. Milky juice is extracted by making a groove all around the root and collecting the liquid that runs in the hollow. The juice is stronger than the milky juice. The roots do not have milky juice in every place. It is experience that teaches that sort of thing.

**7.** Some note that there is yet another *morion* that grows in shady places and around caves, having leaves like those of white mandrake but smaller, about a span long, white, growing in a circle around the root, which is soft and white, slightly longer than a span, and thick as a thumb; they say that it stupefies when as much as one *drachma* is drunk or when eaten in a lump of barley or in prepared food; for the person falls asleep in whatever posture he was when he ate it, feeling nothing for three or four hours from the time it was offered to him. Physicians about to perform surgery or cautery use this one, too. They say that the root is also an antidote when drunk with thorn apple.

### IV, 76 ἀκόνιτον, ~ *Doronicum pardalianches* Jacq., Leopard's bane

Leopard's bane, but some call it *pardalianches,* others *cammaron*, others *thelyphonon*, others *cynoctonon*, and others *myoctonon*: it has three or four leaves like the leaves of cyclamen or of the cucumber, but smaller and not as rough; the stem is a span tall; the root is like a scorpion's tail and shining like alabaster.

They say that when the root is brought near a scorpion it paralyzes it and that it stirs again when white hellebore is set before it. It is mixed with analgesic medications for the eyes and it kills leopards, swine, wolves, and every wild animal when placed on slices of meat and thrown to them.

**IV, 77 ἀκόνιτον ἕτερον, *Aconitum napellus* L., Wolfsbane**

Wolfsbane, which some call *lycoctonon*: it grows in large quantities in Italy, on the mountains called Vestini, and it is different from the one before it. It has leaves like the leaves of the plane tree, but more incised and a great deal smaller and darker, and a stem like the shoot of a male fern, smooth, a cubit tall or even taller. It has fruit in somewhat elongated pods and roots like black legs of shrimp, which they use for hunting wolves, placing them on raw meats: for they are deadly to the wolves that eat them.

**IV, 78 κώνειον, *Conium maculatum* L., Hemlock**

**1.** Hemlock: it sends up a large stem, knotty like fennel, leaves resembling those of giant fennel but narrower and oppressive in scent; at the top it has side-shoots and umbels of whitish flowers; it has seed like that of anise but whiter, and a root that is hollow and not deep.
This one, too, belongs to the plants that are deadly, killing by chilling through and through; unmixed wine, however, does come to the rescue. Before the seed has dried out, juice is extracted from the top foliage. After it is cut, it is pressed, and the juice is condensed in the sun.
**2.** Having been dried, the juice is highly useful for restoring health when mixed carefully with analgesic salves and it quells shingles and erysipelas when plastered on. The plant ground up with its foliage and applied on the testicles come to the aid of those emitting their semen during sleep; plastered on, they relax the genitalia, they dry up the milk, they prevent maidenly breasts from growing big, and they make boys' testicles wither. Most potent are the Cretan, Megarian, Attic, and those growing in Chios and Cilicia.

**IV, 79 σμῖλαξ, *Taxus baccata* L., Yew**

Yew: but some call it *smilos,* others [*tithymalos*,] and the Romans *taxus.* It is a tree that nearly resembles the fir in foliage and size, growing in Italy and in Narbonne next to Spain. Little birds choke when they eat the fruit of the one growing in Italy and people who eat it come down with diarrhea. But the one that grows in Narbonne possesses such great strength that even those who sit or fall asleep under it are harmed, and they often even die. It is mentioned so that one guards against it.

### IV, 80 ἀπόκυνον, *Cynanchum acutum* L. and for the Orient, *Marsdenia erecta* R. Br. = *Cynanchum erectum* L., Dogbane

Dogbane, but some call it *cynanchon,* others *pardalianches*, others *cynomoron*, and others *cynocrambe*: it is a sprout that has long rods, willow-like and hard-to-break, and leaves like those of ivy but softer and more pointed at the tip, oppressive in scent, somewhat slippery, and full of quince-yellow juice. The fruit is like a bean pod; it is about a finger long and it resembles a bag containing small, hard, black seedlets.

Its leaves, molded into patties with suet and thrown out as bait, kill dogs, wolves, foxes, and leopards; it immediately paralyzes their hips.

### IV, 81 νήριον, *Nerium oleander* L., Oleander

**1.** Oleander: but some call it *rhododendron* and others *rhododaphne*. It is a familiar shrub having longer, thicker, and rougher leaves than those of the almond tree, a rose-like flower, fruit like a horn, which when open is full of a wool-like substance resembling the down of thistles; the root is tapering and long and tastes salty. It grows in gardens, by the seaside, and along rivers.

**2.** And while its flower and leaves have a property that is poisonous to asses, mules, and to most quadrupeds, it protects human beings from bites of wild beasts when they are drunk with wine, and especially if <a touch> of rue was mixed with them. But the weaker animals, like goats and sheep, die even if they should drink their infusion.

### IV, 82 μύκητες, Mushrooms

**1.** Mushrooms fall into two categories, for they are either edible or poisonous. They become poisonous for many reasons: namely, either because they are growing next to rusty nails or next to rotting rags or next to nests of reptiles or next to particularly harmful trees. These sorts of mushroom have also a glutinous crust and should they be stored after it has been removed, they rot away and quickly spoil. But the mushrooms that are not of this kind are sweet and are used for

soups. Yet, even these are harmful when eaten in large quantities because they are difficult to digest and cause choking or nausea.
**2.** But all are helped when given to drink soda and olive oil, or sand with vinegar and brine sauce, or a decoction of savory or oregano, or bird dung with vinegar, or a great deal of honey to suck. They are nourishing and hard to dissolve and, by and large, they are evacuated whole with the excrements.

### IV, 83 Κολχικόν, *Colchicum* L. sp., Meadow saffron

**1.** Meadow saffron: but some call it *bolbos agrios* and others *ephemeron*. At the end of autumn it sends out a white flower like the flower of saffron; later it bears leaves very nearly like those of purse tassels but fatter, it has a stem that is a span tall, having red fruit, and a root which has a pale-yellow, somewhat darkish skin. When its skin is peeled, the root is found to be white, soft, sweet, and full of juice. The bulb has a moderate crevice through which it sends forth its flower.
**2.** It grows abundantly in Colchian lands and in Messenia. When eaten, it kills by choking, as do the mushrooms. And I have described it lest it be eaten unwittingly instead of purse tassels: for it is so pleasing that it is uncommonly alluring to the inexperienced. All antidotes that help those who have eaten mushrooms also help those who have eaten meadow saffron, as does also drinking cow's milk, so that when milk is available there is no need of any other help.

### IV, 84 ἐφήμερον, *Polygonatum multiflorium* All. and *P. verticillatum* All., *Ephemeron*

*Ephemeron*: but others call it *iris agria.* Its has leaves and a stem like the white lily's, but more delicate; it has small, white flowers, and soft fruit. The root lies below ground, single, and thick as a finger, long, astringent, and fragrant. It grows in thickets and shady places.
Its root, used as a rinse, is a medicine for toothache, and its leaves, boiled in wine and plastered on, dissipate swellings and growths that do not have pus.

### IV, 85 ἑλξίνη, *Parietaria officinalis* L., Pellitory

**1.** Pellitory: but some call it *parthenion*, others *perdicion*, others *sideritis*, others *Heracleia*, others *hygieine agria*, others *clybatis*, and

others *polyonymon*. It grows around copings and walls. It has delicate reddish little stems and leaves similar to the leaves of mercury, rough; around the stems there are prickly seedlets, so to speak, that attach themselves onto clothing.
The leaves have cooling and astringent properties; this is why when plastered on they treat erysipelas, callous lumps, fiery inflammations, incipient swellings of the glands, and all inflammations and swellings.
**2.** Its juice, smeared on with white lead, is good for erysipelas and shingles, also for gout when made up with cerate of henna or with goat's fat. About one *cyathos* of juice when swallowed helps for chronic coughs, is a useful gargle and salve for inflamed tonsils, and it is beneficially instilled with unguent of roses for earaches.

### IV, 86 ἀλσίνη, *Thelygonum cynocrambe* L. = *Cynocrambe prostrata* Gaertn., Lichwort

Lichwort: some call it *myos ota*[29] from the similarity of its leaves to mouse ears, but it is called *alsine*[30] because it favors shady places and woodlands. It is an herb resembling the pellitory, but it is shorter and it has smaller leaves that are not rough and smell of cucumbers when bruised.
It has cooling and astringent properties that are suitable for inflammations of the eyes when applied with barley groats and for earaches when its juice is instilled. In general, it is capable of the same cures as the pellitory.

### IV, 87 φακὸς ὁ ἐπὶ τῶν τελμάτων, *Lemna minor* L., Duckweed

The duckweed that is on marshlands is found on stagnant waters; it is a plant like the lentil, and, since it has a cooling property, it is a suitable plaster by itself as well as with barley groats for every kind of inflammation, for erysipelas, and for gout. It also heals children's hernias.

---

[29] μυὸς ὦτα, "mouse ears" or "rat ears." The Greeks did not have nor do they still have separate words for mouse and rat. The distinction between the two is made by the adjective μέγας/μεγάλος, "big."
[30] ἀλσίνη, akin to ἄλσος, "grove."

**IV, 88 ἀείζῳον μέγα, *Sempervivum arboreum* L., Houseleek**

**1.** Houseleek: it was named so because its petals are evergreen,[31] but some call it *bouphthalmon*, others *zoophthalmon*, others *stergethron*, and others *ambrosia*. It sends up stems that are a cubit long or even longer, thick as a thumb, fatty, vigorous, incised like those of the wood spurge. Its leaves are fatty, having the size of a thumb and they are tongue-like towards the tip; the lower leaves turn themselves backwards, but the ones toward the top rest on each other forming an eye-like circle. It grows on mountainous and loamy places. Some people plant it on their houses.

**2.** It has cooling and astringent properties that are beneficial for erysipelas, shingles, spreading ulcers, inflammations of the eyes, burns, and gout when the leaves are plastered on either by themselves or with barley groats. Its juice is poured on with unguent of roses for headaches, it is given in a drink to people bitten by venomous spiders, to those who suffer from diarrhea and dysentery, and it expels round intestinal worms when drunk with wine. Used in a pessary it also stems leucorrhea. The juice is smeared beneficially also on people suffering from ophthalmia.

**IV, 89 ἀείζῳον τὸ μικρόν, *Semper vivum tectorum* L., Houseleek**

Houseleek: it grows on walls, rocks, copings, and shady graves. It has many little stems growing from one root, which are full of leaflets that are round, fatty, and pointed at the tip. It also grows a stem in the middle, about a span long, having an umbel and pale-green, delicate flowers.

Its leaves have the same properties as the one mentioned before.

**IV, 90 τρίτον εἶδος ἀειζῴου, *Sedum* L. sp., Third kind of Houseleek = Stonecrop**

But there seems to be a third kind of houseleek = stonecrop that some called *andrachne agria*, others *Telephion*, and the Romans *illecebra*. It has broader leaves, tending toward the leaves of purslane, and they are rough. It grows on rocks.

---

[31] ἀείζῳον, "everliving" or "evergreen."

It has properties that warm, that are sharp, that ulcerate, and that disperse scrofulous swellings of the glands when plastered on with lard.

### IV, 91 κοτυληδών, *Umbilicus pendulinus* DC., Navelwort

Navelwort: but some call it *scytalion* and others *cymbalion*. It has a leaf like a saucer, round, and imperceptibly shallow, and a little short stem whereon is seed, and a root that is round like an olive.
Its juice and the juice of the leaves smeared on with wine or used as a clyster, ease contractions in the genitalia, and when plastered on assuage erysipelas, chilblains, scrofulous swellings of the glands, and heartburn. The leaves eaten with the root break up stones, set the urine in motion, and are given to those who have edemata with honey mixed with wine. It is used also in love-potions.

### IV, 92 ἕτερον εἶδος κοτυληδόνος, *Saxifrage* L. sp., Another kind of navelwort[32]

There is yet another type of navelwort having wider and fatty leaves; they are like little tongues, closely packed around the root, forming, as it were, an eye in the middle, just like the houseleek, and astringent in taste. It has a slender little stem and on it there are flowers and seedlets similar to those of St. John's wort. It has a rather large root.
It is good for the same conditions as the stonecrop.

### IV, 93 ἀκαλήφη, *Urtica* L. sp., Stinging nettle

**1.** Stinging nettle, but some call it *cnide*: there are two types of this plant. For one is wilder, it has rougher, wider, and darker leaves, and the fruit is like linseed, except smaller. The other has fine seeds and it is not quite as rough.
The leaves of both, applied with salt, treat dog bites, gangrenous, malignant, and filthy sores, sprains, growths, tumors of the parotid glands, swellings of the glands, and abscesses; they are applied with cerate on those with spleen disease. The leaves are also good for nosebleeds when inserted ground up with their juice. Inserted as a

---

[32] See J. Berendes, pp. 420-421 for various identifications by Matthiolus and by Fraas.

pessary ground up with myrrh, they set menstruation in motion and when new leaves are placed around a prolapsed uterus they set it right. **2.** The seed is aphrodisiac and opens the uterus when drunk with grape syrup; used in a lozenge with honey, it is beneficial for orthopnea, pleurisies, and inflammations of the lungs; it also brings up matter from the chest, and it is combined with septic medications. Boiled with cockles, the leaves soften the bowels, stop flatulence, are diuretic, and they bring up matter from the chest when cooked with peeled barley. The decoction of the leaves, drunk with a bit of myrrh, moves the menstrual period, and their juice reduces an inflamed uvula when used as a gargle.

### IV, 94 γαλήοψις *Scrofularia peregrina* L., Brownwort

Brownwort: but some call it *galepsis* and others *galeobdolon.* The entire little shrub together with its stem and leaves resembles the nettle, except that its leaves are smoother and rather foul smelling when ground. It has delicate purple flowers. It grows on fences and around roads and building lots everywhere.

The leaves and stem are capable of dissolving indurations, tumors, scrofulous swellings of the glands, swellings of the glands, and tumors of the parotid glands. One must apply them twice daily with vinegar making the plaster tepid; their decoction, too, is used beneficially as a rinse; plastered on with salt they are good for spreading ulcers, gangrenes, and putrid humors.

### IV, 95 γάλιον, *Galium verum* L., Bedstraw

Bedstraw: but some call it *galairion* and others *galation.* It was named so because it coagulates milk as well as rennet.[33] Its little spray and leaf are very much like those of cleavers, upright, and at the end there is a quince-yellow flower, delicate, compact, and very aromatic. Its flower is plastered on for burns and it is suitable for hemorrhages. It is also mixed with cerate of roses in the sun until it becomes white, and prepared this way it is analgesic. Its root is aphrodisiac. It grows on marshlands.

---

[33] γάλα,"milk," is imbedded in all its names.

**IV, 96 ἠριγέρων, *Senecio vulgaris* L., Groundsel**

**1.** Groundsel: it is a little stalk, a cubit tall, somewhat reddish, having small leaves, cloven at the end like the leaves of rocket, but a great deal smaller. The flowers are quince-yellow, quickly opening up and bursting into what is called down; it is for this reason that it was named *erigeron,*[34] because in the spring the flowers become hoary like hair. The root is useless. It grows mostly on copings and around cities.
**2.** The leaves with the flowers have a cooling property, wherefore, when plastered on with a small amount of grape syrup or even by themselves, they treat testicular and anal inflammations, and in combination with frankincense they cure both other injuries and injuries in the tendons. The down does also the same when plastered by itself with vinegar, but the new down causes choking when drunk.

**IV, 97 θαλίητρον, *Thalictrum flavum* L., *Th. minus* L., Meadow rue**

Meadow rue: it has leaves that nearly resemble those of coriander but fatter, and a little stem of the thickness of rue on which grow the leaves. Ground up and plastered on, they cicatrize sores that are chronic. It grows mostly on plains.

**IV, 98 βρύον θαλάσσιον, Ulva *lactuca* L., *U. latissima* L., etc., Sea lettuce**

Sea lettuce: it grows on rocks and on shells by the sea. It is lettuce-like, slender, stemless, quite astringent, and effective for inflammations and for gouts that need cooling.

**IV, 99 φῦκος θαλάσσιον, *Cystoseira foeniculosa* sp., Seaweed**

Seaweed: there is one kind that is broad, another that is longish and somewhat purple, and another that is curly, growing in Crete, near the shore; it is very colorful and not prone to decay.
All of them have an astringent property and are good in plasters for gout and for the <other> inflammations. But they must be used while moist and before they have dried up. Nicander (*Th.* 845) says that the

[34] Meaning "early-old."

purple is also an antidote for poisonous animals, which some thought to be what women use, that being a tiny root called similarly seaweed.

**IV, 100 ποταμογείτων, *Ottelia alismoides* Pers., Pondweed**

Pondweed: it is a leaf that is like the beet, thick, and emerging slightly above the water. It cools, it is astringent, and it suitable for itching, for spreading ulcers, and for sores of long standing. It was so named because it grows in marshes and wetlands.

**IV, 101 στρατιώτης ὁ ἐπὶ τῶν ὑδάτων φυόμενος, *Pistia stratiotes* L., Water lettuce**

Water lettuce: it, too, was so named from its habit of swimming on water and living without a root. Its leaf is similar to that of the houseleek but larger, having a cooling property, and it is able to stop hemorrhages from the kidneys when drunk; it maintains injuries free of inflammations and treats erysipelas and swellings when plastered on with vinegar.

**IV, 102 στρατιώτης ὁ χιλιόφυλλος, *Achillea millefolium* L., Yarrow or Milfoil**

Yarrow or milfoil: it is a tiny shrub, about a span tall or even taller, having leaves similar to a nestling's down. The outgrowths from the leaves are very short and split, the leaves are very much like wild cumin in their shortness, even shorter, and its umbel is rather thick and fuller. For on top it has little dry stalks on which the umbels are as of the dill and white small flowers. It grows on lands that are fallow, somewhat rough, and especially by the roadside.

This herb is extremely good for hemorrhages, for old and new ulcers, and for fistulas.

**IV, 103 φλόμος, *Verbascum* L. sp., Mullein**

**1.** Mullein: it is of two principal kinds. For one kind of this plant is white and the other is dark, and of the white, one is female and the other male. The leaves of the female very nearly resemble cabbage leaves, but they are a great deal more downy, broader, and white; the stem is a cubit tall or even taller, white, somewhat downy; the flowers are white or pale yellow; the seed black, and the root is long, astringent, and having the thickness of a finger. It grows in plains. The other one, which is called male, also has white leaves, but the leaves are longish, and narrower, and the stem is more slender.

**2.** The dark is similar to the white in every respect, except that it has wider and darker leaves. There is also the mullein called wild, bearing tall, tree-like shoots and leaves similar to sage. All around, in a circle, it has shoots, just like the horehound; it has a quince-yellow, gold-like flower. There are also little mulleins that are double, downy, low-growing, having leaves that are round, and a third little mullein, called *lychnitis,* but some call it *thryallis,* having three or four or even more little leaves that are thick, downy, fatty, and good for lamp-wicks.

**3.** The root of the first two is astringent, that is why an amount of the size of a vertebra is profitably given in a drink with wine to those suffering from diarrhea; its decoction is helpful for ruptures, spasms, bruises, and old coughs; it also assuages a toothache when used as a mouthwash. The one with gold-like flowers dyes hair and attracts cockroaches[35] wherever it is placed. The leaves, boiled in water, are plastered on for swellings and for inflammations of the eyes, also for gangrened ulcers with honey or with wine, but with vinegar they treat injuries and help people stung by scorpions. The leaves of the wild are a plaster for burns and they say that the leaves of the female when placed between dry figs keep them from spoiling.

### IV, 104 Αἰθιοπίς, *Salvia aethiopis* L., *S. argentea* L., Silver sage

Silver sage: it, too, has leaves closely resembling the mullein, very rough and thick, growing in a circle around the base of the root. It has a quadrangular, rough, and thick stalk that resembles that of the balm or of the bearwort and that puts out many branches. The seed is roughly the size of a bean, two seeds growing together is one vessel; it has many long thick roots from the same stock that taste gluey; as they dry up, they become black and dark like horns. A great deal of it grows in Messenia and on Ida.

Its root boiled and drunk helps for hip disease, pleurisy, spitting of blood, and roughness of the trachea; it is taken with honey as a lozenge.

---

[35] Or "bookworms."

**IV, 105 ἄρκτιον, ~ *Inula candida* L., ~ *Celsia orientalis* L., ~ *C. acaulis* Bory, etc., Bearwort**

Bearwort: but some call it *arctouros*. It, too, has leaves like those of the mullein except rougher and rounder and a soft, white, and sweet root; it has a long, soft stem and seed like small cumin.

Its root and fruit boiled down in wine assuage toothaches when held in the mouth and it is a rinse for burns and chilblains. They are also drunk with wine for hip disease and for difficult micturition.

**IV, 106 ἄρκιον, *Arctium lappa* L., Burdock**

Burdock, but some call it *prosopis* and others *prosopion*: it has leaves similar to those of the round gourd but larger, tougher, darker, and rough. The plant is without a stalk and the root, which is large and white, helps those who spit blood and who suffer from abscesses when an amount of one *drachma* is drunk with pine nuts; ground up and plastered on, it also stops the pains around the joints that stem from twistings. Also the leaves are applied beneficially on old ulcers.

**IV, 107 πετασῖτις, *Petasitis officinalis* Moench, Butterbur**

Butterbur: it is a shoot, taller than a cubit and thick as a thumb, bearing large, hat-shaped leaves, as if they were mushrooms, and which are good for malignant and cancerous ulcers when applied ground.

**IV, 108 ἐπιπακτίς, *Herniaria glabra* L. sp., Rupturewort**

Rupturewort, but some call it *elleborine*: it is a tiny little shrub having very few tiny leaves. It is drunk to counteract poisons and for diseases associated with the liver.

**IV, 109 καπνὸς ὁ ἐν ταῖς κριθαῖς φυόμενος, *Fumaria officinalis* L., Fumitory**

Fumitory: it is a small, shrub-like little herb resembling coriander, very tender, and abounding in rather pale, ash-colored leaves. The flower is purple.

Its juice is sharp, it promotes sharp-sightedness, and it produces tears, whence it was named.[36] Smeared on with gum it also can prevent hair pulled from the eyebrows from growing back. The plant drives bile through the urine when eaten.

**IV, 110 λωτὸς ὁ ἐν τοῖς παραδείσοις φυόμενος, *Melilotus,* sp. Adans., Italian melilot**

Italian melilot, which some call *triphyllon*, made into juice and mixed with honey clears away albugo, cloud-like opacities on the eyes, leucomas, and the elements that cast a shadow over the pupils of the eyes.

**IV, 111 λωτὸς ἄγριος, *Trigonella elatior* Sibth. sp., *T. gladiata* L. sp., Wild fenugreek**

Wild fenugreek: it grows extensively in Libya, bearing a stem that is two-cubits tall or even taller that has many axils; it has leaves like the three-leaved clover that grows in meadows, seed resembling the fenugreek but a great deal smaller and tasting like medicine. It has properties that warm, that are mildly astringent, and that remove facial blemishes and freckles when smeared on with honey; drunk all by itself ground up or even with seed of mallow and wine or grape syrup, it helps for pains in the area of the bladder.

**IV, 112 κύτισος, *Medicago arborea* L., Tree medick**

Tree medick: it is a shrub that is entirely white, sending up twigs a cubit tall or even taller that are surrounded by leaves like those of fenugreek or the three-leaved clover, but they are smaller and they have a mid-rib. When crushed with the fingers they smell of broth but they taste of fresh chick peas.

Ground up and plastered on with bread, the leaves have the ability to cool and to disperse incipient swellings; their decoction also sets micturition in motion when drunk. Some plant it near beehives as it attracts bees.

---

[36] καπνός, means "smoke."

**IV, 113 λωτὸς ὁ ἐν Αἰγύπτῳ γεννώμενος, *Nelumbo nucifera* Gaertn., Egyptian lotus**

The Egyptian lotus that grows in the water when the fields are flooded:[37] it has a stalk that resembles that of the bean, having a white flower like a white lily. They say that the flower opens at sunrise and closes at sunset when the entire head hides itself in the water then it pops up again around sunrise. The head resembles a very large poppy, wherein is seed, just like millet, which the people who live in Egypt after drying, grind for making bread. The root is similar to the root of quince; it, too, is eaten both boiled and raw. Boiled, it corresponds in texture to egg yolk.

**IV, 114 μυριόφυλλον,[38] *Myriophyllum spicatum* L., Water milfoil**

Water milfoil: it is a tiny, tender stalk, single stemmed, of a single root, surrounded by countless smooth leaves resembling those of the fennel. It is for this reason that it was so named. The stem is somewhat yellow and quite hollow, as if it had been bored on purpose. It grows in marshlands.

Plastered on with vinegar, either fresh or dry, it keeps fresh injuries free from inflammations; it is also given to drink with water and salt for falls.

**IV, 115 μυρρίς, *Myrrhis odorata* Scop., Sweet cicely**

Sweet cicely, but some call it *myrra*: in stem and foliage it is like the hemlock, but it has a root that is somewhat long, soft, round, aromatic, and pleasant to eat; the root helps those bitten by poisonous spiders when drunk with wine. It also cleanses off the menstrual period and the discharges following childbirth, and it is profitably given boiled down to tuberculars to sip. Some report that, during epidemics, it helps those who drink it with wine two or three times a day stay healthy.

---

[37] This is the Nile water lily.

[38] μυριόφυλλον, "countless leaves."

**IV, 116 μύαγρον, ~ *Chamaelina sativa* Crantz. var. *microcarpa* Andrtz., Ball mustard**

Ball mustard, but some call it *melampyron*: it is a plant that belongs to the class of undershrubs, two-cubits tall, having leaves that resemble the leaves of the madder, and seed like that of fenugreek, greasy, which they use chopped up slightly roasted, plaster on rods, and employ as candles.

Their grease seems to smooth and soften roughnesses of the body.

**IV, 117 ὀνάγρα, *Epilobium angustifolium* L., Oleander**

The oleander that some call *onotheras* and others *ono<tho>uris*: it is a tree-like shrub, of a good size, having leaves nearly resembling the leaves of the almond tree, but broader and resembling the leaves of the white lily. It has large, rose-like flowers, and a long white root that smells like wine when dry. It grows in mountainous places.

The infusion of its root has the property of taming wild animals when they drink it. Applied as a plaster, the root assuages malignant sores.

**IV, 118 κρίσσιον, ~ *Carduus tenuiflorus* Curtis, ~ *C. pycnocephalus* L., Thistle**

Thistle: it is a tender little stalk, about two-cubits tall, triangular at its lower part, having on it at intervals soft little thorns. The leaves are like those of bugloss, moderately rough and smaller, whitish, and prickly at the ends; but the topmost part of the stalk is round, rough, and on it there are purple-tipped heads that become plumed.

Andreas writes that its root, fastened over the place that hurts, stops pains from varicose veins.[39]

**IV, 119 ἀστὴρ Ἀττικός, *Aster amellus* L., Blue daisy**

Blue daisy: but some call it *boubonion.* It is a woody little shoot, having at the top a purple or quince-yellow flower like that of the chamomile, a little head slit all around, and the little petals are like a star. The leaves surrounding the stem are longish and rough.

[It helps for heartburn, for inflammations of the eyes, and for prolapses of the anus. They say also that the purple flower, when

---

[39] Or "pains from varicocele."

drunk with water helps for sore throats and for epilepsy in children.][40] Plastered on moist, it is suitable for inflammations of the groin and picked up dry with the left hand of someone who hurts and tied to the groin it relieves his pain.

**IV, 120 ἰσόπυρον, *Corydalis claviculata* Pers., Fumitory**

Fumitory: but some call it *phaselion*[41] *from* its resemblance to the bean that has a tendril toward the upper leaf. At the top of the stem there are small delicate heads full of little seeds, tasting very much like black cumin, but the leaf tastes like anise.

Its seed is a remedy for ailments around the chest, for a cough, for liver disease patients, and for those spiting blood when drunk with hydromel.

**IV, 121 ἴον, *Viola odorata* L., Violet**

Violet: it has a smaller and a more delicate leaf than the ivy but it is darker, yet it is not unlike it, and it has a little stem from the middle of the root, on which there is a small, very aromatic, purple flower. It grows in shady and rough places.

The leaves have a cooling property when plastered by themselves as well as with barley groats; they help for heartburn, inflammations of the eyes, and prolapses of the anus. And they say that the purplish part of the flower helps for sore throats and for epilepsy in children when drunk with water. [42]

**IV, 122 κακκαλία, ~ *Senecio thapsoides* DC., ~ *Mercurialis tomentosa* L., *Caccalia***

*Caccalia*: but some call it *leantice*: it has large white leaves; their stem, however, is middling, upright, and white, having a flower that resembles bryony. It grows in mountains.

---

[40] Following Saracenus, Max Wellmann, *Pedanii Dioscuridis Anazarbei De Materia Medica,* Bk. IV, p. 269, brackets this passage and points out that it was copied from Dsc. Bk. IV, 121 below.

[41] φασήλιον, "small bean."

[42] See Dsc. Bk. IV, 119 and n. 40 above for the similarities between these two chapters.

Its root, soaked in wine like tragacanth and sucked like a lozenge or chewed all by itself, treats coughs and roughnesses of the trachea. And the seeds that grow after the flowers have faded, ground up, compounded with cerate, and smeared on keep the face taut and wrinkle-free.

**IV, 123 βούνιον, Bunium *ferulaceum* Sibth. and Sm., Earthnut**

Earthnut, but some call it *action*: it sends up a stem that is quadrangular, of good length, and thick as a finger. The leaves are similar to the celery's but a great deal more delicate, nearer those of coriander. The flower is like that of anise and the seed is fragrant and smaller than that of henbane.

It is diuretic, it warms, it draws out the afterbirth, and it is suitable for the spleen, kidneys, and bladder. It is used moist and dry as well as converted into juice with its roots, stems, and leaves and with honey and water.

**IV, 124 ψευδοβούνιον, *Pimpinella cretica* L., Cretan pimpinel**

Cretan pimpinel: it is a shrub tall as the palm of a hand, growing in Crete, and having leaves like those of earthnut.

About four of its little sprays can treat colic, difficult micturition, and pains of the side when drunk with water. It dissipates also scrofulous swellings of the glands when plastered on tepid with salt and wine.

**IV, 125 χαμαίκισσος, *Glechoma hederacea* L., Ground ivy**

Ground ivy: it has many leaves that are like the wheat's but longer and thinner, five or six small sprays, a span long and full of leaves from the ground, and flowers that are like gillyflowers but smaller and very bitter in taste. The root is white, delicate, and useless. It grows in tilled lands.

About one *triobolon* of leaves, when drunk for 40 or 50 days in three *cyathoi* of water, is suitable for people suffering from hip ailments; the leaves also clear away jaundice when similarly drunk for six or seven days.

**IV, 126 χαμαιπεύκη, *Chamaepeuce mutica*, Fishbone thistle**[43]
Fishbone thistle: ground up and drunk with water it is beneficial for lower back pain.

**IV, 127 βούγλωσσον, *Anchusa italica* Retz., Bugloss**
Bugloss: it resembles the mullein. Its foliage lies on the ground and it is jagged, darker, and smaller, resembling a cow's tongue. It is thought to make people mirthful when dropped into their wine.

**IV, 128 φύτευμα, *Reseda phyteuma* L., Montpellier rocket**
Montpellier rocket: it has leaves similar to those of soapwort but smaller, a great deal of seed that has holes, and a small, delicate, and superficial root. Some people write that the root is suitable for love potions.

**IV, 129 ὑπόγλωσσον, *Ruscus hypoglossum* L., Horse tongue**[44]
Horse tongue: it is a small shrub having leaves similar to those of the small butcher's broom, prickly foliage, and on top it has next to the leaves small offshoots resembling tiny tongues.
The foliage seems to be a useful amulet for people with headaches. It is also mixed with emollients.

**IV, 130 ἀντίρρινον *Antirrhinum orontium* L., Calf's snout**
Calf's snout, but some people have called it *anarrinon* and others have called this one, too, *lychnis agria.* It is an herb resembling the pimpernel in foliage and stem; but its flowers are like gillyflowers except smaller and purple, and it is for this reason that it has been called also *agria lychnis.* It bears fruit similar to the snout of a calf.
It is said that it guards against poisons when worn, and that it makes a person alluring when smeared on with oil of lily.

---

[43] Jacques André, *Les noms des plantes dans la Rome anrique,* p. 60, says that the absence of descriptions for this plant makes it impossible to identify it. Its botanical name here is from LSJ.
[44] The English name of this plan, "horse tongue," derives from a false etymology of ὑπόγλωσσον : ὑπό, "below" and γλώσσα, "tongue." The ὑπό element, however, seems to have been confused with ἵππο-, "horse."

**IV, 131 καταναγκη, *Ornithopus compressus* L., Vetch**

Vetch: one kind has small leaves like those of the hartshorn plantain, a delicate root like that of camel hay, and six or seven heads like those of the bitter vetch, containing fruit similar to that of the bitter vetch. As it dries, it bends over the ground simulating the talon of a dead kite. The other kind … and of the size of a small apple, a root that is small like an olive, leaves that in shape and color resemble an olive but are softer, small fruit perforated in many places, resembling a chick-pea, and purple.

Some report that both kinds are suitable for love potions and that the Thassalian women use them.

**IV, 132 τριπόλιον, ~ *Aster tripolium* L., ~ *Limonium* L. sp., Sea starwort**

Sea starwort: it grows on coastal areas where the sea ebbs and flows, neither on dry land nor in the sea. It has leaves closely resembling the leaves of woad but thicker, and a stem that is a span tall and split on top. Its flower reportedly changes color three times a day; in the morning it is white, around noon purple, and late in the day red.[45] The root is white, fragrant, and warms him who tastes it; a quantity of two *drachmai* of it being drunk in wine drives down the abdomen water and urine. It is also cut for witchcraft.

**IV, 133 κῆμος ~ *Evax pygmaea* Pers., ~ E. *asterifolia* Pers., ~ *Plantago cretica* L., ~ *Gnaphalium leontopodium* L., etc., *Cemos***

*Cemo*s: it is a tiny herb, two fingers tall, having narrow, strong little leaves, about four- or three-fingers long, and they are rough; the ones growing near the root are woollier and whitish. At the ends of the stems, there are little heads, as if perforated, containing fruit hard to see because of the surrounding down. The root is small. They say that it is useful for love potions.

---

[45] According to Jacques André, *Les noms des plantes dans la Rome antique*, p. 265 this statement is based on some folk tradition and does not conform to reality. See P. Fournier, Bull. Soc. Bot. Fr., 96, 1949, p. 189 where he suggests that τριπόλιον may be a species of λειμώνιον.

**IV, 134 ἀδίαντον, *Adiantum capillus Veneris* L., Maidenhair**

**1.** Maidenhair: but some call it *polytrichon.* It has little leaves similar to coriander, split at the end, and the small shoots on which they grow are quite dark, delicate, and a span long. It has neither little stalk nor flower nor seed. The root is useless.

When drunk, the decoction of this plant can help asthmatics, the jaundiced, those with spleen disease, and those who have difficult micturition. It breaks up stones, it stops diarrhea, it helps those bitten by wild animals, and it stems fluid discharges from the stomach when drunk with wine; it also moves both the menstrual period and the discharges that follow childbirth, and it stems blood spitting.

**2.** It is plastered on for malignant sores, it restores hair on bald spots, it dissipates scrofulous swellings of the glands, and when used with soap powder it wipes clean dandruff and scurf. With gum ladanum and with oil of myrtle or with unguent of lilies or with hyssop and wine, it prevents hair from falling, as does its decoction when used as a cleanser with wine and soap powder. It makes cocks and quails belligerent when mixed with their feed. It is cultivated in enclosed places for the benefit of sheep. It grows in shady spots, on humid walls, and around fountains.

**IV, 135 τριχομανές, *Asplenium trichomanes* L., Waterwort**

Water wort: but some call this one also *adianton;* it grows around the same places. It is like the male fern, tiny, having slender, lentiform leaves in a row, opposing each other on both sides on little rods that are slender, stiff, gleaming, and somewhat black.

It is thought to be capable of the same activities as the above.

**IV, 136 ξάνθιον, *Xanthium strumarium* L., Broad-leaved burweed**

**1.** Broad-leaved burweed: but some have called it *phasganon,* others *antithesion*, others *chascanon*, others *choiradolethron,* and others have called this one, too, *aparine.* It grows in fertile lands and in marshes that have dried up. It has a stem a cubit tall, shiny, and angular, and from it grow many axils; its leaves are like those of orach, notched, and nearly resembling nose-smart in scent; it has round fruit, like a large olive, prickly like the globular catkin of the plane tree, and adhering to clothing on contact.

**2.** The fruit, collected before it is fully dried, pounded, and stored in a clay vessel, can dye hair blond if one, at the time of using it, took a quantity of one *tryblion*, diluted it in tepid water, and after cleaning the head with soda, plastered it on; but some store it also after beating it with wine. The fruit is plastered advantageously also on swellings.

**IV, 137 αἰγίλωψ, *Aigilops ovata* L., Haver grass**
Haver grass: it is a small herb having leaves similar to those of wheat but softer. The fruit is at the top of the head, having two or three seed capsules on which grow beards as if they were hair.
Plastered on with meal, this plant treats lachrymal fistulas and dissipates indurations. Its juice is stored for the same purposes after it has been mixed with meal and dried.

**IV, 138 γλαύξ, ~ *Coronopus procumbens* Gilib., Wart cress**
Wart cress: its little leaves are like those of the tree medick or the lentil; its lower leaves are rather white but the upper pale-green. It sends out from the root along the ground five or six slender little twigs, a span long. The blossoms are similar to gillyflowers but smaller and purple. It grows near the sea.
This plant, boiled with barley meal, salt, and oil, and sipped, restores milk that is drying up.

**IV, 139 πολύγαλον, *Polygala venulosa* Sibth., Milkwort**
Milkwort: it is a small stalk, a span tall, having lentiform leaves, somewhat astringent in taste. This plant, too, is thought to increase milk production when drunk.

**IV, 140 ὄσιρις, *Osiris alba* L., Poet's cassia**
Poet's cassia: it is a small underbrush, dark, slender, a little twig that is hard to break, surrounded by leaflets like those of the flax; they are dark; at first <the seedlets are dark> but they change becoming reddish.
Its decoction helps for jaundice when drunk. They also make brooms from this plant.

**IV, 141 ἐχῖνος, *Echinos***

*Echinos*: it grows near rivers and springs. It has leaves similar to those of basil but smaller and split from the upper parts, five or six little stems, a span long, white flowers, and fruit that is black, small and astringent. The stem and petals are full of juice.

An amount of two *drachmai* of its fruit mixed with four *drachmai* of honey and used as ointment stems fluxes from the eyes. The juice stops earaches when instilled with native sulfur and soda.

**IV, 142 μῖλαξ τραχεῖα, *Smilax aspera* L., Rough bindweed**

Rough bindweed: it has leaves like those of honeysuckle and many twigs that are thin and thorny like the Christ's thorn or the bramble, and it spirals around trees, spreading itself up and down. It has fruit like a bunch of grapes, red when ripe and mildly biting in taste, and a tough and thick root. It grows in marshy and rough places.

Drunk beforehand as well as afterwards, its leaves and fruit are antidotes to deadly poisons. And according to tradition they protect against all poisonous substances if after pounding some leaves one gave them to a newly born child to swallow. They are also cut for witchcraft.

**IV, 143 μῖλαξ λεία, *Convolvulus sepium* L., Great bindweed**

Great bindweed: it has leaves similar to the ivy's but softer and thinner, and its twigs are just like the twigs of the one before, although they do not have thorns and they are smooth; it spirals around trees just like the other one. It has fruit like the lupine, black and small, having on top many white round flowers along the entire calyx. They even make arbors with it in the summer; it does, however, shed its leaves in the fall.

Its seed when drunk with *dorycnion,*[46] one Attic *triobolon* of each, is reported to cause many nightmares.

**IV, 144 μυρσίνη ἀγρία, *Ruscus aculeatus* L., Butcher's broom**

**1.** Butcher's broom: but some call it *oxymyrsine,* others *myrtacanthos,* others *acairon*, others *cine*, others *leichene*, others *chamaimyrsine*,

---

[46] See Dsc. Bk. IV, 74.

and the Boeotians *gorgynthia.* It has foliage that is similar to myrtle but wider, lanceolate, pointed at the tip, and fruit that is round, growing between the leaves, red as it ripens, having a bony inner part. It has many withy twigs growing from the same root, hard to break, a cubit tall, full of leaves, and a root that nearly resembles that of dogtooth grass, harsh in taste, and somewhat bitter. It grows in rough and precipitous places.

**2.** Drunk in wine, the leaves and fruit have the ability to move the urine, to bring on the menstrual periods, and to break stones in the bladder. They treat jaundice, difficult micturition, and headaches. The decoction of the root, too, when drunk with wine does the same. The newly sprouted stems are even eaten as potherbs instead of asparagus. They are bitter and diuretic.

### IV, 145 δάφνη Ἀλεξάνδρεια, *Ruscus hypophyllum* L., Daphne Alexandreia

But some people call it *Idaia,* others *Danae*, others *hypoglotton,* others *zaleia*, and others *stephanos.* Its has leaves similar to those of butcher's broom but larger, softer, and whiter, red fruit between the leaves, the size of chick-peas, branches that grow from the ground, a span tall or even taller, and a root closely resembling that of butcher's broom but larger, fragrant, and softer; it grows in mountainous places.

The root has the property of helping those having difficulty giving birth and patients of strangury when a quantity of six *drachmai* is drunk with sweet wine. It also draws blood.

### IV, 146 δαφνοειδές, *Daphne laureola* L., Spurge laurel

Spurge laurel: but some call it *eupetalon,* others *chamaidaphne*, and others <*eu*>*peplon.* It is a small shrub, a cubit tall, having many fibrous branches that bear leaves toward the upper half — the bark around the shoots being very sticky — leaves resembling those of the laurel but softer and thinner, not easily broken, biting and burning the mouth and throat. It has white flowers and the fruit is black when ripe. The root is useless. It grows in mountainous places.

Its dry or fresh leaf when drunk drives through the bowels substances full of phlegm. It induces vomiting and menstruation, and it purges away phlegm when chewed; it does also cause sneezing. Its fruit also purges when a quantity of 15 berries is drunk.

**IV, 147 χαμαιδάφνη, *Ruscus ramosus*, L., Chamaidaphne**

Chamaidaphne: but some call this plant, too, *Alexandreia.* Is sends up shoots that are a cubit tall, single-stemmed, thin, and smooth; the leaves of this one, too, are like those of the laurel, although they are a great deal thinner and paler. It has a round, red fruit growing on the leaves.

Ground up and plastered on, its leaves assuage headaches and heartburn and they stop colic when drunk with wine; their juice gets the menses and the urine going when given to drink with wine and it does the same when inserted in a pessary.

**IV, 148 ἐλλέβορος λευκός, *Veratrum album* L., White hellebore**

**1.** White hellebore: it has leaves similar to the leaves of the plantain or of the wild beet but shorter, darker, and red in color; it has a stem that is a span tall and hollow and that loses its outer layer all around as it begins to dry up. The roots are below ground, many, delicate, and growing together from a small and longish head as from an onion. It grows in mountainous places.

One must dig up the roots around the time wheat is harvested. The best is moderately long and white, friable, fleshy, not tapering or stringy, releasing fine down when broken, having a tender pith, not burning the taste much nor drawing the spittle all at once. For this kind causes choking.[47]

**2.** The best is the Anticyrinian; but the Galatian, [the *Gallicos,*] and the Cappadocian are whiter, thinner, and more likely to cause choking. It purges through vomiting, bringing up matter that is of different colors; it is mixed with eye medications that can cleanse those substances which cast a shadow over the pupils and it both draws the menstrual period and destroys embryos/fetuses when inserted as a

---

[47] The "choking" appears to be due to the effect it has on the salivary glands which causes them to be hyperactive and which appear to be one of the side effects of some white hellebores. In general, *veratrum album* is highly toxic because of the alkaloidal steroids it contains, some of which are teratogenic in sheep. See *Phytochemical Dictionary,* B. Harborne et al., Eds. Pp. 972, 329, 331-332, and 335.

pessary; it also provokes sneezing, it kills mice when kneaded with honey and barley groats, and it dissolves meats when cooked together with them. It is given on an empty stomach by itself and with fruit of black hellebore, juice of deadly carrot, fish-sauce, hydromel or with gruel or lentils or porridge. It is also kneaded into bread and baked.

**3.** Those who wrote principally about its dosage worked out its administration and subsequent regulation in the diet; and we are very much in agreement with Philonides the Sicilian from Enna. For in an account that deals chiefly with the tradition of herbal remedies, it is tiresome to put down dosages. Some give it with much porridge, or with a large quantity of juice, or they even offer the hellebore after first offering some food, especially in cases where they suspect the patients may choke, or when their constitution is weak. For the purging does no harm to those who take it in this manner because the medication is put into their bodies tempered. Even the suppositories that are made from it cause vomiting when applied to the seat with vinegar.

### IV, 149 σησαμοειδὲς τὸ μέγα, *Reseda alba* L., Bastard rocket

Bastard rocket which the people in Anticyra call *elleboros* because it is mixed in their purgings with white hellebore. The plant resembles the groundsel or the rue. The leaves are long, the flower is white, the root is thin and ineffectual, and the seed is like sesame and bitter in taste; it purges upward phlegm and bile when an amount of three-fingers[48] is taken ground up together with three *obols* of white hellebore and hydromel.

### IV, 150 σίκυς ἄγριος, *Ecballium elaterium* Rich., Squirting cucumber

**1.** Squirting cucumber, which some call *pherombron*, differs from the cultivated cucumber only in its fruit, which is a great deal smaller and resembles longish acorns; but its leaves and twigs are like those of the cultivated cucumber and the root is white and large. It grows on building lots and in sandy places; the entire shrub is bitter.

---

[48] A finger is a measure of length. A quantity of a finger = a finger's breadth, about 7/10 of an inch.

The juice of its leaves is suitable to instill for earaches. The root, plastered on with barley groats, disperses all old indurations, breaks up tumors when applied with resin of terebinth, and when boiled with vinegar is beneficial to plaster on gout. Its decoction is both a clyster for hip ailments and a rinse for toothaches.

**2.** When ground up dry it cleanses dull-white leprosies, leprosies, lichen-like eruptions, and it removes both dark scars and facial blemishes. Both the juice of its root, at least three half-*obols,* and its bark, about a quarter of an *oxybaphon*, purge phlegm and bile, especially of people who have edemata, without harming their stomach. Taking a *hemilitron* of root, one must triturate it with two *xestes* of wine, preferably resinated wine, and give three *cyathoi* of it on an empty stomach for three days until the distention is sufficiently reduced.

**3.** The so-called *elaterion* is made from the fruit of the squirting cucumber this way: having chosen squirting cucumbers that spring back when squeezed, set them aside, leaving them for one night. On the following day, place on a bowl a finely meshed sieve, outfit it with a small knife lying on its back, its cutting edge on top, and taking one by one the squirting cucumbers with both hands, cut them into two and squeeze the liquid into the underlying vessel, squeezing also the fleshy part which falls on the sieve so that it, too, passes through; then place the strained part of the cucumbers into a basin lying near by.

**4.** Heap up on the sieve the pieces that have been squeezed, dowse them with fresh water, press them, and discard them. Then stir the liquid that is in the vessel, cover it with a linen cloth, set it in the sun, and when it has settled, pour out all the liquid that floats on top together with the scum, and repeat the process many times, and when the surface water comes to a standstill, decanting it carefully, put the sediment in a mortar, triturate it, and shape it into troches. But some, in order that the liquid evaporates quickly, spread sifted ashes on the ground, make a hole in the middle, stretch on top a triple layer of linen cloth, and pour over it the *elaterion* together with its moisture, and after it has dried, triturate it in a mortar as described above.

**5.** And some wash it by pouring seawater instead of fresh water, while others pour hydromel for the last wash.

The best, in addition to being white, seems to be somewhat moist, smooth, light, very bitter in taste, and burning easily when placed near a lamp. But that which is greenish, rough, turbid in appearance, and full of dirt and ashes is both heavy and bad. Some mix in also the juice of the cucumber while others add even starch to imitate *elaterion* that is white and light. That which is two years old is suitable for purgatives up to ten years. The ideal dose is one *obol,* the minimum is one-half *obol*, and for children one *dichalcon*. For it is risky to give more.

**6.** It activates purging both upwards and downwards, driving out phlegm and bile. It is an excellent purgative for people who suffer from dyspnea. But if you wish to purge someone down the bowel, after mixing twice as much salt and enough kohl to color it, give it with water as a little pill the size of a bitter vetch, but that person should also swallow one *cyathos* of tepid water. To induce vomiting, after dissolving it in water, smear as far as possible with a feather the areas under the tongue; and if the patient has difficulty vomiting, dissolve it either in olive oil or in unguent of iris and do not let him fall asleep.

**7.** You must keep offering wine with oil to those who are overpurged; for by vomiting they are restored. But should the vomiting not stop, you must offer them cold water, barley groats, sour wine mixed with water, fruit, and as many substances as can thicken the stomach. *Elaterion* sets menstruation in motion, kills embryos/fetuses when used in a pessary, purges jaundice and relieves chronic headaches when poured into the nostrils with milk, and it is a useful ointment with aged olive oil or honey or bile of bull for people with sore throats.

**[IV, 151 ἡμέρου σικύου ἡ ῥιζα, *Cucumis sativus* L., Root of the cultivated cucumber**

One *drachma* of ground cultivated cucumber root drunk with hydromel causes vomiting; and if one wishes a mild after-dinner emetic, two *obols* are sufficient.][49]

---

[49] This chapter may have been moved here from Dsc. Bk. II, 135, where the cultivated cucumber is discussed. See Max Wellmann, *Pedanii Dioscuridis Anazarbei De Materia Medica*, Bk. IV, p. 296.

**IV, 152 σταφὶς ἀγρία, *Delphinium staphisagria* L., Stavesacre**

**1.** Stavesacre: it has leaves that are jagged just like the leaves of the wild grapevine and stems that are upright and black. The flower it bears is like that of woad; the seed is in little pale-green capsules like the seed of the chick-pea, triangular, rough, somewhat yellow on black, but internally it is white, and sharp in taste.

If one gave 15 seeds, triturated in hydromel, he would purge thick substances by means of vomiting; but people who take the potion must keep on walking. Care must be taken, indeed, to give them continuously honey and water because of the risk of suffocation and of burning their throat.

**2.** Brayed either by itself or with red sulfide of arsenic and anointed with olive oil, it is suitable for infestations of lice, itching, and mange, it brings up much phlegm when chewed, it is beneficial for toothaches when boiled with vinegar and when used as a rinse, and with honey it both staunches rheumy gums and treats oral thrush. It is also mixed with heating emollients.

**IV, 153 θαψία, *Thapsia garganica* L., Deadly carrot**

**1.** Deadly carrot: it was so named from the belief that it was first found on Thapsos, the island of the same name. In its entire nature it resembles the giant fennel, although its stem is thinner; its leaves, too, are like the fennel's. At the top, at each side-shoot, there are little umbels resembling the dill's, upon which is a quince-yellow flower. The seed is somewhat broad, resembling that of the giant fennel but smaller and the root is white, large, thick-skinned, and pungent. After digging the root up, they extract its juice by scratching the skin or by hollowing it out conically and covering it with a lid so that the milky juice stays clean. The following day they must come to collect the milky juice that flowed out.

**2.** Juice is extracted from the root also by cutting it, pressing it out through a strainer [with an implement] and drying it in the sun using a thick clay vessel. Some press together also the leaves. But this kind is weak. You can tell the juice extracted from the root because it smells rather foul and remains moist, but that from the leaves dries up and becomes worm-eaten. Those who extract the milky juice must not face the wind; on the contrary, they must do the extraction when there is no wind: for it causes severe facial swelling, and the uncovered parts do blister from the sharpness of the emanation. Therefore, they must first anoint the exposed parts of the body with liquid cerates that bind.

**3.** The skin of the root as well the juice and the milky extract, taken in a drink with honey and water, have a cathartic property, both upward and downward. Of the root, one *tetrabolon* is given with three *drachmai* of dill seed, of the juice one *triobolon*, and of the milky extract, one *obol*. For it is dangerous to give more. Purging with it is suitable for asthmatics, chronic pains of the sides, and for expectorations, but to those who do not vomit easily, it is given in cereals or boiled vegetables. Both the milky juice and the root possess properties that alter the state of pores more than all other drugs that have the same properties, wherever one needs to draw something from deep inside or to change the state of the pores.

**4.** It is for this reason that the juice when anointed or the green root when rubbed on causes bald spots to grow hair, and that the ground root or the juice with equal amounts of frankincense and wax removes black eye and livid spots; but they must stay on no more that two hours then washed with warm seawater. The juice removes freckles, lifts leprous scales when anointed with honey, and breaks up tumors when smeared on with sulfur. It is profitably smeared on those with chronic conditions of the side or lung or feet or joints. It is also useful for the foreskin, raising a swelling on people whose lack of foreskin is not due to circumcision, for as the defective part of the phallus is bathed and softened by the ointments, it fills up.

### IV, 154 σπάρτιον, *Spartium junceum* L., Spanish broom

Spanish broom: it is a shrub producing long, leafless, solid, and hard to break shoots with which they tie grapevines; it bears pods like those of the calavance bean wherein lie lentiform seedlets and a quince-yellow flower like the gillyflower.

An amount of five *obols* of its seed and flowers when drunk with honey and water purges upward with much retching, just like the hellebore, risk free. But the fruit activates also the downward purging. The juice of the shoots themselves, extracted after soaking them in water and braying them, helps people with hip disease when a quantity of one *cyathos* is drunk on an empty stomach. And some people, after soaking them in brine or seawater, treat with clysters those with hips ailments; it also drives out bloody matter and debris.

**IV, 155 σίλλυβον, *Silybum marianum* Gaertn., Milk thistle**

Milk thistle: it is a broad thorn, having leaves that nearly resemble those of the pine thistle. When newly grown, it is eaten boiled with oil and salt. About one *drachma* of the root's milky juice drunk with water and honey induces vomiting.

**IV, 156 βολβός ὁ ἐμετικός, ~ *Narcissus tazetta* L., Narcissus tazetta**

Narcissus tazetta has more fibrous and far longer leaves than the purse tassels and a root like a bulb that is surrounded by black skin.
The root eaten by itself and its decoction when drunk induce vomiting.

**IV, 157 βάλανος μυρεψική, *Moringa* sp.[50] Ben**

**1.** Ben: it is the fruit of a tree that resembles the tamarisk and it is similar to the nut called Pontic. Its inner part when pressed just like bitter almonds releases a liquid that is used instead of olive oil in the manufacture of costly unguents. It grows in Ethiopia, Egypt, Arabia, and in Judean Petra. It is best when fresh, full, white, and when it peels easily. About one *drachma* ground up and drunk with sour wine mixed with water reduces the spleen.

**2.** It is also plastered, with meal of darnel and honey mixed with water, on people suffering from spleen disease and on the gouty. With vinegar, it wipes off mange, leprosy, dull-white leprosies, and black scars; with urine, it removes birthmarks, facial eruptions, freckles, and facial pimples, and with hydromel, it induces vomiting and loosens the bowel. It is, however, quite bad for the stomach and its oil purges the bowel. Its skin is quite astringent. After the liquid has been pressed out of the nut, the pulpy mass that is left is mixed with medications suitable for roughnesses and itching.

---

[50] I am thankful to O. Wenskus for suggesting that I use *Moringa* sp. instead of *Moringa Arabica,* the binomial I used for ben in the first edition. Otta Wenskus, Anzeiger für die Altertumswissenschaft, LXIII, Band, Juli/Oktober 2010, 3./4. Heft, p. 159.

**IV, 158 νάρκισσος, *Narcissus poeticus* L., Narcissus**

**1.** Narcissus: some people have called this plant, too, *leirion,* just like the white lily. Its leaves are like the leek's, but slender and a great deal smaller, it has a hollow and leafless stem, longer than a span, on which grows a white flower, the center of which is saffron-colored, but on some it is purplish; the root is white, round, and bulb-like; the fruit, as if encapsulated, is dark and elongated. It grows most beautiful in mountainous areas, and it is fragrant. The rest of the plant, however, smells like leeks and emits an herb-like odor.

**2.** Its root, when eaten boiled and when drunk, causes vomiting. Ground up and plastered on with honey, it is suitable for burns and it mends gashes around the tendons; plastered on ground up with honey, it helps for sprains of the ankles and for chronic ailments around the joints; with nettle seed and vinegar, it removes both freckles and dull-white leprosies, and, with bitter vetch and honey, it cleanses filthy sores and opens abscesses that do not ripen easily. It also draws out splinters when plastered on with meal of darnel and honey.

**IV, 159 ἱπποφαές, *Euphorbia acanthothamnos* Heldr. and Sart, Spurge**

**1.** Spurge, but some call it *hippophaos.* It is used to full cloth. It grows in coastal and sandy places. It is a bush that belongs to the class of undershrubs, thick, wide-spreading, having long leaves tending toward the leaves of the olive tree but narrower and softer, and between them, at a distance from each other, it has thorns that are dry, somewhat white, and angular. The flowers resemble clusters of ivy fruit, lying on each other like small clusters of grapes, but they are smaller and soft, white with a touch of red. The root is thick, soft, full of juice, and bitter in taste; juice is extracted from it in the same manner as from the deadly carrot.

**2.** Its juice is stored neat as well as blended with meal of bitter vetch and dried. One *obol* of unblended juice purges bilious, phlegm-like and watery elements downward, but of the one combined with the bitter vetch, one *tetrobolon* mixed with honey and water is needed. The shrub, too, dried up with its roots, is chopped and given ground up in the amount of one and one-half *cotyle* with honey and water.

They also make juice from the root and the herb the way they make it from the deadly carrot. One *drachma* of this is given for purges.

**IV, 160 ἱππόφαιστον, *Centaurea spinosa* L., *Hippophaiston***

*Hippoohaiston*: it grows in the same places as does the spurge *hippophaes* and it, too, is a kind of fuller's thorn. It is low growing, having only spongy little heads and tiny little leaves. It has neither flower nor stem; it has a thick and soft root.

After extracting the juice from its leaves, head, and root, dry it, and give an amount of one *triobolon* with honey and water when you wish to remove water and phlegm. Purging by this means is particularly well suited for orthopnea, epilepsy, and for ailments associated with the tendons.

**IV, 161 κίκι, *Ricinus communis*, L., Castor oil tree**

**1.** Castor oil tree: but some people call it *sesamon agrion*, others *seseli Cyprion,* and others *croton*[51] because of the similarity of its seed to the tick. It is a tree that has the size of a small fig tree, and its leaves are like those of the plane tree but larger, smoother, and darker; its limbs and boughs are hollow like reeds, and the fruit, which is in bunches that are rough and grape-like, resembles the insect tick when peeled. The so-called castor oil is extracted from it. And while it is inedible, it is quite useful for lamps and plasters.

**2.** About thirty seeds in number, cleaned and drunk ground up, drive through the bowels phlegm, bile, and water; they also cause vomiting. That sort of purging is very unpleasant, difficult, and greatly upsets the stomach. Triturated and applied as a plaster, the seeds remove facial eruptions and freckles, and the leaves, ground together with fine meal of barley groats, stop swellings and inflammations of the eyes, also breasts from swelling, and they quench erysipelas when smeared on by themselves or with vinegar.

[51] κρότων, "tick," *Ixodes ricinus.*

**IV, 162 ἑλλέβορος ὁ μέλας, *Helleborus cyclophyllus* R. Br., Black hellebore**

**1.** Black hellebore: but some call it *Melampodion,* others *ectonon*, and others *polyrrhizon*; and they call it *Melampodion* because it seems that a certain Melampus, a goatherd, purged and cured with it the daughters of Proitus who were stricken with madness.[52] It has pale-green leaves closely resembling those of the plane tree, but smaller by comparison to the leaves of cow parsnip, much more cloven, darker, and somewhat rough. The stem is short, the flowers white, inclining to purple, resembling grape clusters in configuration, and containing fruit nearly resembling the safflower. The inhabitants of Anticyra call this one also *sesamoeides,* using it for purgings. The roots are black and slender, seemingly hanging from an onion-like little head, of which also there is use. It grows in rough, hilly, and very dry places.

**2.** The best is harvested from places such as these. The hellebore of Anticyra is like this, for black hellebore grows best there. Choose the kind that is sturdy and fleshy, having its innermost part thin, sharp and hot in taste. Such are the ones growing on Mount Helicon, on Mount Parnassus and in Aitolia; but the Heliconian is the best.

It purges the lower abdomen driving downward phlegm and bile when given in the amount of one *drachma* or one *triobolon* either by itself or with scammony and salt. But it is also boiled with lentils and with broths that are taken for purging.

**3.** It is good for epileptics, the atrabilious, the insane, arthritics, and paralytics; inserted as a suppository, it draws the menstrual period and destroys embryos/fetuses, it cleanses fistulas when inserted into them and removed after the third day, and it is similarly inserted into the ear of the hard of hearing and left there for two or three days. It also treats mange when smeared with frankincense, wax, and the watery part of wood tar or oil of cedar; and when daubed on either with vinegar or by itself it treats dull-white leprosies, lichen-like eruptions on the skin, and leprosies. Boiled in vinegar and used as a mouthwash it assuages

---

[52] Melampus was reputed to have cured the daughters of Proitus/Proetus from the madness they suffered because of some impiety they committed against Dionysus or Hera. He kept goats in Messenia, where he settled coming from Thessaly and was known for his prophetic powers.

toothaches, it is mixed with putrefactive medications, and with barley meal and wine it is a useful plaster for those with edemata.

**4.** Planted near the roots of grapevines, it makes their wine purgative. They even sprinkle it around houses because they believe that it purifies. Wherefore, even when digging it up they stand facing east, praying to Apollo and Aesculapius and watching out for the eagle; for they say that the eagle that flies overhead is fraught with danger. For this bird brings death if it should witness the digging of the hellebore. Moreover, one must dig it fast because the emanations cause headaches; it is for this reason that diggers in order to protect themselves eat garlic beforehand and drink wine, becoming less vulnerable. The pith is removed the way the pith of the white hellebore is removed.

### IV, 163 σησαμοειδὲς τὸ μικρόν, *Aubrieta deltoides* L., Purple rock cress

Purple rock cress: the little stems are a span long and they have leaves similar to crow's foot but rougher and smaller; at the end of the little stems there are little heads of purplish flowers with white centers; they contain seed which resembles sesame and which is bitter and yellowish. The root is delicate.

About half an *oxybaphon* of seed, ground up and drunk with hydromel, purges downwards phlegm and bile. Applied as a plaster with water it dissipates tumors and swellings. It grows in rough places.

### IV, 164 τιθύμαλλος, *Euphorbia* L. sp. Spurge

**1.** There are seven kinds of spurges, of which the male is called *characias*, but some call it *cometes* or *amygdalites* or *cobios*; and there is a kind called female or *myrsinites*,[53] which they call also *caryites*; and there is *paralios*, which some called *tithymallis*;[54] and there is *helioscopios*,[55] *cyparissios*,[56] *dendroides*,[57] and *platypthyllos*.[58]

[53] "Myrtle spurge."
[54] "Sea spurge."
[55] "Sun spurge."
[56] "Cypress spurge."
[57] "Tree-like spurge."

The stems of the one called *characias* are over a cubit long, red, and full of a milky juice that is sharp and white. The leaves surrounding the shoots are like those of the olive tree but longer and narrower and the root is stout and woody. At the tips of the stems there is foliage from rush-like little twigs, and on them there are hollows that resemble little cups, wherein is the fruit. It grows in rough and mountainous places.

**2.** A quantity of two *obols* of the milky juice taken with sour wine mixed with water has the property of purging the lower abdomen, expelling phlegm and bile, and, with a mixture of honey and water, it is also emetic. Milky juice is extracted from shoots collected and chopped up around harvest time. They must be kept in a vessel. Some, mixing the milky juice with flour of bitter vetch, form pills the size of bitter vetches; some dribble three or four drops of milky juice on figs that are drying and store them after drying them; it is also pounded by itself in a mortar, molded, and stored.

**3.** In extracting the milky juice, one must neither stand against the wind nor touch his eyes with his hands, but even before starting the extraction one must anoint his body with suet or with oil combined with wine, especially the face, scrotum, and neck. It also chafes the throat; it is for this reason that one must coat the little pills with wax or with boiled honey, and thus administer them. Taking two or three dry figs is definitely enough for purging. The newly made juice, when smeared on with olive oil in the sun, removes hair and makes the hair that grows afterwards blond and fine; in the end it destroys it entirely.

**4.** It is also inserted into the cavities of teeth, allaying the aches. But one must surround the teeth with wax, lest, spilling over, it may harm the throat or tongue. When smeared on, it also removes warts that spread under the skin, warts that have a neck, warty excrescences, and lichen-like eruptions on the skin. It is also suitable for membranes that grow over the eyes from the inner corners, for carbuncles, for cankers, for gangrenes, and for fistulas. Its fruit, too, collected during the fall, dried in the sun, cut up a bit, and after its bran is removed, it is stored clean; similarly are stored also the dry leaves. The fruit and leaves given to drink in the amount of half an *oxybaphon* effect the same

---

[58] "Broad-leaved spurge."

results as the milky juice. Some even preserve them, combining them by means of milk with pepperwort and chopped cheese.

**5.** The root, too, purges the bowel when one *drachma* of it is sprinkled with hydromel and drunk, and it helps for toothaches when boiled with vinegar and used as a rinse.

The female, which some called *myrsinites* or *caryites,* resembles spurge laurel; it is white in nature and it has leaves like laurel but bigger and strong, sharp and thorny at the tip. It sends up twigs from the root, about a span long, and it bears fruit every other year that resembles a nut, biting mildly the tongue. It, too, grows in rough terrains.

**6.** Its milky juice, root, fruit, and leaves have the same properties as the previous one. But the former is a more powerful emetic than this one.

The one called *paralios tithymallos,* which some called *tithymallis* or *mycon,* grows in places near the sea. It has twigs a span long, erect, and reddish, five or six growing from the same root; the leaves around the twigs are in a row; they are small, somewhat narrow, oblong, and they resemble those of flax. At the tip they have a dense and round head wherein lies the fruit like a bitter vetch; it is pied. The flowers are white.

**7.** The entire shrub and root are full of much white milky juice. The use and storage of this one, too, is the same as of the ones previously mentioned.

The one called *helioscopios* has leaves like the purslane's but thinner and more rounded, and it sends up from the root four or five twigs that are a span long, delicate, red, and full of a great deal of white juice; the head is dill-like, and its fruit as if it were in little sacs. Its foliage turns as the sun sets; hence it was named *helioscopios.*[59] It grows mostly among ruins and around cities.

**8.** The milky juice and fruit are collected just as from the other spurges; they have the same properties but not the intensity.

*Cyparissias* sends up a stem a span tall or even taller, reddish, from which grow leaves similar to the leaves of the *pitys* pine, but they are tenderer and more slender, and, in general, it resembles a newly grown

[59] From ἥλιος, "sun" and the suffix σκοπ- of σκοπεύω, "look toward."

pine and whence it was named.[60] It, too, is full of white juice. It has the same properties as the ones before it.

**9.** The one that grows among rocks and that is called *dendroeides* spreads widely on top, it is full of foliage and of milky juice, and it has reddish twigs that are surrounded by leaves that resemble those of slender myrtle; the fruit is similar to that of *characias*. It, too, is put up and operates like the ones mentioned before.

*Platyphyllos* resembles the mullein. Its root, milky juice, and leaves drive down the bowel watery elements; it also kills the fish when chopped up and released in the water. The ones described above also do the same.

**IV, 165 πιτυοῦσα, *Euphorbia pityusa* L., Quacksalver's spurge**

Quacksalver's spurge: but some call it *clema*, others *crambion*, others *paralion*, and others *Canopicon*. It does not seem to differ in kind from spurge *cyparissias*, therefore, it, too, is counted as a species of *cyparissias*. It sends up a stem longer than a cubit which has many joints and which is covered by pointed and delicate little leaves like those of *pitys* pine. It has small purplish flowers, fruit that is flat like a lentil, and a root that is white, thick, and full of milky juice. In some places the shrub is very large.

The root purges downward. Two *drachmai* of it are given with honey mixed with water; but of the fruit, one *drachma*, and of the milky juice about a spoonful made into a little pill with meal, as indicated, and of the leaves three *holcai*.

**IV, 166 λαθυρίς, *Euphorbia lathyris* L., Caper spurge**

**1.** Caper spurge: some people count even this one among the spurges. It sends up a stem a cubit tall, hollow, thick as a finger, and on top of it there are axils. The leaves on the stem are longish, like the leaves of the almond tree but they are broader and smoother; those at the end of the small branches are smaller; they are like the leaves of the long birthwort or of the ivy.

---

[60] This is a wood spurge and derives its name, κυπαρισσίας, from κυπάρισσος, "cypress" and not from πίτυς, "pine."

**2.** At the end of the branches its has a tripartite fruit, round like a caper, containing three round seedlets kept separate from each other by capsules, bigger than bitter vetches, white, and sweet-tasting when peeled. The root is thin and useless. The entire shrub is full of milky juice just like a spurge.
The seeds have the property of purging the bowel when about seven or eight in number are taken in a pill or are eaten or drunk then followed by a draught of cold water. They also draw phlegm, bile, and water. The milky juice, too, compounded like the milky juice of spurge, does the same. The leaves are cooked with either fowl or vegetables for the same effect.

**IV, 167 πέπλος, *Euphorbia peplus* L., Wartweed**
Wartweed: but some call it *syce* and others *mecon aphrodes*. It is a small shrub full of white juice, having a small leaf like that of the rue but broader. Its entire foliage is about a span, globular, spreading out on the ground, and underneath the leaves there is small round fruit, smaller than that of the white poppy. The plant is full of fruit; it has a single, useless root from which the entire shrub grows. It grows in gardens and vineyards. The fruit is gathered when wheat is harvested, dried in the shade, and turned over frequently. After it has been chopped and winnowed, it is stored.
A quantity of one *oxybaphon* drunk with one *cotyle* of hydromel drives out phlegm and bile; even when mixed with side dishes, it stirs up the belly. It is preserved in brine.

**IV, 168 πεπλίς, *Euphorbia peplis* L., Wild purslane**
Wild purslane: but some call it *andrachne agria* and Hippocrates[61] calls it *peplion*. It is a widespread shrub growing mostly by the seaside, it is full of milky juice, it has leaves similar to those of the garden purslane but they are round and reddish below. Its fruit, too, is round, lying underneath the leaves just like that of the wartweed, and it tastes hot. The root is delicate, single, and useless. It is collected, stored, and administered just like the wartweed; it is also cured.
It has the same property.

---

[61] VII 184 L.

**IV, 169 χαμαισύκη, *Euphorbia chamaisyce* L., Thyme spurge**

Thyme spurge: but some call it *syce*. It sends out twigs, four-fingers long, prostrate in a circle and full of milky juice. It has small, delicate, lentoid leaves, similar to the leaves of the wartweed, and close to the ground. The fruit is under the leaves, round, like that of the wartweed. It has neither flower nor stalk, and it has a thin and useless root.

Triturated with wine, the twigs have the property of ending pains in the area of the uterus when applied instead of a pessary; plastered on they remove swellings, thin-necked warts, and warts that spread below the skin, and they relax the bowel when eaten boiled. Their milky juice, too, accomplishes the same and it helps people stung by scorpions when smeared on. It is also suitable to smear for dim-sightedness, misting eyes, incipient cataracts, scars, and cloud-like opacities on the eyes. It grows in rocky and dry places.

**IV, 170 σκαμμωνία, *Convolvulus scammonia* L., Scammony**

**1.** Scammony: it sends up many twigs from a single root that are three-cubits tall, greasy, and that seem to be somewhat rough; the leaves, too, are rough, resembling those of *helxine*[62] or of ivy, softer, to be sure, and triangular in shape. The flowers are white, round, hollow like baskets, and oppressive in smell. The root is of a good length, thick as an arm, white, oppressive in smell, and full of milky juice. The milky juice is extracted by removing the head of the root and cutting the root out conically into a hollow. For the milky juice flows into it and it is thus recovered into receptacles.

**2.** And some, dig the ground in the shape of a mortar, line it with walnut leaves, pour the milky juice into it, and remove it after it has dried. It is of good quality if translucent, light, thin, having the color of bull-glue, slender-quilled, and spongy. Such is the one exported from Asian Mysia. And one must not pay attention only to whether it turns white when the tongue touches it—for this happens also when it has been mixed with the milky juice of spurge—but rather to what has been said above and that it must not burn the tongue too much, which happens when spurge has been added.

---

[62] ἑλξίνη, "pellitory" or "bindweed."

**3.** But the Syrian and the one produced in Judea are the worst; they are heavy, thick, and adulterated with a mixture of spurge and meal.
An amount of one *drachma* or of one *triobolon* of its milky juice, taken either with honey mixed with water or with water, can purge phlegm and bile downward. But to loosen the bowel, two *obols* taken with sesame seed or with some other kind of seed are enough. For a more vigorous purging, four *obols* of the milky juice, two *obols* of black hellebore, and a <quantity> of one *drachma* <of bitter aloes> and of salt are given.
**4.** They also make cathartic salts by mixing 20 *holcai* of the milky juice of scammony with six *cyathoi* of salts. They are taken in proportion to one's strength: three spoons being the full measure, an average is two, and the minimum is one. One or two *drachmai* of the root combined with the ingredients that were mentioned are also cathartic, and some people drink it after boiling it. Boiled with vinegar and triturated with barley meal, it is a plaster for people with hip ailments. The milky juice applied to the uterus with a wool pad destroys embryos/fetuses and it dissolves even growths when anointed with honey or oil; boiled with vinegar and smeared on it removes leprosies, and in combination with vinegar or unguent of roses it is a lotion for chronic headaches.

## IV, 171 χαμελαία, *Daphne oleides* L. and *D. oleafolia* L., Spurge olive

Spurge olive: but some call it *pyros achne* or *acneston* or *coccos Cnidios*. It has twigs that are a span long, and the shrub belongs to the class of undershrubs, having leaves closely resembling those of the olive tree but thinner and bitter, dense, pungent in taste, and irritating the throat.
Its leaves purge phlegm and bile downward, especially when taken in the form of a little pill, two parts of wormwood *Artemisia absinthium* being mixed with one part of spurge olive. But make sure that they are blended with water or honey into little pills. They are insoluble because they pass through the system as big as they were when taken. The leaves ground up and prepared with honey clean filthy and scabby sores.

**IV, 172 θυμελαία ἢ χαμελαία, *Daphne gnidium* L., Spurge flax**

**1.** Spurge flax: but some call it *pyros achne,* or *cnestron* or *cneoron.* From it the Cnidian berry, which is its fruit, is collected. The Euboeans call it *apolinon*, but others call it *linon*[63] because the shrub is like in nature to cultivated linen. It sends out many beautiful shoots, about two cubits tall. Its leaves are like those of spurge olive except narrower and shinier, somewhat tough and glutinous when chewed. The flowers are white and among them is the fruit, small as myrtle-berries, rounder, initially pale-green, thereafter red.

**2.** The shell of the fruit is hard and black and the inside is white; the inside of about 20 berries purges downward water, bile, and phlegm when drunk; but it does burn the throat; it is for this reason that it must be give either with meal or with barley groats, and that one must swallow it either in a grape or coated with boiled honey, also people who have difficulty sweating must be rubbed with oil together with soda and vinegar. The leaves, which are commonly called *cneora,* must be collected around wheat-harvest time, dried in the sun, and stored; in administering them one must chop them up and remove their ribs.

**3.** A quantity of one *oxybaphon,* molded with diluted wine, purges by driving out watery matter, but it effects a gentler purging when mixed with boiled lentils or with puréed vegetables. They ground them up, mold them with juice of unripe olives into little pills, and store them. But this herb is bad for the stomach and it destroys embryos/fetuses when used as a pessary. It grows in mountainous and rough places. Those who think that the Cnidian berry is the fruit of the spurge olive are wrong. They are misled by the similarity of their leaves.

**IV, 173 ἀκτη, *Sambucus nigra* L., Elder**

**1.** Elder: it is of two kinds. For one is tree-like, having reed-like branches that are round, whitish, and quite long; its leaves, three or four spaced around the shoot, are similar to the leaves of the walnut tree, but they are oppressive in scent and smaller; at the end of the branches it has round umbels that have white flowers, and fruit like

[63] From λίνον, "linen."

that of the terebinth, purplish tending toward black, resembling a bunch of grapes, and containing much wine-like juice.

**2.** The other kind of this plant is called *chamaiacte* and by some *heleios acte.*[64] It is smaller and more like an herb, having a quadrangular stem with many joints. The leaves, spaced around each joint, are pinnatifid; they are similar to the leaves of the almond tree but notched all around and longer, and of a heavy scent. The umbel at the tip is like that of the previous one, as are the flower and fruit. The root is below ground, long, and of the thickness of a finger.

The properties and uses of both are the same: they cool and they drive out water, but they are definitely bad for the stomach. The leaves, boiled as one boils vegetables, purge phlegm and bile, and the soft stems taken boiled in a dish do the same.

**3.** Its root, boiled with wine and given as part of the diet, benefits those with edemata and helps those bitten by vipers when similarly drunk. Boiled with water and used in a sitz bath, it softens and opens the uterus and it corrects conditions associated with it. The fruit also accomplishes the same when drunk with wine and it also dyes the hair black when smeared on it. With barley groats, the leaves that are young and soft assuage inflammations and they are suitable to apply as a plaster on burns and on people bitten by dogs. They also seal together fistulas and they help the gouty when plastered on with suet or with goat fat.

## IV, 174 πυκνόκομον ~ *Leonurus cardiaca* L., ~ *L. marrubiastrum* L., ~ *Valeriana tuberosa* L., Motherwort [65]

Motherwort: it has leaves similar to the rocket's, rough, pungent, and thicker, a quadrangular stem, a flower that is like the flower of the basil, seed as of the leek, and a dark root that is round like a small apple and that smells of earth. It grows in rocky places.

---

[64] This is the deadwort, *Sambucus ebulus* L.

[65] According to Jacques André, *Les noms des plantes dans la Rome antique,* p. 211, the possible identifications of this plant with either *Leonurus cardiaca* L. or *L. marrubiastrum* L., are incorrect since their leaves are not like those of the rocket nor do they have a round root like a small apple. It is P. Fournier R. E. A. 60 (1958), p. 484 who suggests *Valeriana tuberosa* L.

When drunk in the amount of one *drachma*, the fruit can cause many disturbing dreams and when applied as a plaster with barley groats, it disperses swellings and extracts splinters and thorns; also the leaves dissolve tumors and small abscesses when plastered on. Its root loosens the bowel and sets bile in motion. Give two *drachmai* with a mixture of honey and water.

**IV, 175 ἄπιος, *Euphorbia apios* L., Tuberous spurge**

Tuberous spurge: but some people call it *ischas,* others *chamaibalanon,* others *rhaphanos agria*, and others *linozostis*. It sends up from the ground two or three stringy little twigs, thin, red, and rising slightly above ground. The leaves resemble those of the rue but they are longer and pale-green. The fruit is small. The root closely resembles that of the asphodel but it is rounder, tending toward being pear-shaped, full of milky juice, and it has skin that is black on the outside, but inside the root is white.

The upper part of this root when ingested brings up bile and phlegm by vomiting, but the part that is toward the bottom purges downward, and the entire root when taken sets in motion both purgings. Should you wish to extract the milky juice, chop the roots up and after placing them in a bowl of water, stir them and removing with a feather the milky juice that floats on top, dry it. Three *hemiobolia* of it purge upward and downward when drunk.

**IV, 176 κολόκυνθα ἀγρία, *Citrullus colocynthis* Schrad., Colocynth**

**1.** Colocynth: but some people call it *sicya picra* and others *colocynthis*. It sends out little twigs and leaves that are strewn on the ground. They are similar to those of the cucumber and they are split. It has round fruit like a medium-size ball and very bitter. It must be harvested as it begins to change into a paler color.

An amount of four *obols* of the fruit's pulp made into little pills with soda, myrrh, and boiled honey has a purging property when taken with hydromel.

**2.** The gourds themselves, dry and ground up, are beneficially mixed in clysters for people with hip ailments, paralysis, and colic, removing phlegm, bile, and loose shreds, and, at times, even bloody matter; they also destroy embryos/fetuses when inserted as a pessary. And it is a rinse for toothaches if one removed the interior of the gourd, wrapped it with clay, boiled it in vinegar, and gave the vinegar to be used as a mouthwash. And if one after boiling in it honey mixed with water or else grape syrup and after putting it out in the sun gave it to drink, it does remove thick masses and particles. But it is very bad for the stomach. They also insert suppositories made from it to get rid of excrements. The juice of fresh colocynth is suitable to rub on people with hip ailments.

**IV, 177 ἐπίθυμον, *Cuscuta epithymum* L., *Epithymon*[66]**

*Epithymon*: it is the flower of the tougher thyme and of the one that resembles savory. The little heads are fine and light, having hair-like stems.

When drunk it purges phlegm and black bile downward and it is especially suitable for melancholiacs and for those afflicted with flatulence when they take a cupful of four *drachmai* with honey, salt, and a bit of vinegar. It grows plentiful in Pamphylia and Cappadocia.

**IV, 178 ἄλυπον, *Globularia alypum* L., Herb terrible**

Herb terrible: It is a shrubby plant, reddish, having thin twigs and thin leaves, and a soft and unsubstantial flower. The root is like that of the beet, full of sharp juice, and the seed is like that of *epithymon.* It grows plentiful in coastal areas, especially in the coastlands of Libya as well as in other places.

The seed, taken in the same quantities as *epithymon* with salts and vinegar, purges black bile downward but it ulcerates somewhat the intestines.

**IV, 179 ἔμπετρον, *Frankenia hirsuta* L. and *F. pulverulenta* L., Sea heath**

Sea heath: but some call it *phacoeides.* It grows on mountainous and maritime rocks. It is salty in taste, but the one that grows more inshore is bitterer. Given in a broth or with hydromel, it removes phlegm, bile, and watery elements.

[66] A parasitic plant.

**IV, 180 κληματίς, *Clematis vitalba* L., *C. cirrosa* L., *C. flammula* L., Traveler's joy**

Traveler's joy: it sends out a vine-twig, reddish, and willowy, and a leaf that is very sharp in taste and ulcerative. It entwines itself around trees just like bindweed.

Its fruit, ground up and drunk with water or with hydromel, removes downward phlegm and bile. The leaves remove leprosies when plastered on them. They are also cured with pepperwort for eating.

**IV, 181 ἄμπελος ἀγρία, *Vitis silvestris* Gmel., Wild grapevine**

Wild grapevine: it sends out long vine twigs like those of the cultivated grapevine, woody, rough, and with bark that cracks, leaves like those of the hound's berry but wider and smaller, hair-like and catkin-like flowers, and fruit like small grape clusters and red when ripe. The shape of its pips is round.

Its root, boiled in water and drunk with wine mixed with seawater in the amount of two *cyathoi*, purges watery elements; it is given to those with edemata. The grape clusters remove freckles and all blemishes. The young boughs of this plant also are cured for eating.

**IV, 182 ἄμπελος λευκή, *Bryonia dioica* Jacq., Bryony**

**1.** Bryony: but some call it *bryonia,* others *ophiostaphylon,* others *chelidonion,* others *<mados>* or *melothron* or *psilothron* or *archezostis* or *agrostis* or *cedrostis*. Its twigs, leaves, and tendrils are similar to those of the cultivated grape, except that all of them are rougher; it, too, entwines itself around the nearby shrubs seizing hold of them with its tendrils. Its fruit is in bunches and it is red. It is used to remove hair from pelts. Its shoots, when they first come out, are eaten boiled, setting in motion micturition and bowel movement.

**2.** Its leaves, fruit, <stem>, and root have a sharp property, wherefore, when plastered on with salt they are effective for sores that are malignant, gangrenous, cancerous, and that cause rotting of the legs. The root cleanses the skin and frees it of wrinkles; and with bitter vetch and fenugreek, it removes freckles, facial eruptions, birthmarks, and dark scars. Boiled with olive oil until it becomes soft, it is suitable for the same purposes. Plastered on with wine it removes black eye, it shrinks the fleshy excrescences that grow on the fingers, it dissipates inflammations, and it breaks abscesses; ground up it even draws out bones when plastered on, and it is compounded advantageously with septic medications.

**3.** One *holce* is drunk daily for one year for epilepsy, it is good for paralytics and for people who suffer from dizziness when similarly taken, and a weight of two *drachmai* when drunk helps those bitten by vipers and destroys embryos/fetuses. At times, however, it addles the mind. Inserted as a pessary into the uterus it also draws out embryos/fetuses and the afterbirth. It is diuretic when drunk; a lozenge made from it with honey is given to people who choke, to those who have dyspnea, who cough, who have a pain in the side, for ruptures, and for spasms; it also reduces the spleen when a weight of one *triobolon* is drunk with vinegar for thirty days.

**4.** It is also plastered profitably with a fig for the same purposes. It is boiled for sitz baths, too, being a cleanser of the uterus and abortifacient. Juice is extracted from its root in the spring; the juice is drunk with hydromel for the same purposes, removing phlegm. The fruit is good for mange and leprosies when rubbed on and when plastered on. The juice of its fruit also draws out milk when taken in a drink with boiled wheat.

**IV, 183 ἄμπελος μέλαινα, *Tamus communis* L., Black bryony**

**1.** Black bryony, which some call idiomatically *bryonia* and others *Cheironios ambelos*. Its leaves are like those of the ivy tending more toward those of bindweed, as are its stems, but these are larger. It, too, attaches itself to trees by means of its tendrils. The fruit is in clusters, at first pale-green but after ripening it becomes black. The root is outwardly black but inside it has the color of boxwood.

**2.** Its stems, too, when first sprouting, are used as vegetables. They are diuretic, they set the menses going, they reduce the spleen, and they are well suited for epileptics, paralytics, and for those suffering from dizziness. The root possesses the same properties as the bryony and it is appropriate for the same purposes, although it is less effective. The leaves made into a poultice with wine are good for the ulcerated napes of draught animals and they are similarly applied for sprains.

**IV, 184 πτερίς, *Polystichum filix mas* Roth., Male fern**

Male fern, which some people call *blechron* and others *polyrrhizon.* The leaves are without stems, without flowers, and without fruit, growing from one petiole about a cubit in size; they are incised, they open like a wing, and they are somewhat rank smelling. It has a superficial root, which is black, somewhat long, having many offshoots, and it is somewhat astringent in taste. It grows in mountainous and stony places.

Four *drachmai* of its root taken with honey mixed with water expel the flat intestinal worm. But it is better if one gave it with two *drachmai* of scammony or black hellebore. Those who take it must first eat garlic.

**IV, 185 θηλυπτερίς, *Pteris aquiline* L., Bracken**

Bracken: but some call it *nymphaia pteris.* Its leaves are like those of the male fern, although they are not from a single petiole as are the leaves of that one, but they have many rather tall off-shoots. The roots are below, oblique and long; many are yellowish tending toward a dark color, but some are red.

They, too, expel the flat intestinal worm when taken in a lozenge with honey and they cast out the round worm when drunk in the amount of three *drachmai* with wine. When given to women they cause barrenness, and should a pregnant woman take them, she aborts. They are sprinkled dry over difficult to cure and very purulent sores, and they repair the napes of draught animals. Its young leaves soften the bowel when boiled as potherbs then eaten,

**IV, 186 πολυπόδιον, *Polypodium vulgare* L., Polypody**

Polypody: it grows on moss-covered rocks and on the mosses on stumps of old trees. It is as tall as span, it resembling the male fern, it is somewhat rough and sectioned but the sections are not quite as narrow. The root below is thick, having tentacles like an octopus; it is as thick as the little finger, and when scraped it is pale inside; it tastes astringent and somewhat sweet and it has a cathartic property. It is given boiled together with chicken or fish or beet or mallow. When sprinkled dry with honey mixed with water, it draws phlegm and bile.

Ground up and plastered on, the root is good also for sprains and for fissures between the fingers.

**IV, 187 δρυπτερίς, ~ *Asplenium onopteris* L., ~ *Dryopteris* L. sp., Black oak fern**

Black oak fern: it grows on the mossy parts of old oaks, it resembles the male fern, but it is a great deal smaller and delicately slit. It has roots that are matted, sharp, and taste somewhat sweet.

This plant removes hair when applied ground up with its roots. One must, however, wipe clean the first application after it has moistened the skin and make a fresh application.

**IV, 188 κνῆκος, *Catharmus tinctorius* L., Safflower**

**1.** Safflower: it has leaves that are longish, slit, rough, and prickly, stems that are two-cubits tall, on which there are little heads about the size of an olive, a flower similar to the saffron, and seed that is white and red, longish, and angular. They use its flower in side dishes.

Juice from the chopped seed with hydromel or chicken broth purges the bowel. But it is bad for the stomach.

**2.** Lozenges that soften the bowel are also made from it by braying it in a mortar and mixing it with almonds, soda, anise, and boiled honey. Dividing them into four parts the size of a walnut, you must take two or three before dinner. You must prepare them this way: one *xestes* of white safflower, three *cyathoi* of roasted almonds, their skins removed, one *drachma aphronitron*,[67] one *drachma* anise, <enough honey>,[68] and the flesh of 30 figs. The juice of the seed also curdles milk and makes it more laxative.

**IV, 189 λινόζωστις, *Mercurialis annua* L., Mercury**

**1.** Mercury: but some call it *parthenion* and others *Hermou botanion.* Its leaf is similar to that of basil, tending toward the leaf of *helxine*[69] but smaller; it has little sprays that have two joints and many closely packed axils. The female plant has much fruit in bunches, but the male

[67] A form of native sodium carbonate.

[68] Namely, a sufficient amount to enable one to shape them.

[69] Dioscorides calls ἑλξίνη two plants, 1) pellitory, IV, 89 and 2) bindweed, IV, 39.

has small fruit hard by the leaves, round, lying in pairs like testicles. The entire little shrub is a span tall or taller.
**2.** Prepared like vegetables and eaten, both set the bowel going; and when boiled in water and their water is drunk, they remove bile and watery matter. And it is thought that the ground leaves of the female plant, when drunk and when applied to the genitalia after the menstrual period, cause the conception of a girl, and that those of the male plant, similarly used, promote the conception of males.

**IV, 190 ἡλιοτρόπιον τὸ μέγα, *Heliotropium europaeum* L., *H. villosum* L., *H. supinum* L., Large heliotrope**
**1.** Large heliotrope that some call *scorpiouron*[70] from the shape of its flower and *heliotropion* because its leaves follow the sun to its setting. It has leaves nearly resembling those of basil except they are rougher and darker, two or three small twigs that grow from the root, and from them many axils. At the ends there is a white flower, slightly purple, and curling like a scorpion's tail; the root is thin and useless. It grows in rough places.
**2.** A handful of it, boiled with water and drunk, removes phlegm and bile through the bowel. It is also suitable for people stung by scorpions when drunk with wine and when plastered on. Some bind the root on people stung by scorpions to free them from pain. And they say that four grains of fruit, drunk with wine one hour before an attack, get rid of quartan fevers and that three grains get rid of tertian fevers. Applied as a plaster, the fruit dries up warts that spread under the skin, warts that have a neck, large warts, and pustules that are most painful at night, and the leaves are beneficially plastered on for gout, sprains, and on children suffering from heatstroke. Inserted ground up as a pessary, they move both the menstrual period and embryos/fetuses.

[70] I.e. scorpion-tailed.

**IV, 191 ἡλιοτρόπιον τὸ μικρόν, *Chrozophora tinctoria* Juss., Small heliotrope**

Small heliotrope: it grows in swampy places and near marshes, having leaves closely resembling the leaves of the above but rounder, and round fruit hanging like thin-necked warts.

The plant with the fruit when drunk with soda, hyssop, garden cress, and water can expel the flat and the round intestinal worms. It also lifts up warts that have thin necks when plastered on with salt.

**IV, 192 σκορπιοειδές, *Coronilla scorpioides* Koch, Scorpionwort**

Scorpionwort: it is a small herb that has few leaves and seeds that resemble tails of scorpions. They help people stung by scorpions when plastered on.

# BOOK V

Dear Areios,
In the previous four books I discussed aromatics, oils, unguents, trees, their fruits and saps; also animals, honey, milk, what are called grains and potherbs, and I rendered a full account of roots, herbs, juice extracts, and seeds. In this one, which is the last of my entire treatise, I shall discuss wines and what are called minerals, beginning with an account of the grapevine.

### V, 1 ἄμπελος οἰνοφόρος, *Vitis vinifera* L., Grapevine

**1.** Ground up and plastered on, the leaves and tendrils of the grapevine assuage headaches and, since they are astringent and possess a cooling property, they relieve inflammations of the stomach and heartburn when plastered on either with barley groats or by themselves. When drunk, their juice helps dysenterics, people who spit blood, those with stomach ailments, and pregnant women who crave for strange foods; even its tendrils do the same when soaked in water and drunk.
**2.** Its sap, which is similar to gum and congeals around the trunks, when drunk with wine expels stones. It also treats lichen-like eruptions of the skin, leprosies, and mange when smeared on. But you must first clean the area with soda. Smeared on repeatedly with olive oil it is depilatory, especially that sap that exudes from the green vine-twig when it burns. This sap also gets rid of warts that spread below the skin. But the ashes of the vine-twigs and of the grape pressings, plastered on with vinegar, treat excised callous lumps around the anus, large warts, sprains, and when plastered on with unguent of roses, rue, and vinegar they help people bitten by vipers and for inflammations of the spleen.

### V, 2 ἄμπελος ἀγρία, *Vitis silvestris* L., Wild grapevine

Wild grapevine: it is of two sorts: for one produces grapes that do not ripen but throughout the blooming time puts out the so called

*oinanthe;*[1] the other produces perfect fruit, although the grape is small, black, and astringent.
Its leaves, tendrils, and stems have the same properties as those of the cultivated.

**V, 3 σταφυλή, Grape**
**1.** Grape: all fresh grapes trouble the belly and produce stomach gas, but grapes that have been hanging for some time partake slightly of these characteristics because much of their moisture has dried up and they are wholesome, they restore the appetite, and they are well suited to the sick. Grapes from the pressings and from the vats are tasty, wholesome, and can check diarrhea, but they attack the bladder and head. They are suitable also for people who spit blood. So are also the grapes that are put in must; but grapes from concentrated must and from grape syrup are rather bad for the stomach.
**2.** They are also put up in rainwater having been first made into raisins; such as these do become mildly winy in flavor, but they quench thirst and they are useful for persistent high fevers. The mass of their pressings that was stored, <ground up> with salt, is plastered on inflammations, indurations, and distension of the breasts. And the decoction from the mass of pressings benefits dysenterics, the colicky, and women suffering from discharges when used as a clyster; it is also used for sitz baths and rinses. Their seeds are astringent, wholesome, and when roasted and sprinkled ground up instead of barley groats they are suitable for dysenterics, the colicky, and for people with an upset stomach.
**3.** White raisins are more astringent. Their flesh benefits the trachea, a cough, the kidneys, the bladder, and dysentery when consumed with the seeds by itself, also when combined with meal of millet and egg then fried and taken with honey. It is also good for purging phlegm and it stops testicular inflammations when plastered on with meal of beans and cumin. Ground up without the seeds and applied with rue, it treats pustules that are most painful at night, carbuncles, impetigo contagiosa, putrid humors around the joints, and gangrenes. With gum

[1] Οἰνάνθη is the inflorescence of the grapevine, *vitis vinifera* L. as well as of the wild grapevine, *vitis silvestris* L.

of Hercules' woundwort, it is a suitable plaster for gout and it removes loosened nails rather quickly when smeared on them.

### V, 4 οἰνάνθη, *Oinanthe*

**1.** *Oinanthe* is called the flower of the wild grapevine when in bloom. After harvesting it and drying it in the shade on a linen cloth, it must be stored in an unpitched clay vessel. The best grows in Syria, Cilicia, and Phoenicia.

It has an astringent property, wherefore, it is wholesome and diuretic when drunk, stopping diarrhea and blood spitting when applied dry; it is also beneficial for a nauseous and sour stomach.

**2.** With vinegar and unguent of roses it is also an embrocation for headaches; both fresh and dried it is an anti-inflammatory plaster for bleeding wounds, for incipient lachrymal fistulas, for mouth sores, and for spreading genital ulcers when triturated with honey, saffron, unguent of roses, and myrrh; it is mixed in pessaries for staunching blood and it is plastered on with fine meal of barley groats and wine for running eyes and for heartburn. Burned in a clay vessel on top of red-hot coals, it is good for eye medications, and with honey it treats whitlow, fleshy excrescences over the inner corners of the eyes, and flaccid and bleeding gums.

### V, 5 ὀμφάκιον, *Omphacion*

**1.** *Omphacion* is the juice of the unripe Psithian or Aminnaian grape. Having pressed the grapes before the arrival of the Dog Star's days, you must set the juice out in the sun in a copper vessel covered with a linen cloth until all of it thickens, always mixing thoroughly the thickened part with the liquid, and at night you must take it indoors; for the dews prevent it from setting. Choose it yellow or red, quite astringent, and biting the tongue. But some people thicken the juice by boiling it.

**2.** It is good with honey or grape syrup for inflammations of the tonsils, the uvula, for thrush, flaccid gums, and for purulent ears, and with vinegar, for fistulas, old sores, and spreading ulcers. It is also used as a clyster for dysenterics and for women suffering from discharges. It promotes sharp-sightedness and it is suitable both for roughness on the eyes and for ulcerations of the corners of the eyes. It is drunk for spitting uncoagulated blood that is due to a rupture. But it must be used sparingly, diluted with a great deal of water, because it is highly caustic.

**V, 6 οἶνοι, Wines**

**1.** Wines: old wines are harmful to the nerves and to the other sense organs although they taste very pleasant; it is for this reason that people who have some weak area must avoid them; even so, they are consumed tempered and sparingly for good health. But new wine causes flatulence, it is difficult to digest, it gives bad dreams, and it is diuretic.

**2.** Wine of average age is free of the shortcomings of both; consequently its use is recommended both in health and in sickness.

Furthermore, white wine is delicate, easy to digest, and wholesome. But red wine[2] is thick and difficult to digest, engendering drunkenness and fleshiness. The tawny, being in between, has also middling strength in relation to each of these two. Nevertheless, white wine is preferable both in health and in sickness.

They differ, moreover, even in quality. For sweet wine is coarse and slow to evaporate, distending the stomach, upsetting the belly and bowels as does also the sweet new wine, although it inebriates less, and it is suitable for the bladder and kidneys.

**3.** Dry wine is more diuretic and causes headaches and drunkenness. Wine that is astringent is most suitable for the digestion of foods and it halts a runny bowel and other discharges. Wine that is weak affects less the nervous system and is less diuretic. But wine that has been mixed with seawater is bad for the stomach, thirst making, bad for the nerves, loosens the bowels, and it is not recommended for people recovering from a long illness.

**4.** But the wine that is made from sun-dried grapes or from grapes that were baked on the vines then pressed, and the one called Cretan or the

---

[2] Homer, *Od.* 5. 265, 9.196, sings of μέλας οἶνος, literally, "black wine," but of course, meaning red wine. In *Od.* 5. 165 and 9. 163 he also speaks of ἐρυθρός οἶνος, "red wine" and in *Il.* 1. 462 and 4. 259 of αἰθίοψ οἶνος, "sparkling" or "fiery wine." Dioscorides in this chapter, apart from such adjectives as sweet, dry, etc. talks of μέλας οἶνος, which I have translated as "red wine" not "black wine," of λευκός οἶνος, "white wine," and κιρρός οἶνος, "tawny wine."

*protropos wine* or the Pramneios wine, or the wine made from sweet new wine that is boiled down, which is called *siraios* or *epsema*, are sweet. The red one called *melampsithio,* is thick and very nourishing, but the white is more delicate, and that in the middle[3] has also a middling quality. All wines, moreover, are astringent, good for getting back the pulse, good for all poisons that destroy by ulceration when drunk with oil and vomited, and they are good for opium, for *pharicon*,[4] for arrow poison, for hemlock, for curdled milk, and for irritated and ulcerated bladder and kidneys.

**5.** But they do cause a great deal of flatulence and they are bad for the stomach. Melampsinthios is particularly well suited to people who have intestinal diarrhea, and white wine softens the bowel more that the rest. Wine containing gypsum is bad for the nervous system, causes headaches, inflames, and is unsuitable for the bladder but it is more suitable for deadly poisons than the rest. Those containing pitch or *pitys* pine resin warm and promote digestion but they are unsuitable for people inclined to vomiting. The wines that are unblended, having concentrated must mixed in them, attack and heat the head, engender drunkenness, cause flatulence, are slow to evaporate, and are bad for the stomach.

**6.** The wine that seems to be best among the Italian wines, called Phalerian, after it has aged is very easy to digest, it is good for getting back the pulse, it binds the bowel, it is good for the stomach, it is unsuitable for the bladder, it weakens the sight, and it is unsuitable for hard-drinking. The Albanian is coarser than the Phalerian: it is somewhat sweet, it inflates the stomach, it softens the bowel, and it does not assist digestion the same way, but it is less harmful to the nervous system. However, this wine, too, becomes dry when aged.

**7.** The Caicoubos, being sweet, is coarser than the Albanian; it engenders both fleshiness and good complexion, but it is unsuitable for the digestion. The Syrentine is quite dry, wherefore it stops intestinal and stomach discharges and it attacks the head less because it consists of fine parts. It becomes more wholesome and sweeter after it ages. The Adriatic and the Mamertine produced in Sicily are equally

[3] This is the tawny wine referred to earlier.
[4] Name of a poison.

hearty, mildly astringent, and age rather fast; they have a lesser effect on the nervous system because of their smoothness.

**8.** The Praitytian, this wine, too, is brought from places down the Adriatic, is fragrant and rather smooth; wherefore one drinks much without realizing it and remains inebriated for a long time. The wine called Istrian resembles the Praitytian, although it is more diuretic. The Chian, <which is called Ariousios>, is smoother than the aforesaid wines, easy to drink, nutritious, less apt to inebriate, capable of checking discharges, and useful in the preparation of eye medications.

**9.** The Lesbian is easy to digest, lighter than the Chian, and easing the bowel. The wine from around Ephesus, which is called Phygelites, has the same properties as the Lesbian. But the Mesogites from Asia, which comes from mount Tmolos, gives headaches and is harmful to the nerves. The Coan and Clazomenean wines, because they contain a great deal of seawater, spoil easily, inflate, upset the belly, and harm the nerves.

**10.** Shared properties of wine. In general, every pure, unmixed, and naturally dry wine warms, is easily digested, wholesome, stimulates the appetite, is nutritious, soporific, strengthens, and gives a good complexion. Drunk in sufficient amounts, it helps people who have taken hemlock or coriander or pine thistle[5] or *pharicon*[6] or opium or litharge or yew[7] or hemlock or leopard's bane or mushrooms; it also helps for bites of serpents and strokes of all creatures whose stroke or bite kills by chilling or upsets the stomach. It is also good for chronic flatulence, for gnawing of the hypochondrium, for distention and loosening of the stomach or bowel, and for diarrhea. Wines are also suitable for people who perspire and who are weakened, especially the white, aged, and fragrant wines.

**11.** It should be pointed out that aged and sweet wines are more suitable for conditions associated with the bladder and kidneys as well as for injuries and inflammations when applied with greasy wool, <and> they are poured beneficially over malignant, cancerous, and

---

[5] See Dsc. Bk. III, n. 11.

[6] Some kind of poison.

[7] See Dsc. Bk. IV, 79.

running sores. Suitable to use for good health are the wines that are free of seawater, dry, and white. Best among them are the Italian, as for instance the Phalerian, the Syrentine, the Caicoubos, the Signinan and many others from Campania, also the Praitytian <that comes> from the Adriatic, and <the> Sicilian called Mamertine; and of the Greek wines, <the> Chian, the Lesbian, and the Phygelites, which is produced in Ephesus.

**12.** But wines that are heavy and dark are bad for the stomach, they cause flatulence, and they are definitely fattening. On the other hand, wines that are light and dry are good for the stomach and less fattening; but very old, white, [and light] wines are more diuretic and they give headaches; consumed to excess they affect the nervous system. Wines of average age are best for drinking, as are those over seven-years old. Amounts should be based on the age of the wine, the time of the year, the customs, and the quality of the wine. Not being thirsty and moistening the food moderately are both excellent rules.

**13.** All drunkenness is dangerous but especially continuous drunkenness: for nerves that are assailed every day, finally give up, and daily drinking binges create severe health problems; on the other hand, drinking moderate amounts of wine for a few days is beneficial and especially if one drank water first. For wine does alter somewhat the state of pores, clearing out completely the palpable secretions as well as opening imperceptibly the pores. Of course, one must also drink water after drinking a great deal of wine because it does afford the constitution some means for recovery.

**14.** *Omphacites*. The wine called *omphacites* is made especially in Lesbos from grapes which are not entirely ripe but still sour; they are dried in the sun for three or four days until the clusters become wrinkled, and, after pressing them, the wine is fermented in clay vessels.

It has astringent and wholesome properties that are suitable for people with indigestion, for those with stomach problems, for those hankering after strange foods, and for those suffering from intestinal obstructions. It is believed, moreover, that drinking it even helps people suffering from fatal diseases.

**15.** But wines such as these need many years, otherwise they are unfit to drink.

*Deuterias*. The wine called *deuterias*, which some call *potimos*, is made this way: into masses of grape pressings from which you have squeezed 30 *metretai* of wine add three *metretai* of water, and after mixing and trampling them, strain and boil down to one third. For each *chous* of the *metretai* that remains mix two *xestes* of salt, and at the end of the winter pour into clay vessels. But use it up after a year because it quickly becomes weak.

**16.** It is suitable for those to whom we hesitate to give wine yet we are forced to do so because the patient hankers for it; it is also suitable for those recovering from a long illness.

*Adynamos*. There is also a wine called *adynamos* that has the same properties as *deuterias*. Mixing equal parts of water and must, you need to boil the mixture slowly over a gentle fire until the water has evaporated then, after cooling it, you must put it into a pitched vessel.

**17.** But some, after mixing equal amounts of seawater, rainwater, honey, and must, and after bottling this mixture, ferment it for 40 days; they use it after a year for the same purposes.

*Agriostaphylites*: the red wine of the wild grape, being astringent, is suitable for diarrhea and for a rheumy stomach as well as for all the other conditions that need astringency and contraction.

### V, 7 μελιτίτης, *Melitites*

**1**. The wine called *melitites* is given in cases of chronic fevers to those who have a weak stomach: for it gently softens the stool, it is diuretic, it purges the stomach, and it is suitable for arthritics, nephritics, and for those of weak constitution. It is useful also to women who drink water: for it is fragrant and nutritious.

**2.** It differs from *oinomeli*[8] in that *oinomeli* is made from aged dry wine and a little honey, while *melitites* takes for every five *choes* of hard must one *chous* of honey and one *cyathos of* salt. It must be prepared in a large vessel in order to have room to ferment thoroughly, sprinkling on it the salt mentioned earlier, a little at a time, until it ferments, and after it has stopped bubbling, it must be bottle in clay vessels.

[8] A kind of mead.

**V, 8 οἰνόμελι, Wine and honey mixture**

**1.** Mixture of wine and honey: it is best when made of aged dry wine and good honey, for this sort causes less flatulence and it quickly becomes fit for drinking. When aged, it is nutritious, when moderately old, it eases the bowel and it is diuretic; it is harmful if taken after the meal, but it is pleasant at the beginning of a meal and thereafter it stimulates the appetite.

**2.** It is generally prepared by mixing with every two *metretai* of wine one *metretes* of honey. But others, in order to make it faster, boil the honey together with the wine and thus bottle it. And some, for the sake of economy, mixing six *xestes* of seething must with *one xestes* of honey, bottle it after the fermenting ceases. It does stay sweet.

**V, 9 μελίκρατον, Mixture of honey and water = Hydromel**

**1.** Mixture of honey and water = hydromel has the same properties as mixture of wine and honey. We use it not boiled down on people whose stool we want to soften or whom we want to make vomit, as for instance people who drunk deadly poisons, administering it with olive oil; but boiled down, we use it on people whose pulse is weak, who are sickly, who cough, who have lung inflammations, and who are weakened from perspiration. That which is prepared and stored, which some call properly *hydromeli,* when of average age corresponds to the wines *deuterias*[9] and *adynamos*[10] in as much as it does restore strength; wherefore it is more convenient than *deuterias* for people who have an inflammation somewhere.

**2.** But that which is rather old is unsuitable for those with inflammations and for those who are constipated; on the other hand, it is useful for those with stomach problems or rheums, or who have no appetite, or who are weakened by perspiration. They prepare it by mixing and fermenting one part honey with two parts stale rainwater. But some mix in spring water, boil it down to one third, and store it. Some call *apomeli* the mixture of honey and water they make by washing the honeycomb with water, which they then store. But it must

---

[9] See Dsc. Bk. V, 6,15.

[10] See Dsc. Bk. V, 6,16.

be made rather pure. Some boil down this one, too. It is, however, unsuitable for the sick because it contains too much beebread.

**V, 10 ὕδωρ, Water**

Generally speaking it is difficult to assess water due to the peculiarities and specific nature of its provenience, the winds, and several other factors; but on the whole, it is excellent if it is clean and sweet, free of any quality whatsoever, tarrying in the abdomen not even for the shortest period of time, and passing through painlessly and easily, causing neither flatulence nor becoming spoiled.

**V, 11 θαλάττιον ὕδωρ, Seawater**

**1.** Seawater is harsh, warms, is bad for the stomach, upsets the belly, and removes phlegm. Used as a warm rinse, it draws to itself and dissipates, and it is suitable for conditions associate with the tendons and for chilblains before they become ulcerated; it is mixed conveniently with bruised meal of raw corn, it is well suited for plasters and resolvent emollients, it is used warm in clysters to cleanse the bowel and hot for colic, and it is a wash for mange, itching, lichen-like eruptions on the skin, nits, and for breasts swollen with milk.

**2.** It disperses livid spots when used as a fomentation and it is good for bites of all wild animals that cause tremblings and chills, but especially for bites of scorpions, poisonous spiders, and asps. And should one step into hot seawater, bathing in it benefits both chronically unwell bodies and nerves, and vaporized seawater relieves those with edemata, headaches, and hardness of hearing.

**3.** Seawater that is pure and that was not mixed with drinking water, when laid aside becomes free of smell. But some boil it first and put it up this way. It is also given neat for purging or with sour wine mixed with water or with wine or with vinegar mixed with honey, and after the purge chicken or fish broth is given to allay the severity of the gnawing.

**V, 12 θαλασσόμελι, Seawater mixed with honey**

Seawater mixed with honey is thought to purge vigorously. It is prepared with equal parts honey, rainwater, and seawater, strained, and fermented in a pitched vessel during the burning heat of the Dog Star.

But some, after mixing two parts boiled seawater and one part honey, bottle it. This is gentler and milder than seawater.

**V, 13 ὄξος, Vinegar**

**1.** Vinegar cools and contracts; it is good for the stomach, it stimulates the appetite, and it staunches all hemorrhages when drunk and when used in a sitz bath. Boiled with food, it is suitable for abdominal diarrhea and it treats bleeding wounds and inflammations when applied with greasy wool or sponges. It shrinks the uterus, a prolapsed anus, and flaccid and bleeding gums. Mixed with some suitable compound, it is good for spreading ulcers, erysipelas, shingles, leprosies, lichen-like eruptions on the skin, and membranes that grow over the inner corner of the eyes. Used as a continuous fomentation, it checks both cancerous sores and spreading ulcers.

**2.** Used as a warm rinse with sulfur, it is good for the gouty; smeared on with honey, it removes black eye; for heatstroke it is used with unguent of roses and with greasy wool or with a sponge, and it is good for those with edemata, for hardness of hearing, and for ringing and singing in the ears when vaporized hot. Instilled, it kills earwigs; it checks cancerous sores when used tepid as a rinse or when applied with sponges; it allays itching, and it is used as a warm rinse for all animal bites that cause chills, but for poisonous bites that burn, it is used cold.

**3.** It is good for deadly poisons, being drunk warm and vomited; it is especially good for those who drank opium, leopard's bane, and hemlock, and for blood and milk clots in the chest; for mushrooms, pine thistle,[11] and yew[12] it is good with salt, it expels swallowed leeches when drunk, and it soothes an old cough but exacerbates a new one. When drunk warm it is suitable also for orthopnea. As a gargle it checks discharges in the throat, it is suitable for sore throats, for a slackened uvula, and for toothaches <when held> warm in the mouth and when used as a rinse.

---

[11] See Dsc. Bk. III, n.11.

[12] See Dsc. Bk. IV, 79.

**V, 14 ὀξύμελι, Oxymel**
Oxymel is prepared this way: taking five *cotylai* of vinegar, one *mna* sea salt, ten *mnai* honey, ten *cotylai* water, and after mixing them together, boil until the mixture has bubbled up ten times, then cool and bottle.
When taken it is thought to drive out thick masses, to benefit people with hip ailments, with arthritis, and epileptics; it comes to the aid of those bitten by the viper called *seps*, to those who took opium or pine thistle, and it is a useful gargle for sore throats.

**V, 15 ὀξάλμη, Brine vinegar**
Brine vinegar is a good fomentation for spreading ulcers, putrid humors, dog bites, and for bites of venomous animals. It stems the hemorrhaging of those who were operated for stones when injected warm immediately following the surgery, it draws in a prolapsed anus when used as a sitz bath, and it is administered in a clyster to dysenterics that have spreading ulcers; afterwards, however, one must treat them with a milk clyster. When drunk and as a gargle, it expels leeches. It clears up both dandruff and scurf.

**V, 16 θυμοξάλμη, Brine vinegar flavored with Cretan thyme**
The ancients used brine vinegar flavored with Cretan thyme on those with a weak stomach; they mixed with warm water about three or four *cyathoi* of brine vinegar flavored with Cretan thyme and gave it to them; they also used it on arthritics and the flatulent: for it does drive out thick and black humors. It is prepared this way: placing one *oxybaphon* of ground Cretan thyme, an equal amount of salt, a little of each barley groats, rue, and pennyroyal into a vessel, pour over them six *cotylai* of water and half a *cotyle* of vinegar, and, after covering the vessel with a linen cloth, expose it to the sun and air.

**V, 17 τὸ σκιλλητικὸν ὄξος, Vinegar flavored with squill**
**1.** Vinegar flavored with squill is prepared this way: after cleaning, cutting up, and threading white squill with a linen thread so that the sections do not touch each other, dry them in the shade for 40 days; then taking one *mna* of it drop it into 12 *xestes* of good vinegar and let it steep for 60 days in the sun, having sealed carefully the vessel. Then

scoop up and squeeze the squill, discard it, and after straining the vinegar bottle and store it.

**2.** Some, however, mix <one> *mna* with five *xestes* of vinegar and some, right after cleaning it and without drying it, add the same amount of vinegar and leave it for six months: this sort becomes more biting.

Used as a rinse, it is good for gums afflicted with pyorrhea, tightening them and making them firmer, for loose teeth and for bad breath, eliminating it quite nicely, and it makes both the trachea firm and hard and the voice vigorous and clear when drunk.

**3.** It is used for stomach problems, for indigestion, for people with epilepsy, for dizziness, for people who are of melancholic temperament, for people who become delusive, also for uterine suffocation, for overgrown spleens, and for hip ailments. It also restores those that are quite weak and makes their body healthy and of good complexion. It does promote sharp-sightedness, and it is capable of resisting hardness of hearing when instilled. And, in general, it is effective for everything except for internal ulcerations. Give it to drink daily on an empty stomach, at first in small quantities, but shortly thereafter increase the amount to one *cyathos*. But some people give two *cyathoi* or even more.

**V, 18 ὁ ἀπὸ τῆς σκίλλης οἶνος, Wine from squill**

**1.** Wine from squill is made this way: having cut up the squill, as I described, dry it in the sun, then bray one *mna* of it and after sifting it through a fine sieve and wrapping it in a loosely woven linen cloth, drop it into 20 *xestes* must of good quality and let it steep for three months. Then decant the wine into another vessel, seal carefully, and store.

**2.** But it is possible to use the squill also moist, paring it around and around and doubling the quantity; but you must put it out in the sun for 40 days and age it for a long time. The above wine is also made this way: take three *mnai of* cleaned and chopped squill, drop them into one Italian *metretes* of good quality must, stop up the vessel, and put it aside for six months, then filter, decant, and store.

**3.** It is good for indigestion, for food poisoning, for people who vomit their food, for those whose stomach or abdomen contains gross humors, for splenetics, for the jaundiced, for people with cachexia, with edemata, for those with difficult micturition, for the colicky, for the flatulent, for paralytics, for those suffering from dizziness, for long-lasting chills, and for spasms; it is also emmenagogic. It does not vex the tendons at all. That which is more aged is better. You must guard, however, against using it when patients run a fever or when they have an internal sore.

**V, 19 οἱ διὰ θαλάττης οἶνοι, Wines made with seawater**

**1.** Wines made with seawater are prepared in various ways: for some mix seawater immediately after the grapes are harvested, others dry them first in the sun and thus step on them mixing seawater, still others after turning the grapes into raisins, soak them in large wine jars with seawater and thus treading on them squeeze them out; this kind of wine does become sweet.

**2.** But the ones that are made drier for drinking are good for curing fevers, if Aminnaian wines[13] are unavailable, for purging the bowel, for people suffering from abscesses, for the constipated, and for those whose head is affected by Aminnaian wines; even these, however, are bad for the stomach and cause flatulence.

**3.** And we think that it is also useful to describe for amateur physicians the preparation of composite wines so that this treatise becomes comprehensive. Not that they are used much or that it is necessary to use them, but rather so that I may in no way appear to have omitted anything. Some of them are no trouble to make and are applied to medicinal uses, for instance, wines from quinces, pears, fruit of the carob tree, and even from myrtles.

**V, 20 ὁ κυδωνίτης, Wine flavored with quinces**

Wine that is flavored with quinces, which some call *melites,* is prepared as follows: after removing the seed of quinces and cutting them the way one cuts up turnips, soften for 30 days in one *metretes* of must 12 *mnai* of quinces, then strain and store. It is also prepared another way: after chopping and squeezing out the quinces you must mix one *xestes* of honey with 12 *xestes* of their juice, then store. It is

[13] An Italian wine made from a grape of that name.

astringent, wholesome, suitable for dysenteries, for people with liver disease, kidney disease, and for difficult micturition.

**V, 21 μηλόμελι, Honey flavored with quinces**

Honey flavored with quinces, which is called also *cydonomeli,* is prepared by placing quinces from which the seeds were removed into as much honey as needed to cover them. It becomes smooth after a year, it resembles wine mixed with honey, and it is suitable for the same purposes as the preparation mentioned before this.

**V, 22 ὑδρόμηλον, Water and honey flavored with quinces**

Water and honey lavored with quinces is made by mixing one *metretes* of honey flavored with quinces with two *metretai* of boiled water and setting it out in the sun during the Dog Star days. The properties of this one, too, are the same.

**V, 23 ὀμφακόμελι, Unripe grapes and honey drink**

Unripe grapes and honey drink is made this way: taking sour grapes that have not yet begun to turn dark, put them in the sun for three days, then after you have squeezed them, add to three parts of the juice one part skimmed honey of excellent quality and placing it into a ceramic bottle sun it.

It has astringent and cooling properties, wherefore it is suitable for people with stomach problems and for the colicky. It is used after a year.

**V, 24 ἀπίτης, Pear wine**

Pear wine is prepared the same way as quince wine, but the pears should not be too ripe. Similarly prepared is also wine of carobs, of medlars, and of sorb apples. All are astringent, sour, wholesome, and they keep in check internal fluxes.

**V, 25 οἰνάνθινος, Wine flavored with flowers of the wild grape**

Wine flavored with flowers of the wild grape is made this way: having taken the inflorescence of wild grape that is teeming with blooms, place two *mnai* into one *metretes* of must for 30 days, then after straining store.

It is good for slackness of the stomach, for lack of appetite, for the colicky, and for dysenterics.

**V, 26 ῥοίτης, Pomegranate wine**

Pomegranate wine is prepared this way: taking ripe, pipless pomegranates, and after squeezing the juice out of the globules, store it, or after boiling it down to one third, store it this way.
It is good for internal fluxes and for very high fevers. It is wholesome, it staunches the bowels, and it is diuretic.

**V, 27 ῥοδίτης, Wine flavored with roses**

Wine flavored with roses is prepared this way: wrapping in a linen cloth one *mna* dried, chopped roses of this year drop them into 20 *xestes* must and seal tightly. Three months later, strain, decant, and store.
It is useful to the feverless for stomachaches and for the digestion when drunk after a meal; also for diarrhea and for dysentery.
The so-called *rhodomeli* is made from rose juice mixed with honey; it is suitable for roughness of the throat.

**V, 28 μυρτίτης, Myrtle wine**

In preparing myrtle wine, you must take black myrtles that are past their prime, pound them, press out their juice through a sieve, and decant. Some even boil the juice down to one-third. But others first dry them in the sun, and after drying them mix with every *choinix* of chopped berries three *cotylai* water and an equal amount of old dry wine and thus strain and store.
It is quite astringent and good for the stomach; it is useful both for a rheumy stomach and diarrhea, also for internal ulcerations and fluxes; it also blackens hair on the head.

**V, 29 μυρσινίτης, Wine flavored with myrtles**

Wine flavored with myrtles is prepared this way: after taking the branches and leaves of black myrtles together with the myrtles, you must chop them, then place into three *choes* of must 10 *mnai* of the chopped myrtle, boil until two *choes* are left, and after straining store.

This wine is good both for scurf and dandruff, for pustules, gums, tonsils, and for purulent ears; it also checks perspiration.

**V, 30 ὁ σχίνινος, Mastic wine**

Mastic wine, too, is prepared like wine flavored with myrtles, as is also wine flavored with **terebinth**: for the branches of these plants, too, are gathered full of fruit.

Additionally, they are even of about equal strength, and they are astringent, wholesome, and suitable for fluxes from the stomach, the intestines, the bladder, and for hemorrhages. Used as a rinse, they cicatrize all running sores, and if administered in sitz baths they stop fluxes from around the uterus and anus.

**V, 31 φοινικίτης, Date palm wine**

**1.** Date palm wine: taking ordinary dates that are ripe, place them in a vessel that has a hole at the bottom and that is stoppered with a pitched reed; plug the hole with linen. Pour over ten *choinices* of dates three *choes* of water, but should you wish it to be not very sweet, pour over the dates five *choes* of water. Set aside for 10 days.

**2.** On the eleventh day, after removing the linen cloth that is in the reed, collect the sweet thick wine and store.

While it is sweet, it does give headaches. It is effective for fluxes because it binds and it is for this reason that it is suitable for the colicky and for those who spit blood. But some mixing the same amount of water a second time, collect it and repeat the process a third, fourth, and fifth time when it then grows sour.

**V, 32 ὁ τροχίτης, Fig wine**

**1.** Fig wine, which some call *sycites,* is prepared in Cyprus the same way as date wine, but it differs in that some instead of the water add the same amount of an infusion of freshly pressed grapes. They use the figs called *chelidonioi* or Phoenician—they are black—and they soak them as indicated above. After 10 days, they collect the liquid and pour a second infusion of freshly pressed grapes and even a third one in the same proportions.

**2.** The fourth and fifth infusions are collected at similar intervals; however, since they are acidic they use them for vinegar.

It is fine-bodied, it causes flatulence, it is bad for the stomach, and it spoils the appetite, but it does ease the bowel and it is diuretic. It draws down the menstrual period and it increases milk production; however, it makes blood bad and it causes elephantiasis, just like beer.
**3.** Some also add 10 *ceramia* of salt to six *xestes* of liquid; others add one *ceramion* of seawater, thinking that it will make it harder to change and that it will be laxative. And others put first at the bottom of the receptacle Cretan thyme and fennel then the dried figs, and repeat the process until they fill the vessel.

### V, 33 ὁ ἐκ τῶν συκομόρων, Wine of sycamore figs

Wine of sycamore figs is prepared the same way. But it turns into sharp vinegar because their strength cannot hold onto the sweetness streaming from them.

### V, 34 ὁ ῥητινίτης, Wine flavored with resin

**1.** Wine flavored with resin is made throughout the world <in various ways>. It abounds in Galatia, because its wine turns sour unless it is mixed with <resin of> *peuce* pine since the grapes do not ripen due to the cold. The resin is brayed with the bark and one-half of a *cotyle* is mixed with a *ceramion* of wine. Some strain the wine at the end of the fermentation process, removing the resin, but others leave the resin in it. As these wines age, they become sweet.
**2.** All such wines cause headaches and dizziness, although they aid digestion and they are diuretic; they are suitable for people who have catarrhs and who cough, for the colicky, the dysenterics, those with edemata, and for women suffering from discharges; they are also a clyster for those with deep internal ulcerations. Keep in mind that the one that is darkish is more astringent than the white.

### V, 35 ὁ στροβιλίτης, Wine flavored with *strobilos* pine cones

Wine flavored with *strobilos* pine cones is prepared by soaking in must crushed *strobilos* pine cones that have been freshly harvested. It accomplishes the same results as wine flavored with resin. But if one after soaking the cones of the *strobilos* pine in grape syrup should boiled it, then it is suitable also for tuberculars when drunk in large quantities.

**V, 36 ὁ κέδρινος ἢ ἀρκεύθινος ἢ κυπαρίσσινος ἢ δάφνινος ἢ πιτύινος ἢ ἐλάτινος, Wine flavored with cedar or juniper or cypress or sweet bay or *pitys* pine or fir**

**1.** Wine flavored with cedar or juniper or cypress or sweet bay or *pitys* pine or fir is prepare the same way: having split wood newly hewn from these trees at the time they bear fruit, it is necessary to place it in the sun or in a bathroom or near a fire so that it sweats and to mix one *mna* wood with one *chous* must; and, having done so, to allow two months to go by then to decant, and after setting it out in the sun to store it. Bottles of medicinal wines must be filled to the brim because if not quite full the wines become sour.

**2.** Medicinal wines are definitely not recommended for the healthy. All of them warm, are diuretic, and are somewhat astringent; in fact, sweet bay wine warms more than the rest.

There is also a wine made from the fruit of Syrian cedars. You must mix one-half *mna* chopped Syrian cedar berries with one *chous* must, set it out in the sun for 40 days then strain and bottle. In a fashion similar to wine flavored with oil of Syrian cedar, there is also a wine made from juniper berries that does the same.

**V, 37 κεδρίτης, Wine flavored with resin of Syrian cedar**

They make wine flavored with resin of Syrian cedar this way: after washing resin of Syrian cedar with fresh water, they pour into each jar one *cyathos* and so fill the jar with must.

This wine, too, warms and attenuates; it is suitable for old coughs, provided the patients are free of fever, for chest and side pains, for colic, for abdominal and intestinal ulcers, for those suffering from abscesses, from edemata, and for uterine suffocation. It is good both for intestinal worms and for shiverings, it helps those bitten by wild animals, it kills reptiles, and it treats earaches when instilled.

**V, 38 οἶνος πισσίτης, Wine flavored with pitch**

**1.** Wine flavored with pitch is made with raw pitch and must. You must first wash the raw pitch for quite a while either with seawater or brine until it becomes white and the seawater flows clean, then with fresh water, then mix into every eight *choes* of must two *oungiai* of

pitch and leave it alone. After it has bubbled up and settled you must decant.
**2.** It warms, aids digestion, cleanses, promotes vomiting, is suitable for pains around the chest, abdomen, liver, spleen, and uterus, provided the patient is free of fever, and for chronic discharges and deep internal ulcerations. It is also efficacious for coughs, bradypepsia, inflations, and asthma, and it is more efficacious for sprains than vinegar when applied with greasy wool.

### V, 39 ἀψινθίτης, Wine flavored with wormwood *artemisia absinthium*

**1.** Wine flavored with wormwood *artemisia absinthium* is prepared in a variety of ways: some, mixing one *litra* of Pontic wormwood with 48 *xestes* <must>, boil the mixture down until one-third is left; then they pour over it 90 *xestes* must and one-half *litra* wormwood *artemisia absinthium, <and>* after careful mixing, bottle it; after it has settled, they strain and store. Others soak one *mna* of wormwood *artemisia absinthium* in one *metretes* of must for three months; others, after chopping and tying in a loosely woven linen cloth one *mna* of wormwood, drop it into a *ceramion* of must for two months.
**2.** Some, after chopping in a mortar three *oungiai* wormwood *artemisia absinthium,* but others after chopping four, and two *oungiai* each of Syrian nard, cinnamon, cassia, sweet flag, flower of camel hay, and date palm inflorescence. drop them into one *metretes* of must and tightening the lid, they leave it alone for two months. Then after straining and decanting it, store it. Others place into one *metretes* of must 14 *drachmai* of Celtic spikenard and 40 *drachmai* of wormwood *artemisia absinthium* tied together in a linen cloth and after 40 days decant.
**3.** Others put one *litra* of wormwood *artemisia absinthium* and two *oungiai* of dry *pitys* pine resin into 20 *xestes* of must; 10 days later they strain and store.
It is wholesome, diuretic, useful to people with liver disease, kidney disease, and jaundice; also for those suffering from bradypepsia, lack of appetite, stomach ailments; also for chronic abdominal tension and flatulence, for round intestinal worms, for menstrual periods that have

stopped, and for drinking pine-thistle[14] when a great deal of it is drunk and vomited.

**V, 40 ὑσσωπίτης, Wine flavored with hyssop**

**1.** Hyssop wine flavored with Cilician hyssop is excellent; it is prepared the same way as wine flavored with wormwood. You must add to one *ceramion* of must one *litra* chopped leaves of hyssop wrapped in a loosely woven linen cloth; pebbles are dropped along with it so that the bundle settles at the bottom. After 40 days, strain and decant.

**2.** It is suitable for chest, side, and lung conditions, and for old coughs and asthma. It is diuretic and it is fit for the colicky and for shiverings during intermittent fevers; it also sets the menses going.

**V, 41 ὁ χαμαιδρυίτης, Wine flavored with germander**

Wine flavored with germander is made like wine flavored with hyssop. It warms and relaxes. It is suitable for spasms, jaundice, inflations of the uterus, bradypepsia, and for incipient edemata. It improves with age.

**V, 42 <ὁ > στοιχαδίτης, Wine flavored with French lavender**

Wine flavored with French lavender is similarly made.

You must add one *mna* of French lavender to six *choes* of must. It does away with thick masses, inflations, pains of the side and tendons, and chills; it is also given successfully with pellitory and *sagapenon*[15] to epileptics.

**V, 43 ὄξος διὰ στοιχάδος, French lavender vinegar**

They even make vinegar with French lavender that is good for the above conditions by soaking the plant in vinegar, as previously stated. It is good for the same ailments.

---

[14] See Dsc. Bk. III, n. 11.

[15] Perhaps *Ferula persica.*

**V, 44 ἐκ κέστρου τοῦ ψυχροτρόφου οἶνος,Wine made from betony**

Wine is also made from betony. You must take this plant when full of ripe seed together with the branches, place one *mna* into two *choes* of wine, and after seven months simply decant.

It is effective for many internal conditions for which the shrub is also effective. In general, all medicinal wines acquire the strength of their components; it is for this reason that those who know the nature of the components can also infer easily the properties of the wines. Of course, the use of wines is for people who do not run a fever. They also make vinegar from it that is useful for the same ailments.

**V, 45 τραγοριγανίτης, Wine flavored with goat's marjoram**

Wine flavored with goat's marjoram: drop four *drachmai* goat's marjoram wrapped in a linen cloth into four *xestes* of must and after three months decant. It is suitable for colic, spasms, ruptures, pains on the side, intestinal rumblings, and indigestion.

**V, 46 οἶνος διὰ βουνίου, Wine flavored with earthnuts**

Wine flavored with earthnuts: having chopped two *drachmai* earthnuts drop them into four *cotylai* of must and do the rest the same way. It is suitable for people with disorders of the stomach and for those exhausted from fighting with heavy weapons or from much horseback riding.

**V, 47 δικταμνίτης, Wine flavored with dittany of Crete**

Wine flavored with dittany of Crete: soak similarly four *drachmai* dittany of Crete in eight *cotylai* must. It is good for those who feel nauseous from over eating and it draws both the menstrual period and the discharges following childbirth.

**V, 48 ὁ διὰ πρασίου, Wine flavored with horehound**

Wine flavored with horehound: after chopping two *choinices* of fully grown horehound leaves, drop them into one *metretes* of must and do the rest the same way. It is suitable for chest conditions and for all the things for which horehound is suitable.

**V, 49 θυμίτης, Wine flavored with Cretan thyme**

Wine flavored with Cretan thyme: drop into one *ceramion* of new wine 100 *drachmai* Cretan thyme, chopped, sifted, and tied in a linen cloth.

It is suitable for indigestion, lack of appetite, lassitude of tendons, pains of the tendons, abdominal pains, winter shiverings, and for venoms that cause chills and stiffness.

**V, 50 θυμβρίτης, Wine flavored with savory**

Wine flavored with savory is similarly prepared and it is good for the same purposes as wine flavored with Cretan thyme.

**V, 51 οἶνος ὀριγανίτης, Wine flavored with oregano**

Wine flavored with oregano is made with Heracleotic oregano the same way as wine flavored with Cretan thyme and it is good for the same purposes.

**V, 52 οἶνος καλαμινθίτης, γληχωνίτης, ἀβροτονίτης, Wines flavored with catmint, pennyroyal, wormwood *artemisia abrotonon***

Wines flavored with catmint, pennyroyal, and wormwood *artemisia abrotonon* are prepared the same way as wine flavored with Cretan thyme and they are good for people with stomach ailments, for those having no appetite, and for jaundice, for they are diuretic.

**V, 53 οἶνος κονυζίτης, Wine flavored with fleabane**

Wine flavored with fleabane is similarly prepared and it is the most effective wine of all against venomous bites.

**V, 54 οἶνος ἀρωματίτης, Wine made with aromatics**

**1.** Wine made with aromatics is prepared this way: triturate one *chous* of each date fronds, camel's-thorn, sweet flag, and Celtic spikenard, make a paste with grape syrup, shape it into sizable patties, place them into 20 *xestes* of hard must, seal the vessel, and set aside for 40 days; then strain and store. Or, triturate six *holcai* sweet flag, seven *drachmai* Cretan spikenard, two *drachmai* costusroot, six *drachmai* Syrian spikenard, eight *drachmai* cassia, four *drachmai* saffron, five *drachmai* Nepal cardamom, and four *drachmai* hazelwort; drop them

tied in a linen cloth into one *metretes* of hard must and decant the wine when the fermentation stops.
**2.** It is good for pains in the chest, side, lung, for difficult micturition, for shiverings, for interrupted menstrual periods and it is a <suitable> drink both for those who travel in icy cold weather and for those who produce thick humors. It does also achieve good complexion, it is soporific and analgesic, and it is appropriate for ailments associated with the bladder and kidneys.

### V, 55 οἶνος πρὸς κατάρρους, Wine for catarrhs

There is a wine that is made for catarrhs, coughs, indigestion, flatulence, and for an abundance of stomach liquids. Cast into six *xestes* of wine two *drachmai* myrrh, one *drachma* white pepper, six *drachmai* iris, and three *drachmai* dill, all coarsely pounded and tied in a linen cloth; after three days strain, store in a flask, and give one *cyathos* to drink unmixed, after a walk.

### V, 56 ὁ νεκταρίτης, Wine flavored with elecampane

Wine flavored with elecampane is prepared with the elecampane that some call *medice*, others *symphyton,* others *Idaios phlomos*, others *Orestion*, and others *nectarion*. Cast into six *choes* of must 50 *drachmai* dry root of elecampane, tied in a linen cloth, and three months later decant. It is good for the stomach and chest. It is also diuretic.

### V, 57 ὁ διὰ Συριακῆς νάρδου καὶ Κελτικῆς καὶ μαλαβάθρου, Wine flavored with Syrian spikenard, Celtic spikenard, and leaf of malabar

Wine flavored with Syrian spikenard, Celtic spikenard, and leaf of malabar is prepared this way: take of each of these one-half *mna,* cast into two *choes* of must, and after two months strain. Give one *cyathos* mixed with three of water to people with kidney disease, jaundice, liver disease, difficult micturition, to people who are pale, and to those who have stomach problems. But some make it with two *oungiai* sweet flag and three *oungiai* Celtic spikenard in a *ceramion* of must.

**V, 58 ἀσαρίτης, Wine flavored with hazelwort**

Wine flavored with hazelwort: cast similarly three *drachmai* hazelwort into 12 *cotylai* must. It is diuretic, suitable for people with edemata, jaundice, liver disease, and hip ailments.

**V, 59 ὁ διὰ τῆς ἀγρίας νάρδου, Wine flavored with Cretan spikenard**

Wine flavored with Cretan spikenard: similarly soak for two months into one *chous* of must eight *drachmai* of fresh root of Cretan spikenard, ground up and sifted. It is useful to people with liver disease, to those having difficult micturition, stomach problems, and to the flatulent.

**V, 60 δαυκίτης, Wine flavored with *daucos*[16]**

Wine flavored with *daucos*: similarly soak 60 *drachmai* of coarsely chopped root of *daucos* in one *ceramion* must then decant. It is good for pains in the chest, hypochondrium, and uterus; it draws the menstrual periods, it is eructative and diuretic; it is suitable for coughs, spasms, and ruptures.

**V, 61 ἐλελισφακίτης, Wine flavored with sage**

Wine flavored with sage is similarly made. Into one *amphoreus* of must, which is a *ceramion,* cast 70 *drachmai* of sage. It is good for pains of the kidneys, bladder, and sides, for coughing up blood, for coughs, ruptures, spasms, bruises, and for when menstruation has stopped.

**V, 62 πανακίτης, Wine flavored with allheal**

Wine flavored with allheal. Cast 10 *drachmai* of allheal into one *chous* must then decant the same way. It is good for spasms, ruptures, bruises, orthopnea, and it reduces the thickness of the spleen. It is also good for colic, hip ailments, and bradypepsia, it draws down the menstrual period and embryos/fetuses, and it suitable for those with edemata and for those bitten by wild animals.

---

[16] See Dsc. Bk. III, 72.

**V, 63 ἀκορίτης καὶ ὁ ἀπὸ γλυκυρρίζης, Wine flavored with yellow flag and wine flavored with licorice**

Wine flavored with yellow flag and wine flavored with licorice are made the same way. For after soaking 80 *drachmai* of each into six *choes* of must for three months, you must decant. They are good for the side and chest and they set micturition in motion.

**V, 64 σελινίτης, Wine flavored with celery**

Wine flavored with celery. Similarly place into one *ceramion* of must 70 *drachmai* of celery seed that is ripe, new, sifted, and wrapped in a linen cloth. It stimulates the appetite and it is suitable both for people who have stomach problems and for those with difficult micturition. It is also a breath sweetener.

**V, 65 μαραθίτης καὶ ἀνήθινος καὶ πετροσελινίτης, Wine flavored with fennel, wine flavored dill, and wine flavored parsley**

Also wines flavored with fennel, dill, and parsley are similarly prepared and effective for the same purposes.

**V, 66 δι' ἁλὸς ἄνθους <οἶνος>, Wine from salt-water froth**

They also make a wine from salt-water froth which is more purgative than that made from seawater. However, it harms the throat, kidneys, bladder, and stomach; therefore, this sort of wine is useful neither for health nor in sickness.

**V, 67 φθόριος ἐμβρύων οἶνος, Abortifacient wine**

There is also an abortifacient wine. For hellebore or squirting cucumber or scammony is planted together with grapevines and the grapes, absorbing the properties of these plants, produce a wine that is abortifacient. An amount of one *cyathos* is given diluted to women who have vomited, on an empty stomach.

**V, 68 θυμελαίτης, Wine flavored with spurge flax**

Wine flavored with spurge flax. Place 30 *drachmai* of the little branches together with the leaves and fruit into three *choes* of must, cover, and cook gently until two *choes* are left, then strain and store. It cleanses watery matter and it reduces the spleen.

**V, 69 χαμελαίτης, Wine flavored with spurge olive**
Wine flavored with spurge olive. When the shrub is in bloom chop it with its leaves, sift, place 12 *drachmai* into one *chous* must, and after two months decant. It is good for people with edemata, with liver disease, for the weary, and for women that are hard to purge after childbirth.

**V, 70 χαμαιπιτύινος, Wine flavored with ground pine**
Wine flavored with ground pine:[17] it is similarly prepared and it is suitable for the same conditions, being diuretic.

**V, 71 μανδραγορίτης, Wine flavored with mandrake**
Wine flavored with mandrake: cut into pieces the skin of its root, thread half a *mna* with a linen thread, and place it into one *metretes* of must for three months then decant. The average potion is one half *cotyle*; however, twice this quantity is drunk when grape syrup is added. They say that it is soporific and that it plunges an entire dinner party into deep sleep if one *cotyle* of it was mixed with one *chous* of wine; one *cyathos* drunk with one *xestes* of wine is lethal. Its moderate use, however, allays pain and thickens discharges. Both when smelled and when used as a clyster it does the same.

**V, 72 ἐλλεβορίτης, Wine flavored with hellebore**
**1.** Wine flavored with hellebore. Place 12 *drachmai* of ground black hellebore, wrapped in a loosely woven linen cloth, in one *chous* of must diluted with seawater; decant when it bubbles up. Or place in one *chous* of must that was not diluted with seawater 15 or 14 *drachmai* of coarsely crushed black hellebore and after a few days strain and use. For loosening the bowel, offer a drink of one *cyathos* with water after the bath to those who vomited after dinner.
**2.** Or, having sifted 20 *drachmai* of hellebore, 12 *drachmai* of camel hay, and 13 *drachmai* of Syrian base horehound place them wrapped in a linen cloth in 14 *cotylai* Coan wine for 40 days. Then strain and give three *hemicotylia* to drink. Or macerate in one *ceramion* of must and two *xestes* of boiled seawater for 40 days one half *litra* white

---

[17] See Dsc. Bk. III, 158.

hellebore then after straining use. Or soak for 15 days in 12 *cotylai* must 12 *drachmai* hellebore and four *drachmai* soda then filter and use after six months. This wine also causes miscarriages.

**3.** Or take one *metretes* of must made from grapes that were dried in the sun and place 20 *drachmai* chalk into the wine and leave it for two days, then drop a bag of 30 *drachmai* black hellebore, 30 *drachmai* camel hay, 30 *drachmai* sweet flag, one-half *choinix* and a quarter of juniper berries, and suspend one *drachma* each of myrrh and saffron wrapped in a linen cloth for 40 days; then filter and give three or two *cyathoi* to drink diluted with water. It purges from childbirth and miscarriages, it destroys embryos/fetuses, and it is good for uterine suffocation.

### V, 73 σκαμμωνίτης, Wine flavored with scammony

Wine flavored with scammony: 15 *drachmai* scammony root, dug up at the time of wheat harvest and ground, are placed wrapped in a linen cloth in one *chous* of must for 30 days. It purges the bowels driving out bile and phlegm.

### V, 74 καδμεία, Calamine

**1.** The best calamine is the Cyprian, surnamed *botryitis*; it is dense, moderately heavy and inclined more toward lightness, botryoid in surface, and ash-colored, but when crumbled, it is ash- and rust-colored inside. The next best is that which is bluish outside but rather white inside, having cracks very much like those of onyx stone. These kinds of calamine are mined from old quarries. There is also a kind that is called *placote*, having crevices resembling belts from which they named it *zonitis*.[18] And there is one called *ostracitis*, it is thin and, by and large, black, of an earth-like or clayish surface. But the white is inferior.

**2.** *Botrytes* and the one called *onychites*[19] are useful for eye medications, the rest are useful for salves and for dry medicines that can cicatrize as is also the Cyprian; those brought from Macedonia,

---

[18] From ζώνη, "belt."

[19] This is the calamine which Dioscorides says in the first paragraph of this chapter has "cracks very much like those of onyx stone."

Thrace, and Spain are useless. It has properties that are astringent, fill up hollows, and cleanse filth. It stops up, desiccates, dries thoroughly, controls fleshy excrescences, and cicatrizes the malignant elements of sores.

**3.** Calamine is formed as copper is heated in furnaces and soot settles on the walls and roof of the furnaces. Right there, there are <iron> bars of enormous size, which the miners call *acestides*; they are joined together at the top so that the particles that rise from the copper settle on them and form deposits. As more and more particles are deposited they solidify, and sometimes one kind of calamine is produced and sometimes two or every kind.

**4.** It is also mined from the mountain that is situated above Soli, from the burned ore called copper pyrites.[20] In this same mountain one finds some veins, as it were, of rock-alum, copper ore, ferrous sulfate, shoemaker's black, blue copper carbonate, basic copper carbonate, copper sulfate, and baked clay. Some say that calamine is found even in stone quarries, being deceived by stones that are very similar to it, as for instance the stone found in Cumae, which exhibits no strength whatsoever; these stones are easily recognized because they are lighter than calamine and not mild in taste when chewed.

**5.** Also, if it is stone, it vexes the teeth when chewed, but if it is calamine, it can be chewed because it tolerates the chewing since it gives. Moreover, calamine is discernable because it effervesces when triturated with vinegar and dried in the sun, but this does not happen to stone. Additionally, one can decide whether it is calamine because triturated stone that is placed on a fire jumps up and the smoke it emits is of the same nature as that of the fire, but calamine does not jump up and emits soot that is quince-yellow and appearing like copper, as if it were some kind of a multicolored belt.

**6.** The stone, moreover, if burned then cooled, will change in color and will become lighter, but calamine will not change at all, unless one burned it for quite a few hours. It is also formed in silver furnaces, being whiter, lighter, and inferior in strength.

The calamine discussed above must be burned, buried in coals, until it becomes translucent and bubbles up like slag of iron then quenched

---

[20] On copper pyrites see Dsc. V, 125.

with Aminnaian wine. But if it is to be used for itch-salves, it is quenched with vinegar.

**7.** Some, however, after triturating with wine calamine that was burned this way bray it again in an unbaked clay pot until it crumbles like pumice, then after triturating it again with wine, burn it for a third time until it is completely reduced to ashes, having no roughness whatsoever, and use it instead of ash.

It is washed in a mortar, rubbing it with water that is poured off until there is no filth standing on top, it is then molded and stored.

### V, 75 πομφόλυξ, *Pompholyx*

**1.** *Pomholyx* differs from *spodos* in form,[21] for there is no generic difference between them. For *spodos,* on the one hand, is somewhat dark, heavier, and for the most part full of twigs, hair, and dirt, as if it were some refuse and litter from the floors and ovens of foundries. *Pompholyx*, on the other hand, is greasy and white; moreover, it is so very light that it can float in the air. There are two kinds of it: one is pale blue and somewhat fatty and the other is very white and extremely light.

**2.** The white *pompholyx* is produced when, in processing and finishing copper, metallurgists, wishing to improve it, sprinkle it generously with triturated calamine. For the smoke that rises from it, which is very white, forms bubbles. But *pompholyx* is produced not only when working with copper and copper materials but also from calamine that is blasted on purpose to create *pompholyx*.

**3.** It is made this way: in a building of two chambers a flue is built and at the upper chamber a hole is made of equivalent dimensions as the flue opening from the parts above. The wall of the chamber close to the flue is bore through with a small hole level to the melting pot to receive the bellows. The chamber has also a door of proper size built by the craftsman to get in and out.

**4.** Attached to this building is another room wherein are the bellows and where the bellows blower works. So, coals are placed in the

---

[21] Both *Pompholyx* and *spodos* are zinc oxides. *Pompholyx* is pure zinc oxide that has sublimated to the top of the furnace while *spodos* is impure, collected from the bottom of the furnace.

furnace and lit, then the attending craftsman sprinkles the calamine finely crushed from stations above the top of the furnace and the helper does the same and at the same time throws continuously coal until all the charge is consumed.

**5.** For as it burns, the part that is thin and that is composed of light particles is borne to the upper story and settles on its walls and ceiling; then it solidifies and becomes at first like bubbles that rise from rushing waters; then, as more particles are added, it becomes like fleeces of wool.

**6.** But the heavier stuff falls down, and some spreads itself around the furnace and some on the floor of the chamber; this must be considered inferior to the one made of fine particles because it is earth-like and full of impurities as one gathers it. Some believe that this is the only way that the *spodos* mentioned above is made.[22]

**7.** The Cyprian must be thought to be the best; when kneaded with vinegar, it emits a smell of copper and it is somewhat rust in color; moreover, it has a muddy taste. Also, if pure *pompholyx* should be placed on red-hot coals, it effervesces, becoming light blue in color. You must pay close attention to the above criteria. For some adulterate it with bull's glue or with lamb's lungs or with lungs of sea creatures or with burned figs and with certain other similar things. But it is easy to decide, for on close examination none of the criteria mentioned above is met by such as have been adulterated.

**8.** In general, you must wash *pompholyx* this way: having wrapped it either dry or softened in water in a linen cloth of moderately tight weave, drop it in a bowl containing rainwater and rinse it out by moving the bag hither and thither. This way its slimy and valuable part will run out and all the useless stuff will remain in the linen cloth. Then, allowing it to settle, strain out the water containing the *spodos* and again pouring new water, stir, and decant; and do these things both straining and adding water until no sandy substance deposits. Then squeeze out the water, and, after drying the *spodos,* store it.

**9.** But some, after drying <it> thoroughly, triturating it with water by hand and making it of a honey-like consistency, strain it through a

---

[22] See Wyndham Hulme E., *Notes and Queries*, March 24, 1945 p.123, citation in R. J. Forbes, *Studies in Ancient Technololy*, VIII, p. 263.

linen cloth that they spread over the receiving vessel tying it loosely. <And> in order to allow it to pass through easily, they pour much water over it and stir the *spodos*.

**10.** Then they scoop up immediately with a spoon that part which passed through and swims in the vessel on top like foam, transfer it to a new clay pot, and stirring the lees gently, they decant into another vessel leaving the sandy element at the bottom; then, allowing again the stony elements to settle, they strain into another clean vessel and repeat the process often until the *spodos* becomes clean and free of sand.

**11.** But others, just as it is in large pieces, sprinkle it lightly on water, thinking that the sand mentioned above and the stony elements will sink by their own weight to the bottom of the vessel, while the hair, twigs, and the like will rise to the top because of their lightness. Then separating the *spodos* that is in the middle and placing it into a mortar, they wash it like calamine. It is also washed with Chian wine containing seawater by the methods described above; it becomes more astringent than that washed with water.

**12.** *Pompholyx* has astringent, cooling, filling, purging, adhesive, and somewhat desiccative properties. It is also one of the substances that are mildly caustic. But should it be necessary to bake the *spodos*, after triturating it carefully, mixing it into a paste with water, <and> shaping it into little lozenges, place them on a new clay vessel — place this vessel on a small and gentle coal-fire — and keep turning around the lozenges until they become dry and red-hot.

**13.** You must know that *spodos* is formed also from gold and silver, as well as from lead, and that next to the one from copper, that from lead is the best.

And because *antispoda*,[23] too, are quite useful, *spodos* being frequently unavailable, it is necessary to point out what substances possess the same properties as *spodos*, what they are, and how they should be used.

**14.** Taking, therefore, myrtle leaves with their flowers and their berries still unripe, place them in an unbaked clay vessel to cook in a potter's kiln, covering the vessel with a lid perforated with many holes

---

[23] ἀντίσποδα, "instead of *spodos*".

and luted all around. After the clay vessel is baked, pour its contents into another unbaked vessel, and after it has been thoroughly baked, removing the contents of the second vessel, wash, and use.

**15.** Use even olive foliage that you prepared the same way; let it be, however, from the wild olive. But if wild olive is unavailable, you can take the foliage of the cultivated together with the flowers or quinces all cut up and with their seeds removed or oak-galls or linen rags or unripe white mulberries that were previously dried in the sun or mastic or terebinth or wild vine inflorescence or the tender leaves of bramble or the foliage of boxwood or what is called bastard galingale together with its flower.

**16.** Some prepare similarly branches of fig tree that were dried in the sun; others burn bull's glue, and others shaggy and greasy wool smeared with either pitch or honey.

### V, 76 κεκαυμένος χαλκός, Burned copper

**1.** Burned copper is good when red and of the color of cinnabar when rubbed; but if it is black, it was burned more than it should have been. It is made from ships' nails placed in an unbaked vessel and strewn alternately below and above with sulfur and salt in equal amounts. The vessel, lidded and sealed with potter's clay, is put in a kiln until it is thoroughly baked.

**2.** But some sprinkle alum instead of sulfur. Others, placing the nails in the vessel without the sulfur and salts, burn them for several days. Others use only the sulfur, but they do become sooty. Others, after rubbing the nails with split alum, burn them with sulfur and vinegar in an unbaked clay vessel. Still others, after sprinkling them with vinegar in a copper pot, cook them in the kiln this way and, after they have burned, they repeat the process three times then store. The best is that burned in Memphis then that burned in Cyprus.

**3.** It is able to contract, dry, attenuate, reduce, draw, cleanse wounds and cicatrize them, clear off impurities in the eyes, reduce overgrown flesh, and check spreading ulcers. It is also emetic when drunk with hydromel or when sucked with honey or when one's mouth is washed with it. It is washed just like calamine, the water being changed four times a day until there is no scum on it whatsoever. Its slag, which is also washed the same way, has the same properties, although weaker.

**V, 77 χαλκοῦ ἄνθος, Flower of copper**

**1.** Flower of copper, which some ancient writers have called nail-scrapings, is excellent if it crumbles, if it is very red when brayed, and if it is like grains of millet in size, heavy, and moderately shining; moreover, it should be free of copper filings with which it is adulterated. But one can detect their presence because they are flattened when crushed by the teeth.

**2.** It is made this way: when the copper that was smelted in the ore furnaces flows down through the strainers of the conveying ducts into the receptacles, the attendants, after removing the dirt, pour on it very fresh water, their purpose being to cool it. And so, from the sudden condensation and contraction, the above-mentioned is formed on the surface, as if it were spat out.

It, too, contracts, reduces excrescences, and purges those elements that cast a shadow over the pupils of the eyes, stinging quite a bit. Given in the amount of four *obols*, it draws out gross humors, it reduces fleshy excrescences both in the nostrils and on the anus, it checks pustules with wine, and the kind that is white is blown, ground up, through a tube for chronic hardness of hearing. Applied ground up with honey, it shrinks both uvulas and tonsils.

**V, 78 λεπίς, Flake [of copper ore]**

**1.** The flake of copper ore that is thick, called *helitis*, is good; but the one from bronze is bad because it is thin and weak. We reject it as worthless, choosing that which is thick, yellow, and growing rusty when vinegar is sprinkled on it.

It has astringent, staunching, attenuating, and putrefactive properties; it is capable of checking spreading ulcers and of cicatrizing; when drunk with hydromel it draws out water.

**2.** Some, after mixing it with flour, administer it as a little pill. It is also mixed with ophthalmic medicines, drying up watery eyes and reducing rough eyelids.

**3.** It is washed this way: after cleaning one *hemimnaion* of dried flakes, place them in a mortar with clear water and stir them carefully by hand. When the flakes have settled down, removing what floats on top, pour out the water, pour in one *cyathos* of rainwater, and with the palm of your hand rub them against the mortar as if you were scraping them.

**4.** When they begin to release some stickiness, little by little, pour over them up to six *cyathoi* of water and rub them rigorously. Then take the flakes up with your hand, rub them hard against the side of the mortar, squeeze them out, and take up the run off into a copper box. For this is, as it were, the flower of the flakes; it is both strong in its efficacy and useful for eye medications, but the remaining is weak.

**5.** Washing similarly even the remainder, take it up until it secretes no stickiness whatsoever; then you must cover it with a linen cloth and leave it undisturbed for two days; then you must pour out the water that stands on top, dry, and store in a box. But some wash this one also like calamine then store.

Flake of hammered iron has the same properties as flake of copper and is similarly washed and stored, but it is not as effective for purging the bowel as that of copper.

### V, 79 ἰὸς ξυστός, Verdigris

**1.** You must prepare verdigris this way: after pouring very sharp vinegar into a cask or into another similar container, cover it with an inverted copper vessel; it is good if the cover were concave, but if not, it may be flat. It should also be clean and tight fitting. After ten days, removing the cover, scrape off the verdigris that coats it. Or, making a thin blade of the same copper, hang it over the container so as not to touch the vinegar and after the same number of days scrape it.

**2.** Or having stashed among grape pressings that are not fresh and that are growing sour a lump of copper or a thin blade or even several thin blades, dig them up after the same number of days. But it is also possible to make it from shavings, or from the thin blades between which gold leaves are placed when they are being hammered out, if one sprinkled them with vinegar and turned them upside down three or four times a day until fully covered with verdigris.

**3.** And they say that verdigris is also formed in Cypriot mines, one type forming on the surface of some stones that contain copper and the other drips from a certain cave during the burning heat of the Dog Star. They also say that while the former is scarce and of excellent quality, the one deriving from the cave, while it flows plentiful and it is nicely colored, it is, nevertheless, inferior because it contains many stony elements.

**4.** It is adulterated with many different things but especially with these: for some mix it with pumice stone, others with marble, and others with copper sulfate. We shall detect the pumice stone and marble by wetting the thumb of our left hand and rubbing against it a bit of verdigris with the other thumb. It happens that the unadulterated verdigris dissolves, while that with pumice stone or marble does not and becomes finally all white from much rubbing and from the absorption of moisture.

**5.** And that is not all; we shall detect adulterants also from the pressure teeth exert on it: for that which is pure gives, being smooth and not rough. Copper sulfate is detected with fire. For if one, having sprinkled verdigris that had been adulterated in this manner on a thin blade or on a potsherd, should place either of these on warm ashes or coals, the copper sulfate would change and grow red because it naturally has that kind of color when burned.

**6.** *Ios scolycos.* There are two types of the so called *ios scolycos*,[24] for one is mined and the other is prepared this way: after pouring into a mortar of Cyprian copper equipped with a pestle made of the same material one-half *cotyle* white harsh vinegar, beat it until it becomes sticky, then add four *drachmai* of round alum and of mined salt that is translucent or of very white and solid sea salt, otherwise an equal amount of soda. Then beat it in the sun, <during> the heat of the Dog Star, until it becomes rusty in color and wrinkled in appearance and thus shape it into worms similar to the Rhodian and store.

**7.** It does become very strong and very well colored if one part vinegar and two parts urine of a child[25] were added and everything else was done as indicated. But some, mixing gum with verdigris that did not pass muster, mold it <and sell> it; you must reject it because it is ineffective. There is also a kind that goldsmiths make with a mortar and a pestle of Cyprian copper and with a child's urine, which they use to solder gold.

[24] This is *aerugo vermicularis*, which is shaped like worms.

[25] All other readings have "old urine" for "urine of a child."

**8.** In general, the verdigris mentioned above are equivalent to burned copper and have formidable strength. But one must know that verdigris that was mined is the best among them; next best is that which was scraped, and then the artificial. Even this one is, indeed, rather biting and binding, while the one of the goldsmiths' corresponds to the scraped.
**9.** All verdigris can bind, warm, wipe off and thin out eye scars, cause tears, control spreading ulcers, maintain injuries free of inflammations, and, with oil and wax, cicatrize old wounds. Boiled with honey, they clear completely calluses and the sordid elements of sores.
**10.** Compounded with gum ammoniac into salves, they melt away fistulous sores and calluses and they are useful for growths and bumps on the gums. Smeared on with honey, they thin the eyelids quite a bit; but after the smearing, one must foment the eyelids with hot water, using a sponge. Compounded with turpentine and copper sulfate or soda, they get rid of leprosies.
**11.** You must burn whichever verdigris you have chosen this way: breaking it into large pieces and placing it in a clay pan, rest it on very hot coals and stir until it changes color and becomes somewhat ashen; then, after cooling it, store and use it. Some burn it in an unbaked pot as described earlier, but it does not always change into the same color when burned.

**V, 80 ἰὸς σιδήρου, Iron rust**
**1.** Iron rust binds and stems leucorrhea when applied and causes barrenness when drunk. Smeared on with vinegar, it effectively treats erysipelas and pustules; it is useful for whitlow, for membranes that grow over the inner corners of the eye, for rough eyelids, and for callous lumps. It strengthens the gums, it is beneficial to the gouty when smeared on, and it restores hair on bald patches on the head.
**2.** The water or wine in which red-hot iron was quenched is a suitable drink for people with colic, dysentery, spleen disease, cholera, and for a slackened stomach. Iron slag can accomplish all the things that iron rust accomplishes but to a lesser degree; drunk with oxymel it helps also for leopard's bane.

**V, 81 πεπλυμένος μόλυβδος, Washed lead**

**1.** Washed lead is prepared this way: place water in a lead mortar, beat it with a leaden pestle until the water turns black and becomes turbid, then filter it through a linen cloth, pouring additional water, so that all the dissolved matter passes through, and repeat the process until you think you have enough. Next, letting the washed lead settle, pour out the water, pour on new, wash as one washes calamine until no more blackness stands on it, then shape into small lozenges and store.

**2.** But some, filing down clean lead, beat it with water in a stone mortar with a stone pestle or with their hands, decanting at once the blackened material, which, having allowed to settle <and> having poured off the water, shape immediately into lozenges. That which is rubbed for quite some time becomes like white lead. Some people add to the filings a touch of galena, maintaining that lead that is washed this way is better.

**3.** It can contract, cool, stop up, soften, fill up hollows, and stop running eyes and sores that grow fungous. It also stops bleeding, it is good, in combination with unguent of roses, for anal sores, callous lumps, hemorrhoids, and for sores that are hard to heal, and, in general, it accomplishes everything that ashes do without being caustic. Pure lead helps for the stroke of the sea scorpion and the great weever when rubbed on.

**4.** Lead is burned this way: taking sheets of lead that are as thin as possible, place them on a new flat dish, and after sprinkling over them sulfur, place on top again new leaves of lead and sprinkle them with sulfur, and again place new sheets, and repeat the process until you have filled the dish; then light a fire underneath. When the lead catches fire, move it about with an iron rod until it has turned fully to ashes and no lead element is left and lift the dish, shielding your nostrils because the fumes are harmful.

**5.** Or, after placing lead shavings and sulfur in a flat dish, simply burn them. But some after placing the sheets of lead in an unbaked clay pot, as indicated, put it in an oven or on top of coals, having luted the lid and given it a small air hole. Others sprinkle on them white lead or barley instead of sulfur.

**6.** Others, after placing the flakes without adding anything to them, use a high flame and stir them vigorously with an iron rod until they

turn to ashes. But this type of burning is difficult and if the lead is burned more than it should have been burned, it acquires the color of lead monoxide. I definitely prefer the first method of burning. It must be washed like calamine and stored.
It has the same properties as washed lead but far stronger.

**V, 82 σκωρία μολύβδου, Lead dross**
Lead dross that looks like white lead, that is thick and difficult to break, that contains nothing lead-like, but that is quince-yellow and glassy is excellent.
It is good for the same things as burned lead, but it is more astringent.
It is washed in a mortar into which water is poured and the quince-yellow film on top is poured out. The process is repeated many times until the dross is consumed. Then, letting it settle, we pour out the water and simply mold it.

**V, 83 ὁ μολυβδοειδὴς λίθος, Leadstone**
Leadstone has properties that are comparable to those of lead dross and it is similarly washed.

**V, 84 στίβι, Antimony**
**1.** Antimony is excellent if it glitters and shines, if it is laminated when broken, containing neither soil nor dirt, and if it is easily broken. Some have called this kind *platyophthalmon* and others *larbason.*
**2.** It has properties that stop the pores, that are astringent, that cool, check overgrown flesh, cicatrize sores, and cleanse the sordid elements and ulcers in the eyes. It also stems hemorrhages from the membranes, and in general its properties are similar to those of burned lead. But it prevents especially burns from forming scabs when anointed with fresh suet and it cicatrizes burns that have formed scabs when mixed with wax and white lead.
**3.** It is cooked wrapped in dough and buried in coals until the dough turns to ash; and after it has been dug out, it is quenched with milk from a woman who gave birth to a boy or with old wine. It is burned, placed on coals and blown until it catches fire: for if it should burn too much, it melts like lead. It is washed like calamine and <burned> copper. But some people wash it the same way as lead dross.

### V, 85 μολύβδαινα, Galena

**1.** Galena that looks like litharge, that is blond, somewhat shining, orange-tawny when triturated, and liver-colored when cooked in oil, is of excellent quality. But it is bad when it is grey or leaden. It is made from silver and from gold. There is also a kind that is mined, found around Sebastes and Corycos; of this one, too, the best is neither dross-like nor pebbly but blond and shiny.

**2.** It has the same properties as litharge and lead dross and it is similarly washed and burned. But this one is mixed more conveniently with oily plasters and it is combined advantageously with plasters that do not require a bandage, making flesh grow and causing it to heal. It is not suitable, however, for cleansing medicines.

### V, 86 ἡ τοῦ ἀργύρου σκωρία, Silver dross

Dross from silver is called *helcysma*. It has the same properties as galena, whereof it is mixed <both> with grey plasters and with plasters that cicatrize, being astringent and causing adherence.

### V, 87 λιθάργυρος, Litharge

**1.** Litharge: there is one type that is produced from the sand called *molybditis* when it is smelted until its complete calcination, another from silver, and another from lead. The best is the Attic, second best is the Spanish, after them those produced in Dicaiarchia and in Sicily. For in <these> places it is produced in large quantities during the firing of lead plates.

**2.** The one that is golden and shining is called *chrysitis*; it is the best. The dull one is called *argyritis*, and the one made from silver is called *scalauthritis*.

It has properties that are astringent, emollient, that cool, that are capable of stopping the pores, of filling up hollows, of controlling fleshy excrescences, and of healing.

**3.** You will burn it this way: cutting it up into pieces the size of walnuts <and> placing it on coals, then fanning it until burned, and after wiping the dirt that surrounds it, store it. But some after quenching it three times with vinegar or wine burn it again, and then store it. It is washed like calamine.

**4.** It is bleached this way: taking one Attic *choinix* of the one called *argyritis*, although if it is unavailable you may surely take another kind, break it up into pieces the size of beans, and placing it in a new clay container pour water over it, adding one *choinix* white wheat, and tying separately in a clean loosely woven linen cloth a handful of barley, hang it from the handle of the container and boil until the barley cracks.

**5.** Then, after pouring everything into a wide-mouthed bowl, remove and discard the wheat, and pouring water over the litharge, wash it, rubbing it at the same time vigorously with your hands; then taking it out and drying it, pound it in a Theban mortar, pouring over it hot water until it dissolves, then straining out the water, pound it again all day long. In the evening, pour over it hot water and leave it alone, and in the morning strain, and pour on new water and strain three times a day. Do this for seven days.

**6.** Then mixing with one *mna* litharge five *drachmai* mined salt, and pouring in also hot water, pound it three times a day, straining and adding water. When it has become white, pouring over it hot water, repeat the process until it has no appearance of saltness whatsoever, then squeeze out the moisture, dry it under a piercing sun, and store.

**7.** Or take one *mna* of *argyritis*, pound it carefully and after pounding it mix it with three times as much pulverized mined salt and place it in a new clay pot; then pouring on water to cover, stir it every day, morning and evening, adding on water, pouring out none of the first water, and do so for 30 days; for unless it is stirred, it becomes dry like a potsherd.

**8.** Then gently pouring out the brine, pound the litharge in a Theban mortar, and placing it in a clay pot and pouring over it water, stir it carefully with your hands, pouring out the first water and adding new until there is no trace whatsoever of saltiness. Then decanting the white of the litharge into another vessel, shape into little wheels, and store in a leaden box.

**9.** Others, however, after breaking the litharge into pieces the size of beans and placing it into a raw swine's belly, boil it in water until the belly is softened; then taking it out and rubbing it with an equal amount of salt, wash it as previously described. Still others taking one *litra* salt and as much litharge, rub it in the sun with water, pouring it out continuously, until it becomes white.

**10.** Or it is bleached even this way: taking as much litharge as you may wish and wrapping it in white wool, set it in a new clay pot, and, after adding water and a handful of clean new beans, boil. When the beans crack and the wool has turned black, removing the litharge and wrapping it in fresh wool, boil for a second time, adding clean water and the same quantity of beans.

**11.** Do the same things as described above for a third time, and, in general, do so until the wool no longer gets dyed; then pouring it out into a mortar, mix with 80 Attic *drachmai* of litharge one *litra* of mined salt and pound. Letting some time pass, add 47 *holcai* of very white soda dissolved in water and again pound it until the litharge becomes quite white; and thus pouring it into a broad-mouthed clay vessel, adding plenty of water, and allowing it to settle, strain, add new water, and stirring it with your hands allow it again to settle and strain.

**12.** Do the above again and again until the water that runs off is very clear, sweet, and free of saltiness. Finally, pouring it into a fresh clay platter, gently strain the liquid, set it under the Dog Star's sun for 40 days, and after drying it use it.

**13.** That which was washed seems to be good for eye medications, for unseemly scars, and for faces full of wrinkles and blemishes.

**V, 88 ψιμύθιον, White lead**

**1.** White lead is made this way: pouring into a wide-mouthed jar or into a pot-bellied clay jar very strong vinegar, and after lining the mouth of the jar with a mat of reeds, place on the jar's mouth a lead block and throw ever it coverings to prevent the vinegar from evaporating. When the lead block sinks down crumbling, you must, on the one hand, strain the clean liquid that floats on top and, on the other hand, you must pour the viscous part into a container and dry it in the sun.

**2.** Next you must grind it with a hand-mill or triturate it somehow and sift it; and after you have done that, you must grind fine and sift the balance of what is hard, repeating the procedure a third and a fourth time. Best is that which was sifted first; it must be used in eye medications. The next is second best; and the rest in the order they were sifted.

**3.** But some, fixing a piece of <wood> in the middle of the jar, place the reed-mat on top in such a manner as not to touch the vinegar, then stopping the opening and greasing it all around, they leave it alone. Ten days later, uncover and take a look. When it is dissolved, they do the rest just as described.

**4.** And should one wish to mold it, he must mix it with strong vinegar and simply shape and dry it in the sun. Moreover, the above preparations must be conducted in the summer. This way it becomes white and efficacious. But it is also made in the winter, by placing the jars on top of the furnaces of baths or on top of ovens. For the rising heat acts on it the same way as does the sun. That made in Rhodes or in Corinth or in Lacedaimon must be deemed the best and the one from Dicaiarchia second.

**5.** It must be baked this way: placing a new clay container, preferably one from Attica, on very hot coals, sprinkle on it ground white lead and stir continuously. When it has become ashen in color, take it up, cool and use it. But if you wish to burn it, placing it ground fine in a hollow vessel and setting it on top of the coals, stir it with a stick of giant fennel until it becomes like red sulfide of arsenic in color, then take it and use it.

**6.** Some call that which was prepared this way *sandyx.* White lead is washed the same way as calamine.

It has properties that cool, cause adhesion, soften, fill up, and thin; moreover, they control excrescences to some degree and they cicatrize when mixed with cerates, oily plasters, and troches. But it is also one of the poisonous substances.

### V, 89 χρυσοκόλλα, Basic copper carbonate

**1.** The best basic copper carbonate[26] is the Armenian, being intensely green in color; second best is the Macedonian, then the Cyprian. You must choose that which is clean and reject the one that is full of earth and stones.

---

[26] Also known as gold-solder and as malachite. See Dsc. Bk. V, 74,4.

**2.** The above mentioned must be washed this way: after breaking it up, place it in a mortar and pouring over it water, rub it vigorously against the mortar with the palm of your hand; then allowing it to settle, strain, and after adding fresh water rub again. Repeat these steps until it becomes clean and pure, then after drying it in the sun, store and use.
**3.** If you wish to burn it, burn it this way: pounding a sufficient amount of it, place it in a pan, and after setting the pan on coals, do the rest the way described on the subject in the chapter before this one. Chrysocolla has properties that cleanse scars, check fleshy excrescences, and promote vomiting; it is astringent, it warms, and it is mildly septic with a touch of stinging; it belongs to the medications that cause vomiting and that can kill.

**V, 90 Ἀρμένιον, Azurite**
Azurite: you must choose it smooth, of a deep and very even blue color, without stones, easily broken, and as thick as chrysocolla. It accomplishes the same results as chrysocolla, falling short of it only in efficacy.
It also promotes the growth of eyelashes.

**V, 91 κύανος, Lapis lazuli**[27]
Lapis lazuli is produced in Cyprus from copper mines, but most is produced from the coastal sand found along certain cavern-like underminings of the sea. This one is also the best. You must choose it deeply colored, burn it like rock-alum,[28] and wash it like calamine.
It has repressing, mildly stringent, escharotic, and ulcerative properties.

**V, 92 Ἰνδικόν, Indigo**
Of the so called indigo, some occurs naturally, as if it were an excretion of Indian reeds,[29] but the so called *baphicon* is scum from

---

[27] There are two types of lapis lazuli, this one, κύανος, and the one in Dsc. Bk. V, 139, λίθος σάπφειρος. Theophrastus, *Lap.* 23 and 37, also mentions two, κυανή and χρυσή.
[28] See Dsc. Bk. V, 99.
[29] *Indigofera tinctoria.*

purple murex[30] floating on the copper cauldrons, which the craftsmen skim off and dry in the sun. The one that is deep blue, juicy, and smooth must be considered to be the best.
It belongs to the group of preparations that mildly cool and shrivel inflammations and swellings. It cleanses and represses ulcers.

**V, 93 ὦχρα, Yellow ocher**
You must select yellow ocher that is very light, quince-yellow throughout, of a deep color, free of stones, easily broken, and of Attic provenience. It, too, must be burned and washed like calamine.
It has properties that are astringent, septic, and dispersive of inflammations and growths, it reduces fleshy excrescences, in combination with a cerate, it fills up hollows, and it breaks up chalkstones.[31]

**V, 94 κιννάβαρι, Cinnabar**
**1.** Some are wrong in thinking that cinnabar is the same as that which is called *minion*: for *minion* is made in Spain from a certain stone that is mixed with sand containing silver-ore. This stone is otherwise unknown and in the furnace changes into a very bright and flaming color. It does have a suffocating smell among minerals. At any rate, the natives there place around their faces bags to enable them to see but not to breathe the air.
**2.** Painters use it in their costly wall-decorations. Cinnabar, on the other hand, is brought from Libya. It is very expensive and so scarce that there is hardly enough for painters to variegate lines. It is also of a deep-color, wherefore some people thought that it is dragon's blood.
**3.** Cinnabar has the same properties as hematite, but it is a great deal more suitable for eye medications, for it is more astringent. Wherefore, it also staunches blood and it treats burns and pustules when compounded with cerate.

---
[30] Which yields the purple dye.
[31] Formed in the joints.

### V, 95 ὑδράργυρος, Mercury

**1.** Mercury is made from what is called *minion*, which is wrongly called also cinnabar: for placing an iron spoon that has cinnabar on a clay vessel, they turn over it a cup, lute it with clay, and burn it on coals. For the soot that settles on the cup becomes mercury when scraped off.

**2.** It is also found condensed in drops from the ceiling when silver ore is processed. Some people report that mercury occurs even naturally in the mines. It is kept in glass or lead or tin or silver containers because it eats through all other materials and flows away.

**3.** It has deadly properties when drunk, eating away the inner parts with its weight. Large quantities of milk drunk and vomited help, as does wine with wormwood *artemisia absinthium* or seed of celery or of clary or oregano or hyssop with wine.

### V, 96 μίλτος Σινωπική, Sinopic red earth

**1.** Sinopic red earth is excellent if dense and heavy, liver-colored, free of stones, evenly colored, and capable of much diffusion in solution. It is collected in Cappadocia, in certain caves, and after it is refined it is brought to Sinope and sold, whence it also received its surname.

**2.** It has astringent, desiccative, and adhesive properties on account of which it is compounded with plasters for wounds and with troches that dry and make costive. It stops diarrhea when taken with egg and when used in a clyster. It is given also to patients with liver disease.

**3.** τεκτονικὴ <μίλτος>, Builders' red earth is in every respect inferior to Sinopic red earth, although those from Egypt and from Carthage, being stone free and crumbly, are first-rate. It is also produced in the western part of Spain when yellow ocher is burned and changes into builder's red earth.

### V, 97 Λημνία γῆ, Lemnian earth

**1.** What they call Lemnian earth is brought up from a certain cavernous underground passage and mixed with goat's blood; the people there after molding it and stamping it with the figure of a goat call it *sphragis*.

**2.** It is an uncommonly effective antidote for deadly poisons when drunk with wine, and, when taken ahead of time, it forces one to vomit the poisons. It is suitable both for the strokes of venomous animals and for their bites. It is mixed with antidotes. Some use it even in mystic rites.

### V, 98 χαλκανθές, Copper sulfate, Vitriol

**1.** There is a single kind of copper sulfate: for it is a congealed liquid. It does come, however, in three specific types. One kind of copper sulfate is formed as a stalactite from liquids that filter into certain underground conduits and this is why the people who work the copper mines call it *stalacton.* [32] Then there is another that filters abundantly in caves and after it is poured into troughs it becomes compacted; this is why it is called idiomatically also *pecton.*[33]

**2.** The third kind is called *ephthon*[34] and it is made in Spain. This is how they make it and it is both very pale and very weak: after diluting it in water, they boil it, pour it out into basins, and leave it alone. It congeals after a certain number of days have passed, dividing into cubical shapes that touch each other like grape-clusters.

**3.** The best is blue and heavy, dense, clean and translucent; such is the *stalacton,* which some call *lonchoton.*[35] Then comes the *pecton*; but the *ephthon* is popular for dying and for black hair dyes; experience has proven, however, that it is very weak for medical <use>.

**4.** It can contract, warm, form eschars, and remove flat intestinal worms when one *drachma* of it is drunk or sucked with honey. It causes vomiting, it helps people who have eaten poisonous mushrooms when drunk in water, and it clears the head when diluted in water and dripped from a wool wad into the nostrils. It is burned, as we shall demonstrate forthwith on the chapter on rock-alum.

### V, 99 χαλκῖτις, Rock alum

**1.** You must choose rock alum that is copper-colored and easily breakable, free of stones and not old; moreover, you must choose it with longish and shiny veins.

---

[32] Meaning “dripping.”
[33] Meaning “compacted.”
[34] Meaning “boiled.”
[35] “Lanceolate.”

It has properties that contract, warm, form eschars, and cleanse impurities around the corners of the eyes and around the eyes.

**2.** It belongs to that class of substances that contract moderately. It is good for erysipelas, shingles, and for uterine and nose bleedings with leek juice, but it is good dry for growths on the gums, for spreading ulcers, and for inflammation of the tonsils, and when burned it is highly useful ground up with honey for eye medicines, reducing calloused and rough eyelids. It also shrinks fistulas when it is inserted, having been given an oblong shape.

**3.** The so-call *psoricon*[36] is made from it by mixing two parts rock alum with one part calamine and pounding them together with vinegar. It must, however, be buried in a clay vessel in dung for 40 days during the heat of the Dog Star. It does become rather sharp and it is capable of all the things that rock alum is also capable. But some, combining equal amounts, pound them with wine and do the same things. You must burn it by placing it on a fresh clay vessel and setting it over very hot coals.

**4.** Let the standard for burning be this: if the samples contain a great deal of moisture, they should have no bubbles and should become nicely dry, but the rest should change into a brighter color. When the sample becomes red throughout like the color of red earth, you must lift it, blow off the dirt that covers it, and store. It is cooked on coals, blowing on it until it becomes light yellow, or on a clay container on top of very hot coals, turning it frequently until it catches fire and changes color.

### V, 100 μίσυ, *Misy*[37]

You must choose *misy* that is Cyprian, shining like gold, hard, and when broken into pieces golden and shining like a star.

Its properties and burning are the same as of rock alum, except that *psoricon* cannot be made from it and that is more or less where it differs. The Egyptian is superior to the others, being very strong, but for eye medications it falls a great deal short of the one mentioned before.

---

[36] "Itch-salve."

[37] A copper ore that is found on Cyprus.

## V, 101 μελαντηρία, Shoemaker's black

There is a shoemaker black that solidifies like salt scum at the mouth of copper mines, another that comes from the upper surface of the places mentioned above and it is earth-like, and there is even one kind that is mined in Cilicia as well as in many other places. The best among them is sulfur-colored, smooth, even, clean, and rapidly turning black at the touch of water.
It has the same properties and burning as *misy*.

## V, 102 σῶρι, Melanterite[38]

**1.** Some assumed wrongly that melanterite is shoemakers' black: for melanterite is *sui generis,* although somewhat like shoemaker's black, and it is more foul smelling and nauseating. It is found in Egypt and in other places, as in Libya, Spain, and Cyprus. The Egyptian is to be preferred and when it appears rather black when broken, when it has many small holes, when it is somewhat shiny, astringent and malodorous when swallowed or smelled, and when it upsets the stomach.
**2.** But the one glowing like *misy* when shattered must be judged to be something different and ineffectual.
It has the same properties and it is burned the same way as the ones spoken of above. It does treat toothaches when placed on the teeth's cavities, it strengthens loose teeth, it helps those suffering from hip ailments when employed in a clyster with wine, and it checks facial eruptions when smeared on with water.
**3.** It is also mixed with black hair dyes. In general, however, regarding these substances and nearly all the rest, the unburned must be considered to be stronger than those that were burned, except for salts, lees,[39] soda, chalk, and the like, which are weak when raw: these do become more effective when burned.

---

[38] The identification in LSJ of σῶρυ, "ferrous sulfate" or "melanterite" is tentative.
[39] These are of wine or vinegar. See Dsc, Bk. V, 114 on how lees were burnt and on their benefits.

**V, 103 διφρυγές,[40] Pyrites**

**1.** One must suppose that pyrites from copper mines is of three kinds: for one is a mineral, occurring, in fact, only in Cyprus. For being clay-like, it is brought up from the depths of some <cave> there and, after it has been carried up, it is dried in the sun, then burned surrounded by kindling; it is for this reason that it was named 'twice roasted', because it is parched and roasted by the sun and by the kindling.

**2.** The second kind is like some sort of sediment and dross of wrought copper. For after the cold water, of which we spoke above in discussing flower of copper,[41] has been poured and the copper has been removed, it is found at the bottom and it has both the astringency and taste of copper. The third kind is made this way: the attendants at these projects, place into the furnace the ore called copper pyrites and burn it for quite a few days like chalk. When it acquires the color of red earth, they remove and store it

**3.** But some say that the above is produced only from the substance that makes copper ore when, having been baked in the so-called threshing floors, it is carried up into the pits and burned there. For it spreads all around the area of these pits and it is found even after the removal of the ores. You must choose that which has a coppery taste, a rusty appearance, and which binds and dries the tongue quite a bit, characteristics that burned earth, which people sell as pyrites from copper mines, does not have.

**4.** It has astringent, highly desiccative, emetic, and cleansing properties. It is fit for controlling overgrown flesh and for cicatrizing pernicious and spreading ulcers. It also dissolves abscesses when combined with turpentine or with cerate.

**V, 104 ἀρσενικόν, Yellow orpiment**

Yellow orpiment is formed in the same mines as red sulfide of arsenic. That which is laminated, golden in color, with laminas that flake off and are as if lying on one another, and which is pure must be thought to be excellent. Such is the one formed in Mysia, at the Hellespont. There are two kinds of it. The one is as described above; the other is

---

[40] διφρυγές, "twice roasted."

[41] See Dsc. Bk. V, 77.

lumpy, bright red in color, and it is brought from Pontus and Cappadocia. This kind ranks second. It is baked this way: after putting it in a fresh clay vessel, place it on red-hot coals and stir it continuously until it becomes red-hot and changes color; then cool, pound, and store.
It has putrefactive and escharotic properties with burning and intense biting. It belongs to the group of astringents. It is also depilatory.

### V, 105 σανδαράκη, Arsenic sulfide

**1.** You must select arsenic sulfide that is deep red, [friable,] easily triturated and clean, having the color of cinnabar, and also smelling like sulfur.
It has the same properties and it is baked the same way as yellow orpiment. But in combination with pine resin it also treats bald spots, with pitch it removes psoriatic nails, with olive oil it is good for pediculosis, and with animal fat it dissolves tumors.
**2.** It is also suitable for sores in the nose, mouth, and for the rest of sores, for pustules with unguent of roses, and for callous lumps. It is given with honey mixed with wine to people who suffer from internal abscesses, it is burned with pine resin to produce smoke from below and the steam is drawn with the mouth through a siphon for an old cough, it clears the voice if sucked with honey, and it is given to asthmatics with pine resin as a little pill.

### V, 106 στυπτηρία, Alum

**1.** Nearly every kind of alum is found in the same mines in Egypt. But alum also occurs in other places, as in Melos, Macedonia, Lipari, Sardinia, Hierapolis of Phrygia, Libya, Armenia, and in many other places, just like red earth.
There are many kinds of it, but for medicinal purposes they use that which is cloven, round, and moist.
**2.** Outstanding is the cloven, and of this one, that which is fresh, very white, oppressive in smell, powerfully astringent, and free of stones; moreover, it should not be compressed like a clump of earth nor spindly, but it should be arranged in strands resembling gray hairs; the

one called *trichitis,*[42] which occurs in Egypt, is of that sort. There is, however, a stone that resembles it a great deal which you must identify by the criterion of taste because it is not astringent. Of the round, the one that is man-made is unsatisfactory. It is recognizable from its shape.

**3.** You must use that which is naturally round and which is like bubbles, whitish, and extremely astringent; moreover, it should have a touch of paleness and at the same time some glitter; in addition to these characteristics it should be free of stones, crumbling, and either Melian or Egyptian of origin. But of the moist you must choose that which is very translucent and milky, smooth and moist throughout; moreover, you must choose it free of stones and emanating heat.

**4.** They have properties that warm, that are astringent, that clear off the elements that cast a shadow over the pupils of the eyes, and that reduce both the flesh on the eyelids and other overgrown fleshes. The one that is cloven must be regarded more effective than the round. Alums are calcined and baked like rock alum. They stem both putrid humors and hemorrhages, they tighten flaccid gums, and with vinegar or honey they strengthen loose teeth.

**5.** They are beneficial with honey for thrush and for pustules, <and> with the juice of *polygonon*[43] for ear rheums. They are suitable for leprosies and for itches when boiled with cabbage juice or with honey, and they are poured with water over scaly nails, fleshy excrescences, and chilblains. They are suitable for cancerous conditions smeared on with vinegar lees and with an equal amount of burned oak galls.

**6.** For spreading ulcers, they are anointed with twice as much salt, for dandruff, with the watery part of wood-tar, and <they are helpful> when rubbed on with water for nits, pediculosis, and burns; they are also used as ointments for swellings and for the bad odors of armpits and groins. They help to induce menstruation and for barrenness when placed at the mouth of the uterus prior to sexual intercourse, and they expel embryos/fetuses. They are also suitable for growths on the

[42] Akin to θρίξ, τριχός, "hair."

[43] Ordinarily πολύγονον is qualified by ἄρρεν, "knot-grass," *Polygonum aviculare*, or θῆλυ, "mare's tail" *Hippuris vulgaris.*

gums, for swollen uvulas, for the tonsils, the mouth, and they are also smeared with honey for the ears and the genitalia.

**V, 107 θεῖον, Sulfur**

**1.** Sulfur that has not been burned must be judged to be excellent when it is of a shiny color, transparent, and free of stones, but of the sulfur that has been burned, it is the pale green and very fat that is excellent. Much sulfur is produced on Melos and on the Lipari islands. The sulfur mentioned first, warms, disperses, causes quick ripening, is good for coughs, for people who suffer from abscesses, and for asthmatics when taken in an egg and when burned so as to produce smoke.

**2.** In addition to these uses, it does draw embryos/fetuses when burned so as to produce smoke from below; moreover, it removes leprosies, lichen-like eruptions of the skin, and psoriatic nails when mixed with turpentine resin. Smeared on with vinegar, it is good for leprosies and it removes dull-white leprosies. Mixed with pine resin, it treats the strokes of scorpions and assuages the stroke of the great weever and of the sea scorpion when laid on with vinegar. Used as a wash with soda, it stops itching throughout the body.

**3.** It clears away jaundice when an amount of one spoonful is sprinkled on a drink or is taken with an egg that can be supped up. It is good both for a running nose and for catarrh, it controls perspiration when used like dusting powder, it benefits the gouty when smeared on with soda and water, and it is beneficial for hardness of hearing when, as it smolders, its smoke is siphoned into the ears. It even treats people affected by lethargic fever when burned to produce smoke, and it stems hemorrhages and heals bruised ears when anointed with wine and myrrh.

**V, 108 κίσηρις, Pumice stone**

**1.** One must prefer pumice stone that is very light and porous, cloven and free of stones. Additionally, it should be friable and white. You must burn it this way: after taking as much of it as you wish, burry it among very hot coals. When it has caught fire, take it out and quench it with fragrant wine, and after burning it again, quench it. After you have done so three times, let it cool by itself, store, and use.

**2.** It has properties that contract, clean the gums, purge the elements that cast a shadow over the pupils of the eyes by way of warming, fill up and cicatrize sores, also reduce excrescences, clean the teeth and the body when used as a powder, and are suitable for the removal of hair. Theophrastus[44] reports that if one dropped pumice stone into a boiling cask of wine, the boiling immediately stops.

### V, 109 ἅλς, Salt

**1.** The most effective salt is that which is mined and of this kind, in general, that which is white, free of stones, translucent, dense, smooth in its formation, particularly the Ammonian[45] in origin, that can be split, and that has straight cracks. But you must select sea salt that is dense, white, and smooth. Excellent is salt produced in Cyprus, especially in Salamis of Cyprus, and in Megara, then that produced in Sicily and Libya, and among the above mentioned, salt from marshlands is preferable. Of this type, the Phrygian, which is called *Tattaion,* is very strong.

**2.** The salts mentioned above, which are highly useful and differ in varying degrees, have in common properties that are astringent, detersive, that cleanse, and that dissolve; furthermore, they are capable of suppressing and of forming eschars. They can also stop putrid humors and they are mixed with itch salves; they check small protuberances on the eyes, they draw in membranes that grow over the eyes from their inner corners and the other types of flesh overgrowths, they are suitable to put in clysters, they relieve weariness when smeared on with olive oil, they are good for the swellings of the dropsical, and a hot compress of salts in little bags allays pains.

**3.** They also stop itching when smeared on by the fire with olive oil and vinegar until the patients sweat. When laid on with honey, vinegar, and olive oil they relieve likewise leprosies, lichen-like eruptions on the skin, itching, and sore throats. But for tonsillitis and for inflammations of the uvula they are plastered on with honey, and for thrush, flaccid gums, and cankers they are applied burned with barley groats.

---

[44] Theophrastus, *H. P.*, IX, 17, 3.

[45] This is rock salt mined near the temple of Jupiter Ammon, in Libya.

**4.** For strokes of scorpions, they are laid on with linseed; for viper stings, with oregano, honey, and hyssop; for the sting of the asp, with pitch or with oil of Syrian cedar or with honey; for the bite of the millipede, with vinegar and honey, also for the sting of wasps and of earth-wasps; but for pimples on the head, warty excrescences, and growths, they are combined with calf's suet.

**5.** With raisins or with beef suet or with honey, they dissolve small abscesses and testicular swelling; with oregano and leaven, they cause <small abscesses> to mature faster. Tied ground up in a linen cloth and dipped in vinegar, they help those bitten by crocodiles, the bitten parts being constricted with tourniquets; they also help those bitten by wild animals, and for facial bruises with honey, and for drinking opium juice, and for mushrooms when drunk with a mixture of vinegar and honey.

**6.** They are good with flour and honey for sprains, they prevent burns from blistering if plastered on with oil, they are similarly applied on the gouty, they are applied with vinegar for earaches, and they check erysipelas and shingles when plastered on with vinegar or when smeared on with hyssop.

You must burn them by placing them in a clay vessel, seal it carefully so that they do not fly off, and bury the vessel in coals until completely burned.

**7.** But some wrap quarried salt in dough, bury it in coals, and leave it until the dough is thoroughly burned. It is possible to burn even common salt this way: after rinsing it with water once and letting it dry out, place it in a vessel and, covering it with a lid, burn it from below, moving about the pot until the salt no longer leaps up.

### V, 110 ἁλὸς ἄχνη, Salt froth

Salt froth is the foamy scraping of salt found on the small stones; it has the same properties as salt.

### V, 111 ἅλμη, Brine

Brine has the same activity as salt; it is astringent, detersive, and it thins; it is a clyster for dysenterics, for those who have spreading ulcers as well as chronic hip ailments, and it is suitable to use as rinses on those to whom seawater is useful.

**V, 112 ἄνθος ἁλός, Salt efflorescence/Salt scum**

**1.** Salt efflorescence/salt scum flows down the river Nile and settles on top of certain marshes. You must take it saffron colored, smelling somewhat rank like *garum*, occasionally smelling even more foul, biting in taste, and being somewhat greasy. But if it is tinged with red or if it is lumpy, it must be considered inferior. Moreover, when pure it is soluble only in oil, but the adulterated is partly soluble even in water.

**2.** It is good for malignant and cancerous sores, for spreading ulcers in the genitalia, for purulent ears, for dim-sightedness, for scars, and for leucomas. It is mixed with plasters and with unguents for coloration, as it is also mixed with unguent of roses. It sets perspiration in motion, it upsets the bowel when taken with wine and water, and it is bad for the stomach. It is mixed with analgesics and with soaps for thinning hair, and, in general, it is harsh and burns like salt.

**V, 113 νίτρον, Soda**

**1.** One must choose soda that is light and either rosy or white in color, having holes, as if it were a spongy substance. Such is the one from Bryges.[46]

ἀφρὸς νίτρου. Foam of soda seems to be of excellent quality if it is very light, flaky, crumbly, inclining to purple, foamy, and biting. Such is the one brought from Philadelphia in Lydia. The Egyptian is ranked second. It occurs also in Magnesia of Caria.

**2.** Both it and soda have the same properties and they are burned the same way as salt; however, soda can to a far greater degree stop colic when triturated with cumin and drunk with hydromel or with must or with any of the substances that can dissipate flatulence, such as rue or dill. It is also an ointment for intermittent fevers before their anticipated attack. It is mixed with plasters that are capable of dispersing, that draw, and that are good for leprosies.

**3.** Infused with water or wine, it treats inflations, ringing of the ears, and purulent discharges; poured on with vinegar, it cleanses also filth,

---

[46] There are various readings of this passage for Bryges, which may be a place name. Among them there are also βουνῶν, "*from* mountains" and νησῶν, "from islands."

and with ass's or pig's fat, it treats those bitten by dogs. Compounded with turpentine, it opens up small abscesses. With figs, it is a plaster for those with edemata; smeared on with honey, it promotes sharp-sightedness; it is suitable to drink with vinegar and water for mushrooms, with water for the poisonous beetles, and with laserwort for bull's blood.
**4.** It is a useful plaster for those who waste away and with cerate it abates suffering from tetanic recurvation and sprains. It is mixed beneficially also with bread for those whose tongue is paralyzed.
Some burn the above by placing them in a new clay vessel on very hot coals until they become red-hot.

### V, 114 τρύξ, Wine lees

**1.** You must use preferably the wine lees of an old Italian wine but if unavailable you may even use those of another similar wine. Those from vinegar, however, are much too strong.
You must burn them like bastard sponge, having first dried them carefully. Some place them on a new clay vessel and burn them with a big fire until reduced to ashes. Others bury a lump in red-hot coals and do the same.
**2.** Proof that they were burned sufficiently is their white or gray color and apparent burning of the tongue when placed on it. Vinegar lees are burned the same way also.
They have strongly burning and detersive properties, also properties that are suppressive, astringent, highly putrefactive, and desiccative. You must use lees when they are fresh, for they quickly loose their strength by evaporation; it is for this reason that you must store them neither uncovered nor before putting them into a container.
**3.** They are washed like zinc oxide. Lees that have not been burned, reduce swellings by themselves as well as with myrtle, bind the bowel and a rheumy stomach when plastered on, assuage leucorrhea when smeared on the lower part of the abdomen and the genitalia, dissolve non-ulcerated swellings of the glands and tumors, and dry up breasts that are swollen with milk. Burned lees remove scaly nails with pine resin and dye hair blond when anointed with oil of mastic for the whole night. Washed lees are mixed into eye medications like ashes. Lees such as these eliminate scars and misting in the eyes.

### V, 115 ἄσβεστος, Unslaked lime

**1.** Unslaked lime is made this way: taking the shells of trumpet-shells, bury them into hot embers, or after placing them in a red-hot *clibanos* leave them alone overnight. The following day, if they should have become very white, remove them; otherwise burn them again until they become sufficiently white. Then after dipping them into cold water, place them into a new clay pot and covering them carefully with rags, leave them there for a night. In the morning, having been fully processed, take them out and store them.

**2.** It is also made from riverine pebbles and from common marble, which is even preferable to the other unslaked limes.

**3.** All unslaked limes have in common properties that heat, bite, burn, and that further the formation of eschars. But when combined with certain other ingredients, such as suet or olive oil, they can further maturation, soften, disperse, and cicatrize. That which is fresh and not wet must be considered the most effective.

### V, 116 γύψος, Gypsum

Gypsum has astringent, adhesive, antihemorrhagic, and antiperspirant properties. But if drunk, it kills by suffocation.

### V, 117 τέφρα κληματίνη, Ash of vine twigs

Ash of vine twigs has a caustic property. Plastered on with lard or with olive oil, it benefits bruised ribs, sprained joints, and twisted tendons; with soda and vinegar it reduces fleshy excrescence of the scrotum. Plastered on with vinegar it treats bites of snakes and dogs, and it is mixed with plasters that form incrustations. Its powder also is drunk with salt and vinegar for injuries due to falls and for mushrooms.

### V, 118 ἀλκυόνιον, *Alcyonion*[47]

**1.** You must know that there are five kinds of *alcyonia.* One kind is thick, sponge-like in structure and heavy; moreover, it is malodorous

---

[47] Berendes, p. 541, n. 1, says that these are types of corals that live especially in the Red Sea and the Mediterranian. They consist of gelatine, calcium, and native salts to which they owe their use for diseases of the bladder. LSJ defines it as "bastard sponge."

and smells of fish; it is found in large quantities on beaches. The next one is similar in shape to a membrane growing from the inner corner of the eye or to a sponge; it is light, it has many hollows, and it releases a smell that is like seaweed.

**2.** The third is vermicular and of a purplish color; some call it Milesian. The fourth is like greasy wool, it has many holes, and it is light. And the fifth is like a mushroom in shape, it is odorless and not smooth inside, resembling somewhat pumice stone, but on the outside it is smooth and jagged; much of it grows on the Propontis, around the island called Besbicos. The locals call it salt foam.

**3.** The first and second of them are used in women's cleansers, and for birthmarks, lichen-like eruptions, leprosies, dull-white leprosies, black spots, blemishes in the face and in the rest of the body. The third is good for people with difficult micturition and for patients with renal disease who collect gravelly substances in their bladder, for those with edemata, and for the spleen. Burned and smeared on with wine, it treats bald spots.

**4.** The last can whiten teeth; it is also used mixed with salts for other cleansers and depilatories.

If you wish to burn any of them, place it into an unbaked clay pot and, after luting the opening of the pot with clay, place it in an oven. After the clay has been baked, take it out, store, and use. It is washed like calamine.

### V, 119 ἀδάρκης, *Adarces*[48]

What they call *adarces* occurs in Galatia; it is an incrustation, as it were, somewhat salty, forming in wet and marshy places during draught and attaching itself on reeds and grasses. Its color resembles that of the flower on Assian stone,[49] but in its overall impression it resembles the *alcyonion* that is light and that has many hollows, and it is an *alcyonion* of the marshes, as it were.

It is useful for the removal of leprosies, freckles, lichen-like eruptions on the skin, birthmarks, and the like. On the whole it is sharp, capable of altering the state of the pores, benefiting also hip ailments.

---

[48] This is the salt inflorescence on marsh herbs.

[49] See Dsc. Bk. V, 124 and n. 55.

### V, 120 σπόγγοι, Sponges

**1.** Some people called the sponges that have small holes and that are dense *arenes*[50] among which the ones that are very hard they named *tragoi*[51] and the ones that are the exact opposite of the ones just mentioned *theleis.*[52] Sponges are burned like bastard sponges.
Sponges that are empty and devoid of any fatty substance can treat wounds, repress swellings, glue fresh wounds with water or with water and vinegar, and with boiled honey glue old hollows. But old sponges are useless.
**2.** When <applied> parched with a linen bandage, they open up closed sores and calluses, also when applied dry like pledgets. Applied dry and empty, they dry out the discharges of ulcers that contain a great deal of fluids, that spread, and that are chronic, and with vinegar they stop hemorrhages. Those that have been burned are <suitable> for blepharitis sicca and whenever one needs to clean or contract something. But for eye medications they are more effective if they have been washed. Burned with pitch they are suitable for hemorrhaging.
**3.** The ones that are very soft are bleached during the burning heat of summer. They fill them with the salt froth that settles on rocks and sun them. Make sure that their hollow part faces up and the cut side down. And if the weather is clear, they are even set out under the moon filled with salt froth or with seawater. <Such as these> do not become very white.

### V, 121 τὸ κουράλιον, Coral

**1.** It seems that the coral, which some have called *lithodendron*,[53] is a sea plant and becomes hard when pulled from the bottom of the sea as our ambient air touches it. A great deal of it is found at the promontory called Pachynos near Syracuse.
**2.** Of excellent quality is that which is red in color and which resembles lead oxide or a deep red sandalwood, crumbly, as if of its

[50] I. e. males.
[51] I. e. he-goats.
[52] I. e. females.
[53] "Stonetree."

own accord, smooth through its entire formation, smelling like moss and seaweeds, and in addition to these characteristics, if it is ramose and like the cassia that is in the shape of small shrubs. But that which is like stone in formation, looks rough, and is hollow and porous must be presumed inferior.

**3.** It has properties that bind and gently cool. It reduces excrescences and it clears eye scars; it fills up hollows, it cicatrizes, it treats quite effectively blood spitting, it is suitable for people with difficult micturition, and it reduces the spleen when drunk with water.

### V, 122 ἀντιπαθές, *Antipathes*

Also that which is called *antipathies* must be supposed to be coral, although it has a distinct difference. It is black in color but it, too, is tree-like and quite ramose.

It has the same properties as the above.

### V, 123 λίθος Φρύγιος, Phrygian stone[54]

**1.** Phrygian stone, which the dyers in Phrygia use and from where it was named, is formed in Cappadocia. Best is that which is pale and moderately heavy, not uniformly colored, and having white crevices just like calamine.

**2.** It is burned this way: after wetting it with the best possible wine, bury it in red-hot coals and keep fanning it. When it has changed color becoming more orange-tawny, take it out, quench it with the same kind of wine, and repeat the process, burying it again in the coals. Then burn it a third time, taking care that it does not break nor becomes sooty.

**3.** Unfired as well as fired it has properties that are highly astringent; additionally, they are detersive, escharotic, curative of burns with cerate, and mildly putrefactive. It is washed like calamine.

### V, 124 Ἄσσιος λίθος, Assian stone

**1.** You must use Assian stone of a pumice color, porous and light, crumbly, and with deep, quince-yellow crevices. Its flower is the salt that rises on the surface of the stones; it is fine in structure, some is

[54] A kind of aluminous pumice-stone.

white in color, some resembles somewhat the color of pumice tending towards quince-yellow, and it bites slightly when placed on the tongue.

**2.** Each has properties that are mildly putrefactive and dispersive of growths when taken with turpentine or pitch. But the flower must be regarded as the stronger of the two. The latter, when it has dried, treats marvelously well sores that are old and hard to cicatrize and reduces sores that are overgrown, mushroom-like, and malignant. With honey it also fills up the concavities of ulcers and cleanses them, and with cerate it controls spreading ulcers.

**3.** Used in plasters with bruised corn, <it is good> for the gouty, with vinegar and unslaked lime, for people with spleen disease, and when sucked with honey it benefits the tuberculars. From this stone they also make tubs that help gout sufferers who place their feet into them, and they make flesh-consuming coffins.[55] <Its flower> reduces fleshy as well as obese bodies when applied as a plastered in the bath, instead of soda. If one wishes to wash the above, he should wash them like calamine.

### V, 125 πυρίτης λίθος, Copper pyrites

**1.** Copper pyrites is a type of stone from which copper is mined. You must choose that which is copper-colored and which emits sparks readily. You must burn it this way: after coating it with honey, place it on gently burning coals and fan it continuously until it becomes orange-tawny in color. But some people, after moistening it well with honey, bury it among many very hot coals.

**2.** When it is about to become more orange-tawny, remove it and, after blowing off the ash again, burn it moistened until it becomes uniformly quite brittle. For it is often burned only on the surface. After burning it then this way and drying it, they store it. And if it is needed washed, it must be washed like calamine.

---

[55] Celsus, 4,31,7, Pliny, *N. H.*, 2.211, 36.131 also mention this stone for its remarkable ability to eat the flesh of corpses laid in sarcophagi constructed from it and to allay pain. It gets its name from Assos, a town of the Troad, where excellent Assian stones were quarried.

**3.** Both burned and not burned it is capable of warming, purging, cleansing the elements that cast a shadow over the pupils of the eyes, and of dissolving and softening indurations when compounded with pine resin. It also reduces overgrown flesh with some degree of warmth and astringency. Some call the one that was burned this way *diphryges*.[56]

### V, 126 αἱματίτης λίθος, Hematite

**1.** Hematite is of excellent quality when it breaks easily as if of its own accord and when it is hard, uniformly strong, and free of any dirt or veins.

It has properties that are astringent, that warm somewhat, that thin, and, with honey, that wipe off scars and roughnesses in the eyes. With woman's milk it is good for ophthalmia, for rents,[57] and for bloodshot eyes.

**2.** It is drunk with wine for difficult micturition and for leucorrhea and with the juice of pomegranate for blood spitting. They make from it both salves and medications suitable for eye diseases.

It is burned like Phrygian stone but without the wine. Let the standard for burning it be that it becomes moderately light and full of bubbles.

**3.** Some fake the above this way: taking a lump of talc that is dense and round — such are its so-called 'roots' — bury it in a clay pot that contains hot ashes then after a while they remove it and rub it against a whetstone testing whether it acquired the color of hematite.

**4.** And if it has that color, they store it, otherwise they again bury it, constantly checking and testing it: for if it is left alone for a long time in the ashes, it changes color and it even disintegrates. The counterfeit is refuted first from its divisions. For it breaks off in layers right away, but hematite does not break so.

**5.** <Then> it is refuted also from its color because the counterfeit has a fresh-looking color, but hematite is of a deeper color and it resembles cinnabar.

It is found in Sinopic red earth, it is also made from magnet that was burned for a while, but natural hematite is mined in Egypt.

---

[56] "Twice roasted."

[57] Probably, in the eyes.

**V, 127 σχιστὸς λίθος, ~ Talc[58]**

**1.** Talc is formed in the western part of Spain and it seems to be excellent when it is somewhat saffron-colored and breakable and when it splits easily, as if of its own accord. Because of its composition and of the close texture of its layers it resembles rock salt.

**2.** It has the same properties as hematite, falling short of it only in strength. It fills up hollows when diluted with woman's milk and it is very effective both for rents and for prolapses of the eyes, also for roughness of the eyelids and for defects inside the cornea.

**V, 128 Γαγάτης, Lignite**

**1.** You must choose lignite that catches fire quickly and that smells like asphalt. It is generally black and dry and it is flaky and very light. It has softening and dissolving properties; it is a test for epileptics when burned as to produce smoke from below, and it revives women in a state of uterine suffocation.

**2.** It drives away serpents when burned as to produce smoke and it is combined with medications that are good for the gouty. It occurs in Lycia, being found along the issue of a certain river that empties itself into the sea. The place is called Gagai.

**V, 129 Θρακίας, Thracian stone**

The stone called Thracian is formed in Sintia, in the river called Pontos. It can do the same things as lignite. It is reported that it is set on fire with water and that it is quenched with oil, something that happens also to asphalt.

**V, 130 μαγνῆτις λίθος, Magnet**

The best magnet attracts iron easily, is bluish in color, dense, and not too heavy. It has a property that drives out thick masses when given in the amount of one *triobolon* with hydromel. Some people burn it and sell it as hematite.

---

[58] Conjecture in LSJ.

**V, 131 Ἀραβικὸς λίθος, Arabian stone**

The stone called Arabian resembles flawless ivory.

This stone dries up hemorrhoids when applied ground up and after it is burned it becomes dentifrice.

**V, 132 γαλακτίτης, Milkstone**

Milkstone was named from the milk-like solute it releases. Otherwise it is really ash-colored and sweet in taste.

It is suitable to smear on for running eyes and for eye sores. After reducing it into powder you must store it in water, in a leaden box, for the starchy element surrounding it.

**V, 133 μελιτίτης, Honeystone**

Honeystone resembles milkstone in every respect, differing only in that the juice it releases is very sweet. It is good for all the things that milkstone is also good.

**V, 134 λίθος μόροχθος, Pipe clay**

Pipe clay, which some people have called *galaxias* or *leucographis*, is produced in Egypt. The weavers of linen use it to whiten linens, being soft and easy to dissolve.

It is thought to stop the pores. It is suitable for people who spit blood, for the colicky, for bladder ailments when drunk with water, and similarly for women who suffer from discharges and in a pessary. It is also mixed into soft eye medications. For it does fill up hollows and it stems discharges. Compounded with cerate, it cicatrizes the tender parts of ulcers.

**V, 135 λίθος ἀλαβαστρίτης, Alabaster**

The alabaster called onyx, compounded with pine resin or pitch after it has been burned, dissolves indurations, and with cerate it assuages stomach pains. It also tightens the gums.

### V, 136 θυίτης, *Thyites*[59]

The stone called *thyites* is produced in Ethiopia. It is greenish-yellow, it is jasper-like, it appears milky when broken, and it bites a great deal. It has a property that cleanses the elements that cast a shadow over the pupils of the eyes.

### V, 137 Ἰουδαικὸς λίθος, Judaic stone

Judaic stone is produced in Judea. It is shaped like an acorn; it is white, quite smooth, with parallel lines as if made on a turning lathe, and tasteless when dissolved.

An amount in size like a bean, dissolved like a little pill on a whetstone with three *cyathoi* of hot water and drunk, can help for difficult micturition and break bladder stones.

### V, 138 λίθος ἀμίαντος, Asbestos

Asbestos is produced in Cyprus, it resembles cleft alum, and, because it is fibrous, the <people> who work with it there make fabrics from it for shows. Thrown into a fire, while it does flare up, it comes out brighter, not burned.

### V, 139 λίθος σάπφειρος, Lapis lazuli

Lapis lazuli seems to help people stung by scorpions when drunk. It is drunk for internal ulcerations and it shrinks excrescences, defects inside the cornea and pustules on the eyes, and it joins together the rents of their membranes.

### V, 140 λίθος Μεμφίτης, ~ Memphitic stone[60]

Memphitic stone is found in Egypt, around Memphis. It is of the size of a pebble, shiny, and pied.

Ground up and smeared on areas about to be operated or cauterized, this stone is reported to induce harmless anesthesia.

---

[59] "Turquoise," John Goodyer, *The Greek herbal of Dioscorides*, p. 654. No identification in LSJ.

[60] Identified as *retinasphaltum* in John Goodyer, *op. cit.* p. 655 and described by Charles Hatchett, *Trans. Linn. Soc.* iv, p. 140.

**V, 141 λίθος σεληνίτης, Selenite**

Selenite, which some people have called *aphroselenos*[61] because it is found at night when the moon waxes, occurs in Arabia. It is white, transparent, and light.

It is given as a drink to epileptics and women use it as a protective amulet. It also seems to make trees fruitful when attached to them.

**V, 142 λίθος ἴασπις, Jasper**

There is a jasper which is emerald green, another like crystal, resembling phlegm, another light blue,[62] another smoky, as if it were blackened with smoke, one which has cracks that are quite white <and> shining and which is called *astrios*, and there is one called *terebinthizon*, resembling turquoise in color.

All seem to guard against evil when hung on a person and to promote a speedy birth when tied around the thigh.

**V, 143 λίθος ὀφίτης, Serpentine**

There is a serprntine that is sturdy and black, another ash-colored and spotted, and another that has white lines.

All are useful when tied on people stung by vipers or on those who have headaches. The one that has the lines is reported to be particularly helpful for lethargic fever and headaches.

**V, 144 λίθοι οἱ ἐν τοῖς σπόγγοις, The stones in the sponges**

When drunk with wine, the stones found in sponges break stones in the bladder.

**V, 145 λιθοκόλλα, Stone glue**

Stone glue, which is a mixture of marble or of Parian stone and bull's hide glue, when used with a very hot probe, can glue back eyelashes.

**V, 146 λίθος ὀστρακίτης, Clay stone**

Clay stone is like a shell, it is easy to split, and it is flaky. Women use it instead of pumice for hair removal. An amount of one *drachma*

---

[61] "Moon-foam."

[62] Or perhaps, "grey" or "cloudy."

drunk with wine stops the menstrual period and a weight of two *drachmai* drunk for four days following menstruation causes barrenness. Applied with honey on inflamed breasts, it soothes them and it also stops spreading ulcers.

**V, 147 σμύρις, Emery**

Emery is a stone that lapidaries use to clean their gems. It is useful for putrefactive and caustic medications, for flaccid gums, and as a dentifrice.

**V, 148 ἄμμος, Sand**

Sand that has been heated by the sun at the beach draws out moisture from edematose bodies when heaped over them up to the head. It is also roasted instead of millet or salts for dry fomentations.

**V, 149 ἀκόνης Ναξίας ἀπότριμμα, Naxian whetstone powder**

The powder from Naxian whetstone produced when iron is honed against it causes hair to grow on bald spots and prevents maiden breasts from growing big when smeared on them. It reduces the spleen and it benefits epileptics when drunk with vinegar.

**V, 150 λίθος γεώδης, Earth-like stone**

The earth-like stone binds, dries, and cleanses the elements that cast a shadow over the pupils of the eyes. Smeared on with water, it stops inflammations of the breasts and testicles.

**V, 151 γῆ, Earth**

All earths employed in medicine have properties that cool to the utmost and stop the pores. They differ from each other in kind and they are used, after some preparation, for different purposes.

**V, 152 Ἐρετριάδος γῆ, Eretrian earth**

**1.** One kind of Eretrian earth is exceedingly white, another ashen. The best is ash-colored, very soft, and when drawn against brazen objects, it leaves behind a rust-colored line.

It is washed like white lead or as follows: after triturating as much of it as you may wish by itself as well as with water, let it settle. Then strain out the liquid, and after drying the earth in the sun, pound it again during the day, adding water, and, letting it settle during the night, around dawn strain, and, pounding it in the sun, shape small troches if you can.

**2.** But if there is need for it to be cooked, take bean-size pieces of this earth, place in a perforated earthen vessel, seal its mouth carefully, place on red-hot coals, and fan continuously. When it becomes somewhat like sooty ash, remove and store.

It has astringent and cooling properties, gently softening, filling hollows, and gluing together bleeding wounds.

### V, 153 Σαμία γῆ, Samian earth

**1.** You must choose Samian earth that is very white, light, and when it touches the tongue it sticks to it like glue; also, you must choose it easily soluble, soft, and crumbly. Such is the Samian earth which some call *collourion.* There are two kinds of it: the one just mentioned and the one called *aster,* which is crusty and dense like whetstone.

**2.** Its properties, burning, and washing are similar to those of Eretrian earth. It stops blood spitting, it is given with flower of wild pomegranate to women who suffer from discharges, it represses inflammations of the testicles, of the breasts, and sweats when rubbed on with water and unguent of roses, and it helps those bitten by wild animals and for poisons when drunk with wine.

### V, 154 ἐν τῇ Σαμίᾳ γῇ λίθος, Stone found in Samian earth

There is a stone found in Samian earth which goldsmiths use for smoothing and polishing. It is excellent when white and massive.

It has astringent and cooling properties. It benefits, in a drink, those suffering from stomach ailments and it dulls the senses. It is good with milk both for rheums in the eyes and for sores. It seems to speed childbirth and to protect pregnant women when hung as an amulet.

### V, 155 Χία γῆ, Chian earth

**1.** And of the Chian earth you must take that which is white, somewhat ash-colored, and resembling Samian earth. It is laminated, fine, and it comes in various shapes.

It has the same properties as Samian earth. It makes the face and the entire body smooth, shiny, and healthy looking, and in the bath it cleanses like soda.

**2**. Selinus earth also accomplishes the same things. That which is very white, shiny, crumbly, and dissolves quickly if it should get wet is excellent.

### V, 156 Κιμωλία γῆ, Cimolian earth

**1.** One kind of Cimolian earth is white and the other purplish, having some inherent greasiness and being quite cold to the touch; it must be judged the best.

Both kinds dissolve tumors of the parotid glands and the other growths when diluted in vinegar, and they operate on burns so that they maintain the afflicted areas free of blisters if smeared on them right away.

**2.** They reduce both testicular indurations and inflammations all over the body; additionally, they prevail over erysipelas. In general, genuine Cimolian earths are extremely useful unless one used the counterfeit.

### V, 157 πνιγῖτις γῆ, *Pnigitis* earth

The earth called *pnigitis* is somewhat similar to the Eretrian earth in color, but it comes in large clods, it cools the hands that touch it, and it sticks so tightly to the tongue as to hang from it.

It has the same properties as Cimolian earth, although it falls slightly short of it in strength.

Some sell it as Eretrian earth.

### V, 158 ὄστρακα, Potsherds

When thoroughly burned potsherds from furnaces cicatrize. Therefore, when plastered on with vinegar they treat itching and pustules, they are beneficial to the gouty, and when compounded with cerate they dissolve scrofulous swellings of the glands.

Even the dried-up red earth from the furnaces has the same properties as the potsherds.

### V, 159 Μηλία γῆ, Melian earth

Melian earth also resembles Eretrian earth in color, that is to say the Eretrian earth that is ash-colored, but it is coarse, and when rubbed between the fingers it makes something like a whisper resembling a pumice stone being reduced into small pieces. It has the same properties as alum but quite milder, as is evident also from its taste. It also dries moderately the tongue.

It can cleanse the body and give it a nice color, thin the hair, and cleanse dull-white leprosies and leprosies. It is also useful to painters in prolonging the life of colors and operates as a fixative of greens.

This one, and in general all clays, must be chosen free of stones, fresh, soft, and crumbly, and they should dissolve easily when water touches them.

### V, 160 ἀμπελῖτις γῆ, *Ampelitis* earth[63]

**1.** Of the earth *ampelitis*, which some people call *pharmacitis* and which is produced in Seleucia of Syria, you must choose that which is black, resembling elongated pine coals, tending to splinter, and quite shiny. Furthermore, it should not dissolve slowly when some oil is poured over it during trituration. You must judge as unacceptable that which is light, ash-like, and insoluble.

**2.** It has relaxing and cooling properties. It is used for painting eyelids and eyelashes, for coloring hair, and for smearing on vines at budding time, killing the worms that grow on them.

### V, 161 ἀσβόλη, Soot

The soot that painters use is taken from glass-making factories, for this is the best.

It has putrefactive and astringent properties. It also cicatrizes burns when used with rose cerate.

### V, 162 μέλαν, Black ink

**1.** The black ink with which we write is made from soot collected from torches. Three *oungiai* of soot are combined with one *oungia* of

---

[63] A bituminous earth, See Pliny, *N. H.*, 35. 194.

gum. It is also made from soot of pine resin and from the painters' soot mentioned above. You must take one *mna* of soot, one and one-half *litra* gum, one and one-half *litra* bulls' hide glue, and one and one-half *litra* copper sulfate.

**2.** It is good for putrefactive medications and for burns, being smeared on thick with water and left alone until cicatrization; for it automatically falls off once the sores have healed.

And now, dear Areios, this should be enough, since I think that both the length of my composition and the quantity of medicinal materials and remedies are quite adequate to set this work aside.

And now, dear Areios, this should be enough, since I think that both the length of my composition and the quantity of medicinal materials and remedies are quite adequate to set this work aside.

# BIBLIOGRAPHY

André, Jacques. *Les noms des plantes dans la Rome antique*. Paris: Société d' Edition "Les Belles Lettres," 1985.

Aufmesser, Max. *Etymologische und wortgeschichtliche Erläuterungen zu De materia medica des Pedanius Dioscurides Anazarbeus.* Altertumswissenschaftliche Texte und Studien. Band 34. Hildesheim: Olms–Weidmann, 2000.

____, *Pedanius Dioscurides aus Anazarba. Fünf Bücher über die Heilkunde.* Altertumswissenschaftliche Texte und Studien. Band 37. Hildesheim: Olms–Weidmann, 2002.

Berendes, J. *Des Pedanios Dioskurides aus Anazarbos Arzneimittellehre in Fünf Büchern.* Stuttgart: Ferdinand Enke, 1902.

Bisset, Norman Grainger. Ed. and trans. *Herbal Drugs and Phytochemicals* of the second German ed. by Max Wichtl. Stuttgart: Medpharm Scientific Publishers, 1994.

Brummitt, R. K. and C. E. Powell, eds. *Authors of Plant Names*. Royal Botanic Gardens: Kew, 1992. Repr., 1996.

Celsus. *De medicina*. Ed. and trans. W. G. Spenser. 3 vols. Cambridge, Mass.: Harvard University Press; London: Heinemann: 1935-1938.

*Comicorum atticorum fragmenta*. Ed. Theodor Kock. 3 vols. Suppl. ed. J. Demianczuk. Leipzig: Teubner, 1880-1888; 1912.

Curtis, Robert I. *Garum and Salsamenta. Production and Commerce in Materia Medica*. Leiden: Brill, 1991.

Davidson, James N. *Courtesans and Fishcakes*. New York: St. Martin's Press, 1998.

Forbes, R. J. *Studies in Ancient Technology*. 9 vols. Leiden: Brill, 1964-1966.

Galen. *Claudii Galeni Opera Omnia.* Ed. C. G. Kühn. 20 vols. Leipzig: Cnoblochii, 1821-1833.

Gennadios, P.G. Λεξικόν Φυτολογικόν. Athens: Trochalia, 1914. First Photo Offset, August 1997.

Goodyer, John. *The Greek Herbal of Dioscorides*: Illustrated by a Byzantine A. D. 512. Ed. Robert T. Gunther. London and New York: Hafner, 1934; repr. 1968.

Gunther, Robert T. See Goodyer, John.

Harborne, Jeffrey B., Baxter, Herbert, and Moss, Gerald, P. Eds. *Phytochemical Dictionary. A Handbook of Bioactive Compounds from Plants*. London and Philadelphia, Pa: Taylor & Francis, 1999.

Jacoby, F. *Die Fragmente der griechischen Historiker*. Berlin: Leiden, 1923 -.

Langenheim, Jean H. *Plant Resins*: *Chemistry, Evolution, Ecology, and Ethnobotan*y. Portland: Timber Press, 2003.

Liddell, Henry George and Scott, Robert. *A Greek English Lexicon*. Revised by Jones, Henry Stuart. Oxford: Clarendon Press. First ed. 1843. Ninth ed. 1940; repr. 1953.

Mabberly, D. J. *The Plant Book*. Second ed. Cambridge: Cambridge University Press, 2000.

Miller, J. Innes. *The Spice Trade of the Roman Empire, 29 B. C. to 641 A. D.* Oxford: Clarendon Press, 1969.

Nutton, Vivian. See Scarborough, John.

Paulus Aegineta. *Seven Books of Paulus Aegineta*. Trans. Francis Adams. 3 vols. London: Syndenham Society, 1844.

Pauly-Wissowa-Kroll. *Realencyclopädie der classischen Altertums-wissenschaft*. Stuttgart: Metzler, 1894-.

Pausanias. *Description of Greece*. Trans. W. H. S. Jones, H. A. Ormerod. 4 vols. With a companion vol. containing maps, plans, and indices prepared by R. E. Wycherley. London: Heinemann; Cambridge, Mass.: Harvard University Press, 1918-1935.

Plato, *Timaeus, Critias, Cleitophon, Menexenus, Epistles*. The Rev. R. G. Bury. Cambridge, Mass: Harvard University Press; London: Heinemann, 1981.

Pliny. *Natural History*. Eds. H. Rackham, W. H. S. Jones, and D. E. Eichholz. 10 vols. Cambridge, Mass.: Harvard University Press; London: Heinemann, 1938-1963.

Plutarch. *Moralia. Isis and Osiris*. Trans. Frank Cole Babbitt. London: Heinemann, Cambridge, Mass.: Harvard University Press, 1936.

Powell, C. E. See Brummitt, R. K.

Riddle, John. *Dioscorides on Pharmacy and Medicine*. Austin: University of Texas Press, 1985.

Sarton, George. *Introduction to the History of Science*. 2 vols. Cambridge, Mass.: Harvard University Press, 1959-1960.

Scarborough, John. "Crateuas." Oxford Classical Dictionary. Third ed. Oxford: Clarendon Press, 1996.

____ and Nutton, Vivian. "The Preface of Dioscorides' *De materia medica:* Introduction, Translation, Commentary." *Transactions and Studies of the College of Physicians in Philadelphia* 4, no. 3 (1982): 187-227.

Singer, Charles. "The Herbal in Antiquity and its Transmission to Later Ages." *Journal of Hellenic Studies* 47 (1927): 1-52.

Soranus. *Gynecology*. Trans. Oswei Temkin. Baltimore: Johns Hopkins University, 1956.

Sprengel, Kurt Polycarp Joachim. *Pedanii Dioscoridis Anazarbei De materia medica libri quinque*. C. G. Kühn. ed. Medicorum graecorum opera quae exstant, vols. 25-26. Leipzig: Cnoblochii, 1829-1830.

Strabo. *Geography*. Trans. Horace Leonard Jones. 8 vols. Cambridge, Mass.: Harvard University Press; London: Heinemann, 1917-1935.

Theophrastus. *Enquiry into Plants*. Trans. Arthur Hort. 2 vols. Cambridge, Mass.:Harvard University Press; London: Heinemann, Vol. 1, 1916. Repr. 1968. Vol. 2, 1926. Repr. 1977.

_____. *De lapidibus*. Ed. intro. translation, and commentary by D. E Eichholz. Oxford: Clarendon, 1965.

Veith, Ilza. *Hysteria: The History of the Disease*. Chicago: University of Chicago Press, 1965.

Webster's *New International Dictionary*. Springfield, Mass.: G. & C. Merriam Company, 1950.

Wellmann, Max. *Pedanii Dioscuridis Anazarbei De materia medica libri quinque*. 3 vols. Berlin: Weidmann, 1906-1914; repr. 1958.

______."Dioskurides." No. 12, P.W. 5 (1903): 1131-1142.

______."Λεκάνιος Ἄρειος." No. 13, P. W. 2 (1896): 626.

______. *Krateuas*. Abhandlungen der königlichen Gesellschaft der Wissenschaften zu Göttingen, Phil-Hist. Klasse, Neue Folge, 2: no. 1. Berlin:Weidmann, 1897.

______. "Zur Geschichte der Medizin im Alterthum." *Hermes* 23 (1888): 556-566.

Wenskus, Otta. "Pedanius Dioscorides of Anazarbus: *De materia medica.*" Trans. by Lily Y. Beck. *Anzeiger für die Altertumswissenschaft.* LXIII, Band, Juli-Oktober 2010, 3./4., pp. 158-159.

Wichtl, Max. See Bisset, Norman Grainger.

| **Botanical Name** |
|---|
| *Achillea millefolium* L. (A. p. 238) |
| *Achillea millefolium* . (A. p. 3) |
| *Quercus* L. sp. (A. p. 32) |
| *Polyporus* sp. (A. p. 7) |
| *Agrimonia eupatoria* L. (A. p. 99) |
| *Carum copticum* B. and H. (A. p. 81) |
| *Carum copticum* B. and H. (A. p. 14) |
| *Carum copticum* B. and H. (A. p. 81) |
| *Smyrnium olusatrum* L. (A. p. 124) |
| *Smyrnium olusatrum* L. |
| *Smyrnium olusatrum* L. (A. p. 124) |
| *Smyrnium olusatrum* L. (LSJ) |
| *Smyrnium olusatrum* L. (LSJ) |
| *Medicago sativa* L. (A. p. 157) |
| *Anchusa tinctoria* L. (A. p. 178) |
| *Anchusa tinctoria* L. (A. p. 46) |
| *Anchusa tinctoria* L. (A. p. 16) |
| *Echium diffusum* Sibth. (A. p. 178) |
| *Echium diffusum* Sibth. (A. p. 16) |
| *Echium diffusum* Sibth. (A. p. 16) |
| *Lithospermum fruticosum* L. (A. p. 16) |
| ~*Plantago Bellardii* All., ~ *P. albicans* L. (A. p. 125) |
| *Ferula galbaniflua* Boiss. & Buhse (A. p. 58) |
| *Ferula galbaniflua* Boiss. & Buhse (A. p. 160) |
| *Prunus amygdalus* Stokes esp. var. *sativa* Asch. (A. p. *15)* |
| *Prunus amygdalus* Stokes, var. *amara* Schn. (A. p. 15) |
| *Aloe vera* L. (A. p. 11) |
| *Aquilaria agallocha* Roxb. (A. p. 7) |
| |
| *Artemisia maritima* L. (A. p. 37) |
| *Artemisia maritima* L. (A. p. 26) |
| *Artemisia maritima* L. (A. p. 13) |
| |
| *Anemone coronaria* L. (A. p. 96) |
| *Anemone coronaria* L. |
| *Pimpinella anisum* L. (A. p. 17) |
| *Cressa cretic*a L. (A. p. 18) |
| *Ajuga iva* Schreb. (A. p. 18) |
| |

| **Botanical Name** |
|---|
| |
| |
| *Pirus malus* L. (A. p. 115) |
| *Prunus armeniaca* L. |
| *Prunus armeniaca* L. (A. p. 157) |
| *Lepidium draba* L. (A. p. 90) |
| ~*Ferula nodosa* L. vel ~*Echinophora tenuifolia* L. (A. p. 186) |
| |
| |
| |
| |
| *Asparagus aspartilis* L. (A. p. 126) |
| *Asparagus officinalis* L. (A. pp. 28 and 166) |
| *Asphodelus* L. sp.. (A. pp. 29-30) |
| *Securigera securidaca* L. (A. p. 191) |
| *Securigera securidaca* (A. p. 117) |
| *Meum athamanticum* Jacq. (A. pp. 160-161) |
| ~*Chamaelina sativa* Crantz, var. *microcarpa* Andrz. (A. p. 166) |
| ~*Chamaelina sativa* Crantz, var. *microcarpa* Andrz. (A. p. 157) |
| *Melissa officinalis* L., *M. altissima* Sibth. and Sm. (A. p. 158) |
| *Melissa officinalis* L., *M. altissima* Sibth. and Sm. (A. p. 158) |
| *Hordeum* L. sp. |
| *Stachys* L. sp. (A. p. 247) |
| *Ocimum basilicum* L. sp. (A. p. 175) |
| *Reseda alba* L. (A. p. 237) |
| *Reseda alba* L. (A. p. 94) |
| *Commiphora mukul* Engl. (A. p. 151) |
| *Commiphora mukul* Engl. (A. p. 38) |
| *Commiphora mukul* Engl. (A. p. 34) |
| *Nelumbo nucifera* Gaert. (A. p. 82) |
| *Nelumbo nucifera* Gaert. (A. p. 82) |
| *Vicia faba* L. (LSJ) |
| *Acanthus mollis* L. (A. p. 185) |
| *Acanthus mollis* L. (A. p. 157) |
| *Acanthus mollis* L. (A. p. 2) |
| *Acanthus spinosus* L. (A. p. 2) |
| *Scorpiurus vermiculatus* L. (A. p. 69) |
| ~*Inula candida* L. ~*Celsia* sp.., ~*C. acaulis* Bory (A. p. 23) |
| ~*Inula candida* L.,~*Celsia* sp. ~*C. acaulis* Bory (A. p. 23) |
| *Galium verum* L. (A. p. 108) |

| **Botanical Name** |
|---|
| *Galium verum* L. |
| *Galium verum* L. |
| |
| |
| *Beta maritima* L. (LSJ) |
| *Moringa* sp. |
| *Mentha silvestris* L., M. viridis L. (A. p. 241) |
| *Mentha silvestris* L., *M. viridis* L. (A. p. 122) |
| *Stachys officinalis* L. (A. pp. 209-210) |
| *Stachys officinalis* L. (A. pp. 209-210) |
| *Convolvulus arvensis* L. (A. p. 67) |
| *Convolvulus arvensis* L. (A. p. 119) |
| *Convolvulus arvensis* L. (LSJ) |
| |
| *Aristolochia clematitis* L. (A. p. 25) |
| *Aristolochia longa* L. (A. p. 25) |
| *Aristolochia rotunda* L. (A. p. 25) |
| *Aristolochia longa* L. (A. p. 25) |
| *Aristolochia rotunda* L. (A. p. 25) |
| *Aristolochia longa* L. (A. p. 25) |
| *Aristolochia* L. (A. p. 25) |
| ~*Commiphora kataf* Forsk., ~*Styrax benzoin* Dryand. (A. p. 47) |
| *Vicia ervilia* Willd. (A. p. 182) |
| *Tamus communis* L. (A. p. 39) |
| *Tamus communis* L. (A. p. 14) |
| *Tamus communis* L. (A. p. 14) |
| *Nigella sativa* L. (A. p. 157) |
| *Helleborus cyclophyllu* s R. Br. (A . p. 205) |
| *Helleborus cyclophyllus* R. Br. (A. p. 157) |
| *Helleborus cyclophyllus* R. Br. |
| *Helleborus cyclophyllus* R. Br. (A. p. 93) |
| *Helleborus cyclophyllus* R. Br. |
| *Ballota nigra* L. |
| *Ballota nigra* L. (A. p. 33) |
| ~ *Asplenium onopteris* L. (LSJ) ~ *Dryopteris* L. sp. (A. p. 91) |
| *Populus nigra* L. (A. p. 6) |
| *Vincetoxicum nigrum* Moench (LSJ) |
| *Vincetoxicum nigrum* Moench (LSJ) |
| *Leontice chrysogonon* L. sp. (A. p. 64) |
| *Leontice chrysogonon* L. sp. (LSJ) |

| **Botanical Name** |
|---|
| *Leontice chrysogonon* L. sp. (LSJ) |
| *Amaranthus blitum* L. (A. p. 36) |
| *Aster amellus* L. (A. p. 39) |
| *Aster amellus* L. (A. p. 29) |
| Unidentified |
| *Lagenaria vulgaris* Ser. (A. p. 71) |
| *Rhamnus cathartica* L. (A. p. 217) |
| *Buxus sempervirens* L. (A. p. 42) |
| *Pteris aquilina* L.(A. p. 174) |
| *Pteris aquilina* L. (A. p. 258) |
| *Rubus ulmifolius* Schott (LSJ) |
| |
| |
| |
| *Xanthium strumarium* L. |
| *Xanthium strumarium* L. |
| *Xanthium strumarium* L. (A. p. 196) |
| *Xanthium strumarium* L. (A. p. 278) |
| *Xanthium strumarium* L. (A. p. 19) |
| *Xanthium strumarium* L. |
| *Scrofularia peregrina* L. |
| *Scrofularia peregrina* L. (A. p. 108) |
| *Scrofularia peregrina* L. (A. p. 108) |
| *Bryonia dioica* Jacq. (A. p. 209) |
| *Bryonia dioica* Jacq. (A. p. 62) |
| *Bryonia dioica* Jacq. (A. p. 179) |
| *Bryonia dioica* Jacq. (A. p. 159) |
| *Bryonia dioica* Jacq. (A. p. 151) |
| *Bryonia dioica* Jacq. |
| *Bryonia dioica* Jacq. (A. p. 39) |
| *Bryonia dioica* Jacq. (A. p. 23) |
| *Bryonia dioica* Jacq. (A. p. 14) |
| *Bryonia dioica* Jacq. |
| *Anchusa italica* Retz. (A. p. 40) |
| *Sparganium ramosum* Curtis, *S. simplex* Huds. (A. p. 244) |
| *Arctium lappa* L. (A. p. 208) |
| *Arctium lappa* L. (A. p. 208) |
| *Arctium lappa* L. (A. p. 23) |
| *Sanguisorba minor* Scop. = *Poterium sanguisorba* L. (A. p. 238) |
| *Ruscus aculeatus* L. (A. p. 60) |

| **Botanical Name** |
|---|
| *Ruscus aculeatus* L. (A. p. 183) |
| *Ruscus aculeatus* L. (A. p. 167) |
| *Ruscus aculeatus* L. |
| *Ruscus aculeatus* L. |
| *Ruscus aculeatus* L. |
| *Ruscus aculeatus* L. |
| *Ruscus aculeatus* L. |
| *Petasites officinalis* Moench (A. p. 194) |
| *Brassica oleracea* L. (A. p. 77) |
| *Brassica oleracea* L. ~var. *silvestris*, ~*B. cretica* (A. p. 38) |
| ~*Senecio thapsoides* DC., ~*Mercurialis tomentosa* L. (A. pp. 140-141) |
| ~*Senecio thapsoides* DC., ~*Mercurialis tomentosa* L. (A. p. 43) |
| |
| ~*Calamagrostis epigeios* Roth, ~*Sorgum halepense* L. (A. p. 44), |
| ~*Dactyloctenium aegyptiacum* Willd. = *Cynosurus aegyptius* L. (A. p. 44) |
| *Antirrhinum orontium* L. (A. p. 149) |
| *Antirrhinum orontium* L. (LSJ) |
| *Antirrhinum orontium* L. (A. (LSJ) |
| *Tribulus terrestris* L. (A. p. 263) |
| *Cymbopogon schoenanthus* Spreng. (A. p. 257) |
| *Cymbopogon schoenanthus* Spreng. sp.(.A. p. 229) |
| Cymbopogon schoenanthus Spreng. sp. (A. p. 229) |
| *Cymbopogon schoenanthus* Spreng. (A. p. 229) |
| *Cymbopogon schoenanthus* Spreng. (A. p. 229) |
| *Alhagi maurorum* L. (A. p. 244) |
| *Alhagi maurorum* L. (A. p. 98) |
| *Alhagi maurorum* L. (A. p. 88) |
| *Alhagi maurorum* L. (A. p. 28) |
| *Anthemis tinctoria* L. (A. p. 64) |
| *Anthemis tinctoria* L. (A. p. 63) |
| *Matricaria chamomilla* L. (A. p. 60) |
| *Matricaria chamomilla* L. (A. p. 157) |
| *Matricaria chamomilla* L. |
| *Chamomilla* L. sp. |
| *Matricaria chamomilla* L. (A. p. 96) |
| *Chamomilla* L. sp.. |
| *Phalaris canariensis* L. (A. p. 195) |
| *Linaria spuria* Miller (A. p. 93) |
| *Capparis spinosa* L. |
| *Capparis spinosa* L. |

| Botanical Name |
|---|
| *Capparis spinosa* L. (A. p. 179) |
| *Capparis spinosa* L. (A. p. 179) |
| *Capparis spinosa* L. |
| *Capparis spinosa* L. |
| *Capparis spinosa* L. (A. p. 84) |
| *Capparis spinosa* L. |
| *Capparis spinosa* L. (A. p. 48) |
| *Capparis spinosa* L. |
| *Capparis spinosa* L. (A. pp. 123-124) |
| *Capparis spinosa* L. (A. p. 258) |
| *Capparis spinosa* L. |
| *Euphorbia lathyris* L. (A. p. 139) |
| *Carum carvi* L. (A. p. 51) |
| *Elettaria cardamomum* White & Maton et al. spp. (A. p. 49) |
| *Ceratonia siliqua* L. (LSJ) |
| *Daucus carota* L. (A. p. 248) |
| *Daucus guttatus (* LSJ) |
| Cinnamomum cassia Blume sp. |
| Cinnamomum cassia Blume sp. |
| *Cinnamomum cassia* Blume (A. p. 52) |
| Cinnamomum cassia Blume sp. |
| Cinnamomum cassia Blume sp. |
| Cinnamomum cassia Blume sp. |
| Cinnamomum cassia Blume sp. |
| Cinnamomum cassia Blume sp. |
| *Ricinus communis* L. (A. p. 237) |
| *Ricinus communis* L. (A. p. 237) |
| *Ricinus communis* L. (A. p. 79) |
| *Ricinus communi* s L. (A. p. 66) |
| *Silene gallica* L. (A. p. 175) |
| *Silene gallica* L. |
| *Silene gallica* L. (A. p. 92) |
| *Calamintha nepeta* Savi (A. p. 171) |
| *Calamintha* Lmk. sp. (A. p. 44) |
| *Calamintha* Lmk. sp. (A. p. 44) |
| ~*Caucalis grandiflora* L. (A. p. 53) |
| *Caucalis grandiflora* L. (A. p. 87) |
| *Juniperus* L. (LSJ) |
| *Citrus medica* Risso (A. pp. 68, 153) |
| *Chelidonium majus* L. (A. p. 62) |

| **Botanical Name** |
|---|
| *Chelidonium majus* L. |
| *Apium graveolens* L. (A. p. 234) |
| *Apium graveolens* L. var. *silvestre* (A. p. 118) |
| *Valeriana celtica* L. (A. p. 170) |
| ~*Evax pygmaea* Pers., ~*E. asterifoli* a Pers., ~*Plantago cretic* a L., (A. p. 55) |
| ~*Gnaphalium leontopodium* L. (A. p. 55) |
| *Centaurea centaurium* L. (A. p. 169) |
| *Centaurea centaurium* L. (A. p. 55) |
| *Centaurea centaurium* L. (A. p. 109) |
| *Sedum cepaia* L. (A. p. 56) |
| *Ruscus racemosus* L. (A. p. 59) |
| *Ruscus racemosus* L. (A. p. 9) |
| *Cardopatium corymbosum* Pers. (A. p. 175) |
| *Cardopatium corymbosum* Pers. (A. p. 60) |
| *Cardopatium corymbosum* Pers. (A. pp. 59-60) |
| *Cardopatium corymbosum* Pers. (A. p. 275) |
| *Cardopatium corymbosum* Pers. (A. p. 84) |
| *Cardopatium corymbosum* Pers. (A. p. 84) |
| *Cardopatium corymbosum* Pers. (A. p. 60) |
| *Raphanus raphanistrum* L. (A. p. 138) |
| *Raphanus raphanistrum* (LSJ) |
| *Vitex agnus-castus* L. (A. p. 150) |
| *Vitex agnus-castus* L. (A. p. 8) |
| *Prunus avium (* LSJ) |
| *Castanea vulgaris* Lam. (A. p. 52) |
| *Castanea vulgaris* Lam. |
| *Castanea vulgaris* Lam. (A. p. 52) |
| *Castanea vulgaris* Lam. (A. p. 32) |
| *Castanea vulgaris* Lam. (A. p. 32) |
| *Cicer arietinum* L. (A. p. 182) |
| *Cicer arietinum* L. (A. p. 78) |
| *Cicer arietinum* L. (A. p. 96) |
| *Cichorium endivia* L. (A. p. 236) |
| *Cichorium intybus* L. (LSJ) |
| *Hypericum olympicum (* LSJ) |
| *Orobanche crenata* Forsk. (A. pp. 181-182) |
| *Orobanche crenata* Forsk. (A. p. 141) |
| *Orobanche crenata* Forsk. (A. p. 84) |
| *Orobanche crenata* Forsk. (A. p. 260) |
| *Paliurus australis* Gaertn. = *P. spina Christi* Mill.(A. p. 185) |

| English Name | Greek Name | References |
|---|---|---|
| Cinnamon | Μόσυλον | I, 14 |
| Cinnamon | κινάμωμον | I, 14 |
| Cinnamon | ψευδοκινάμωμον | I, 14 |
| Cinnamon | ξυλοκινάμωμον | I, 14 |
| Cinnamon | ζιγγιβέρι | I, 14 |
| Cinquefoil | ψευδοσέλινον | IV, 42 |
| Cinquefoil | πεντέφυλλον | IV, 42 |
| Cinquefoil | πεντάτομον | IV, 42 |
| Cinquefoil | πενταπετές | IV, 42 |
| Cinquefoil | πενταδάκτυλον | IV, 42 |
| Cinquefoil | ξυλοπέταλον | IV, 42 |
| Cinquefoil | ξυλόλωτον | IV, 42 |
| Cinquefoil | καλλιπέταλον | IV, 42 |
| Citrons | Περσικά | I, 115 |
| Citrons | Μηδικά | I, 115 |
| Citrons | κίτρια | I, 115 |
| Citrons | κεδρόμηλα | I, 115 |
| Clary | ὅρμινον | III, 129 |
| Cleavers | φιλάνθρωπον | III, 90 |
| Cleavers | ὀμφαλόκαρπον | III, 90 |
| Cleavers | ἀπαρίνη | III, 90 |
| Cleavers | ἀμπελόκαρπον | III, 90 |
| Club-rush | ὁλόσχοινος | IV, 52 |
| Cock's head | ὀνοβρυχίς | III, 153 |
| Colocynth | σικύα πικρά | IV, 176 |
| Colocynth | κολοκυνθίς | IV, 176 |
| Colocynth | κολόκυνθα ἀγρία | IV, 176 |
| Coltsfoot | πίθιον | III, 112 |
| Coltsfoot | πήχιον | III, 112 |
| Coltsfoot | πετρώνιον | III, 112 |
| Coltsfoot | βήχιον | III, 112 |
| Comfrey | σύμφυτον ἄλλο | IV, 10 |
| Comfrey | πηκτή | IV, 10 |
| Coriander | κόριον | III, 63 |
| Corn cockle | λυχνὶς ἀγρία | III, 101 |
| Corn flag | φασγάνιον | IV, 20 |
| Corn flag | ξίφιον | IV, 20 |
| Corn flag | μαχαιρίων | IV, 20 |
| Corn poppy | μήκων ῥοιάς | IV, 63 |
| Cornelian cherry tree | κρανία | I, 119 |

| **Botanical Name** |
|---|
| *Cinnamomum tamala* Nees, *C. iners* Blume for India (A. p. 67) |
| *Cinnamomum tamala* Nees, *C. iners* Blume for India (A. p. 67) |
| *Cinnamomum* sp. (A. p. 209) |
| *Cinnamomum* sp. (A. p. 278) |
| *Cinnamomum tamala Nees, C. iners* Blume for India sp. |
| *Potentilla reptans* L. (A. p. 209) |
| *Potentilla reptans* L. (A. p. 191) |
| *Potentilla reptans* L. (A. p. 191) |
| *Potentilla reptans* L. (A. p. 191) |
| *Potentilla reptans L.* (A. p. 191) |
| *Potentilla reptans* L. |
| *Potentilla reptans* L. (A. p. 278) |
| *Potentilla reptans* L. (A. p. 278) |
| *Citrus medica* Risso (A. p. 68) |
| *Citrus medica* Risso (A. p. 153) |
| *Citrus medica* Risso (A. pp. 68, 153) |
| *Citrus medica* Risso (A. pp. 68, 153) |
| *Salvia horminum* L. (A. p. 126) |
| *Galium aparine* L. (A. p. 196) |
| *Galium aparine* L. (A. p. 177) |
| *Galium aparine* L. (A. p. 19) |
| *Galium aparine* L. |
| *Scirpus holoschoenus* L. (A. p. 125) |
| *Onobrychis caput galli* Link. and *O. viciaefolia* Scop. (A. p. 178) |
| *Citrullus colocynthis* Schrad. (A. p. 238) |
| *Citrullus colocynthis* Schrad. (A. p. 71) |
| *Citrullus colocynthis* Schrad. *(* A. p. 71*)* |
| *Tussilago farfara* L. |
| *Tussilago farfara* L. |
| *Tussilago farfara* L. |
| *Tussilago farfara* L. (A. p. 35) |
| *Symphytum bulbosum* (LSJ) |
| *Symphytum bulbosum* (LSJ) |
| *Coriandrum sativum* L. (A. p. 75) |
| *Agrostemma githago* L. (A. p. 149) |
| *Gladiolus segetum* Gawler (A. p. 196) |
| *Gladiolus segetum* Gawler (A. p. 278) |
| *Gladiolus segetum* Gawler (A. p. 151) |
| *Papaver rhoeas* L. (A. p. 156) |
| *Cornus mas* (LSJ) |

| **Botanical Name** |
|---|
| *Saussurea lappa* Clarke (A. p. 76) |
| *Onopordum acanthium* L., *O. illyricum* (A. p. 2) |
| *Gnaphalium* L. sp., *Filago* L. sp. (A. p. 112) |
| |
| *Heracleum sphondylium* L. (A. p. 244) |
| *Pyrus acerba* (LSJ) |
| *Geranium tuberosum* L. (A. p. 110) |
| *Erodium malacoides* Willd. (A. p. 110) |
| *Smyrnium perfoliatum* Mill. (A. p. 242) |
| *Smyrnium perfoliatum* Mill. .(A. p. 1 95) |
| *Athamanta cretensis* L. (LSJ) |
| *Tordylium officinale* L. (A. p. 262) |
| *Tordylium officinale* L. (A. p. 237) |
| *Pimpinella cretica* L. (A. p. 209) |
| *Valeriana phu* L. (A. p. 170) |
| *Valeriana phu* L. (A. p. 170) |
| *Satureia thymbra* L. (A. p. 260) |
| |
| *Colocasia antiquorum* Schott |
| *Colocasia antiquorum* Schott (A. p. 26) |
| *Cucumis sativus* L. (A. p. 80) |
| *Cucumis sativus* L. (A. p. 80) |
| *Cucumis sativus* L. (A. p. 80) |
| *Cuminum cyminum* L. (A. p. 81) |
| *Myrtus communis* L. (LSJ) |
| *Olea europaea* L. var. *sativa* Hoffm. and Lk. (A. p. 176) |
| *Rumex crispus* L. (A. p. 183) |
| *Cyclamen graecum* Link. (A. p. 82) |
| *Lonicera periclymenum* L. (A. p. 82) |
| *Lonicera periclymenum* (A. p. 67) |
| *Cupressus sempervirens* L. (LSJ) |
| *Ruscus hypophyllum* L. (LSJ) |
| *Ruscus hypoglossum* L. (LSJ) |
| *Ruscus hypoglossum* L. (A. p. 130) |
| *Ruscus hypophyllum* L. (LSJ) |
| *Ruscus hypophyllum* L. (LSJ) |
| *Ruscus hypophyllum* L. (LSJ) |
| *Lolium temulentum* L. (A. p. 6) |
| *Phoenix dactylifera* L. (LSJ) |
| ~*Athamanta cretensis* L. (A. p. 87) |

| **Botanical Name** |
|---|
| *Lamium album* L. (A. p. 143) |
| *Thapsia garganica* L. (A. p. 258) |
| *Sambucus ebulus* L. (A. p. 59) |
| *Sambucus ebulus* L. |
| *Anethum graveolens* L. (A. p. 17) |
| *Origanum dictamnus* L. (A. p. 88) |
| *Origanum dictamnus* L. (LSJ) |
| *Origanum dictamnus* L. (LSJ) |
| *Rumex conglomeratus* L. (LSJ) |
| *Rumex aquaticus* L. (A. p. 123) |
| *Mercurialis perennis* L. (A. p. 198) |
| *Cynodon dactylon* Pers. (A. p. 8) |
| *Cynanchum acutum* L., for the Orient: *Marsdenia erecta* Br. (A. p. 189) |
| *Cynanchum acutum* L., for the Orient: *Marsdenia erecta* Br. |
| *Cynanchum acutum* L., for the Orient: *Marsdenia erecta* Br. (A. p. 83) |
| *Cynanchum acutum* L., for the Orient: *Marsdenia erect* a Br. |
| *Cynanchum acutum* L., for the Orient: *Marsdenia erecta* Br. (A. p. 21) |
| *Convolvulus oleaefolius* Desr. |
| *Convolvulus oleaefolius* Desr. (A. p. 90) |
| *Convolvulus oleaefolius* Desr. (A. p. 116} |
| *Arum dracunculus* L. (A. p. 90) |
| *Spiraea filipendula* L. (A. p. 177) |
| *Lemna minor* L. (A. p. 141) |
| *Rhamnus petiolaris* , *Rh. lycoides* , *Rh. punctata* Boiss. (A. p. 212) |
| *Rhamnus petiolaris, Rh. lycoides, Rh. punctata* Boiss. (A. p. 149) |
| *Aquilaria agallocha* Roxb. (A. p. 7) |
| *Bunium ferulaceum* Sibth. and Sm. (A. p. 41) |
| *Bunium ferulaceum* Sibth. and Sm. (A. p. 4) |
| *Erucaria aleppica* (LSJ) |
| *Diospyrus ebenum Koenig* , *D . melanoxylon* Roxb. (A. p. 92) |
| Unidentified |
| *Echium plantagineum* L., *E. rubrum* L. (A. p. 92) |
| *Echium plantagineum* L., *E. rubrum* L. (A. p. 90) |
| *Echium plantagineum* L., *E. rubrum* L. (A. p. 9) |
| *Arum dracunculus* L. (A. p. 90) |
| *Nelumbo nucifera* Gaert. (A. p. 148) |
| |
| *Sambucus nigra* L. (A. p. 4) |
| *Sambucus nigra* L. (A. p. 4) |
| *Sambucus nigra* L. (A. p. 4) |

| **Botanical Name** |
|---|
| *Inula helenium* L. (A. p. 69) |
| Inula helenium L. (A. p. 253) |
| *Inula helenium* L. (LSJ) |
| *Inula helenium* L. (A. p. 181) |
| *Inula helenium* L. (A. p. 157) |
| *Inula helenium* L. (A. p. 253) |
| *Inula helenium* L. (A. p. 181) |
| *Inula helenium* L. (A. p. 118) |
| *Inula helenium* L. (A. p. 171) |
| *Thymus incanus* L. (A. p. 118) |
| *Ulmus glabra* (LSJ) |
| *Cichorium endivia* L. (LSJ) |
| Unidentified |
| *Polygonatum multiflorum* All. and *P. verticillatum* All. (A. p 133) |
| *Polygonatum multiflorum* All. and *P. verticillatum* All. (A. p. 95) |
| Unidentified |
| *Cuscuta epithymum* L. (A. p. 95) |
| *Eryngium campestre* L. |
| *Eryngium campestre* L. (A. pp. 97-98) |
| *Eryngium campestre* L. (A. pp. 97-98) |
| *Bupleurum fruticosum* L. (A. p. 237) |
| *Foeniculum vulgare* Gaertn. (A. p.155) |
| *Trigonella fenum graecum* L. (A. p. 256) |
| *Trigonella fenum graecum* L. (A. p.148) |
| *Trigonella fenum graecum* L. |
| *Trigonella fenum graecum* L. (A. p. 51) |
| *Trigonella fenum graecum* L. (A. p. 39) |
| *Trigonella fenum graecum* L. (A. p. 6) |
| *Chrysanthemum parthenium Bernh.* (A. p. 189) |
| *Erythraea centaurium* L. (A. p. 145) |
| *Chrysanthemum parthenium* Bernh. (A. p. 143) |
| *Erythraea centaurium* L. (A. p. 55) |
| *Erythraea centaurium* L. (A. p. 55) |
| *Chrysanthemum parthenium* Bernh. (A. p. 189) |
| *Zizyphora capitata* L. (A. p. 203) |
| *Cotoneaster pyracantha* Spach. (A. p. 212) |
| *Cotoneaster pyracantha* Spach. (A. p. 211) |
| *Cotoneaster pyracantha* Spach. (A. p. 183) |
| *Ficus carica* L. (A. p. 104) |
| *Scrofularia lucida* L. (A. p. 238) |

| English Name | Greek Name | References |
|---|---|---|
| Figwort | Ἡρακλεία | IV, 35 |
| Filbert | λεπτοκάρυον | I, 125 |
| Filbert | κάρυον Ποντικόν | I, 125 |
| Fish thistle | κόνυζα μείζων | III, 121 |
| Fish thistle | ἄκανθα λευκή | III, 12 |
| Fishbone thistle | χαμαιπεύκη | IV, 126 |
| Fleabane | κόνυζα, τρίτον εἶδος | III, 121 |
| Fleabane | κόνυζα μικρά | III, 121 |
| Fleabane | κόνυζα | III, 121 |
| Fleawort | ψύλλιον | IV, 69 |
| Fleawort | κυνόμυια | IV, 69 |
| Fleawort | κυνοκέφαλον | IV, 69 |
| Fleawort | κρυστάλλιον | IV, 69 |
| Frankincense | λίβανος | I, 68 |
| Frankincense | Συάγριος | I, 68 |
| Frankincense, Kind of | σταγονίας | I, 68 |
| Frankincense, Kind of | σμιλιωτό ς | I, 68 |
| Frankincense, Kind of | ἀμωμίτης | I, 68 |
| French lavender | στοιχάς | III, 26 |
| French turnip | βουνιάς | II, 111 |
| Frothy poppy | μήκων ἀφρώδης | IV, 66 |
| Frothy poppy | Ἡρακλεία | IV, 66 |
| Fumitory | φασήλιον | IV, 120 |
| Fumitory | καπνός | IV, 109 |
| Fumitory | ἰσόπυρον | IV, 120 |
| Galbanum | χαλβάνη | III, 83 |
| Galbanum | μέτωπον | III, 83 |
| Galingale | κύπερος | I, 4 |
| Galingale | ἐρυσίσκηπτρον | I, 4 |
| Galingale, Another | κυπὲρου ἕτερον | I, 5 |
| Gangitis | Γαγγῖτις | I, 7 |
| Garden cress | κάρδαμον | II, 155 |
| Garlic | σκόρδον | II, 152 |
| Garlic | μῶλυ | III, 47 |
| Garlic germander | σκόρδιον | III, 111 |
| Garlic leek | σκορδόπρασον | II, 153 |
| Gentian | γεντιανή | III, 3 |
| Giant fennel | νάρθηξ | III, 77 |
| Giant fennel, Kind of, Juice | μέτωπον | III, 83 |
| Gillyflower | λευκόιον | III, 123 |

| **Botanical Name** |
|---|
| *Scrofularia lucida* L. (LSJ) |
| *Corylus avellana* L. |
| *Corylus avellana* L. |
| *Inula graveolens* Desf., *I. viscosa* Aiton, *I. Britannica* L. (A. p. 74) |
| ~*Cnicus ferox* L. or ~*C. acarna* (A. p. 2) |
| Unidentifiable (A. p. 60,) *Chamaepeuce mutica* (LSJ) |
| *Inula Britannica* L. (A. p. 74) |
| *Inula graveolens* Desf. (A. p. 74) |
| *Inula* sp. |
| *Plantago psyllium* L. and *P. cynops* L. (A. p. 210) |
| *Plantago psyllium* L. and *P. cynop* s L. (A. p. 84) |
| *Plantago psyllium* L. and *P. cynops* L. |
| *Plantago psyllium* L. and *P. cynops* L. (A. p. 79) |
| *Boswellia* sp. (LSJ) |
| |
| |
| |
| |
| *Lavendula stoechas* L. (A. p. 250) |
| *Brassica napus* L. (A. p. 41) |
| *Silene inflata* Sm., *S. muscipula* L. (A. p. 156) |
| *Silene inflata* Sm., *S. muscipula* L. (A. p. 120) |
| *Corydalis claviculata* Pers. |
| *Fumaria officinalis* L. (A. p. 48) |
| *Corydalis claviculata* Pers. (A. p. 133) |
| *Ferula galbaniflua* Boiss. and Buhse (A. p. 108) |
| *Ferula galbaniflua* Boissa and Buhse (A. p. 160)) |
| *Cyperus rotundus* L. (A. p. 85) |
| *Cyperus rotundus* L. (A. p. 98) |
| *Curcuma longa* L. (A. p. 85) |
| *Nardostachys jatamansi* DC. (A. p. 109) |
| *Lepidium sativum* L. (A. p. 49) |
| *Allium sativum* L. (A. p. 232) |
| ~*Allium nigrum* L. (A. p. 163) |
| *Teucrium scordium* L. (A. p. 231) |
| *Allium descendens* (LSJ) |
| *Gentiana lutea* L., *G. purpurea* L. (A. p. 109) |
| *Ferula communis* L. (A. p. 170) |
| *Ferula galbaniflua* L. (A. p. 160) |
| *Matthiola incana* L. (A. p. 142) |

| English Name | Greek Name | References |
|---|---|---|
| *Gingiberi* | ζιγγίβερι | I, 14 |
| Ginger | ζιγγίβερι | II, 160 |
| *Gingidion* | γιγγίδιον | II, 137 |
| Gladwyn | ξυρίς | IV, 22 |
| Gladwyn | ξιρίς | IV, 22 |
| Gladwyn | ἶρις ἀγρία | IV, 22 |
| Gladwyn | γλαδίολος | IV, 22 |
| *Glaucion* | γλαύκιον | III, 86 |
| Goat's marjoram | τραγορίγανος | III, 30 |
| Goat's marjoram | πράσιον | III, 30 |
| Goat's thorn | φρύνιον | III, 15 |
| Goat's thorn | ποτίρριον | III, 15 |
| Goat's thorn | νευράς | III, 15 |
| Goat's thorn | ἀκιδωτόν | III, 15 |
| Gold flower | χρυσάνθεμον | IV, 57 |
| Gold flower | ἑλίχρυσον | IV, 57 |
| Gold flower | ἀμάραντον | IV, 57 |
| Golden cow-parsnip | αέσελι τό ἐν Πελοποννήσῳ | III, 53 |
| Golden thistle | σκόλυμος | III, 14 |
| Grape | σταφυλή | V, 3 |
| Grape, Inflorescence of Wild | οἰνάνθη | V, 2; V, 4 |
| Grapes, Unripe, Honey Drink | ὀμφακόμελι | V, 23 |
| Grapevine | ἄμπελος οἰνοφόρος | V, 1 |
| Grass of Parnassus | ἄγρωστις ἡ ἐν τῷ Παρνασσῷ | IV, 31 |
| Great bindweed | μῖλαξ λεία | IV, 143 |
| Great sea-rush | ὀξύσχοινος | IV, 52 |
| Green mint | μίνθη | III, 34 |
| Green mint | ἡδύοσμον | III, 34 |
| Groats | χόνδρος | II, 96 |
| Groomwell | λιθόσπερμον | III, 141 |
| Groomwell | Ἡρακλεία | III, 141 |
| Groomwell | ἐξώνυχον | III, 141 |
| Groomwell | Διὸς πυρός | III, 141 |
| Groomwell | ἀετώνυχον | III, 141 |
| Ground ivy | χαμαίκισσος | IV, 125 |
| Ground pine | χαμαίπιτυς | III, 158 |
| Ground pine | σιδηρῖτις | III, 158 |
| Ground pine | ὀλόκυρος | III, 158 |
| Ground pine | ἰωνία | III, 158 |
| Ground pine, Another | χαμαίπιτυς | III, 158 |

| **Botanical Name** |
|---|
| (see A. p. 67 s. v. cinnamomum) |
| *Zingiber officinale* Roscoe (A. p. 279) |
| *Malabaila sekakul* Russ. (A. p. 110) |
| *Iri* s L. sp. (A. p. 278) |
| *Iris* L. sp. (A. p. 278) |
| *Iris* L. sp. (A. p. 278) |
| *Iris* L. sp. (A. p. 278) |
| *Glaucium corniculatum* Curtis (A. p. 112) |
| *~Thymus graveol.Sibth. sp.,~Th. tragoriganum L. sp.Origanum heracleoticum Richb. sp* |
| See Bk. III, n. 25 |
| *Astagalus poterium* Labill. (A. p. 198) |
| *Astagalus poterium* Labill. (A. p. 207) |
| *Astagalus poterium* Labill. (A. p. 171) |
| *Astagalus poterium* Labill. |
| *Helichrysum orientale* L., *H. stoechas* L., *H. siculum* L. (A. p. 63) |
| *Helichrysum orientale* L., *H. stoechas* L., *H. siculum* L. (A. p. 118) |
| *Helichrysum orientale* L., *H. stoecha* s L., *H. siculum* L. (A. p. 13) |
| *Malabaila aurea* Sibth. (A. p. 237) |
| *Scolymus maculatus* L. and *S. hispanicu* s L. (A. p. 231) |
| |
| *Vitis silvestris* Gmel. (A. p. 176) |
| |
| *Vitis vinifera* L. (LSJ) |
| *Parnassia palustris* L. (A. p. 8) |
| *Convolvulus sepium* L. (A. p. 161) |
| *Juncus acutus* L. (A. p. 184) |
| *Mentha* L. |
| *Mentha* L. |
| |
| *Lithospermum officinale* L. (A. p.147) |
| *Lithospermum officinale* L. (A. p. 120) |
| *Lithospermum officinale* L. (A. p. 100) |
| *Lithospermum officinale* L. (A. p. 89) |
| *Lithospermum officinale* L. |
| *Glechoma hederacea* L. (A. p. 59) |
| *Ajuga chia* Schreb. (A. p. 60) |
| *Ajuga hamaepitys* L. (A. p. 258) |
| *Ajuga hamaepitys* Schreb. (A. p. 125) |
| *Ajuga hamaepitys* Schreb. |
| *Ajuga hamaepitys* Schreb. (A. p. 60) |

| **Botanical Name** |
|---|
| *Ajuga iva* Schreb. (A. p. 60) |
| *Senecio vulgaris* L. (A. p. 96) |
| |
| *Ferula marmarica* L. (A. p. 116) |
| *Ferula marmarica* L. (A. p. 7) |
| *Cistus creticus* L., *C. cyprius* L. (A. p. 137) |
| *Chondrilla juncea* L. (LSJ) |
| *Chondrlla ramosissima* L. (LSJ) |
| |
| |
| |
| |
| |
| |
| *Bupleurum fruticosum* L. (A. p. 237) |
| *Trifolium arvense* L. (A . p. 137) |
| *Scolopendrium officinale* L. sp. (A. p. 105) |
| *Plantago coronopus* (LSJ) |
| *Tordylium officinale* L. (A. p. 237) |
| *Aegilops ovata* L. (A. p. 6) |
| *Asarum europaeum* L. |
| *Asarum europaeum* L. (A. p. 27) |
| *Sisymbrium officinale* Scop., *S. iri* o L. (A. p. 98) |
| *Conium maculatum* L. (A. p. 73) |
| *Cannabis sativa* L. (A. p. 47) |
| *Althaea cannabina* L. (A. p. 47) |
| *Hyoscyamus* L. sp ( A. p. 127) |
| *Hyoscyamus* L. sp. (A. p. 5) |
| *Lawsonia inermis* L. (A. p. 85) |
| *Ajuga iva* Schreb. (A. p. 60) |
| *Globularia alypum* L. (A. p. 12) |
| *Opoponax hispidus* Grisb. (A. p. 186) |
| *Centaurea spinosa* L. (A. p. 124) |
| *Quercus ilex* L. (A. p. 207) |
| *Aspidium lonchitis* L. (A. p. 147) |
| *Verbena officinalis* L. (A. p. 193) |
| *Verbena officinalis* L. (A. p. 123) |
| |
| |
| |

| **Botanical Name** |
| --- |
| |
| |
| |
| |
| *Lonicera etrusca* L. (A. p. 247) |
| *Lonicera etrusca* L. (A. p. 192) |
| *Lonicera etrusca* L. (A. p. 69) |
| *Arisarum vulgare* Targ.-Tozz., *A. proboscideum* Savi (A. p. 24) |
| *Marrubium vulgare* L., *M. creticum* Miller (A. p..196) |
| *Marrubium vulgare* L. (LSJ) |
| *Hypecoum procumbens* L. (A. p. 128) |
| *Glaucium flavum* Crantz (A. p. 188) |
| *Glaucium flavum* Crantz (A. p. 57) |
| *Glaucium flavum* Crantz |
| ~*Prangos ferulacea* L. sp. (A. p. 124) |
| ~*Bifora testiculata* Rich. (A. p. 124) |
| *Calamintha clinopodium* Moris (A. p. 175) |
| *Calamintha clinopodium* Moris = *Clinopodium vulgare* L. (A. p. 69) |
| *Calamintha clinopodium* L. (A. p. 69) |
| *Calamintha clinopodium* Moris = *Clinopodium vulgare* L. (A. p. 280) |
| *Ruscus hypoglossum* L. (A. p. 128) |
| *Equisetum silvaticum* L. (A. p. 124) |
| *Equisetum silvaticum* L. (A. p. 124) |
| *Equisetum silvaticum* L. (A. p. 15) |
| *Equisetum maximum* Lmk. = *E. telmateia* Ehr. (A. p. 124) |
| *Solanum nigrum* L. (A. p. 251) |
| *Physalis alkekengi* L. (A. p. 251) |
| *Sempervivum arboreum* L. (A. p. 249) |
| *Sempervivum arboreum* L. (A. p. 280) |
| *Sempervivum arboreum* L. (A. p. 41) |
| *Sempervivum arboreum* L. (A. p. 13) |
| *Sempervivum tectorum* L. (A. p. 8) |
| *Sempervivum arboreum* L. (A. p. 8) |
| *Sedum album* L., *S. stellatum* L. (A. p. 256) |
| *Sedum* L. sp. (A. p. 8) |
| *Sedum album* L., *S. stellatum* L. (A. p. 16) |
| *Teucrium creticum* L. (A. p. 303) |
| *Teucrium polium* L. (A. p. 203) |
| |

| **English Name** | **Greek Name** | **References** |
|---|---|---|
| Hypocist | ὑποκυστίς | I, 97 |
| Hypocist | ὀρόβηθρον | I, 97 |
| Hypocist | κύτινος | I, 97 |
| *Hysobryon* | ὑσόβρυον | III, 42 |
| Hyssop | ὕσσωπος | III, 25 |
| *Idaia rhiza* | Ἰδαία ῥίζα | IV, 44 |
| Immortelle | χρυσοκόμη | IV, 55 |
| Immortelle | χρυσῖτις | IV, 55 |
| Indian ebony | Ἰνδική ἔβενος | I, 98 |
| Indian *lycion* | Ἰνδικὸν λύκιον | I, 100 |
| Indian spikenard | Ἰνδικὴ νάρδος | I, 7 |
| Iris | ἶρις | I, 1 |
| Ironwort | σιδηρῖτις | IV, 33 |
| Ironwort | Ἡρακλεία | IV, 33 |
| Italian melilot | τρίφυλλον | IV, 110 |
| Italian melilot | λωτός ἐν παραδείσοις | IV, 110 |
| Italian millet | μελίνη | II, 98 |
| Italian millet | ἔλυμος | II, 98 |
| Ivy | κισσός | II, 179 |
| Jacob's ladder | χιλιοδύναμον | IV, 8 |
| Jacob's ladder | Φιλεταίριον | IV, 8 |
| Jacob's ladder | πολεμώνιον | IV, 8 |
| Juniper | ἄρκευθος | I, 75 |
| Kermes oak | κόκκος βαφική | IV, 48 |
| Kidney bean | σμῖλαξ κηπαία | II, 146 |
| King's clover | μελίλωτος | III, 40 |
| Knotgrass | τευθαλίς | IV, 4 |
| Knotgrass | πολύκαρπον | IV, 4 |
| Knotgrass | πολύγονον ἄρρεν | IV, 4 |
| Knotgrass | μυρτοπέταλον | IV, 4 |
| Knotgrass | κλῆμα | IV, 4 |
| Knotgrass | καρκίνωθρον | IV, 4 |
| Large heliotrope | σκορπίουρον | IV, 190 |
| Large heliotrope | ἡλιοτρόπιον τὸ μέγα | IV, 190 |
| Laserwort | σίλφιον | III, 80 |
| Lavender cotton | ἀβρότονον θῆλυ | III, 24 |
| Leek | πράσον κεφαλωτόν | II, 149 |
| Lentil | φακός | II, 107 |
| *Leontopetalon* | παρδάλιον | III, 96 |
| *Leontopetalon* | λεύκηθρον | III, 96 |

| **Botanical Name** |
|---|
| *Cytinus hypocistis* L. (A. p. 128) |
| *Cytinus hypocistis* L. (A. p. 182) |
| *Cytinus hypocistis* L. (A. p. 85) |
| *Amaracus sipyleus* Rafin. (A. p. 154) |
| *Satureia graeca* L. = *Micromeria graeca* Benth. (A. p. 129) |
| *Ruscus hypoglossum* L. (LSJ) |
| *Aster linosyris* Bernh. (A. p. 64) |
| *Aster linosyris* Bernh. (A. p. 64) |
| *Diospyrus ebenum* Koenig (A. p. 92) |
| *Acacia catechu* Willd. (A. p.149) |
| *Nardostachys jatamansi* DC. (A. p. 170) |
| *Iris florentina* L., *I. germanica* L., *I. pallida* Lamk. (A. p. 133) |
| *Sideritis romana* L. (A. p. 238) |
| *Sideritis romana* L. (A. p. 120) |
| *Melilotus* Adans. sp. (A. p. 264) |
| *Melilotus* Adans. sp. (A. pp.147-148) |
| *Setaria italica* P. B. (A. p. 158) |
| *Parietaria officinalis* L. (A. p. 119) |
| *Hedera helix* L. (A. p. 67) |
| *Polemonium caeruleum* L. or *Hypericum olympicum* L. (A. p. 203) |
| *Polemonium caeruleum* L. or *Hypericum olympicum* L. (A. p. 196) |
| ~*Polemonium caeruleum* L., ~*Hypericum olympicum* L. (A. p. 203) |
| *Juniperus* L. (LSJ) |
| *Quercus coccifera* L. (A. p. 70) |
| *Vigna sinensis* Endl. (A. p.161,) *Phaseolus vulgaris* L. (LSJ) |
| *Melilotus* Adans. sp. (A. p. 158) |
| *Polygonum aviculare* L. |
| *Polygonum aviculare* L. (A. 203) |
| *Polygonum aviculare* L. (A. p. 204) |
| *Polygonum aviculare* L. (A. 168) |
| *Polygonum aviculare* L. (A. 69) |
| *Polygonum aviculare* L. (A. p. 49) |
| *Heliotropium europaeum* L., *H. villosum* L., *H. supinum* L. (A. p. 232) |
| *Heliotropium europaeum* L., *H. villosum* L., *H. supinum* L. (A. p.119) |
| ~*Ferula tingitana* L. (A. p. 240) |
| *Santolina chamaecyparissus* L. (A. p. 115) |
| *Allium porrum* L. (A. pp. 206-207) |
| *Ervum lens* L. (LSJ) |
| *Leontice leontopetalum* L. (A. p. 189) |
| *Leontice leontopetalum* L. (A. p. 143) |

| **Botanical Name** |
| --- |
| *Leontice leontopetalum* L. (A. p. 142) |
| *Leontice leontopetalon* (LSJ) |
| *Leontice leontopetalum* L. (A. p. 259) |
| ~*Doronicum pardalianches* Jacq. (A. p. 189) |
| ~*Doronicum pardalianches* Jacq. |
| ~ *Doronicum pardalianche* s Jacq. |
| ~*Doronicum pardalianches* Jacq. (A. p. 46) |
| ~*Doronicum pardalianche* s Jacq. (A. p. 258) |
| ~*Doronicum pardalianches* Jacq. (A. p. 4) |
| *Lactuca sativa* L. (A. p. 260) |
| *Lactuca scariola* L. (A. p. 260) |
| |
| *Thelygonum cynocrambe* L. = *Cynocrambe prostrata* Gaertn. (A. p. 166) |
| *Thelygonum cynocrambe* L. = *Cynocrambe prostrata* Gaertn. (A. p. 11) |
| *Glycyrrhiza glabra* L. (A. p. 253 |
| *Glycyrrhiza glabra* L. (A. p 233) |
| *Glycyrrhiza glabra* L. (LSJ) |
| *Glycyrrhiza glabra* L. (A. p. 113) |
| *Glycyrrhiza glabra* L. (A. p. 112) |
| *Glycyrrhiza glabra* L. (A. p. 5) |
| *Lilium candidum* L. (A. p. 145) |
| *Lilium candidum* (LSJ) |
| *Phillyrea* L. sp. (A. p. 197) |
| *Linum usitatissimum* (LSJ) |
| |
| *Serapias lingua* L. (A. p. 147) |
| *Lysimachia vulgaris* L. (A. p. 150) |
| *Levisticum officinale* Koch (A. p. 187 ) |
| *Levisticum officinale* Koch (A. p. 145) |
| *Symphytum tuberosum* L. (A. p. 253) |
| *Medicago sativa* L. (A. p. 157) |
| *Lupinus* L. (LSJ) |
| |
| |
| *Holarrhena antidysenterica* Wall. (A. p. 151) |
| *Rubia tinctorum* L. (A. p. 257) |
| *Rubia tinctorum* L., *R. peregrina* L. (A. p. 98) |
| *Rubia tinctorum* L., *R. peregrina* L. (A. p. 96) |
| *Asperugo procumbens* L. (A. p. 166) |
| *Asperugo procumbens* L. (A. p. 1666) |

| English Name | Greek Name | References |
|---|---|---|
| Madwort | ἄλυσσον | III, 91 |
| *Magydaris* | μαγύδαρις | III, 80 |
| Maidenhair | πολύτριχον | IV, 134 |
| Maidenhair | ἀδίαντον | IV, 134 |
| Malabar | μαλάβαθρον | I, 12 |
| Malabar | μαλάβαθρον | I, 12 |
| Male fern | πτερίς | IV, 184 |
| Male fern | πολύρριζον | IV, 184 |
| Male fern | βλῆχρον | IV, 184 |
| Mallow | μολόχη | II, 118 |
| Man orchis | τρίφυλλον | III, 128 |
| Man orchis | σατύριον ἐρυθραϊκόν | III, 128 |
| Man orchis | σατύριον | III, 128 |
| Mandrake | μανδραγόρας | IV, 75 |
| Mandrake | Κιρκαία | IV, 75 |
| Mandrake | βομβόχυλον | IV, 75 |
| Mandrake | ἀντίμιμον | IV, 75 |
| Mandrake, female | θριδακίας | IV, 75 |
| Mandrake, male | μώριος | IV, 75 |
| Manna ash | μελία | I, 80 |
| Mare's tail | πολύγονον θῆλυ | IV, 5 |
| Marjoram | σάμψουχον | III, 39 |
| Marjoram | πάνακες | III, 29 |
| Marjoram | κονίλη | III, 29 |
| Marjoram | Ἡρακλεία | III, 29 |
| Marjoram | ἀμάρακον | III, 39 |
| Marjoram | ἀγριορίγανος | III, 29 |
| *Maron* | μᾶρον | III, 42 |
| Marsh mallow | ἐβίσκος | III, 146 |
| Marsh mallow | ἀλθαία | III, 146 |
| Martagon lily | ἡμεροκατάλλακτον | III, 122 |
| Martagon lily | ἡμεροκαλλές | III, 122 |
| Massilian hartwort | σέσελι Μασσαλιώτικον | III, 53 |
| Mastic | σχῖνος | I, 70 |
| Meadow rue | θαλίητρον | IV, 97 |
| Meadow saffron | Κόλχικον | IV, 83 |
| Meadow saffron | ἐφήμερον | IV, 83 |
| Meadow saffron | βολβὸς ἄγριος | IV, 83 |
| Meal, Barley | ἄλευρον κρίθης | II, 86 |
| Meal, Fenugreek | ἄλευρον τήλεως | II, 102 |

| **Botanical Name** |
|---|
| *Biscutella* L. sp. (A. p. 12) |
| |
| *Adiantum capillus Veneris* L. (A. p. 205) |
| *Adiantum capillus Veneris* L. (A. p. 5) |
| ~*Cinnamomum tamala* Nees, ~*C. iners* Blume,~*C. zeylanicum* Blume, (A. p. 151-152) |
| ~*Pogostemon patchouli Pell. (* A. p. 151-152*)* |
| *Polystichum filix mas* Roth. (A. p. 210) |
| *Polystichum filix mas* Roth. (A. p. 205) |
| *Polystichum filix mas* Roth. (A. p. 36) |
| *Malva silvestris* (LSJ) |
| *Fritillaria graeca* L. (A. p. 265) |
| *Serapias cordigera* L. (A. p. 228) |
| *Fritillaria graeca* L. (A. p. 228) |
| *Mandragora* L. sp. (A. pp. 153-154) |
| *Mandragora* L. sp. (LSJ) |
| *Mandragora* L. sp. (LSJ) |
| *Mandragora* L. sp. (LSJ) |
| *Mandragora autumnalis* Sprengel (A. p. 259) |
| *Mandragora vernalis* Bertol. (A. p. 164) |
| *Fraxinus ornus* L. (LSJ) |
| *Hippuris vulgaris* L. (A. p. 204) |
| *Majorana hortensis* Moench (A. p. 225) |
| ~*Origanum viride* Boiss. (A. p. 187) |
| ~*Origanum viride* Boiss. (A. p. 73) |
| ~*Origanum viride* Boiss. (A. p. 120) |
| *Majorana hortensis* Moench (A. p. 13) |
| ~*Origanum viride* Boiss. sp. |
| *Amaracus sipyleus* Rafin. (A. p.154) |
| *Althaea officinalis* L. |
| *Althaea officinalis* L. (A . p. 12) |
| *Lilium martagon* L. (A. p. 119) |
| *Lilium martagon* L. (A. p. 119) |
| *Seseli tortuosum* L. (A. p. 237) |
| *Pistacia lentiscus* L. (LSJ) |
| *Thalictrum flavum* L., *Th. minus* L. (A. p. 258) |
| *Colchicum* L. sp. (A. p. 71) |
| *Colchicum* L. (A. p. 95) |
| *Colchicum* L. sp. (A. p. 41) |
| |
| |

| **Botanical Name** |
| --- |
| |
| *Commiphora opobalsamum* Engl. (A. p. 33) |
| |
| ~*Campanula lingulata* L. (A. p. 157) |
| *Mespilus germanica* L. (A. p. 237) |
| *Mespilus germanica* L. (A. p. 160) |
| *Mespilus germanica* L. (A. p. 95) |
| *Mespilus germanica* L. |
| *Mercurialis annua* L. (A. p. 189) |
| *Mercurialis annua* L. (A. p. 146) |
| *Mercurialis annua* L. (A. p. 122) |
| (A. p. 160) |
| (A. p. 160) |
| (A p. 160) |
| *Achillea millefolium* L. (A. p. 250) |
| *Silybum marianum* Gaertn. (A. p. 240) |
| *Notobasis syriaca* Cass. = *Cirsium syriacum* Gaertn. (A. p. 2) |
| *Astragalu* s L. sp. (A. p. 29) |
| *Polygala venulosa* Sibth. (A. p. 203) |
| *Panicum miliaceum* L. (LSJ) |
| *Ceterach officinarum* Willd. (A. p. 247) |
| *Ceterach officinarum* Willd. (A. p. 230) |
| *Ceterach officinarum* Willd. (A. p. 210) |
| *Ceterach officinarum* Willd. (A. p. 119) |
| *Ceterach officinarum* Willd. (A. p. 29) |
| *Rumex* L. sp. (A. p. 183) |
| *Rumex* L. sp. |
| *Rumex* L. sp. |
| *Rumex* L. sp. (A. p. 137) |
| *Rumex* L. sp.(LSJ) |
| *Reseda phyteuma* L. (A. p. 199) |
| *Cinnamomum cassia* sp. (LSJ) |
| ~*Leonurus cardiaca* L., ~ *L. marrubiastrum* L. (A. p. 211) |
| *Ajuga chia* Schreb. (A. p. 60) |
| ~*Athamanta macedonica* L. (A. p. 181) |
| *Valeriana tuberosa* L. (A. p. 170) |
| *Valeriana tuberosa* L. (A. p. 170) |
| *Valeriana tuberosa* L. (A. p. 260) |
| *Morus nigra* L. (A. p. 253) |
| *Morus nigra* L. (A. p. 164) |

| **Botanical Name** |
|---|
| *Scolopendrium hemionitis* Lag. (A. p. 247) |
| *Scolopendrium hemionitis* Lag. (A. p. 120) |
| *Verbascum* L. sp. (A. p. 197) |
| *Verbascum* L. sp. (A. p. 197) |
| *Verbascum* L. sp. (A. p. 149) |
| *Verbascum* L. sp. (A. p. 260) |
| *Fungi* |
| *Sinapis alba* L. (A. p. 240) |
| *Sinapis alba* L. (A. 169) |
| |
| *Commiphora myrrha* Engl. (A. p.167) |
| |
| |
| |
| |
| |
| |
| *Euphorbia myrsinites* L. (A. p. 262) |
| *Euphorbia myrsinites* L. (A. p. 167) |
| *Euphorbia myrsinites* L. (A. p. 52) |
| |
| |
| *Narcissus poeticus* L. (A. p. 169) |
| ~*Narcissus tazetta* (LSJ) see also (A. p. 41) |
| Undetermined |
| Underermined |
| *Umbilicus pendulinu* s DC. |
| *Umbilicus pendulinus* DC. |
| *Umbilicus pendulinus* DC. (A. p. 77) |
| *Saxifrage* L. sp. (A. p. 77) |
| *Amomum subulatum* Roxb. (A. p. 14) |
| *Celtis australis* L. (A. p. 147) |
| *Quercu* s L. sp. (A. p. 91) |
| *Hozanthus europaeus* (LSJ) |
| |
| |
| *Chenopodium botry* s L. (A. p. 13) |
| *Avena sativa* L. |
| |
| |

| **Botanical Name** |
| --- |
| |
| |
| |
| |
| |
| |
| |
| |
| |
| |
| |
| |
| |
| |
| |
| |
| |
| |
| |
| |
| |
| |
| |
| *Nerium oleander* L. (A. p. 217) |
| *Nerium oleander* L. |
| *Epilobium angustifolium* L. (A. pp. 178-179) |
| *Epilobium angustifolium* L. (A. p. 179) |
| *Epilobium angustifolium* L. (A. p. 178) |
| *Nerium oleander* L. (A. p. 171) |
| |
| |
| *Olea europaea* L. var. *sativa* Hoffm. and Lk. (A. p. 176) |
| *Olea europaea* L. var. *silvestris* Miller (A. p. 176) |
| |
| |
| |
| |
| *Allium cepa* (LSJ) |
| |
| *Papaver somniferum* L. |

| **English Name** | **Greek Name** | **References** |
|---|---|---|
| Opium poppy | μήκων πιθῖτις | IV, 64 |
| Opium poppy | μήκων θυλακῖτις | IV, 64 |
| Opium poppy | μήκων | IV, 64 |
| *Opobalsamon* | ὀποβάλσαμον | I, 19 |
| Opopanax | ὀποπάναξ | III, 48 |
| Orach | ἀνδράφαξυς | II, 119 |
| *Orbiclata* | ὀρβικλᾶτα | I, 115 |
| Orchid | ὄρχις κυνός | III, 126 |
| Orchid | ὄρχις | III, 126 |
| Orchid, Another | σεράπιας | III, 127 |
| Orchid, Another | ὄρχις ἕτερος | III, 127 |
| Oregano | ὀρίγανος Ἡρακλεωτική | III, 27 |
| Oregano | κονίλη | III, 27 |
| Oriental tamarisk gall | ἀκακαλλίς | I, 89 |
| Oriental tamarisk | μυρίκη ἡ ἐν Αἰγύπτῳ | I, 87 |
| *Orobias* | ὀροβίας | II, 104 |
| *Othonna* | ὀθόννα | II, 182 |
| Oxeye | κάχλα | III, 139 |
| Oxeye | βούφθαλμον | III, 139 |
| Oxymel | ὀξύμελι | V, 14 |
| *Palimpissa* | παλίμπισσα | I, 72 |
| Papyrus | πάπυρος | I, 86 |
| *Pardalion* | λεοντοπέταλον | III, 96 |
| *Paronychia* | παρωνυχία | IV, 54 |
| Parsley | πετροσέλινον | III, 66 |
| Parsnip | σίσαρον | II, 113 |
| Parsnip | ἐλαφοβόσκον | III, 69 |
| Peaches | Περσικὰ μῆλα | I, 115 |
| Pear | ἄπιος | I, 116` |
| Pellitory | ὑγιεινὴ ἀγρία | IV, 85 |
| Pellitory | σιδηρῖτις | IV, 85 |
| Pellitory | πύρεθρος | III, 73 |
| Pellitory | πολυώνυμον | IV, 85 |
| Pellitory | περδίκιον | IV, 85 |
| Pellitory | παρθένιον | IV, 85 |
| Pellitory | κλύβατις | IV, 85 |
| Pellitory | Ἡράκλεια | IV, 85 |
| Pellitory | ἑλξίνη | IV, 85 |
| Peloponnesian hartwort | σέσελι τῷ ἐν Πελοποννήσῳ | III, 53 |
| Pennyroyal | γλήχων | III, 31 |

| **Botanical Name** |
|---|
| *Papaver somniferum* L. |
| *Papaver somniferum* L. |
| *Papaver somniferum* L. (A. p. 156) |
| |
| *Opopanax hispidus* Grisb. (A. p. 179 and p.186 s.v panaces) |
| *Atriplex hortensis* L. (A. p. 16) |
| |
| ~*Orchis papilionacea* L., ~*O. longicruris* L. (A. p. 84) |
| ~*Orchis papilionacea* L., ~*O. longicruris* L. (A. p. 180) |
| *Orchis morio* L. sp. (A. p. 236) |
| *Orchis morio* L. sp. (A. p. 180) |
| *Origanum heracleoticum* Rchb. and *O. vulgare* L. (A. p. 181) |
| *Origanum heracleoticum* Rchb. and *O. vulgare* L. |
| |
| *Tamarix articulata* (LSJ) |
| *Cicer arietinum* sp. |
| |
| *Chrysanthemum coronarium* L. |
| *Chrysanthemum coronarium* L. (A. p. 41) |
| |
| |
| *Cyperus papyrus* L. (A. p. 188) |
| *Leontice leontopetalon* L. (A. p. 189) |
| *Paronychia* Miller sp. (A. p. 189) |
| *Petroselinum hortense* Hoffm. (A. p. 195) |
| *Pastinaca sativa* L. (A. p. 241) |
| *Pastinaca sativa* L. (A. p. 93) |
| *Prunus persica* Sieb. and Z. (A. p. 153) |
| *Pyrus communis* (LSJ) |
| *Parietaria officinalis* L. |
| *Parietaria officinalis* L. (A. p. 238) |
| *Anacyclus pyrethrum* DC. = *Anthemis pyrhethrum* L. (A. p. 212) |
| *Parietaria officinalis* L. (A. p. 204) |
| *Parietaria officinalis* L. (A. p. 192) |
| *Parietaria officinalis* L. (A. p. 189) |
| *Parietaria officinalis* L. (A. p. 69) |
| *Parietaria officinalis* L. (A. p. 120) |
| *Parietaria officinalis* L. (A. p. 119) |
| *Malabaila aurea* Sibth. (A. p. 237) |
| *Mentha pulegium* L. (A. p. 36) |

| English Name | Greek Name | References |
|---|---|---|
| Pennyroyal | βλήχων | III, 31 |
| Peony | πεντόροβος | III, 140 |
| Peony | παιωνία | III, 140 |
| Peony | Ἰδαίοι δάκτυλοι | III, 140 |
| Peony | γλυκισίδη | III, 140 |
| Peony | ἀγλαοφῶτις | III, 140 |
| *Pepon* | πέπων | II, 135 |
| Pepper | πέπερι | II, 159 |
| Pepper, Long | πέπερι μακρόν | II, 159 |
| Pepper, White | πέπερι λευκόν | II, 159 |
| Pepperwort | λεπίδιον | II, 174 |
| Pepperwort | γιγγίδιον | II, 174 |
| Periwinkle | πολυγονοειδές | IV, 7 |
| Periwinkle | μυρσινοειδές | IV, 7 |
| Periwinkle | κληματίς | IV, 7 |
| Periwinkle | δαφνοειδές | IV, 7 |
| Persea | περσαία | I, 129 |
| *Peuce* pine | πεύκη | I, 69 |
| Pilewort | χελιδόνιον τὸ μικρόν | II, 181 |
| Pilewort | πυρὸς ἄγριος | II, 181 |
| Pimpernel | κιχόριον | II, 178 |
| Pimpernel | ἀναγαλλὶς θήλεια | II, 178 |
| Pimpernel | ἀναγαλλὶς ἄρρην | II, 178 |
| Pimpernel | ἀναγαλλίς | II, 178 |
| Pimpinell | τράγιον ἄλλο | IV, 50 |
| Pine nuts | πιτυίδες | I, 69 |
| Pine thistle | χαμαιλέων λευκός | III, 8 |
| Pine thistle | ἰξία | III, 8 |
| Pistachio nut | πιστάκια | I, 124 |
| Pitch | πίσσα | I, 72 |
| Pitch | βοσκάς | I, 72 |
| Pitch-asphalt | πιττάσφαλτος | I, 73 |
| Pitch-asphalt | πισσάσφαλτος | I, 73 |
| Pitch-oil | πισσέλαιον | I, 72 |
| *Pitys* pine | πίτυς | I, 69 |
| Plane tree | πλάτανος | I, 79 |
| Plantain | πολύπλευρον | II, 126 |
| Plantain | ἑπτάπλευρον | II, 126 |
| Plantain | ἀρνόγλωσσον | II, 126 |
| Plum tree | κοκκυμηλέα | I, 121 |

| Botanical Name |
|---|
| *Mentha pulegium* L. (A. p. 112) |
| *Paeonia* L. (A. p. 191) |
| *Paeonia* L. sp. (A. p. 185) |
| *Paeonia* L. |
| *Paeonia* L. sp. (A. p. 112) |
| *Paeonia* L. sp. (A. p. 7) |
| *Citrullus sativus* Schrad. (A. p. 192) |
| *Piper nigrum* L. (A. p. 200) |
| *Piper officinarum* DC. (A. p. 200) |
| *Piper album* L. (A. p. 200) |
| *Lepidium latifolium* L. (A. p. 142) |
| *Lepidium latifolium* L. (A. p. 110) |
| *Vinca minor* L. (A. p. 204) |
| *Vinca minor* L. (A. p.167) |
| *Vinca minor* L. (A. p. 69) |
| *Vinca minor* L. (A. p. 87) |
| *Mimusops Schimperi* L. (A. p. 193) |
| *Pinus* sp. |
| *Ficaria verna* Huds. (A. p. 62) |
| *Ficaria verna* Huds. (A. p. 212) |
| *Anagallis arvensis* L. (A. p. 65) |
| *Anagallis caerulea* Schreb. (A. p. 15) |
| *Anagallis phoenicea* Scop. (A. p. 15) |
| *Anagallis arvensis* L. (A. p. 15) |
| *Pimpinella tragium* Vill. (A. p. 263) |
| |
| *Atractylis gummifera* L. (A. p. 59) |
| *Atractylis gummifera* L. (A. p. 134) |
| *Pistacia vera* L. (LSJ) |
| |
| |
| |
| |
| |
| *Pinus* sp. |
| *Platanus orientalis* L. (LSJ) |
| *Plantago major* L. sp. (A. p. 204) |
| *Plantago* L. sp. (A. p. 120) |
| *Plantago* L. sp. (A. p. 26) |
| *Prunus domestica* L. (A. p. 71) |

| **English Name** | **Greek Name** | **References** |
|---|---|---|
| Poet's cassia | ὄσιρις | IV, 140 |
| Pollen, wheat | γύρις πυρῶν | II, 85 |
| *Polygonon* | πολύγονον | V, 106 |
| Polypody | πολυπόδιον | IV, 186 |
| Pomegranate | ῥοά | I, 110 |
| Pomegranate flower | κυτίνος | I, 110 |
| Pomegranate flower | βαλαύστιον | I, 111 |
| Pomegranate peel | σίδιον | I, 110 |
| Pondweed | ποταμογείτων | IV, 100 |
| Poppy, capsule | κωδύα | IV, 64 |
| Pot marjoram | ἀγήρατον | IV, 58 |
| Propolis | πρόπολις | II, 84 |
| *Pseudocassia* | ψευδοκασσία | I. 13 |
| *Pseudocinamomon* | ψευδοκινάμωμον | I, 14 |
| Purple rock cress | σησαμοειδὲς τὸ μικρόν | IV, 163 |
| Purse tassels | βολβὸς ἐδώδιμος | II, 170 |
| Purslane | ἀνδράχνη | II, 124 |
| Quacksalver's spurge | πιτυούσα | IV, 165 |
| Quacksalver's spurge | παράλιος | IV, 165 |
| Quacksalver's spurge | κράμβιον | IV, 165 |
| Quacksalver's spurge | κλῆμα | IV, 165 |
| Quacksalver's spurge | Κανωπικόν | IV, 165 |
| Quinces | στρούθια | I, 115 |
| Quinces | κυδώνια | I, 115 |
| Radish | ῥαφανίς | II, 112 |
| Raisin | ἀσταφίς | V, 3 |
| Ranunculus | σέλινον ἄγριον ἕτερον | II, 175 |
| Ranunculus | σέλινον ἄγριον | II, 175 |
| Ranunculus | βατράχιον τρίτον | II, 175 |
| Ranunculus | βατράχιον τέταρτον | II, 175 |
| Ranunculus | βατράχιον ἕτερον | II, 175 |
| Ranunculus | βατράχιον | II, 175 |
| Raspberry | βάτος Ἰδαία | IV, 38 |
| Reed mace | τύφη | III, 118 |
| Reed, Cyprian | κάλαμος, Κύπριος | I, 85 |
| Reed, *donax* | κάλαμος, δονάξ | I, 85 |
| Reed, *nastos* | κάλαμος, νάστος | I, 85 |
| Reed, *phragmites* | κάλαμος, φραγμίτης | I, 85 |
| Reed, *syringias* | κάλαμος, συριγγίας | I, 85 |
| Reed, *thelys* | κάλαμος, θῆλυς | I, 85 |

| Botanical Name |
|---|
| *Osiris alba* L. (A. p. 183) |
| |
| See Diosc. Bk. V, 106, n. 43 |
| *Polypodium vulgare* L. (A. p. 204) |
| *Punica granatum* (LSJ) |
| |
| |
| |
| *Ottelia alismoides* Pers. (A. p. 206) |
| |
| *Achillea ageratum* L. (A. p. 7) |
| |
| .(see A. p. 52) |
| *Cinnamomum tamala* Nees sp., *C. iners* Blume sp. (A. p.209) |
| *Aubrietia deltoides* L. (A. p. 237) |
| *Muscari comosum* Miller (A. p. 40) |
| *Portulaca oleracea* L. (A. p. 16) |
| *Euphorbia pityusa* L. (A. p. 262) |
| *Euphorbia pityusa* L. (A. p. 188) |
| *Euphorbia pityusa* L. (A. p. 77) |
| *Euphorbia pityusa* L. (A. p. 69) |
| *Euphorbia pityusa* L. |
| |
| |
| *Raphanus sativus* (LSJ) |
| |
| *Ranunculus* L. sp. |
| *Ranunculus* L. sp. |
| *Ranunculus* L. sp. |
| *Ranunculus* L. sp. |
| *Ranunculus* L. sp. |
| *Ranunculus* L. sp. (A. p. 34) |
| *Rubus idaeus* L. (A. p. 34) |
| *Typha* L. sp. (A. p. 267) |
| *Arundo donax* L. (A. p. 45) |
| *Arundo donax* L. |
| *Arundo pliniana* Turra (A. pp. 45 and 170) |
| *Arundo* sp. (A. p. 45) |
| *Arundo* sp. |
| *Arundo* sp. |

| English Name | Greek Name | References |
|---|---|---|
| Reed(s) | κάλαμος(οι) | I, 85 |
| Resin | ῥητίνη | I, 71 |
| Resin, Cedar | ῥητὶνη κεδρία | I, 77 |
| Resin, Colophonian | ῥητὶνη Κολοφωνία | I, 71 |
| Resin, Cypress | ῥητὶνη κυπαρισσίνη | I, 71 |
| Resin, Fir | ῥητὶνη ἐλατίνη | I, 71 |
| Resin, Mastic | ῥητὶνη σχινίνη | I, 70 |
| Resin, Mastic | ῥητὶνη μαστίχης | I, 70 |
| Resin, *Peuce* pine | ῥητὶνη πευκίνη | I, 71 |
| Resin, *Pitys* pine | ῥητὶνη πιτυίνη | I, 71 |
| Resin, Ship's | ζώπισσα | I, 72 |
| Resin, Ship's | ἀπόχυμα | I, 72 |
| Resin, *Strobilos* pine | ῥητὶνη στροβιλίνη | I, 71 |
| Resin, Terebinth | ῥητίνη τερμινθίνη | I, 71 |
| Resin, Black poplar | ῥητὶνη αἰγείρου | I, 83 |
| Rest harrow | ὀνωνίς | III, 18 |
| Rest harrow | ἀνωνίς | III, 18 |
| *Rhodia rhiza* | ῥοδὶα ῥίζα | IV, 45 |
| *Rhodides* | ῥοδίδες | I, 99 |
| *Rhodomeli* | ῥοδόμελι | V, 27 |
| Rhubarb | ῥῆον | III, 2 |
| Rhubarb | ῥά | III, 2 |
| Rice | ὄρυζα | II, 95 |
| Rice-wheat | ὄλυρα | II, 91 |
| Rock rose | λῆδον | I, 97 |
| Rock rose | κίσσαρος | I, 97 |
| Rock rose | κὶσθου ἕτερον εἶδος | I, 97 |
| Rock rose | κίσθος | I, 97 |
| Rock rose | κίσθαρος | I, 97 |
| Rock rose, female | κὶσθος θῆλυς | I, 97 |
| Rock rose, male | κὶσθος ἄρρην | I, 97 |
| Rocket | εὔζωμον | II, 140 |
| Rose | ῥόδον | I, 99 |
| Rose apples | Ἠπειρωτικὰ μῆλα | I, 115 |
| Rose campion | λυχνὶς στεφανωματική | III, 100 |
| Rose pastilles | ῥοδίδες | I, 99 |
| Rosemary | λιβανωτίς | III, 75 |
| Rosemary frankincense | λιβανωτὶς κάρπιμος | III, 74 |
| Rosemary frankincense | λιβανωτίς | III, 74 |
| Rosemary frankincense | καμψάνεμα | III, 74 |

| **Botanical Name** |
|---|
| *Arundines* (LSJ) |
| |
| |
| |
| |
| |
| |
| |
| |
| |
| |
| |
| |
| |
| |
| *Ononis antiquorum* L. (A. p. 178) |
| *Ononis antiquorum* L. (A. p. 17) |
| *Sedum roseum* Scop., *S. rhodiola* DC. (A. p. 217) |
| |
| |
| *Rheum officinale* (LSJ) |
| *Rheum ribes* L. (A. p. 217) |
| *Oryza sativa* (LSJ) |
| *Triticum dicoccum* (LSJ) |
| *Cistus creticus* L. (A. p. 141) |
| *Cistus* L. sp. (A. p. 68) |
| *Cistus cyprius* (LSJ) |
| *Cistus* L. sp. (A. p. 68) |
| *Cistus* L. sp. (A. p. 68) |
| *Cistus salviaefolius* L. (A. p. 68) |
| *Cistus villosus* L. (A. p. 68) |
| *Eruca sativa Lam* . (A. p. 100) |
| *Rosa* (LSJ) |
| |
| *Lychnis coronaria* Desr. (A. p. 149) |
| |
| *Rosmarinus officinalis* L. (A. p. 144) |
| ~*Cachris libanotis* Koch,~*Lecokia graeca,* ~ *Prangos ferulea* L. (A. p. 144) |
| ~*Cachris libanotis* Koch,~*Lecokia graeca* (Andrews), ~ *Prangos ferulea* L.(A. p. 144) |
| ~*Cachris libanotis* Koch sp. (A. pp. 46 and 144 ) |

| English Name | Greek Name | References |
|---|---|---|
| Rosemary frankincense | ζέα | III, 74 |
| Rosemary frankincense , fr'less | λιβανωτὶς ἄκαρπος | III, 74, 2, l. 9 |
| Rosemary, The other | λιβανωτὶς ἑτέρα | III, 74. 2, l. 6 |
| Rough bindweed | μῖλαξ τραχεῖα | IV, 142 |
| Rue | πὴγανον ὀρεινόν | III, 45 |
| Rue | πήγανον | III, 45 |
| Rush | σχοῖνος Εὐριπική | IV, 52 |
| Rush | ὀξύσχοινος | IV, 52 |
| Rush | ὁλόσχοινος | IV, 52 |
| Rye grass | φοῖνιξ | IV, 43 |
| Rye grass | ῥοῦς | IV, 43 |
| Rye grass | ἀγχύνωψ | IV, 43 |
| Safflower | κνῆκος | IV, 188 |
| Saffron | κρόκος | I, 26 |
| Saffron residuum | κροκόμαγμα | I, 27 |
| *Sagapenon* | σαγάπηνον | III, 81 |
| Sage | σφάγνος | III, 33 |
| Sage | ἐλελίσφακον | III, 33 |
| Sage | ἐλαφόβοσκον | III, 33 |
| Sage of Jerusalem | φλὸμος ἀγρία | IV, 103 |
| Sage of Jerusalem | λυχνῖτις | IV, 103 |
| Sage of Jerusalem | θρυαλλίς | IV, 103 |
| Salsify | τραγοπώγων | II, 143 |
| Salsify | κόμη | II, 143 |
| Sampharitic spikenard | Σαμφαριτικὴ νάρδος | I, 7 |
| Samphire | κρῆθμον | II, 129 |
| Sarcocolla | σαρκοκόλλα | III, 85 |
| Savin | βράθυ | I, 76 |
| Savin | βόρατον | I, 76 |
| Savory | θύμβρα | III, 37 |
| Scammony | σκαμμωνία | IV, 170 |
| Scarlet windflower | ἠρέμιον | II, 176 |
| Scarlet windflower | ἀργεμώνιον | II, 176 |
| Scarlet windflower | ἀνεμὼνη ἀγρία | II, 176 |
| Scilla | σκίλλα | II, 171 |
| *Scolicitis* | στοράξ | I, 66 |
| Scorpionwort | σκορπιοειδές | IV, 192 |
| Sea cole | κράμβη θαλασσία | II, 122 |
| Sea daffodil | σκίλλα | II, 172 |
| Sea daffodil | παγκράτιον | II, 172 |

| **Botanical Name** |
|---|
| ~*Cachrys libanotis* Koch sp. (A. pp 144 and 279) |
| *Rosmarinum sterile (* LSJ; see A. p. 144) |
| *Ferula ferulago* L . = *Ferulago galbanifera* Koch sp. (A. p. 144) |
| *Smilax aspera* L. (A. p. 161) |
| *Ruta chalepensis L. (A. p. 191)* |
| *Ruta graveolens* L. (A. p. 191) |
| *Scirpus* L. sp., *Juncus* L. sp. (A. p. 229) |
| *Juncus acutus* L. (A. p. 184) |
| *Scirpus holoschoenus* L. (A. p. 125) |
| *Lollium perenne* L. (A. p. 197) |
| *Lollium perenne* L. (A. p. 218) |
| *Lollium perenne* L. (A. p. 16) |
| *Cartharmus tinctorius* L. (A. p. 69) |
| *Crocus sativus* L. (A. p. 79) |
| |
| *Ferula persica* Willd. (A. p. 223) |
| *Salvia* L. sp.. |
| *Salvia* L. sp. (A. p. 93) |
| *Salvia.* L. sp. |
| V*erbascum* L. sp.(A. p. 197) |
| *Verbascum* L. sp. (A. p. 149) |
| *Verbascum* L. sp. (A. p. 260) |
| *Tragopogon porrifolius* L. (A. p. 263) |
| *Tragopogon porrifolius* L. (A. p. 73) |
| |
| *Crithmum maritimum* L. (A. p. 78) |
| *Astragalus fasciculifolius* Boiss. sp. (A. p. 227) |
| *Juniperus sabina* L. (A. p. 38) |
| *Juniperus sabina* L. (A. p. 37) |
| *Satureia thymbra* L. sp. (A. p. 260) |
| *Convolvulus scammonia* L. (A. p. 228) |
| *Anemone coronaria* L. |
| *Anemone coronaria* L. |
| *Anemone coronaria* L. (A. p. 17) |
| *Urginea maritima Baker* = *Scilla maritima* L. (A. p. 229) |
| |
| *Coronilla scorpioides* Koch (A. p. 232) |
| *Convolvulus soldanella* L. (A. p. 38 s. v. brassica) |
| *Pancratium maritimum* L. (A. p. 230) |
| *Pancratium maritimum* L. (A. p. 187) |

| **Botanical Name** |
| --- |
| *Frankenia hirsuta* L. and *F. pulverulenta* L. (A. p. 195) |
| *Frankenia hirsuta* L. and *F. pulverulenta* L. (A. p. 94) |
| *Eryngium maritinum* (LSJ) |
| *Beta maritima* L. (A. p. 172) |
| *Beta maritima* L. (A. p. 146) |
| *Ulva lactuca* L., and *U. latissima* L. (A. p. 39) |
| *Acetabularia mediterranea* L. (A. p. 17) |
| ~*Aster tripolium* L., ~*Limonium* L. sp. (A. p. 265) |
| |
| |
| *Posidonia oceanica* Del. (A. p. 198) |
| *Cystoseira foeniculosa* sp. (A. p. 198) |
| *Nithrophyllum punctatum* L. (A. p. 198) |
| |
| *Sorbus domestica* (LSJ) |
| *Sorbus domestica* (LSJ) |
| *Sesamum indicum* L. (A. p. 237) |
| ~*Lunaria alba* L., ~*Sinapis alba* L., ~*Brassica nigra* Koch (A. p. 259) |
| *Capsella bursa pastoris* L. (A. p. 259) |
| *Acacia arabica* (LSJ) |
| *Genista acanthoclada* (LSJ) |
| *Genista acanthoclada* (LSJ) |
| *Salvia aethiopis* L., *S. argentea* L. (A. p. 7) |
| *Withania somnifera* Dun. (A. p. 251) |
| *Withania somnifera* Dun. |
| *Withania somnifera* Dun. (A. p. 115) |
| *Withania somnifera* Dun. (LSJ) |
| *Chrozophora tinctoria* Juss. (A. p. 119) |
| *Polygonum hydropiper* L. (A. p. 127) |
| *Achillea ptarmica* L. (A. p. 210) |
| |
| *Saponaria officinalis* L. (A. p. 251) |
| *Polygonatum verticillatum* All., *P. officinale* All., *P. multiflorum* L. (A. p. 204) |
| |
| |
| |
| |
| |
| |
| |

| **Botanical Name** |
|---|
| |
| |
| |
| |
| *Sorbus domestica* L. (LSJ) |
| *Artemisia fragrans (* LSJ*)* |
| *Sonchus* L. sp. |
| *Sonchus oleraceus* L. (A. p. 243) |
| *Sonchus asper* L. (A. p. 243) |
| ~*Helichrysum sanguineum* Boiss. = *Gnaphalium sanguineum* L. (A. p. 32) |
| *Spartium junceum* L. (A. p. 244) |
| |
| |
| *Triticum* L. sp. |
| *Lloydia graeca* L. (A. p. 195) |
| *Lloydia graeca* L. (A. p. 195) |
| *Lloydia graeca* L. |
| *Meum athamanticum* Jacq. (A. pp. 160-161) |
| *Nardostachys jatamansi* DC. (A. p. 170,) *Patrinia scabiosifolia* Fisch. (A. p. 170) |
| *Carthamus lanatus* L. (A. p. 69) |
| *Carthamus lanatus* L. (A. p. 30) |
| |
| *Euphorbia Sibthorpii* Boiss. (A. p. 61) |
| *Euphorbia* L. (A. p. 261) |
| *Euphporbia parallias* L. (A. p. 262) |
| *Euphorbia platyphyllos* L. (A. p. 262) |
| *Euphorbia paralias* L. (A. p. 261) |
| *Euphorbia myrsinites* L. (A. p. 262) |
| *Euphorbia Sibthorpii* Boiss. (A. p. 70) |
| *Euphorbia cyparissias* L. (A. p. 262) |
| *Euphorbia Sibthorpii* Boiss. (A. p. 73) |
| *Euphorbia myrsinitis* L. (A. p. 52) |
| *Euphorbia acanthothamnos* Heldr. and Sart. (A. p. 124) |
| *Euphorbia acanthothamnos* Heldr. and Sart. (A. p. 124) |
| *Euphorbia dendroides* L. (A. p. 262) |
| *Euphorbia Sibthorpii* Boiss. |
| *Euphorbia helioscopia* L. (A. p. 262) |
| *Euphorbia resinifera* Berg. (A. p. 99) |
| *Daphne gnidium* L. (A. p. 212) |
| *Daphne gnidium* L. |

| **Botanical Name** |
|---|
| *Daphne gnidium* L. (A. p. 70) |
| *Daphne gnidium* L. (A. p. 70) |
| *Daphne gnidium* L. |
| *Daphne gnidium* L. (A. p. 61) |
| *Daphne gnidium* L. (A. p. 260) |
| *Daphne laureola* L. (A. p. 59) |
| *Daphne laureola* L. |
| *Daphne laureola* L. (A. p. 87) |
| *Daphne laureola* L. (A. p. 99) |
| *Daphne oleides* L. and *D. oleafolia* L. (A. p. 61) |
| *Daphne oleide* s L. and *D. oleafolia* L. (A. p. 212) |
| *Daphne oleides* L. and *D. oleafolia* L. (A. p. 70) |
| *Daphne oleides* L. (LSJ) |
| *Urginea maritima* Baker = *Scilla maritima* L. (A. p. 229) |
| *Ecballium elaterium* Rich. |
| *Ecballium elaterium* Rich. |
| *Hypericum perfoliatum* L. (A. p. 27) |
| *Hypericum crispum* L. (A. p. 60) |
| *Hypericum crispum* L. (A. p. 128) |
| *Hypericum empetrifolium* Willd., ~*H. coris* L. (A. p. 128) |
| *Hypericum empetrifolium* Willd., ~*H. coris* L. (A. p. 75) |
| *Hypericum crispum* L. (A. p. 75) |
| *Hypericum perfoliatum* L. (A. p. 89) |
| *Hypericum perforatum* L. (A. p. 27) |
| *Hypericum perforatum* L. (A. p. 27) |
| *Hypericum crispum* L. (A. p. 17) |
| *Hypericum perforatum L. (A. p. 27)* |
| *Hypericum perfoliatum* L. (A. p. 27) |
| |
| |
| *Ornithogalum umbellatum* L. (A. p. 181) |
| *Delphinium staphisagria* L. (A. p. 248) |
| *Urtica* L. (A. p. 70) |
| *Urtica* L. sp. (A. p. 2) |
| *Anagyris foetida* L. (A. p. 16) |
| *Anagyris foetida* L. (A. p. 16) |
| *Anagyris foetida* L. (A. p. 4) |
| *Pistacia palestina* Boiss. (A. pp. 262-263) |
| *Onosma echinoides* L. (A. p. 197) |
| *Onosma echinoides* L. |

| English Name | Greek Name | References |
|---|---|---|
| Stone bugloss | ὄνωνις | III, 131 |
| Stone bugloss | ὄνοσμα | III, 131 |
| Stone parsley | σίνων | III, 55 |
| Stone pine *cembra* | πίτυς | I, 69 |
| Stonecrop | Τηλέφιον | IV, 90 |
| Stonecrop | ἀνδράχνη ἀγρία | IV, 90 |
| Stonecrop | ἀείζῳον, τρίτον εἶδος | IV, 90 |
| Storax | στύραξ | I, 66 |
| Storax ointment | στυράκινον χρῖσμα | I, 66 |
| Strawberry tree | κόμαρος | I, 122 |
| *Strobiloi* nuts | στρόβιλοι | I, 69 |
| *Strobilos* pine | στρόβιλος | I, 69 |
| *Strouthia* | στρούθια | I, 115 |
| Sulphurwort | πευκέδανον | III, 78 |
| Sumac | ῥοῦς ὁ ἐπὶ τὰ ὄψα | I, 108 |
| Sumac | ἐρυθρόν | I, 108 |
| Summer apple | μελίμηλον | I, 115 |
| Sun spurge | ἡλιοσκόπιος | IV, 164 |
| Swallowwort | ἀσκληπιάς | III, 92 |
| Sweet bay | δάφνη | I, 78 |
| Sweet cicely | μυρρίς | IV, 115 |
| Sweet cicely | μύρρα | IV, 115 |
| Sweet flag | κάλαμος ἀρωματικός | I, 18 |
| Sycamore fig | συκόμορον | I, 127 |
| Sycamore fig | συκάμινον | I, 127 |
| Syrian spikenard | νάρδος Συριακή | I, 7 |
| Tamarisk | μυρίκη | I, 87 |
| Tare | ἀφάκη | II, 148 |
| Teasel | δίψακος | III, 11 |
| *Telephonion* | τηλεφώνιον | II, 186 |
| *Telephonion* | βρύον | II, 186 |
| *Telephonion* | ἀνδράχνη ἀγρία | II, 186 |
| *Telephonion* | ἀείζῳον ἄγριον | II, 186 |
| Terebinth | τέρμινθος | I, 71 |
| Thistle | κρίσσιον | IV, 118 |
| Thorn apple | στρύχνον μανικόν | IV, 73 |
| Thorn apple | πέρσειον | IV, 73 |
| Thorn apple | περισσόν | IV, 73 |
| Thorn apple | πεντόδρυον | IV, 73 |
| Thorn apple | ὀρθόγυιον | IV, 73 |

| **Botanical Name** |
|---|
| *Onosma echinoides* L. (A. p. 178) |
| *Onosma echinoides* L. (A. p. 178) |
| *Sison amomum* L. (A. p. 241) |
| *Pinus* sp. |
| *Sedum* L. sp. (A. p. 256) |
| *Sedum* L. sp. (A. p.16) |
| *Sedum* L .sp. (A. p. 8) |
| *Styrax officinalis* L. (A. p. 252) |
| |
| *Arbutus unedo* L. (A. p. 72) |
| |
| Pinus sp. |
| *Cydonia vulgaris* Pers. (LSJ) |
| *Peucedanum officinale* L. (A. p. 195) |
| *Rhus coriaria* L. (A. p. 218) |
| *Rhus coriaria* L. (LSJ) |
| *Pyrus praecox* (LSJ) |
| *Euphorbia helioscopia* L. (A. p. 118) |
| *Vincetoxicum officinale* Moench (A. p. 27) |
| *Laurus nobilis* L. (LSJ) |
| *Myrrhis odorata* Scop. (A. p. 167) |
| *Myrrhis odorata* Scop. (A. p. 167) |
| *Acorus calamus* L. (A. p. 45) |
| *Ficus sycomorus* L. (A. p. 253) |
| *Ficus sycomorus* L. (A. p. 253) |
| *Patrinia scabiosifolia* Fisch. (A. p. 170) |
| *Tamarix tetrandra* Pall. (A. p. 167) |
| *Vicia sativa* var. *angustifolia* L., *V. articulata* Hornem. (A. p. 19) |
| *Dipsacus fullorum* L., *D. silvestris* L. (A. p. 89) |
| *Andrachna telephioides* L. (A. p. 256) |
| *Andrachna telephioides* L. (A. p. 16) |
| *Andrachna telephioides* L. (A. p. 16) |
| *Andrachna telephioides* L. (A. p. 8) |
| *Pistacia terebinthus* L. (A. p. 256) |
| ~*Carduus pycnocephalus* L., ~*C. tenuiflorus* Curtis (A. p. 67) |
| *Datura stramonium* L. (A. p. 251 see also his comments) |
| *Datura stramonium* L . |
| *Datura stramonium* L. |
| *Datura stramonium* L. |
| *Datura stramonium* L. |

| English Name | Greek Name | References |
|---|---|---|
| Thorn apple | θρύον | IV, 73 |
| Thorn apple | ἔνορυ | IV, 73 |
| Thorn apple | ἄνυδρον | IV, 73 |
| Thorny burnet | στοιβή | IV, 12 |
| Thyme spurge | χαμαισύκη | IV, 169 |
| Thyme spurge | συκῆ | IV, 169 |
| Thyme, Tufted | ζυγίς | III, 38 |
| Tragacanth | τραγάκανθα | III, 20 |
| *Tragos* | τράγος | IV, 51 |
| *Tragos* | τάργανον | IV, 51 |
| *Tragos* | σκορπίον | IV, 51 |
| Traveler's joy | κληματίς | IV, 180 |
| Treacle clover | τρίφυλλον | III, 109 |
| Treacle clover | ὀξύφυλλον | III, 109 |
| Treacle clover | μινυανθές | III, 109 |
| Treacle clover | κνήκιον | III, 109 |
| Treacle clover | ἀσφάλτιον | III, 109 |
| Tree germander | Τεύκριον | III, 97 |
| Tree heath | ἐρείκη | I, 88 |
| Tree medick | κύτισος | IV, 112 |
| Tree moss | σπλάχνον | I, 21 |
| Tree moss | βρύον | I, 21 |
| Tree purslane | ἅλιμον | I, 91 |
| Truffle | ὕδνον | II, 145 |
| Tuberous spurge | χαμαιβάλανος | IV, 175 |
| Tuberous spurge | ῥάφανος ἀγρία | IV, 175 |
| Tuberous spurge | λινόζωστις | IV, 175 |
| Tuberous spurge | ἰσχάς | IV, 175 |
| Tuberous spurge | ἄπιος | IV, 175 |
| Tuberous thistle | φύλλον | III, 19 |
| Tuberous thistle | πολυγόνατον | III, 19 |
| Tuberous thistle | λευκάκανθα | III, 19 |
| Tuberous thistle | λάδανον | III, 19 |
| Tuberous thistle | ἰσχιάς | III, 19 |
| Tufted thyme | ζυγίς | III, 38 |
| Tufted thyme | ἕρπυλος | III, 38 |
| Turmeric | κυπὲρου ἕτερον | I, 5 |
| Turnip | γογγύλη | II, 110 |
| Turpentine, Venice | λάριξ | I, 71 |
| Unguent, Onyx | ὀνύχινον | I, 54 |

| **Botanical Name** |
|---|
| *Datura stramonium* L. |
| *Datura stramonium* L. |
| *Datura stramonium* L. |
| *Poterium spinosum* L. (A. p. 250) |
| *Euphorbia chamaesyce* L. (A. p. 61) |
| *Euphorbia chamaesyce* L. (A. p. 253) |
| *Thymus Sibthorpii* (LSJ) |
| *Astragalus gummife* r Labill., *A. microcephalus* Willd. (A. p. 262) |
| *Ephedra distachya* L. sp. (A. p. 263) |
| *Ephedra distachya* L. |
| *Ephedra distachya* L. (A. p. 232) |
| *Clematis vitalba* L., *C. cirrosa* L., *C. flammula* L. (A. p. 69) |
| *Psorolea bituminosa* L. (A. p. 264) |
| *Psorolea bituminosa* L. (A. p. 183) |
| *Psorolea bituminosa* L. (A. p.162) |
| *Psorolea bituminosa* L. (A. p. 319) |
| *Psorolea bituminosa* L. (A. p. 28) |
| *Teucrium flavum* L. (A. p. 257) |
| *Erica arborea* L. (A. p. 96) |
| *Medicago arborea* L. (A. p. 85) |
| *Evernia* L. (A. p. 247) |
| *Evernia* L. (A. p. 39) |
| *Atriplex halimus* L. (A. p. 116) |
| *Tuber cibarium* L. sp. (A. pp. 126 and 266) |
| *Euphorbia apios* L. (A. p. 59) |
| *Euphorbia apios* L. (A. p. 216) |
| *Euphorbia apios* L. |
| *Euphorbia apios* L. (A. p. 133) |
| *Euphorbia apios* L. (A. p. 20) |
| *Cnicus tuberosus* L. or *Cirstium tuberosum* All. (A. p. 199) |
| *Cnicus tuberosus* L. or *Cirstium tuberosum* All. (A. p. 204) |
| *Cnicus tuberosus* L. or *Cirstium tuberosum* All. (A. p. 142) |
| *Cnicus tuberosus* L. or *Cirstium tuberosum* All. |
| *Cnicus tuberosus* L. or *Cirstium tuberosum* All. (A. p. 133) |
| *Thymus Sibthorpii* (LSJ) |
| *Thymus Sibthorpii* (LSJ) |
| *Curcuma longa* L. (A. p. 85) |
| *Brassica rapa* L. (A. p. LSJ) |
| |
| |

| English Name | Greek Name | References |
|---|---|---|
| Unguent, Basil | ὠκίμινον | I, 49 |
| Unguent, Butter | βουτύρινον | I, 54 |
| Unguent, Cinnamon | κιναμώμινον | I, 61 |
| Unguent,Date palm inflorescence | ἐλάτινον | I, 44 |
| Unguent, Dill | ἀνήθινον | I, 51 |
| Unguent, Fenugreek | τήλινον | I, 47 |
| Unguent, *Hedychroun* | ἡδύχρουν | I, 58 |
| Unguent, Henna | κύπρινον | I, 55 |
| Unguent, Iris | ἴρινον | I, 56 |
| Unguent, Lily | σούσινον | I, 52 |
| Unguent, Lily | λείρινον | I, 52 |
| Unguent, Malabar | μαλαβάθρινον | I, 63 |
| Unguent, Marjoram | σαμψούχινον | I, 48 |
| Unguent, Marjoram | ἀμαράκινον | I, 58 |
| Unguent, *Megalleion* | Μεγάλλειον | I, 58 |
| Unguent, *Mendesion* | Μενδήσιον | I, 59 |
| Unguent, Narcissus | ναρκίσσινον | I, 53 |
| Unguent, Quince | μήλινον | I, 45 |
| Unguent, Rose | ῥόδινον | I, 43 |
| Unguent, Saffron | κρόκινον | I, 54 |
| Unguent, Spikenard | νάρδινον | I, 62 |
| Unguent, Storax | στυράκινον | I, 54 |
| Unguent, Sweet new wine | γλεύκινον | I, 57 |
| Unguent, Wild vine | οἰνάνθινον | I, 46 |
| Unguent, Wormwood | ἀβροτόνινον | I, 50 |
| Valonia oak | φηγός | I, 106 |
| Vervain | περιστέριον | IV, 59 |
| Vervain mallow | ἀλκαία | III, 147 |
| Vetch | κατανάγκη | IV, 131 |
| Vinegar | ὄξος | V, 13 |
| Vinegar, Betony | ὂξος κὲστρου ψυχροτρόφου | V, 44 |
| Vinegar, Brine, Cretan thyme | θυμοξάλμη | V, 16 |
| Vinegar, French lavender | ὂξος διὰ στοιχάδος | V, 43 |
| Vinegar, Honey | ὀξύμελι | V, 14 |
| Vinegar, Lees of | ὂξους τρύξ | V, 114 |
| Vinegar, Squill | ὂξος σκιλλήτικον | V, 17 |
| Violet | ἴον | IV, 121 |
| Viper's herb | λυκαψός | IV, 26 |
| Wall barley | κίννα | IV, 32 |
| Wall barley | ἄγρωστις ἡ ἐν Κιλικίᾳ | IV, 32 |

| **Botanical Name** |
| --- |
| |
| |
| |
| |
| |
| |
| |
| |
| |
| |
| |
| |
| |
| |
| |
| |
| |
| |
| |
| |
| |
| |
| |
| |
| |
| *Quercus aegilops* L. (A. p. 196) |
| *Lycopus europaeus* L. (A. p. 193) |
| *Malope malacoides* L. (A. p. 9) |
| *Ornithopus compressu* s L. (A. p. 53) |
| |
| |
| |
| |
| |
| |
| |
| *Viola odorata* L. (A. p. 132) |
| *Echium italicum* L. sp. (A. p. 149) |
| *Hordeum marinum* L. (LSJ) |
| *Hordeum marinum* L. (LSJ) |

| **Botanical Name** |
|---|
| *Teucrium chamaedrys* L. and ~*T. lucidum* L. (A. p. 59) |
| *Teucrium chamaedrys* L. and *T. lucidum* L. (A. p. 59) |
| *Teucrium chamaedrys* L. and *T. lucidum* L. (A. p. 257) |
| *Teucrium chamaedrys* L. and *T. lucidum* L. (A. p. 146) |
| *Juglans regia* L. (A. p. 52) |
| *Juglans regia* L. (A. p. 52) |
| ~*Coronopus procumbens* Gilib. (A. p.112) |
| *Euphorbia peplis* L. (A. 253) |
| *Euphorbia peplis* L. (A. p. 192) |
| *Euphorbia peplis* L. (A. p. 156) |
| *Trapa natans* L. (A. p. 263) |
| *Nasturtium officinale* R. Br. (A. p. 241) |
| *Nasturtium officinale* R. Br. (A. p. 242) |
| *Nasturtium officinale* R. Br. (A. p. 49) |
| *Rumex aquaticus* L. (A. p. 39) |
| *Pistia stratiotes* L. (A. p. 250) |
| *Myriophyllum spicatum* L. (A. p. 167) |
| *Sium angustifolium* L. (A. p. 242) |
| *Alisma plantago* L., *A. arcuatum* Mich. (A. p. 150) |
| *Alisma plantago* L., *A. arcuatum* Mich. (A. p. 86) |
| *Alisma plantago* L., *A. arcuatum* Mich. |
| |
| *Asplenium trichomanes* L. (A. p. 264) |
| *Triticum* L. |
| |
| *Triticum monococcum* L. (A. p. 279) |
| *Triticum dicoccum* Schrek. (A. p. 279) |
| *Triticum monoccocum* Schrek. (A. p. 279) |
| |
| *Veratrum album* L. (A. p. 94) |
| *Populus alba* L. (A. p. 143) |
| *Rosa sempervirens* L. (A. p. 183) |
| *Rosa sempervirens* L. (A. p. 84) |
| *Nymphaea alba* L. (A. p. 174) |
| *Nuphar luteum* Sm. (A. p. 174) |
| ~*Ocinum pilosum* Willd., ~*Thumus acinos.* L. (A. p.4) |
| ~*Ocinum pilosum* Willd., ~*Thumus acinos.* L. (A. p.4) |
| *Daucus guttatus* L. (LSJ; see also A. pp. 57 and 248) |
| *Daucus guttatus* L. (LSJ; see also A. pp. 57 and 248) |
| *Scandix pecten-Veneris* L. (A. p. 229) |

| **Botanical Name** |
|---|
| *Lagoecia cuminoides* L. (A. p. 81) |
| *Nigella arvensis* (LSJ) |
| *Trigonella elatior* Sibth. sp., *T. gladiata* L. sp. (A. p. 148) |
| |
| |
| *Ficus carica* L. (A. pp. 48 and 96) |
| *Vitis silvestris* Gmel (A. p. 14) |
| *Vitis silvestris* L. (LSJ) |
| *Scilla bifolia* L. (A. p. 126) |
| *Allium ambeloprasum* L. (A. p. 206) |
| *Olea europaea* L. var. *silvestris* Miller (A. p. 76) |
| *Olea europaea* L. var. *silvestris* Miller (A. p. 176) |
| *Olea europaea* L. var. *silvestris* Miller (A. p. 176) |
| *Pyrus amygdaliformis* Vill. (A. p. 3) |
| *Euphorbia peplis* L. (A. p. 192) |
| *Euphorbia peplis* L. (A. p. 192) |
| *Euphorbia peplis* L. (A. p. 16) |
| *Raphanus raphanistrum* (LSJ) |
| *Peganum harmala* L. (A. p. 163) |
| *Peganum harmala* L. (A. p. 163) |
| *Peganum harmala* L. |
| *Peganum harmala* L. |
| *Isatis agrestis* L. (A . p.133) |
| *Salix* L. sp. (A. p. 134) |
| *Polygonum persicaria* L. (A. p. 77) |
| *Papaver argemone* L. (A. p. 23) |

| Botanical Name |
| --- |

| **Botanical Name** |
|---|
| |
| |
| |
| |
| |
| |
| |
| |
| |
| |
| |
| |
| |
| |
| |
| |
| |
| |
| |
| |
| |
| |
| |
| |
| |
| |
| |
| |
| *Physalis alkekengi* L. (A. p. 251) |
| *Physalis alkekengi* L. (A. p. 115) |
| *Isatis tinctoria* L. (A. p. 133) |
| *Aconitum napellus* L. (A. p. 149) |
| *Aconitum napellus* L. (A. p. 4) |
| *Artemisia maritima* L. (A. p. 236) |
| *Artemisia maritima* L. (LSJ) |
| *Artemisia maritima* L. (A . p. 1) |
| ~*Artemisia abrotonum* L. |
| ~*Artemisia abrotonum* L. |
| *Artemisia maritima* L. (A . p.1) |
| *Artemisia genipi* Weber (A. p. 26) |

| English Name | Greek Name | References |
|---|---|---|
| Wormwood | ἀρτεμισὶα πλατυτέρα | III, 113 |
| Wormwood | ἀρτεμισὶα λεπτοτέρα | III, 113 |
| Wormwood | ἀρτεμισία | III, 113 |
| Wormwood | ἀβρότονον | III, 24 |
| *Xylobalsamon* | ξυλοβάλσαμον | I, 19 |
| *Xylocinamomon* | ξυλοκινάμωμον | I, 14 |
| Yarrow | στρατιώτης ὁ χιλιόφυλλος | IV, 102 |
| Yellow flag | ἄσπληνον | I, 2 |
| Yellow flag | ἄκορον | I, 2 |
| Yew | τιθύμαλλος | IV, 79 |
| Yew | τάξος | IV, 79 |
| Yew | σμῖλος | IV, 79 |
| Yew | σμῖλαξ | IV, 79 |

| **Botanical Name** |
|---|
| *Artemisia arborescen* s L. (A. p. 26) |
| *Artemisia campestris* L. (A. p. 26) |
| *Artemisia arborescens* L., *A. campestris* L, *A. genipi* Weber, (A. p. 26) |
| *~Artemisia abrotonum(* L. (A. p .115 s.v. *(h)abrotonum)* |
| |
| |
| *Achillea millefolium* L. (A. p. 250) |
| *Iris pseudacorus* L. (A. p. 4) |
| *Iris pseudacorus* L. (A. p. 4) |
| *Taxus baccata* L. |
| *Taxus baccata* L. (A. p. 256) |
| *Taxus baccata* L. (A. p. 161) |
| *Taxus baccata* L. (A. p. 161) |

| **Botanical name** |
|---|
| |
| ~*Artemisia abrotonum* (A. p. 115 s.v (h)abrotonum) |
| *Artemisia fragrans (* LSJ*)* |
| *Santolina chamaecyparissus* (A. p. 115) |
| *Aquilaria agallocha* Roxb. (A. p. 7) |
| *Aquilaria agallocha* Roxb. (A. p. 7) |
| *Polyporus* sp. (A. p. 7) |
| *Ferula marmarica* L. (A. p. 7) |
| *Achillea ageratum* L. (A. p. 7) |
| *Paeonia* L. sp. (A. p. 7) |
| *Vitex agnus-castus* L. (A. p. 8) |
| *Raphanus raphanistrum* (LSJ) |
| *Olea europaea* L. var. *silvestris* Miller (A. p. 176) |
| *Smyrnium olusatrum* L. (LSJ) |
| ~*Origanum viride* Boiss. sp. |
| *Smyrnium olusatrum* L. (LSJ) |
| *Bryonia dioica Jacq. (A. p. 14)* |
| *Cynodon dactylon* Pers. (A. p. 8) |
| *Hordeum marinum* L. (LSJ) |
| *Parnassia palustris* L. (A. p. 8) |
| *Anchusa tinctoria* L. (A. p.16) |
| *Lithospermum fruticosum* L. (A. p. 16) |
| *Echium diffusum* Sibth. (A. p. 16) |
| *Lollium perenne* L. (A. p. 16) |
| *Hyoscyamus* L. sp. (A. p. 5) |
| *Adiantum capillus Veneris* L. (A. p. 5) |
| *Glycyrrhiza glabra* L., G. echinata L.,(A. p. 5) |
| *Andrachna telephioides* L. (A. p. 8) |
| *Sempervivum arboreum* L. (A. p. 8) |
| *Sempervivum tectorum* L. (A. p. 8) |
| *Sedum* L. sp. (A. p. 8) |
| *Sedum* L. sp. (A. p. 8) |
| *Capparis spinosa* L. |
| *Lithospermum officinale* L. |
| |
| *Populus nigra* L. (A. p. 6) |
| *Aegilops ovata* L. (A. p. 6) |
| *Trigonella fenum graecum* L. (A. p. 6) |
| |
| |

| **Botanical name** |
|---|
| |
| *Carum copticum* B. and H. (A. p. 81) |
| *Salvia aethiopis* L., *S. argentea* L. (A. p. 7) |
| *Lolium temulentum* L. (A. p. 6) |
| *Ruscus aculeatus* L. |
| |
| *Acacia arabica* (LSJ) |
| *Genista acanthoclada* (LSJ) |
| *Genista acanthoclada* (LSJ) |
| *Urtica* L. sp. (A. p. 2) |
| *Notobasis syriaca* Cass. = *Cirsium syriacum* Gaertn. (A. p. 2) |
| ~*Cnicus ferox* L. or ~*C. acarna* (A. p. 2) |
| *Onopordum acanthium* L., *O. illyricum* (A. p. 2) |
| *Acanthus mollis* L. (A. p. 2) |
| *Acanthus spinosus* L. (A. p. 2) |
| *Astagalus poterium* Labill. |
| ~*Ocinum pilosum* Willd, ~ *Thymus acinos* L. (A. p. 4) |
| *Daphne oleides* L. (LSJ) |
| ~*Doronicum pardalianches* Jacq. (A. p. 4) |
| *Aconitum napellus* L. (A. p. 4) |
| ~*Ocinum pilosum* Willd, ~ *Thymus acinos* L. (A. p. 4) |
| *Anagyris foetida* L. (A. p. 4) |
| *Iris pseudacorus* L. (A. p. 4) |
| *Sambucus nigra* L. (A. p. 4) |
| *Sambucus nigra* L. (A. p. 4) |
| *Bunium ferulaceum* Sibth. and Sm. (A. p. 4) |
| *Ruscus racemosus* L. (A. p. 9) |
| |
| |
| |
| |
| *Althaea officinalis* L. (A . p.12) |
| *Convolvulus oleaefolius* Desr. (A. p. 116} |
| *Withania somnifera* Dun. (A. p. 115) |
| *Physalis alkekengi* L. (A. p. 115) |
| *Atriplex halimus* L. (A. p. 116) |
| *Alisma plantago* L. *A. arcuatum* Mich. |
| *Malope malacoides* L. (A. p. 9) |
| *Echium diffusum* Sibth. (A. p. 16) |
| *Echium plantagineum* L., *E. rubrum* L. (A. p. 9) |

| Greek name | English name | References |
|---|---|---|
| ἀλόη | Aloe | III, 22 |
| ἀλσίνη | Lichwort | IV, 86 |
| ἄλυπον | Herb terrible | IV, 178 |
| ἄλυσσον | Madwort | III, 91 |
| ἀμαράκινον | Marjoram unguent | I, 58 |
| ἀμάρακον | Feverfew | III, 138 |
| ἀμάρακον | Marjoram | III, 39 |
| ἀμάραντον | Gold flower | IV, 57 |
| ἀμβροσία | Ambrose | III, 114 |
| ἀμβροσία | Houseleek | IV, 88 |
| ἀμβροσία | Oak of Jerusalem | III, 115 |
| ἀμερσίνη | Bindweed | IV, 39 |
| ἄμι | Ajowan | III, 62 |
| ἀμμωνιακόν | Gum ammoniac | III, 84 |
| ἀμόργη | *Amorge* | I, 102 |
| ἀμόργη | Olives,Sediment of pressed | I, 102 |
| ἀμπελόκαρπον | Cleavers | III, 90 |
| ἀμπελόπρασον | Wild leek | II, 150 |
| ἄμπελος ἀγρία | Wild grapevine | V, 2 |
| ἄμπελος ἀγρία | Wild grapevine | IV, 181 |
| ἄμπελος λευκή | Bryony | IV, 182 |
| ἄμπελος μέλαινα | Black bryony | IV, 183 |
| ἄμπελος οἰνοφόρος | Grapevine | V, 1 |
| ἄμπελος Χειρώνιος | Black bryony | IV, 183 |
| ἀμυγδάλη | Almond | I, 123 |
| ἀμυγδαλίτης | Spurge | IV, 164 |
| ἀμύγδαλον πικρόν | Almond, bitter | I, 123 |
| ἄμυλον | Starch | II, 101 |
| ἀμωμίτης | Frankincense, A kind of | I, 68 |
| ἄμωμον | Nepal cardamom | I, 15 |
| ἀναβάσιον | Horsetail | IV, 46 |
| ἀναγαλλίς | Pimpernel | II, 178 |
| ἀναγαλλὶς ἄρρην | Pimpernel | II, 178 |
| ἀναγαλλὶς θήλεια | Pimpernel | II, 178 |
| ἀνάγυρις | Stinking bean trefoil | III, 150 |
| ἀνάγυρος | Stinking bean trefoil | III, 150 |
| ἀναξυρίς | Monk's rhubarb | II, 114 |
| ἀνάρρινον | Calf's snout | IV, 130 |
| ἀνδράφαξυς | Orach | II, 119 |
| ἀνδράχνη | Purslane | II, 124 |

| **Botanical name** |
|---|
| *Aloe vera* L. (A. p. 11) |
| *Thelygonum cynocrambe* L. = *Cynocrambe prostrata* Gaertn. (A. p. 11) |
| *Globularia alypum* L. (A. p. 12) |
| *Biscutella* L. sp. (A. p. 12) |
| |
| *Chrysanthemum parthenium* Bernh. (A. p. 189) |
| *Majorana hortensis* Moench (A. p. 13) |
| *Helichrysum orientale* L., *H. stoecha* s L., *H. siculum* L. (A. p. 13) |
| *Artemisia maritima* L. (A. p. 13) |
| *Sempervivum arboreum* L. (A. p. 13) |
| *Chenopodium botry* s L. (A. p. !3) |
| *Convolvulus arvensis* L. (LSJ) |
| *Carum copticum* B. and H. (A. p. 14) |
| *Ferula marmarica* L. (A. p. 116) |
| |
| |
| *Galium aparine* L. |
| *Allium ambeloprasum* L. (A. p. 206) |
| *Vitis silvestris* L. (LSJ) |
| *Vitis silvestris* Gmel. (A. p. 14) |
| *Bryonia dioica* Jacq. (A. p. 14) |
| *Tamus communis* L. (A. p. 14) |
| *Vitis vinifera* L. (LSJ) |
| *Tamus communis* L. (A. p. 14) |
| *Prunus amygdalus* Stokes esp. var. *sativa* Asch. (A. p. 15) |
| *Euphorbia Sibthorpii* Boiss. |
| *Prunus amygdalus* Stokes, var. *amara* Schn. (A. p. 15) |
| |
| |
| *Amomum subulatum* Roxb. (A. p. 14) |
| *Equisotum silvaticum* L. (A. p. 15) |
| *Anagallis arvensis* L. (A. p. 15) |
| *Anagallis phoenicea* Scop. (A. p. 15) |
| *Anagallis caerulea* Schreb. (A. p. 15) |
| *Anagyris foetida* L. (A. p. 16) |
| *Anagyris foetida* L. (A. p. 16) |
| *Rumex* L. sp... (LSJ) |
| *Antirrhinum orontium* L. (LSJ) |
| *Atriplex hortensis* L. (A. p. 16) |
| *Portulaca oleracea* L. (A. p. 16) |

| **Botanical name** |
|---|
| *Sedum album* L., *S. stellatum* L. (A. p. 16) |
| *Sedum* L. sp. (A. p. 16) |
| *Andrachna telephioides* L. (A. p. 16) |
| *Euphorbia peplis* L. (A. p. 16) |
| *Hypericum crispum* L. (A. p. 17) |
| *Hypericum perforatum* L. (A. p. 27) |
| *Hypericum perfoliatum* L. (A. p. 17) |
| *Acetabularia mediterranea* L. (A. p. 17) |
| *Anemone coronaria* L. (A. p. 17) |
| *Anemone coronaria* L. (A. p. 17) |
| |
| *Anethum graveolens* L. (A. p. 17) |
| *Pimpinella anisum* L. (A. p. 17) |
| *Chamomilla* L. sp. |
| *Cressa cretic* a L. (A. p. 18) |
| *Ajuga iva* Schreb. (A. p. 18) |
| *Xanthium strumarium* L. |
| *Madragora* L. sp. (LSJ) |
| *Antirrhinum orontium* L. (LSJ) |
| |
| *Datura stramonium* L. |
| *Ononis antiquorum* L. (A. p. 17) |
| *Xanthium strumarium* L. (A. p. 19) |
| *Galium aparine* L. (A. p. 19) |
| *Pyrus communis* (LSJ) |
| *Euphorbia apios* L. (A. p. 20) |
| *Cynanchum acutum* L., for the Orient: *Marsdenia erecta* Br. (A. p. 21) |
| *Daphne gnidium* L. |
| |
| |
| *Papaver argemone* L. (A. p. 23) |
| *Anemone coronaria* L. |
| *Anemone coronaria* L. |
| *Arisarum vulgare* Targ.-Tozz., *A. proboscideum* Savi (A. p. 24) |
| *Aristolochia* L. (A. p. 25) |
| *Aristolochia longa* L. (A. p. 25) |
| *Aristolochia rotunda* L. (A. p. 25) |
| *Aristolochia longa* L. (A. p. 25) |
| *Aristolochia rotunda* L. (A. p. 25) |
| *Juniperus* L. (LSJ) |

| **Botanical name** |
|---|
| *Arctium lappa* L. (A. p. 23) |
| ~*Inula candida* L., ~*Celsia* sp., ~*C. acaulis* Bory (A. p. 23) |
| ~*Inula candida* L., ~*Celsia* sp., ~*C. acaulis* Bory (A. p. 23) |
| *Peganum harmala* L. |
| *Plantago* L. sp. (A. p. 26) |
| *Colocasia antiquorum* Schott (A. p. 26) |
| *Artemisia maritima* L. (A. p. 26) |
| *Artemisia arborescens* L., *A. campestris* L., *A. genipi* Weber . (A. p. 26) |
| *Artemisia campestris* L. (A. p. 26) |
| *Artemisia arborescen* s L. (A. p. 26) |
| *Artemisia genipi* Weber (A. p. 26) |
| |
| *Bryonia dioica* Jacq. (A. p. 23) |
| *Mespilus germanica* L. |
| *Asarum europaeum* L. (A. p. 27) |
| |
| *Vincetoxicum officinale* Moench (A. p. 27) |
| *Hypericum perforatum* L. (A. p. 27) |
| *Hypericum perforatum* L. (A. p. 27) |
| *Hypericum perfoliatum* L. (A. p. 27) |
| *Alhagi maurorum* L. (A. p. 28) |
| *Asparagus officinalis* L. (A. pp. 28 and 166) |
| *Iris pseudacorus* L. (A. p. 4) |
| *Ceterach officinarum* Willd. (A. p. 29) |
| |
| *Aster amellus* L. (A. p. 29) |
| *Astragalu* s L. sp. (A. p. 29) |
| |
| *Psorolea bituminosa* L. (A. p. 28) |
| *Asphodelus* L. sp. (A. pp. 29-30) |
| *Carthamus lanatus* L. (A. p. 30) |
| *Vicia sativa* var. *angustifolia* L., *V. articulata* Hornem. (A. p. 19) |
| *Achillea millefolium* L. (A. p.. 3) |
| *Pyrus amygdaliformis* Vill. (A. p. 3) |
| |
| *Artemisia maritima* L. (A . p. 1) |
| *Artemisia maritima* L. (A . p. 1) |
| *Cymbopogon schoenanthus* Spreng. (A. p. 229) |
| *Origanum dictamnus* L. |
| ~*Helichrysum sanguineum* Boiss. = *Gnaphalium sanguineum* L. (A. p. 32) |

| Greek name | English name | References |
|---|---|---|
| βάλανοι Διός | Chestnuts, Sweet | I, 106 |
| βάλανοι Σαρδιαναί | Chestnuts, Sweet | I, 106 |
| βάλανος | Acorn | I, 106 |
| βάλανος μυρεψική | Ben | IV, 157 |
| βαλαύστιον | Pomegranate flower | I, 111 |
| βαλλωτή | Black horehound | III, 103 |
| βάλσαμον | Mecca balsam | I, 19 |
| βασιλικὸν κύμινον | Ajowan | III. 62 |
| βάτος | Bramble | IV, 37 |
| βάτος Ἰδαία | Elecampane | I, 28 |
| βάτος Ἰδαία | Raspberry | IV, 38 |
| βάτος Μοσυλῖτις | Mosilian bramble | I. 13, 2 |
| βατράχιον | Ranunculus | II, 175 |
| βατράχιον ἕτερον | Ranunculus | II, 175 |
| βατράχιον τέταρτον | Ranunculus | II, 175 |
| βατράχιον τρίτον | Ranunculus | II, 175 |
| βδέλλιον | Bdellium | I, 67 |
| βήσσασα | Wild rue | III, 46 |
| βήχιον | Coltsfoot | III, 112 |
| βλῆχρον | Male fern | IV, 184 |
| βλήχων | Pennyroyal | III, 31 |
| βλίτον | Blite | II, 117 |
| βλόχον | Bdellium | I, 67 |
| Βοιωτιακὴ σμύρνα | Boeotian myrrh | I, 65 |
| βολβὸς ἄγριος | Meadow saffron | IV, 83 |
| βολβὸς ἐδώδιμος | Purse tassels | II, 170 |
| βολβὸς ἐμετικός | Narcissus tazetta | IV, 156 |
| βομβόχυλον | Mandrake | IV, 75 |
| βόρατον | Savin | I, 76 |
| βοσκάς | Pitch | I, 72 |
| βότρυς | Ambrose | III, 114 |
| βουβώνιον | Blue daisy | IV, 119 |
| βούγλωσσον | Bugloss | IV, 127 |
| βούκερως | Fenugreek | II, 102 |
| βουνιάς | French turnip | II, 111 |
| βούνιον | Earthnut | IV, 123 |
| βουτύρινον | Butter unguent | I, 54 |
| βούφθαλμον | Houseleek | IV, 88 |
| βούφθαλμον | Oxeye | III, 139 |
| βράθυ | Savin | I, 76 |

| **Botanical name** |
| --- |
| *Castanea vulgaris* Lam. (A. p. 32) |
| |
| *Quercus* L. sp. (A. p. 32) |
| *Moringa* sp. |
| |
| *Ballota nigra* L. (A. p. 33) |
| *Commiphora opobalsamum* Engl. (A. p. 33) |
| *Carum copticum* B. and H. (A. p. 81) |
| *Rubus ulmifolius* Schott (LSJ) |
| *Inula helenium* L. (A. p. 171) |
| *Rubus idaeus* L. (A. p. 34) |
| *Cinnamomum cassia sp.* (LSJJ |
| *Ranunculus* L. sp. (A. p. 34) |
| *Ranunculus* L. sp. |
| *Ranunculus* L. sp. |
| *Ranunculus* L. sp. |
| *Commiphora mukul* Engl. (A. p. 34) |
| *Peganum harmala* L. |
| *Tussilago farfara* L. (A. p. 35) |
| *Polystichum filix mas* Roth. (A. p. 36) |
| *Mentha pulegium* L. (A. p. 112) |
| *Amaranthus blitum* L. (A. p. 36) |
| *Commiphora mukul* Engl. (A. p. 38) |
| Unidentified |
| |
| *Muscari comosum* Miller (A. p. 40) |
| ~Narcissus tazetta (LSJ) see also (A. p. 41) |
| *Mandragora* L. sp. (LSJ) |
| *Juniperus sabina* L. (A. p. 38) |
| |
| *Artemisia maritima* L. (A. p. 37) |
| *Aster amellus* L. (A. p. 39) |
| *Anchusa italica* Retz. (A. p. 40) |
| *Trigonella fenum graecum* L. (A. p. 39) |
| *Brassica napus* L. (A. p. 41) |
| *Bunium ferulaceum* Sibth. and Sm. (A. p. 41) |
| |
| *Sempervivum arboreum* L. (A. p. 41) |
| *Chrysanthemum coronarium* L. (A. p. 41) |
| *Juniperus sabina* L. (A. p. 38) |

| Greek name | English name | References |
|---|---|---|
| βρεκόκκια | Apricots | I, 115 |
| βρεττανική | Water dock | IV, 2 |
| βρόμος | Oats | II, 94 |
| βρύον | *Telephonion* | II, 186 |
| βρύον | Tree moss | I, 21 |
| βρύον θαλάσσιον | Sea lettuce | IV, 98 |
| βρυωνία | Black bryony | IV, 183 |
| βρυωνία | Bryony | IV, 182 |
| Γαβιρὲα λιπαροτάτη | Myrrh | I, 64 |
| Γαγγῖτις | Gangitis | I, 7 |
| γαλαίριον | Bedstraw | IV, 95 |
| γαλάτιον | Bedstraw | IV, 95 |
| γαλεόβδολον | Brownwort | IV, 94 |
| γαλήοψις | Brownwort | IV, 94 |
| γάληψις | Brownwort | IV, 94 |
| γάλιον | Bedstraw | IV, 95 |
| γεντιανή | Centaury | III, 6 |
| γεντιανή | Gentian | III, 3 |
| γεντιανή | Licorice | III, 5 |
| γεράνιον | Cranesbill | III, 116 |
| γεράνιον ἕτερον | Cranesbill, Another | III, 116 |
| γιγγίδιον | *Gingidion* | II, 137 |
| γιγγίδιον | Pepperwort | II, 174 |
| γίζιρ | Cassia | I, 13 |
| γλαδίολος | Gladwyn | IV, 22 |
| γλαύκιον | *Glaucion* | III, 86 |
| γλαύξ | Wart cress | IV, 138 |
| γλεύκινον | Sweet new wine unguent | I, 57 |
| γλήχων | Pennyroyal | III, 31 |
| γλήχων ἀγρία | Catmint | III, 35 |
| γλήχων ἀγρία | Dittany of Crete | III, 32 |
| γλυκισίδη | Peony | III, 140 |
| γλυκύρριζα | Licorice | III, 5 |
| γλυκὺς ἀγκών | Wormwood | III, 24 |
| γναφάλλιον | Cottonweed | III, 117 |
| γογγύλη | Turnip | II, 110 |
| γογγύλη ἀγρία | Eastern cress | II, 110 |
| γοργυνθία | Butcher's broom | IV, 144 |
| γύρις πυρῶν | Pollen, wheat | II, 85 |
| δακτυλῖτις | Birthwort | III, 4 |

| **Botanical name** |
|---|
| *Prunus armeniaca* L. (A. p. 157) |
| *Rumex aquaticus* L. (A. p. 39) |
| *Avena sativa* L. |
| *Andrachna telephioides* L. (A. p. 16) |
| *Evernia* L. (A. p. 39) |
| *Ulva lactuca* L., and *U. latissima* L. (A. p. 39) |
| *Tamus communis* L. (A. p. 39) |
| *Bryonia dioica* Jacq. (A. p. 39) |
| |
| *Nardostachys jatamansi* DC (A. p. 109) |
| *Galium verum* L. |
| *Galium verum* L. |
| *Scrofularia peregrina* L. (A. p. 108) |
| *Scrofularia peregrina* L. (A. p. 108) |
| *Scrofularia peregrina* L. |
| *Galium verum* L. (A. p. 108) |
| *Centaurea centaurium* L. (A. p. 109) |
| *Gentiana lutea* L., *G. purpurea* L. (A. p. 109) |
| *Glycyrrhiza glabra* L., G. echinata L.,(A. p. 109) |
| *Geranium tuberosum* L. (A. p. 110) |
| *Erodium malacoides* Willd. (A. p. 110) |
| *Malabaila sekakul* Russ. (A. p. 110) |
| *Lepidium latifolium* L. (A. p. 110) |
| |
| *Iris* L. sp. (A. p. 278) |
| *Glaucium corniculatum* Curtis (A. p. 112) |
| ~*Coronopus procumbens* Gilib. (A. p.112) |
| |
| *Mentha pulegium* L. (A. p. 36) |
| *Calamintha* Lmk. sp. (A. p. 44) |
| *Origanum dictamnus* L. |
| *Paeonia* L. sp (A. p. 112) |
| *Glycyrrhiza glabra* L., G. echinata L. (A. p. 112) |
| ~*Artemisia abrotonum* L. (A. p. 115 s. v. *(h)abrotonum* ) |
| *Gnaphalium* L. sp., *Filago* L. sp. (A. p. 112) |
| *Brassica rapa* L. (A. p. LSJ) |
| *Erucaria aleppica* (LSJ) |
| *Ruscus aculeatus* L. |
| |
| *Aristolochia longa* L. (A. p. 25) |

| **Botanical name** |
|---|
| *Alisma plantago* L., *A. arcuatum* Mich. (A. p. 86) |
| *Ruscus hypophyllum* L. (LSJ) |
| |
| ~*Athamanta cretensis* L. (A. p. 87) |
| *Caucalis grandiflora* L. (A. p. 87) |
| *Laurus nobilis* L. (LSJ) |
| *Ruscus hypophyllum* L. (LSJ) |
| |
| *Vinca minor* L. (A. p. 87) |
| *Daphne laureola* L. (A. p. 87) |
| *Euphorbia dendroides* L. (A. p. 262) |
| *Alhagi maurorum* L. (A. p. 88) |
| *Origanum dictamnus* L. (A. p. 88) |
| *Hypericum perfoliatum* L. (A. p. 89) |
| *Castanea vulgaris* Lam. |
| *Lithospermum officinale* L. (A. p. 89) |
| *Vincetoxicum nigrum* Moench (LSJ) |
| *Dipsacus fullorum* L., *D. silvestris* L. (A. p. 89) |
| *Convolvulus oleaefolius* Desr. (A. p. 90) |
| *Lepidium draba* L. (A. p. 90) |
| *Arum dracunculus* L. (A. p. 90) |
| *Arum dracunculus* L. (A. p. 90) |
| ~*Asplenium onopteris* L. (LSJ,) ~*Dryopteris* L. sp. (A. p. 91) |
| *Quercu* s L sp. (A. p. 91) |
| *Echium plantagineum* L., *E. rubrum* L. (A. p. 90) |
| *Diospyrus ebenum Koenig* , *D . melanoxylon* Roxb. (A. p. 92) |
| *Althaea officinalis* L. |
| *Helleborus cyclophyllus* R. Br. (A. p. 93) |
| *Olea europaea* L. var. *silvestris* Miller (A. p. 176) |
| *Olea europaea* L. var. *sativa* Hoffm. and Lk. (A. p. 176) |

| **Botanical name** |
|---|
| |
| |
| |
| |
| |
| |
| |
| |
| |
| |
| |
| |
| |
| |
| |
| |
| |
| |
| |
| |
| *Linaria spuria* Miller (A. p. 93) |
| |
| *Pastinaca sativa* L. (A. p. 93) |
| *Salvia* .L sp |
| *Sambucus ebukus* L. |
| *Salvia* L. sp. (A. p. 93) |
| *Inula helenium* L.(A. p. 118) |
| *Thymus incanus* L. (A. p. 118) |
| *Apium graveolens* L. var. *silvestre* (A. p. 118) |
| *Helichrysum orientale* L., *H. stoechas* L., *H. siculum* L. (A. p. 118) |
| *Reseda alba* L. (A. p. 94) |
| *Veratrum album* L. (A. p. 94) |
| *Helleborus cyclophyllus* R. Br. |
| *Convolvulus arvensis* L. (A. p. 119) |
| *Parietaria officinalis* L. (A. p. 119) |
| *Parietaria officinalis* L. (A. p. 119) |
| *Frankenia hirsuta* L. and *F. pulverulenta* L. (A. p. 94) |
| *Datura stramonium* L. |
| *Lithospermum officinale* (A. p. 100) |
| *Cuscuta epithymum* L. (A. p. 95) |

| Greek name | English name | References |
|---|---|---|
| ἐπιμήδιον | *Epimedion* | IV, 19 |
| ἐπιμηλίς | Medlar | I, 118 |
| ἑπτάπλευρον | Plantain | II, 126 |
| ἐράνθεμον | Chamomile | III, 137 |
| ἐρέβινθος ὁ ἥμερος | Chickpea, Cultivated | II, 104 |
| ἐρείκη | Tree heath | I, 88 |
| ἐρευθέδανον | Madder | III, 143 |
| ἐρινεός | Wild fig | I, 128 |
| Ἑρμοῦ βοτάνιον | Mercury | IV, 189 |
| ἕρπυλος | Tufted thyme | III, 38 |
| ἕρπυλος ἄγριος μέγας | Bergamot mint | III, 41 |
| Ἐρυθραικὸν σατύριον | Man orchis | III,128 |
| ἐρυθρόδανον | Madder | III, 143 |
| ἐρυθρόν | Sumac | I, 108 |
| ἐρύσιμον | Hedge mustard | II, 158 |
| ἐρυσίσκηπτρον | Camel's-thorn | I, 20 |
| ἐρυσίσκηπτρον | Galingale | I, 4 |
| εὔζωμον | Rocket | II, 140 |
| Εὐπατόριος | Agrimony | IV, 41 |
| εὔπεπλον | Spurge laurel | IV, 146 |
| εὐπέταλον | Spurge laurel | IV, 146 |
| Εὐριπικὴ σχοῖνος | Euripic rush | IV, 52 |
| εὐφόρβιον | Spurge | III, 82 |
| ἔφεδρον | Horsetail | IV, 46 |
| ἐφήμερον | *Ephemeron* | IV, 84 |
| ἐφήμερον | Meadow saffron | IV, 83 |
| ἐχῖνος | *Echinos* | IV, 141 |
| ἔχιον | Catchfly | IV, 28 |
| ἔχιον | *Echion* | IV, 27 |
| ζαλεία | Daphne Alexandreia | IV, 145 |
| ζέα | Rosemary frankincense | III, 74 |
| ζέα | Wheat *zea* | II, 89 |
| ζὲα δίκοκκος | Wheat *zea* , two-seeded | II, 89 |
| ζὲα μονόκκοκος | Wheat *zea* , one-seeded | II, 89 |
| ζιγγιβέρι | Cinnamon | I, 14 |
| ζιγγίβερι | Ginger | II, 160 |
| ζυγίς | Tufted thyme | III, 38 |
| ζῦθος | Beer | II, 87 |
| ζῳόφθαλμον | Houseleek | IV, 88 |
| ζώπισσα | *Zopissa* | I, 72 |

| **Botanical name** |
|---|
| Unidentified |
| *Mespilus germanica* L. (A. p. 95) |
| *Plantago* L. sp. (A. p. 120) |
| *Matricaria chamomilla* |
| *Cicer arietinum* L. (A. p. 96) |
| *Erica arborea* L. (A. p. 96) |
| *Rubia tinctorum* L., *R. peregrina* L. (A. p. 96) |
| *Ficus carica* L. (A. pp. 48 and 96) |
| *Mercurialis annua* L. (A. p. 122) |
| *Thymus Sibthorpii* (LSJ) |
| *Mentha silvestris* L., *M. viridis* L. (A. p. 122) |
| *Serapias cordiga* L. (A. p. 228) |
| *Rubia tinctorum* L., *R. peregrina* L. (A. p. 98) |
| *Rhus coriaria* L. (LSJ) |
| *Sisymbrium officinale* Scop., *S. iri* o L. (A. p. 98) |
| *Alhagi maurorum* L. (A. p. 98) |
| *Cyperus rotundus* L. (A. p. 98) |
| *Eruca sativa Lam* . (A. p. 100) |
| *Agrimonia eupatoria* L. (A. p. 99) |
| *Daphne laureola* L. |
| *Daphne laureola* L. (A. p. 99) |
| *Scirpus* L. sp., *Juncus* L. sp. (A. p. 229) |
| *Euphorbia resinifera* Berg. (A. p. 99) |
| *Equisetum silvaticum* L. (A. p. 124) |
| *Polygonatum multiflorum* All., P. *verticillatum* All. (A. p. 95) |
| *Colchicum* L. (A. p. 95) |
| Unidentified |
| *Silene gallica* L. (A 92) |
| *Echium plantagineum* L., *E. rubrum* L. (A. p. 92) |
| *Ruscus hypophyllum* L. (LSJ) |
| ~ *Cachrys libanotis* Koch sp. (A. p. 279) |
| *Triticum* L. sp. |
| *Triticum dicoccum* Schrek. (A. p. 279) |
| *Triticum monoccocum* Schrek. (A. p. 279) |
| Cinnamomum tamala Nees, *C. iners* Blume sp. |
| *Zingiber officinale* Roscoe (A. p. 279) |
| *Thymus Sibthorpii* (LSJ) |
| |
| *Sempervivum arboreum* L. (A. p. 280) |
| |

| Greek name | English name | References |
|---|---|---|
| Ζωπύριον | Horse thyme | III, 95 |
| ἡδύοσμον | Green mint | III, 34 |
| ἡδύσαρον | Axweed | III, 130 |
| ἡδύχρουν | *Hedychroun* unguent | I, 58 |
| ἤλεκτρον | Amber | I, 83 |
| ἡλιοσκόπιος | Sun spurge | IV, 164 |
| ἡλιοσκόπιος | Spurge | IV, 164 |
| ἡλιοτρόπιον τὸ μέγα | Large heliotrope | IV, 190 |
| ἡλιοτρόπιον τὸ μικρόν | Small heliotrope | IV, 191 |
| ἡμεροκαλλές | Martagon lily | III, 122 |
| ἡμεροκατάλλακτον | Martagon lily | III, 122 |
| ἡμιόνιον | Miltwaste | III, 134 |
| ἡμιονῖτις | Mule fern | III, 135 |
| Ἠπειρωτικὰ μῆλα | Rose apples | I, 115 |
| Ἡρακλεία | Figwort | IV, 35 |
| Ἡρακλεία | Frothy poppy | IV, 66 |
| Ἡρακλεία | Groomwell | III, 141 |
| Ἡρακλεία | Ironwort | IV, 33 |
| Ἡρακλεία | Marjoram | III, 29 |
| Ἡράκλεια | Pellitory | IV, 85 |
| Ἡράκλειον | Southernwood | III, 24 |
| Ἡράκλειον | Wormwood | III, 24 |
| ἠράνθεμον | Camomile | III, 137 |
| ἠρέμιον | Anemone poppy | II, 176 |
| ἠρέμιον | Scarlet windflower | II, 176 |
| ἠριγέρων | Groundsel | IV, 96 |
| ἠρύγγη | Eryngo | III, 21 |
| ἠρύγγιον | Eryngo | III, 21 |
| θαλασσόμελι | Honey and sea water | V, 12 |
| θαλίητρον | Meadow rue | IV, 97 |
| θαλλία | Caper | II, 173 |
| θαψία | Deadly carrot | IV, 153 |
| θέρμος | Lupine | II, 109 |
| θηλυπτερίς | Bracken | IV, 185 |
| θηλυφόνον | Leopard's bane | IV, 76 |
| θλάσπι | Sheparrd's purse | II, 156 |
| θορύβηθρον | *Leontopetalon* | III, 96 |
| θριδακίας | Mandrake, female | IV, 75 |
| θριδάξ ἀγρία | Lettuce, Wild | II, 136 |
| θριδάξ ἥμερος | Lettuce, Cultivated | II, 136 |

| **Botanical name** |
|---|
| *Calamintha clinopodium* Moris. = *Clinopodium vulgare* L.(A. p. 280) |
| *Mentha* L. |
| *Securigera securidaca* (A. p. 117) |
| |
| |
| *Euphorbia helioscopia* L. (A. p. 118) |
| *Euphorbia helioscopia* L. (A. p. 262) |
| *Heliotropium europaeum* L., *H. villosum* L., *H. supinum* L. (A. p.119) |
| *Chrozophora tinctoria* Juss. (A. p. 119) |
| *Lilium martagon* L. (A. p. 119) |
| *Lilium martagon* L. (A. p. 119) |
| *Ceterach officinarum* Willd. (A. p. 119) |
| *Scolopendrium hemionitis* Lag. (A. p. 120) |
| |
| *Scrofularia lucida* L. (LSJ) |
| *Silene inflata* Sm., *S. muscipula* L. (A. p. 120) |
| *Lithospermum officinale* L. (A. p.120) |
| *Sideritis romana* L. (A. p. 120) |
| ~*Origanum viride* Boiss. (A. p. 120) |
| *Parietaria officinalis* L. (A. p. 120) |
| *Artemisia abrotonon* L. |
| ~*Artemisia abrotonum* L. |
| *Metricaria camomilla* L. (A. p. 96) |
| *Anemone coronaria* L. (A. p. 96) |
| *Anemone coronaria* L. |
| *Senecio vulgaris* L. (A. p. 96) |
| *Eryngium campestre* L. (A, p. 97-98) |
| *Eryngium campestre* L. (A. pp. 97-98) |
| |
| *Thalictrum flavum* L., *Th. minus* L. (A. p. 258) |
| *Capparis spinosa* L. (A. p. 258) |
| *Thapsia garganica* L. (A. p. 258) |
| *Lupinus* L. (LSJ) |
| *Pteris aquilina* L. (A. p. 258) |
| ~*Doronicum pardalianche* s Jacq. (A. p. 258) |
| *Capsella bursa pastoris* L. (A. p. 259) |
| *Leontice leontopetalum* L. (A. p. 259) |
| *Mandragora autumnalis* Sprengel (A. p. 259) |
| *Lactuca scariola* L. (A. p. 260) |
| *Lactuca sativa* L. (A. p. 260) |

| Greek name | English name | References |
|---|---|---|
| θρυαλλίς | Mullein | IV, 103 |
| θρυαλλίς | Mullein | IV, 103 |
| θρυαλλίς | Sage of Jerusalem | IV, 103 |
| θρύον | Thorn apple | IV, 73 |
| θυλακῖτις | Mountain spikenard | I, 9 |
| θύμβρα | Savory | III, 37 |
| θυμελαία | Spurge flax | IV, 172 |
| θυμοξάλμη | Vinegar, Brine, Cretan thyı | V, 16 |
| θύμος | Cretan thyme | III, 36 |
| θυρσῖτις | Chokefitch | II, 142 |
| ἴασπις | Black turnip | IV, 56 |
| Ἰδαία | Daphne Alexandreia | IV, 145 |
| Ἰδαία ῥίζα | *Idaia rhiza* | IV, 44 |
| Ἰδαῖοι δάκτυλοι | Peony | III, 140 |
| ἱερὰ βοτάνη | Holy vervain | IV, 60 |
| ἰλλεκέβρα | Houseleek, Third kind of | IV, 90 |
| Ἰνδικὴ ἔβενος | Indian ebony | I, 98 |
| Ἰνδικὴ νάρδος | Indian spikenard | I, 7 |
| Ἰνδικὸν λύκιον | Indian *lycion* | I, 100 |
| ἰξία | Pine thistle | III, 8 |
| ἰξίας | Chameleon thistle | III, 9 |
| ἰξός | Birdlime | III, 89 |
| ἰξός | Oak mistletoe | III, 89 |
| ἴον | Violet | IV, 121 |
| ἱππολάπαθον | Dock sorrel | II, 115 |
| ἱππομανές | Caper | II, 173 |
| ἱππομάραθον | Horse fennel | III, 71 |
| ἱππομάραθον ἕτερον | Horse fennel, Another | III, 71 |
| ἱπποσέλινον | Alexanders | III, 67 |
| ἵππουρις | Horsetail | IV, 46 |
| ἵππουρις ἑτέρα | Horsetail, Another | IV, 47 |
| ἱπποφαές | Spurge | IV, 159 |
| ἱππόφαιστον | *Hippophaiston* | IV, 160 |
| ἱππόφαος | Spurge | IV, 159 |
| ἴρινον | Iris unguent | I, 56 |
| ἶρις | Iris | I, 1 |
| ἶρις ἀγρία | *Ephemeron* | IV, 84 |
| ἶρις ἀγρία | Gladwyn | IV, 22 |
| ἰσάτις | Woad | II, 184 |
| ἰσὰτις ἀγρία | Wild woad | II, 185 |

| Botanical name |
|---|
| *Verbascum* L. sp. (A. p. 260) |
| *Verbascum* L. sp. (A. p. 260) |
| *Verbascum* L. sp. (A. p. 260) |
| *Datura stramonium* L. |
| *Valeriana tuberosa* L. (A. p. 260) |
| *Satureia thymbra* L. sp. (A. p. 260) |
| *Daphne gnidium* L. (A. p. 260) |
| |
| *Satureia thymbra* L. (A. p. 260) |
| *Orobanche crenata* Forsk. (A. p. 260) |
| *Leontice chrysogonon* L. sp. (LSJ) |
| *Ruscus hypoglossum* L. (A. 130) |
| *Ruscus hypoglossum* L. (LSJ) |
| *Paeonia* L. |
| *Verbena officinalis* L. (A. p. 123) |
| *Sedum* L. sp. (A. p. 8) |
| *Diospyrus ebenum* Koenig (A. p. 92) |
| *Nardostachys jatamansi* DC (A. p. 170) |
| *Acacia catechu* Willd. (A. p.149) |
| *Atractylis gummifera* L. (A. p. 134) |
| *Cardopatium corymbosum* Pers. (A. p. 60) |
| |
| *Hozanthus europaeus* (LSJ) |
| *Viola odorata* L. (A. p. 132) |
| *Rumex aquaticus* L. (A. p. 123) |
| *Capparis spinosa* L. (A. pp. 123-124) |
| ~*Prangos ferulacea* L. sp. (A. p. 124) |
| ~*Bifora testiculata* Rich. (A. p. 124) |
| *Smyrnium olusatrum* L. (A. p. 124) |
| *Equisetum silvaticum* L. (A. p. 124) |
| *Equisetum maximum* Lmk = *E. telmateia* Ehr. (A. p. 124) |
| *Euphorbia acanthothamnos* Heldr. and Sart. (A. p. 124) |
| *Centaurea spinosa* L. (A. p. 124) |
| *Euphorbia acanthothamnos* Heldr. and Sart. (A. p. 124) |
| |
| *Iris florentina* L., *I. germanica* L., *I. pallida* Lamk. (A. p. 133) |
| *Polygonatum multiflorum* All. and *P. verticillatum* All. (A. p 133) |
| *Iris* L. sp. (A. p. 278) |
| *Isatis tinctoria* L. (A. p. 133) |
| *Isatis agrestis* L. (A . p.133) |

| **Greek name** | **English name** | **References** |
|---|---|---|
| ἰσόπυρον | Fumitory | IV, 120 |
| ἰσχάς | Tuberous spurge | IV, 175 |
| ἰσχιάς | Tuberous thistle | III, 19 |
| ἰτέα | Willow | I, 104 |
| ἰωνία | Ground pine | III, 158 |
| ἰωνίτης | Caper | II, 173 |
| κάγκαμον | Bisabol | I, 24 |
| κακκαλία | *Caccalia* | IV, 122 |
| κακκαλία | Sleepy nightshade | IV, 72 |
| καλαμάγρωστις | *Calamagrostis* | IV, 30 |
| καλαμάγρωστις | *Calamagrostis* | IV, 30 |
| καλαμίνθη | Catmint | III, 35 |
| κάλαμος ἀρωματικός | Sweet flag | I, 18 |
| κάλαμος, Κύπριος | Reed, Cyprian | I, 85 |
| κάλαμος, δονάξ | Reed, *donax* | I, 85 |
| κάλαμος, θῆλυς | Reed, *thelys* | I, 85 |
| κάλαμος, νάστος | Reed, *nastos* | I, 85 |
| κάλαμος, συριγγίας | Reed, *syringias* | I, 85 |
| κάλαμος, φραγμίτης | Reed, *phragmites* | I, 85 |
| κάλαμος(οι) | Reed(s) | I, 85 |
| καλλέας | *Dorycnion* | IV, 74 |
| καλλία | Camomile | III, 137 |
| καλλιπέταλον | Cinquefoil | IV, 42 |
| κάλυξ | Alkanet | IV, 23 |
| κάμμαρον | Leopard's bane | IV, 76 |
| καμψάνεμα | Rosemary frankincense | III, 74 |
| κάνναβις | Hemp | III, 148 |
| κάνναβις ἀγρία | Hemp mallow | III, 149 |
| Κανωπικόν | Quacksalver's spurge | IV, 165 |
| καπνός | Fumitory | IV, 109 |
| κάππαρις | Caper | II, 173 |
| καπρία | Caper | II, 173 |
| καρδαμίνη | Water cress | II, 128 |
| κάρδαμον | Garden cress | II, 155 |
| καρδάμωμον | Cardamom | I, 6 |
| καρκίνωθρον | Knotgrass | IV, 4 |
| καρυίτης | Spurge | IV, 164 |
| καρυίτις | Myrtle spurge | IV, 164 |
| κάρυον | Eryngo | III, 21 |
| κάρυον βασιλικόν | Walnut | I, 125 |

| **Botanical name** |
|---|
| *Corydalis claviculata* Pers. (A. p. 133) |
| *Euphorbia apios* L. (A. p. 133) |
| *Cnicus tuberosus* L. or *Cirstium tuberosum* All. (A. p. 133) |
| *Salix* L. sp. (A. p. 134) |
| *Ajuga hamaepitys* Schreb. |
| *Capparis spinosa* L. |
| ~*Commiphora kataf* Forsk., ~*Styrax benzoin* Dryand. (A. p. 47) |
| ~*Senecio thapsoides* DC., ~*Mercurialis tomentosa* L. (A. p. 43) |
| *Withania somnifera* Dun. |
| ~*Calamagrostis epigeios* Roth, ~*Sorgum halepense* L., |
| ~*Dactyloctenium aegyptiacum* Willd. = *Cynosurus aegyptius* L. (A. p. 44) |
| *Calamintha* Lmk. sp. (A. p. 44) |
| *Acorus calamus* L. (A. p. 45) |
| *Arundo donax* L. (A. p. 45) |
| *Arundo dona* x L. |
| *Arundo* sp. |
| *Arundo pliniana* Turra (A. pp. 45 and 170) |
| *Arundo* sp. |
| *Arundo* sp. (A. p. 45) |
| *Arundines* (LSJ) |
| *Convolvulus oleaefolius* Desr. |
| *Chamomilla* sp. |
| *Potentilla reptans* L. (A. p. 278) |
| *Anchusa tinctoria* L. (A. p. 46) |
| ~*Doronicum pardalianches* Jacq. (A. p. 46) |
| ~*Cachris libanotis* Koch sp. (A. p. 46) |
| *Cannabis sativa* L. (A. p. 47) |
| *Althaea cannabina* L. (A. p. 47) |
| *Euphorbia pityusa* L. |
| *Fumaria officinalis* L. (A. p. 48) |
| *Capparis spinosa* L. (A. p. 48) |
| *Capparis spinosa* L. |
| *Nasturtium officinale* R. Br. (A. p. 49) |
| *Lepidium sativum* L. (A. p. 49) |
| *Elettaria cardamomum* White and Maton and other spp. (A. p. 49) |
| *Polygonum aviculare* L. (A. p. 49) |
| *Euphorbia myrsinitis* L. (A. p. 52) |
| *Euphorbia myrsinites* L. (A. p. 52) |
| *Eryngium campestre* L. |
| *Juglans regia* L. (A. p. 52) |

| **Botanical name** |
|---|
| *Juglans regia* L. (A. p. 52) |
| *Corylus avellana* L. |
| *Trigonella fenum graecum* L. (A. p. 51) |
| *Carum carvi* L. (A. p. 51) |
| *Cinnamomum cassia* Blume (A. p. 52) |
| *Castanea vulgaris* Lam. (A. p. 52) |
| *Ornithopus compressu* s L. (A. p. 53) |
| ~*Caucalis grandiflora* L. (A. p. 53) |
| |
| *Chrysanthemum coronarium* L. |
| |
| *Panicum miliaceum* L. (LSJ) |
| |
| *Malus medica* Risso (A. pp. 68, 153) |
| *Juniperus* L. (LSJ) |
| *Bryonia dioica* Jacq., *B. cretica* Fr. (A. p. 54) |
| *Erythraea centaurium* (A. p. 55) |
| *Erythraea centaurium* (A. p. 55) |
| *Centaurea centaurium* L. (A. p. 55) |
| *Daucus guttatus L.* (LSJ; see also A. pp. 57 and 248)) |
| *Trigonella fenum graecum* L. |
| *Prunus avium* (LSJ) |
| *Ceratonia siliqua* L. (LSJ) |
| *Stachys officinalis* L. (A. pp. 209-210) |
| |
| ~*Evax pygmaea* Pers. ,~*E. asterifoli* a Pers., (A. p. 55) ~*Plantago cretica* L., |
| ~*Gnaphalium leontopodium* (A. p. 55) |
| *Sedum cepaia* L. (A. p. 56) |
| *Ricinus communi* s L. (A. p. 66) |
| |
| *Cinnamomum tamala Nees* , *C. iners* Blume (A. p. 67) |
| *Ruscus aculeatus* L. |
| *Hordeum marinum* LSJ) |
| *Vincetoxicum nigrum* Moench (LSJ) |
| *Madragora* L. sp. (LSJ) |
| *Cistus* L. sp. (A. p. 68) |
| *Cistus* L. sp. (A. p. 68) |
| *Cistus villosus* L. (A. p. 68) |
| *Cistus salviaefolius* L. (A. p. 68) |
| *Cistus cyprius* (LSJ) |

| **Botanical name** |
|---|
| *Convolvulus arvensis* L. (A. p. 67) |
| *Lonicera periclimenum* (A. p. 67) |
| *Cistus* L. sp. (A. p. 68) |
| *Hedera helix* L. (A. p. 67) |
| *Citrus medica* Risso (A. pp. 68, 153) |
| |
| *Cichorium intybus* L. (LSJ) |
| *Anagallis arvensis* L. (A. p. 65) |
| *Calamintha clinopodium* L. (A. p. 69) |
| *Inula helenium* L. (A. p. 181) |
| *Polygonum aviculare* L. (A. 69) |
| *Euphorbia pityusa* L. (A. p. 69) |
| *Vinca minor* L. (A. p. 69) |
| *Clematis vitalba* L., *C. cirrosa* L., *C. flammula* L. (A. p. 69) |
| *Aristolochia clematitis* L. (A. p. 25) |
| *Calamintha clinopodium* Moris. = *Clinopodium vulgare* L. (A. p. 69) |
| *Parietaria officinalis* L. (A. p. 69) |
| *Scorpiurus vermiculatus* L. (A. p. 69) |
| *Lonicera etrusca* L. (A. p. 69) |
| *Daphne gnidium* L. (A. p. 70) |
| *Psorolea bituminosa* L. (A. p. 319) |
| *Cartharmus tinctorius* L. (A. p. 69) |
| *Carthamus lanatus* L. (A. p. 69) |
| *Daphne gnidium* L. (A. p. 70) |
| *Urtica* L. (A. p. 70) |
| *Quercus coccifera* L. (A. p. 70) |
| *Daphne oleides* L. and *D. oleafolia* L. (A. p. 70) |
| *Prunus domestica* L. (A. p. 71) |
| *Citrullus colocynthis* Schrad. (A. p. 71) |
| *Lagenaria vulgaris* Ser. (A. p. 71) |
| *Citrullus colocynthis* Schrad. (A. p. 71) |
| *Colchicum* L. sp. (A. p. 71) |
| *Arbutus unedo* L. (A. p. 72) |
| *Tragopogon porrifolius* L. (A. p. 73) |
| *Euphorbia Sibthorpii* Boiss. (A. p. 73) |
| |
| |
| |
| |
| |

| **Botanical name** |
| --- |
| |
| ~*Origanum viride* Boiss. (A. p. 73) |
| *Origanum heracleoticum* Rchb. and *O. vulgare* L. |
| *Inula* sp. |
| *Inula viscosa* Aiton (A. p. 74) |
| *Inula graveolens* Desf. (A. p. 74) |
| *Inula Britannica* L. (A. p. 74) |
| *Coriandrum sativum* L. (A. p. 75) |
| *Hypericum crispum* L. (A. p. 75) |
| *Hypericum empetrifolium* Willd., ~ *H. coris* L. (A. p. 75) |
| *Plantago coronopus* (LSJ) |
| *Saussurea lappa* Clarke (A. p. 76) |
| *Olea europaea* L. var. *silvestris* Miller (A. p. 76) |
| *Umbilicus pendulinus* DC. (A. p. 77) |
| *Saxifrage* L. sp. (A. p. 77) |
| |
| *Brassica oleracea* L. ~ var. *silvestris,* ~ *B. cretica* (A. p. 38) |
| *Brassica oleracea* L. (A. p. 77) |
| *Convolvulus soldanella* L. (A. p. 38 s. v. brassica) |
| *Euphorbia pityusa* L. (A. p. 77) |
| *Cornus mas* (LSJ) |
| *Polygonum persicaria* L. (A. p. 77) |
| *Crithmum maritimum* L. (A. p. 78) |
| *Athamanta cretensis* L. (LSJ) |
| *Hordeum* L. sp. |
| *Chelidonium majus* L. |
| |
| |
| *Lilium candidum* (LSJ) |
| *Cicer arietinum* L. (A. p. 78) |
| ~*Carduus pycnocephalus* L., ~*C. tenuiflorus* Curtis (A. p. 67) |
| |
| *Eryngium maritinum* (LSJ) |
| |
| *Crocus sativus* L. (A. p. 79) |
| *Allium cepa* (LSJ) |
| *Ricinus communis* L. (A. p. 79) |
| *Plantago psyllium* L. and *P. cynops* L. (A. p. 79) |
| *Nelumbo nucifera* Gaert. (A. p. 82) |
| *Vicia faba* L. (LSJ) |

| Greek name | English name | References |
|---|---|---|
| κύαμος Ποντικός | Bean, Egyptian | II, 106 |
| κυδώνια | Quinces | I, 115 |
| κυδωνόμελι | Honey flavored with quinc | V, 21 |
| κυκλάμινος | Cyclamen | II, 164 |
| κυκλάμινος ἑτέρα | Cyclamen, Another | II, 165 |
| κυμβάλιον | Navelwort | IV, 91 |
| κύμινον ἄγριον | Wild cumin | III, 60 |
| κύμινον ἕτερον γένος | Wild cumin, Another | III, 61 |
| κύμινον ἥμερον | Cultivated cumin | III, 59 |
| κύναγχον | Dogbane | IV, 80 |
| κυνόζολον | Chameleon thistle | III, 9 |
| κυνοκέφαλον | Fleawort | IV, 69 |
| κυνοκράμβη | Dogbane | IV, 80 |
| κυνοκτόνον | Leopard's bane | IV, 76 |
| κυνόμαζον | Chameleon thistle | III, 9 |
| κυνομόριον | Chokefitch | II, 142 |
| κυνόμορον | Dogbane | IV, 80 |
| κυνόμυια | Fleawort | IV, 69 |
| κυνόσβατος | Caper | II, 173 |
| κυνόσβατος | White rose | I, 94 |
| κυπαρισσίας | Spurge | IV, 164 |
| κυπάρισσσος | Cypress | I, 74 |
| κύπερος | Galingale | I, 4 |
| κυπὲρου ἕτερον | Turmeric | I, 5 |
| κυπὲρου ἕτερον | Galingale, Another | I, 5 |
| κύπρινον | Henna unguent | I, 55 |
| κύπρος | Henna | I, 95 |
| κυτίνος | Pomegranate flower | I, 110 |
| κύτινος | Hypocist | I, 97 |
| κύτισος | Tree medick | IV, 112 |
| κωβιός | Spurge | IV, 164 |
| κωδύα | Poppy, capsule | IV, 64 |
| κώνειον | Hemlock | IV, 78 |
| λαγώπουν | Hare's foot trefoil | IV,17 |
| λάδανον | Gum ladanum | I, 97 |
| λάδανον | Tuberous thistle | III, 19 |
| λαθυρίς | Caper spurge | IV, 166 |
| λαμψάνη | Charlock | II, 116 |
| λάπαθον | Monk's rhubarb | II, 114 |
| λάπαθον ἄγριον | Dock | II, 114 |

| **Botanical name** |
|---|
| *Nelumbo nucifera* Gaert. (A. p. 82) |
| |
| |
| *Cyclamen graecum* Link. (A. p. 82) |
| *Lonicera periclymenum* L. (A. p. 82) |
| *Umbilicus pendulinus* DC. |
| *Lagoecia cuminoides* L. (A. p. 81) |
| *Nigella arvensis* (LSJ) |
| *Cuminum cyminum* L. (A. p. 81) |
| *Cynanchum acutum* L., for Orient: *Marsdenia erect* a Br. |
| *Cardopatium corymbosum* Pers. (A. p. 84) |
| *Plantago psyllium* L. and *P. cynops* L. |
| *Cynanchum acutum* L., for Orient: *Marsdenia erecta* Br. (A. p. 83) |
| ~ *Doronicum pardalianche* s Jacq. |
| *Cardopatium corymbosum* Pers. (A. p. 84) |
| *Orobanche crenata* Forsk. (A. p. 84) |
| *Cynanchum acutum* L., for Orient: *Marsdenia erecta* Br. |
| *Plantago psyllium* L. and *P. cynop* s L. (A. p. 84) |
| *Capparis spinosa* L. (A. p. 84) |
| *Rosa sempervirens* L. (A. p. 84) |
| *Euphorbia cyparissias* L. (A. p. 262) |
| *Cupressus sempervirens* L. (LSJ) |
| *Cyperus rotundus* L. (A. p. 85) |
| *Curcuma longa* L. (A. p. 85) |
| *Curcuma longa* L. (A. p. 85) |
| |
| *Lawsonia inermis* L. (A. p. 85) |
| |
| *Cytinus hypocistis* L. (A. p. 85) |
| *Medicago arborea* L. (A. p. 85) |
| *Euphorbia Sibthorpii* Boiss. (A. p. 70) |
| |
| *Conium maculatum* L. (A. p. 73) |
| *Trifolium arvense* L. (A . p. 137) |
| *Cistus creticus* L., *C. cyprius* L. (A. p. 137) |
| *Cnicus tuberosus* L. or *Cirstium tuberosum* All. |
| *Euphorbia lathyris* L. (A. p. 139) |
| *Raphanus raphanistrum* L. (A. p.138) |
| *Rumex* L. sp. (A. p. 137) |
| *Rumex conglomeratus* L. (LSJ) |

| **Botanical name** |
| --- |
| |
| *~Senecio thapsoides* DC., *~Mercurialis tomentosa* L. (A. pp. 140-141) |
| *Beta maritima* L. (A. p. 146) |
| |
| *Lilium candidum* L. (A. p. 145) |
| |
| |
| *Ruscus aculeatus* L. |
| *Leontice leontopetalum* (LSJ) |
| *Leontice leontopetalum* L. (A. p. 142) |
| *Lepidium latifolium* L. (A. p. 142) |
| *Corylus avellana* L. |
| *Cnicus tuberosus* L. or *Cirstium tuberosum* All. (A. p. 142) |
| *Lloydia graeca* L. |
| *Matricaria chamomilla* L. |
| *Chrysanthemum parthenium* Bernh. |
| *Lamium album* L. (A. p. 143) |
| *Populus alba* L. (A. p. 143) |
| *Leontice leontopetalum* L. (A. p. 143) |
| *Matthiola incana* L. (A. p. 142) |
| *Orobanche crenata* Forsk. (A. p. 141) |
| *Cistus creticus* L. (A. p. 141) |
| *Boswellia* sp. (LSJ) |
| *~Cachris libanotis* Koch, *~Lecokia graeca (* Andrews), *~Prangos ferulea* L (A. p.144) |
| *Rosmarinus officinalis* L. (A. p. 144) |
| *Rosmarinum sterile (* LSJ, (see A. p. 144) |
| *Ferula ferulago* L . = *Ferulago galbanifera* Koch (A. p. 144) |
| *~Cachrys libanotis* Koch sp. (A. p. 144) |
| |
| |
| |
| |
| |
| |
| |
| *Levisticum officinale* Koch (A. p. 145) |
| *Lithospermum officinale* L. (A. p.147) |
| *Erythraea centaurium* L. (A. p. 145) |
| *Teucrium chamaedrys* L. *and T. lucidum* L. *(A. p. 146)* |
| *Mercurialis annua* L. (A. p. 146) |

| **Botanical name** |
|---|
| *Euphorbia apios* L. |
| *Leontice chrysogonon* L. sp. (LSJ) |
| *Daphne gnidium* L. |
| *Linum usitatissimum* (LSJ) |
| *Serapias lingua* L. (A. p. 147) |
| *Aspidium lonchitis* L. (A. p. 147) |
| *Castanea vulgaris* Lam. |
| *Colocasia antiquorum* Schott |
| |
| *Vitex agnus-castus* L. (A. p. 150) |
| *Echium italicum* L sp. (A. p. 149) |
| *Rhamnus petiolaris, Rh. lycoides, Rh. punctata* Boiss. (A. p.149) |
| *Aconitum napellus* L. (A. p. 149) |
| *Alisma plantago* L., *A. arcuatum* Mich. (A. p. 150) |
| *Lysimachia vulgaris* L. (A. p. 150) |
| *Antirrhinum orontium* L. (A. p. 149) |
| *Agrostemma githago* L. (A. p. 149) |
| *Lychnis coronaria* Desr. (A. p. 149) |
| *Verbascum* L. sp.(A. p. 149) |
| *Verbascum* L. sp. (A. p. 149) |
| *Verbascum* L. sp. (A. p. 149) |
| *Trigonella fenum graecum* L. (A. p.148) |
| *Trigonella elatior* Sibth. sp., *T. gladiata* L. sp. (A. p. 148) |
| *Melilotus Adans*. sp. (A. pp. 147-148) |
| *Nelumbo nucifera* Gaert. (A. p. 148) |
| *Celtis australis* L. (A. p. 147) |
| |
| *Bryonia dioica* Jacq. (A. p. 151) |
| *Holarrhena antidysenterica* Wall. (A. p. 151) |
| |
| ~*Cinnamomum tamala* Nees, ~*C. iners* Blume, , (A. p. 152) |
| ~*C. zeylanicum Blume*, ~*Pogostemon patchouli* Pell. (A. p. 152) |
| ~*Commiphora mukul* Engl. (A. p. 151-152) |
| *Madragora* L. sp. (A. pp. 153-154) |
| *Mandragora vernalis* Bert. (A. p. 154) |
| *Mandragora autumnalis* Sprengel (A. p. 154) |
| *Foeniculum vulgare* Gaertn. (A. p. 155) |
| *Amaracus sipyleus* Rafin (A. p. 154) |
| *Gladiolus segetum* Gawler (A. p. 151) |
| |

| **Botanical name** |
|---|
| *Helleborus cyclophyllus* R. Br. (A. p. 157) |
| *Ballota nigra* L. |
| ~*Chamaelina sativa* Crantz, var. *microcarpa* Andrz. (A. p. 157) |
| *Acanthus mollis* L. (A. p. 157) |
| *Nigella sativa* L. (A. p. 157) |
| |
| *Fraxinus ornus* L. (LSJ) |
| |
| *Melilotus* Adans. sp. (A. p. 158) |
| *Pyrus praecox* (LSJ) |
| *Setaria italica* P. B. (A. p. 158) |
| *Melissa officinalis* L., *M. altissima* Sibth. and Sm. (A. p. 158) |
| |
| *Melissa officinalis* L., *M. altissima* Sibth. and Sm. (A. p. 158) |
| |
| |
| *Mespilus germanica* L. (A. p. 160) |
| |
| (A. p. 160) |
| *Ferula galbaniflua* Boiss. & Buhse (A. p. 160) |
| *Citrus medica* Risso (A. p. 153) |
| *Medicago sativa* L. (A. p.157) |
| *Inula helenium* L. (A. p. 253) |
| *Medicago sativa* L. (A. p.157) |
| ~*Campanula lingulata* L. (A. p. 157) |
| *Papaver somniferum* L. (A. p. 156) |
| *Glaucium flavum* Crantz |
| *Silene inflata* Sm., *S. muscipula* L. (A. p. 156) |
| *Euphorbia peplis* L. (A. p. 156) |
| *Papaver somniferum* L. |
| *Glaucium flavum* Crantz (A. p. 57) |
| *Glaucium flavum* Crantz (A. p. 188) |
| *Papaver somniferum* L. |
| *Papaver rhoeas* L. (A. p. 156) |
| *Papaver somniferum* L. |
| |
| *Prunus armeniaca* L. |
| *Matricaria chamomilla* L. (A. p. 157) |
| *Pirus malus* L. (A. p. 115) |
| |

| **Botanical name** |
|---|
| |
| *Pyrus acerba* (LSJ) |
| Unidentified |
| *Capparis spinosa* L. |
| *Bryonia dioica* Jacq. (A. p. 159) |
| *Meum athamanticum* Jacq. (A. pp. 160-161) |
| *Meum athamanticum* Jacq. (A. pp. 160-161) |
| *Convolvulus sepium* L. (A. p. 161) |
| *Smilax aspera* L. (A. p. 161) |
| |
| *Mentha* L. |
| *Psorolea bituminosa* L. (A. p. 162) |
| *Malva silvestris* (LSJ) |
| *Morus nigra* L. (A. p. 164) |
| *Cinnmomum cassia* sp. |
| *Cinnamomun tamala* Nees, C. *iners* Blume sp. |
| *Castanea vulgaris* Lam. (A. p. 52) |
| ~*Chamaelina sativa* Crantz, var. *microcarpa* Andrz. (A. p. 166) |
| *Fungi* |
| ~*Doronicum pardalianches* Jacq. |
| *Asperugo procumbens* L. (A. p. 166) |
| *Thelygonum cynocrambe* L. = *Cynocrambe prostrata* Gaertn. (A. p. 166) |
| *Asperugo procumbens* L. (A. p. 166) |
| *Tamarix tetrandra* Pall. (A. p. 167) |
| *Tamarix articulata* (LSJ) |
| *Myriophyllum spicatum* L. (A. p. 167) |
| *Myrrhis odorata* Scop. (A. p. 167) |
| *Myrrhis odorata* Scop. (A. p. 167) |
| *Ruscus aculeatus* L. |
| *Myrtus communis* L. (LSJ) |
| *Euphorbia myrsinites* L. (A. p. 167) |
| *Euphorbia myrsinites* L. (A. 262) |
| *Vinca minor* L. (A. p.167) |
| *Ruscus aculeatus* L. (A. p. 167) |
| |
| *Polygonum aviculare* L. (A. p. 168) |
| |
| ~*Allium nigrum* L. (A. p. 163) |
| *Peganum harmala* L. (A. p. 163) |
| *Mandragora vernalis* Bert. (A. p. 164) |

| Greek name | English name | References |
|---|---|---|
| μώριος ἑτέρα | Sleepy nightshade, Another | IV, 75 |
| νᾶπυ | Mustard | II, 154 |
| νάρδινον | Spikenard unguent | I, 62 |
| νάρδος | Spikenard | I, 7 |
| νὰρδος ἀγρία | Cretan spikenard | I, 11 |
| νὰρδος ἀγρία | Hazelwort | I, 10 |
| νὰρδος Ἰνδική | Indian spikenard | I, 7 |
| νὰρδος Κελτική | Celtic spikenard | I, 8 |
| νάρδος ὀρεινή | Mountain sipkenard | I, 9 |
| νὰρδος Συριακή | Syrian spikenard | I, 7 |
| νάρθηξ | Giant fennel | III, 77 |
| νάρκαφθον | *Narcaphthon* | I, 23 |
| νάρκη | Centaury | III, 6 |
| ναρκίσσινον | Narcissus unguent | I, 53 |
| νάρκισσος | Narcissus | IV, 158 |
| νάσκαφθον | *Narcaphthon* | I, 23 |
| νάφθα | Naphtha | I, 73 |
| νεκτάριον | Elecampane | I, 28 |
| νεπέτα | Catmint | III, 35 |
| νευράς | Goat's thorn | III, 15 |
| νευροειδές | Sea lavender | IV, 16 |
| νήριον | Oleander | IV, 81 |
| νυμφαία | White water lily | III, 132 |
| νυμφαὶα ἄλλη | White water lily, Another | III, 132 |
| νυμφαὶα πτερίς | Bracken | IV, 185 |
| ξάνθιον | Broad-leaved burweed | IV, 136 |
| ξιρίς | Gladwyn | IV, 22 |
| ξίφιον | Corn flag | IV, 20 |
| ξυλοβάλσαμον | *Xylobalsamon* | I, 19 |
| ξυλοκινάμωμον | *Xylocinamomon* | I, 14 |
| ξυλόλωτον | Cinquefoil | IV, 42 |
| ξυλοπέταλον | Cinquefoil | IV, 42 |
| ξυρίς | Gladwyn | II, 22 |
| ὀθόννα | *Othonna* | II, 182 |
| οἰνάνθη | Dropwort | III, 120 |
| οἰνάνθη | Grape, Inflo'ce of wild | V, 2; V, 4 |
| οἰνάνθινον | Wild vine unguent | I, 46 |
| οἰνάνθινος | Wine, Wild grape flowers | V, 25 |
| οἶνοι | Wines | V, 6 |
| οἰνόμελι | Wine and honey mixture | V, 8 |

| **Botanical name** |
|---|
| *Withania somnifera* Dun. (LSJ) |
| *Sinapis alba* L. (A. 169) |
| |
| *Nardostachys jatamansi* DC (A. p. 170), *Patrinia scabiosifolia* Fisch. (A. p. 170) |
| *Valeriana phu* L. (A. p. 170) |
| *Asarum europaeum* L. |
| *Nardostachys jatamansi* DC. (A. p. 170) |
| *Valeriana celtica* L. (A. p. 170) |
| *Valeriana tuberosa* L. (A. p. 170) |
| *Patrinia scabiosifolia* Fisch. (A. p. 170) |
| *Ferula communis* L. (A. p. 170) |
| Underermined |
| *Centaurea centaurium* L. (A. p. 169) |
| |
| *Narcissus poeticus* L. (A. p. 169) |
| Undetermined |
| |
| *Inula helenium* L. (A. p. 157) |
| *Calamintha nepeta* Savi (A. p. 171) |
| *Astagalus poterium* Labill. (A. p. 171) |
| *Beta maritima* L. (A. p. 172) |
| *Nerium oleander* L. (A. p. 171) |
| *Nymphaea alba* L. (A. p. 174) |
| *Nuphar luteum* Sm. (A. p. 174) |
| *Pteris aquilina* L.(A. p. 174) |
| *Xanthium strumarium* L. (A. p. 278) |
| *Iris* L. sp. (A. p. 278) |
| *Gladiolus segetum* Gawler (A. p. 278) |
| |
| *Cinnamomum* sp. (A. p. 278) |
| *Potentilla reptans* L. (A. p. 278) |
| *Potentilla reptans* L. |
| *Iri* s L. sp. (A. p. 278) |
| |
| *Spiraea filipendula* L. (A. p. 177) |
| Vitis silvestris Gmel. (A. p.176) |
| |
| |
| |
| |

**Botanical name**

| Greek name | English name | References |
|---|---|---|
| οἶνος κυδωνίτης | Wine, Quince | V, 20 |
| οἶνος κυπαρίσσινος | Wine, Cypress | V, 36 |
| οἶνος μανδραγορίτης | Wine, Mandrake | V. 71 |
| οἶνος μαραθίτης | Wine, Fennel | V, 65 |
| οἶνος μελιτίτης | Wine, Honey | V, 7 |
| οἶνος μηλίτης | Wine, Quince | V, 20 |
| οἶνος μυρσινίτης | Wine, Myrtles | V, 29 |
| οἶνος μυρτίτης | Wine, Myrtle | V, 28 |
| οἶνος ὁ τῶν μεσπίλων | Wine, Medlar | V, 24 |
| οἶνος ὀριγανίτης | Wine, Oregano | V, 52 |
| οἶνος οὔων | Wine, Sorb apple | V, 24 |
| οἶνος πανακίτης | Wine, Allheal | V, 62 |
| οἶνος πετροσελινίτης | Wine, Parsley | V, 65 |
| οἶνος πισσίτης | Wine, Pitch | V, 6 |
| οἶνος πιτύινος | Wine, Pitys pine | V, 36 |
| οἶνος πρὸς βῆχας | Wine, Coughs | V, 55 |
| οἶνος πρὸς ἐμπνευματώσεις | Wine, Flatulence | V, 55 |
| οἶνος πρὸς κατάρρους | Wine, Catarrhs | V, 55 |
| οἶνος πρὸς στομάχου πλάδον | Wine, Stomach fluid | V, 55 |
| οἶνος πρὸς ὠμότητας | Wine, Indigestion | V, 55 |
| οἶνος ῥητινίτης | Wine, Resin | V, 34 |
| οἶνος ῥοδίτης | Wine, Roses, Flavored with | V, 27 |
| οἶνος ῥοίτης | Wine, Pomegranate | V, 26 |
| οἶνος σελινίτης | Wine, Celery | V, 64 |
| οἶνος σκαμμωνίτης | Wine, Scammony | V, 73 |
| οἶνος στοιχαδίτης | Wine, French lavender | V, 42 |
| οἶνος στομάχου πλάδον | Wine, Stomach | V, 55 |
| οἶνος στροβιλίτης | Wine, *Strobilos* pine cones | V, 35 |
| οἶνος συκίτης | Wine, Fig | V, 32 |
| οἶνος συκομόρων | Wine, Sycamore fig | V, 33 |
| οἶνος σχίνινος | Wine, Mastic | V, 30 |
| οἶνος τερεβίνθινος | Wine, Terebinth | V, 30 |
| οἶνος τραγοριγανίτης | Wine, Goat's marjoram | V, 45 |
| οἶνος τροχίτης | Wine, Fig | V, 32 |
| οἰνός τρύξ | Wine, Lees of | V, 114 |
| οἶνος ὑσσωπίτης | Wine, Hyssop | V, 40 |
| οἶνος φθόριος ἐμβρύων | Wine, Abortifacient | V, 67 |
| οἶνος φοινικίτης | Wine, Date palm | V, 31 |
| οἶνος χαμαιδρυίτης | Wine, Germander | V, 41 |
| οἶνος χαμαιπιτύινος | Wine, Ground pine | V, 70 |

| Botanical name |
| --- |

| Greek name | English name | References |
|---|---|---|
| οἶνος χαμελαίτης | Wine, Spurge olive | V, 69 |
| οἶνος, δευτερίας | Wine, *Deuterias* | V, 6 |
| ὀλέσαθρον | Alexanders | III, 67 |
| ὁλόκυρος | Ground pine | III, 158 |
| ὁλόστεον | Allbone | IV, 11 |
| ὁλόσχοινος | Club-rush | IV, 52 |
| ὁλόφυτον | Caper | II, 173 |
| ὄλυνθος | Wild fig | I, 128 |
| ὄλυρα | Rice-wheat | II, 91 |
| ὀμφάκιον | *Omphacion* | V, 5 |
| ὀμφακίτης | *Omphacites* | V, 6 |
| ὀμφακῖτις | Oak gall | I, 107 |
| ὀμφακόμελι | Grapes, Unripe honey drin | V, 23 |
| ὀμφαλόκαρπον | Cleavers | III, 90 |
| ὀνάγρα | Oleander | IV, 117 |
| ὀνό‹θο›υρις | Oleander | IV, 117 |
| ὀνοβρυχίς | Cock's head | III, 153 |
| ὀνοθήρας | Oleander | IV, 117 |
| ὀνόκλεια | Alkanet | IV, 23 |
| ὄνοσμα | Stone bugloss | III, 131 |
| ὀνοχειλές | Alkanet, Another | IV, 24 |
| ὀνύχινον | Onyx unguent | I, 54 |
| ὀνωνίς | Rest harrow | III, 18 |
| ὄνωνις | Stone bugloss | III, 131 |
| ὀξαλίς | Monk's rhubarb | II, 114 |
| ὀξάλμη | Brine vinegar | V, 15 |
| ὄξος | Vinegar | V, 13 |
| ὄξος διὰ στοιχάδος | Vinegar, French lavender | V, 43 |
| ὄξος κέστρου ψυχροτρόφου | Vinegar, Betony | V, 44 |
| ὄξος σκιλλήτικον | Vinegar, Squill | V, 17 |
| ὄξους τρύξ | Vinegar, Lees of | V, 114 |
| ὀξυάκανθα | Fiery thorn | I, 93 |
| ὀξυάκανθα | White rose | I, 94 |
| ὀξυλάπαθον | Curled dock | II, 114 |
| ὀξύμελι | Oxymel | V, 14 |
| ὀξύμελι | Vinegar, Honey | V, 14 |
| ὀξυμυρσίνη | Butcher's broom | IV, 144 |
| ὀξύσχοινος | Rush | IV, 52 |
| ὀξύφυλλον | Treacle clover | III, 109 |
| ὀποβάλσαμον | *Opobalsamon* | I, 19 |

| **Botanical name** |
|---|
| |
| |
| *Smyrnium olusatrum* L. |
| *Ajuga hamaepitys* Schreb. (A. p. 125) |
| ~*Plantago Bellardii* All., ~ *P. albicans* L. (A. p. 125) |
| *Scirpus holoschoenus* L. (A. p. 125) |
| *Capparis spinosa* L. |
| |
| *Triticum dicoccum* (LSJ) |
| |
| |
| |
| |
| *Galium aparine* L. (A. p. 177) |
| *Epilobium angustifolium* L. (A. p. 178) |
| *Epilobium angustifolium* L. (A. p. 179) |
| *Onobrychis caput galli* Link.aAnd *O. viciaefolia* Scop. (A. p. 178) |
| *Epilobium angustifolium* L. (A. pp. 178-179) |
| *Anchusa tinctoria* L. (A. p.178) |
| *Onosma echinoides* L. (A. p. 178) |
| *Echium diffusum* Sibth. (A. p. 178) |
| |
| *Ononis antiquorum* L. (A. p. 178) |
| *Onosma echinoides* L. (A. p. 178) |
| *Rumex* sp. |
| |
| |
| |
| |
| |
| |
| *Cotoneaster pyracantha* Spach. (A. p. 183) |
| *Rosa sempervirens* L. (A. p. 183) |
| *Rumex crispus* L. (A. p. 183) |
| |
| |
| *Ruscus aculeatus* L. (A. p. 183) |
| *Juncus acutus* L. (A. p. 184) |
| *Psorolea bituminosa* L. (A. p. 183) |
| |

| Greek name | English name | References |
|---|---|---|
| ὀποπάναξ | Opopanax | III, 48 |
| ὀρβικλᾶτα | *Orbiclata* | I, 115 |
| ὀρεοσέλινον | Mountain parsley | III, 65 |
| Ὀρέστιον | Elecampane | I, 28 |
| ὀρθόγυιον | Thorn apple | IV, 73 |
| ὀρίγανος Ἡρακλεωτική | Oregano | III, 27 |
| ὅρμινον | Asparagus | II, 125 |
| ὅρμινον | Clary | III, 129 |
| ὄρνιθος γάλα | Starflower | II, 144 |
| ὀροβάγχη | Chokefitch | II, 142 |
| ὀρόβηθρον | Hypocist | I, 97 |
| ὀροβίας | Chickpea, Cultivated | II, 104 |
| ὄροβος | Bitter vetch | II, 108 |
| ὀρρός | Whey | II, 70 |
| ὄρυζα | Rice | II, 95 |
| ὄρχις | Orchid | III, 126 |
| ὄρχις ἕτερος | Orchid, Another | III, 127 |
| ὄρχις κυνός | Orchid | III, 126 |
| ὄσιρις | Poet's cassia | IV, 140 |
| ὀσμάς | Stone bugloss | III, 131 |
| οὐλοφόνιον | Chameleon thistle | III, 9 |
| οὖον | Sorb apple | I,120 |
| ὀφιόσκορδον | Caper | II, 173 |
| ὀφιοστάφυλον | Bryony | IV, 182 |
| ὀφιοστάφυλον | Caper | II, 173 |
| παγκράτιον | Sea daffodil | II, 172 |
| παιδέρως | Bear's-foot | III, 17 |
| παιωνία | Peony | III, 140 |
| παλίμπισσα | *Palimpissa* | I, 72 |
| παλίουρος | Christ's- thorn | I, 92 |
| πάνακες | Lovage | III, 51 |
| πάνακες | Marjoram | III, 29 |
| πάνακες | Allheal | III, 83 |
| πάνακες Ἀσκληπί‹ει›ον | Asculapius' allheal | III, 49 |
| πάνακες Ἡράκλειον | Hercules' woundwort | III, 48 |
| πάνακες Χειρώνιον | Chiron's allheal | III, 50 |
| πάπυρος | Papyrus | I, 86 |
| παράλιος | Quacksalver's spurge | IV, 165 |
| παράλιος | Spurge | IV, 164 |
| παρδαλιαγχές | Dogbane | IV, 80 |

| **Botanical name** |
| --- |
| *Opopanax hispidus* Grisb. (A. p. 179 and p.186 s.v panaces) |
| Unidentified |
| ~*Athamanta macedonica* L. (A. p. 181) |
| *Inula helenium* L. (A. p. 181) |
| *Datura stramonium* L. |
| *Origanum heracleoticum* Rchb. and *O. vulgare* L. (A. p. 181) |
| *Asparagus aspartilis* L. (A. p. 126) |
| *Salvia horminum* L. (A. p. 126) |
| *Ornithogalum umbellatum* L. (A. p. 181) |
| *Orobanche crenata* Forsk. (A. pp. 181-182) |
| *Cytinus hypocistis* L. (A. p. 182) |
| *Cicer arietinum* L. (A. p. 182) |
| *Vicia ervilia* Willd. (A. p. 182) |
| |
| *Oryza sativa* (LSJ) |
| ~*Orchis papilionacea* L., ~ *O. longicruris* L. (A. p. 180) |
| *Orchis morio* . L. sp. (.A. p. 180) |
| ~*Orchis papilionacea* L., ~ O. *longicruris* L. (A. p. 84) |
| *Osiris alba* L. (A. p. 183) |
| *Onosma echinoides* L. |
| *Cardopatium corymbosum Pers.* (A. p. 275) |
| *Sorbus domestica,* L. (LSJ) |
| *Capparis spinosa* L. (A. p. 179) |
| *Bryonia dioica* Jacq. (A. p. 179) |
| *Capparis spinosa* L. (A. p. 179) |
| *Pancratium maritimum* L. (A. p. 187) |
| *Acanthus mollis* L. (A. p. 185) |
| *Paeonia* L. sp. (A. p. 185) |
| |
| *Paliurus australis* Gaertn. = *P. spina Christi* Mill. (A. 185) |
| *Levisticum officinale* Koch (A. p. 187 ) |
| ~*Origanum viride* Boiss. (A. p. 187) |
| *Ferula galbaniflua* Boiss. And Buhse (A. p. 58) |
| ~*Ferula nodosa* L. or ~*Echinophora tenuifolia* L. (A. p. 186) |
| *Opoponax hispidus* Grisb. (A. p. 186) |
| *Hypericum olympicum* (LSJ) |
| *Cyperus papyrus* L. (A. p. 188) |
| *Euphorbia pityusa* L. (A. p. 188) |
| *Euphorbia paralias* L. (A. p. 261) |
| *Cynanchum acutum* L., for the Orient: *Marsdenia erecta* Br. (A. p. 189) |

| Greek name | English name | References |
|---|---|---|
| παρδαλιαγχές | Leopard's bane | IV, 76 |
| παρδάλιον | *Leontopetalon* | III, 96 |
| παρθένιον | Feverfew | III, 138 |
| παρθένιον | Mercury | IV, 189 |
| παρθένιον | Pellitory | IV, 85 |
| παρωνυχία | *Paronychia* | IV, 54 |
| πεδιάσιος λιπαρά | Myrrh | I, 64 |
| πελεκῖνος | Axweed | III, 130 |
| πενταδάκτυλον | Cinquefoil | IV, 42 |
| πενταπετές | Cinquefoil | IV, 42 |
| πεντάτομον | Cinquefoil | IV, 42 |
| πεντέφυλλον | Cinquefoil | IV, 42 |
| πεντόδρυον | Thorn apple | IV, 73 |
| πεντόροβος | Peony | III, 140 |
| πέπερι | Pepper | II, 159 |
| πέπερι λευκόν | Pepper, White | II, 159 |
| πέπερι μακρόν | Pepper, Long | II, 159 |
| πέπλιον | Wild purslane | IV, 168 |
| πεπλίς | Wild purslane | IV, 168 |
| πέπλος | Wartweed | IV, 167 |
| πέπων | Cucumber, ripe | II, 135 |
| πέπων | *Pepon* | II, 135 |
| περδίκιον | Pellitory | IV, 85 |
| περικλύμενον | Honeysuckle | IV, 14 |
| περισσόν | Thorn apple | IV, 73 |
| περιστερεών | Holy vervain | IV, 60 |
| περιστέριον | Vervain | IV, 59 |
| περσαία | Persea | I, 129 |
| πέρσειον | Thorn apple | IV, 73 |
| Περσικά | Citrons | I, 115 |
| Περσικὰ μῆλα | Peaches | I, 115 |
| Περσική | Elecampane | I, 28 |
| Περσικὸν σίνηπι | Sheparrd's purse | II, 156 |
| πετασῖτις | Butterbur | IV, 107 |
| πετραία | Caper | II, 173 |
| πετροσέλινον | Cretan alexanders | III, 68 |
| πετροσέλινον | Parsley | III, 66 |
| πετρώνιον | Coltsfoot | III, 112 |
| πευκέδανον | Sulphurwort | III, 78 |
| πεύκη | *Peuce* pine | I, 69 |

| **Botanical name** |
|---|
| ~ *Doronicum pardalianches* Jacq. (A. p. 189) |
| *Leontice leontopetalum* L. (A. p. 189) |
| *Chrysanthemum parthenium* Bernh. |
| *Mercurialis annua* L. (A. p. 189) |
| *Parietaria officinalis* L. (A. p. 189) |
| *Paronychia* Mill. sp. (A. p. 189) |
| |
| *Securigera securidaca* L. (A. p. 191) |
| *Potentilla reptans L.* (A. p. 191) |
| *Potentilla reptans* L. (A. p. 191) |
| *Potentilla reptans* L. (A. p. 191) |
| *Potentilla reptans* L. (A. p. 191) |
| *Datura stramonium* L. |
| *Paeonia* L. (A. p. 191) |
| *Piper nigrum* L. (A. p. 200) |
| *Piper album* L. (A. p. 200) |
| *Piper officinarum* DC. (A. p. 200) |
| *Euphorbia peplis* L. (A. p. 192) |
| *Euphorbia peplis* L. (A. p. 192) |
| *Euphorbia peplis* L. (A. p. 192) |
| *Cucumis sativus* L. (A. p. 80) |
| *Citrullus sativus* Schrad. (A. p. 192) |
| *Parietaria officinalis* L. (A. p. 192) |
| *Lonicera etrusca* L. (A. p. 192) |
| *Datura stramonium* L. |
| *Verbena officinalis* L. (A. p. 193) |
| *Lycopus europaeus* L. (A. p. 193) |
| *Mimusops Schimperi* L. (A. p. 193) |
| *Datura stramonium* L . |
| Citrus medica Risso |
| *Prunus persica* Sieb. and Z. (A. p. 153) |
| *Inula helenium* L. (LSJ) |
| ~*Lunaria alba* L., ~ *Sinapis alba* L., ~ *Brassica nigra* Koch (A. p. 259) |
| *Petasites officinalis* Moench (A. p. 194) |
| *Capparis spinosa* L. |
| *Smyrnium perfoliatum* Mill. (A. p. 1 95) |
| *Petroselinum hortense* Hoffm. (A. p. 195) |
| *Tussilago farfara* L. |
| *Peucedanum officinale* L. (A. p. 195) |
| *Pinus* sp. |

| Greek name | English name | References |
|---|---|---|
| πήγανον | Rue | III, 45 |
| πήγανον ἄγριον | Wild rue | III, 46 |
| πήγανον ὀρεινόν | Rue | III, 45 |
| πηκτή | Comfrey | IV, 10 |
| πήχιον | Coltsfoot | III, 112 |
| πίθιον | Coltsfoot | III, 112 |
| πίσσα | Pitch | I, 72 |
| πισσάσφαλτος | Pitch-asphalt | I, 73 |
| πισσέλαιον | Pitch-oil | I, 72 |
| πιστάκια | Pistachio nut | I, 124 |
| πιττάσφαλτος | Pitch-asphalt | I, 73 |
| πιτυίδες | Pine nuts | I, 69 |
| πιτυούσα | Quacksalver's spurge | IV, 165 |
| πίτυρον | Bran | II, 85 |
| πίτυς | *Pitys* pine | I, 69 |
| πίτυς | Stone pine *cembra* | I, 69 |
| πλάτανος | Plane tree | I, 79 |
| πλατύφυλλος | Spurge | IV, 164 |
| πολεμώνιον | Jacob's ladder | IV, 8 |
| πόλιον | Hulwort | III, 110 |
| πολύγαλον | Milkwort | IV, 139 |
| πολυγόνατον | Solomon's seal | IV, 6 |
| πολυγόνατον | Tuberous thistle | III, 19 |
| πολυγονοειδές | Periwinkle | IV, 7 |
| πολύγονον | *Polygonon* | V, 106 |
| πολύγονον ἄρρεν | Knotgrass | IV, 4 |
| πολύγονον θῆλυ | Mare's tail | IV, 5 |
| πολύκαρπον | Knotgrass | IV, 4 |
| πολύκνημον | Field basil | III, 94 |
| πολύπλευρον | Plantain | II, 126 |
| πολυπόδιον | Polypody | IV, 186 |
| πολύρριζον | Black hellebore | IV, 162 |
| πολύρριζον | Male fern | IV, 184 |
| πολύτριχον | Maidenhair | IV, 134 |
| πολυώνυμον | Pellitory | IV, 85 |
| Ποντικὴ ῥίζα | Licorice | III, 5 |
| ποταμογείτων | Pondweed | IV, 100 |
| ποτίρριον | Goat's thorn | III, 15 |
| πράσιον | Goat's marjoram | III, 30 |
| πράσιον | Horehound | III, 105 |

| **Botanical name** |
|---|
| *Ruta graveolens* L. (A. p. 191) |
| *Peganum harmala* L. (A. p. 163) |
| *Ruta chalepensis L. (A. p. 191)* |
| *Symphytum bulbosum* (LSJ) |
| *Tussilago farfara* L. |
| *Tussilago farfara* L. |
| |
| |
| |
| *Pistacia vera* L. (LSJ) |
| |
| |
| *Euphorbia pityusa* L. (A. p. 262) |
| |
| *Pinus* sp. |
| *Pinus* sp. |
| *Platanus orientalis* L. (LSJ) |
| *Euphorbia platyphyllos* L. (A. p. 262) |
| ~*Polemonium caeruleum* L. ~*Hypericum olympicum* L. (A. p. 203) |
| *Teucrium polium* L. (A. p. 203) |
| *Polygala venulosa* Sibth. (A. p. 203) |
| *Polygonatum verticillatum* All., *P. officinale* All., *P. multiflorum* L. (A. p. 204) |
| *Cnicus tuberosus* L. or *Cirstium tuberosum* All. (A. p. 204) |
| *Vinca minor* L. (A. p. 204) |
| See Diosc. Bk. V, 106, n. 43 |
| *Polygonum aviculare* L. (A. p. 204) |
| *Hippuris vulgaris* L. (A. p. 204) |
| *Polygonum aviculare* L. (A. 203) |
| *Zizyphora capitata* L. (A. p. 203) |
| *Plantago major* L. sp. (A. p. 204) |
| *Polypodium vulgare* L. (A. p. 204) |
| *Helleborus cyclophyllu* s R. Br. (A . p. 205) |
| *Polystichum filix mas* Roth. (A. p. 205) |
| *Adiantum capillus Veneris* L. (A. p. 205) |
| *Parietaria officinalis* L. (A. p. 204) |
| *Glycyrrhiza glabra* L. (LSJ |
| *Ottelia alismoide* s Pers. (A. p. 206) |
| *Astagalus poterium* Labill. (A. p. 207) |
| See Bk. III, 30, n. 25 |
| *Marrubium vulgare* L. (LSJ) |

| **Botanical name** |
| --- |
| *Allium porrum* L. (A. pp. 206-207) |
| *Quercus ilex* L. (A. p. 207) |
| |
| |
| *Arctium lappa* L. (A. p. 208) |
| *Arctium lappa* L. (A. p. 208) |
| *Achillea ptarmica* L. (A. p. 210) |
| *Ulmus glabra* (LSJ) |
| *Polystichum filix mas* Roth. (A. p. 210) |
| *Ceterach officinarum* Willd. (A. p. 210) |
| ~*Leonurus cardiaca* L., ~ *L. marrubiastrum* L. (A. p. 211) |
| *Rhamnus petiolaris*, *Rh. lycoides*, *Rh. punctata* Boiss. (A. p. 212) |
| *Buxus sempervirens* L. (A. p. 42) |
| *Cotoneaster pyracantha* Spach. (A. p. 211) |
| *Anacyclus pyrethrum* DC. = *Anthemis pyrhethrum* L. (A. p. 212) |
| *Cotoneaster pyracantha* Spach. (A. p. 212) |
| *Valeriana tuberosa* L. (A. p. 170) |
| *Triticum* L. |
| *Ficaria verna* Huds. (A. p. 212) |
| *Daphne gnidium* L. (A. p. 212) |
| *Daphne oleide* s L. and *D. oleafolia* L. (A. p. 212) |
| |
| *Rheum ribes* L. (A. p. 217) |
| *Rhamnus cathartica* L. (A. p. 217) |
| *Raphanus sativus* (LSJ) |
| *Euphorbia apios* L. (A. p. 216) |
| *Rheum officinale* (LSJ) |
| |
| |
| |
| |
| |
| |
| |
| |
| |
| |
| |
| |
| *Punica granatum* (LSJ) |

| **Botanical name** |
|---|
| *Sedum roseum* Scop., *S. rhodiola* DC. (A. p. 217) |
| |
| |
| |
| *Nerium oleander* L. |
| *Nerium oleander* L. (A. p. 217) |
| |
| |
| *Rosa* (LSJ) |
| *Lollium perenne* L. (A. p. 218) |
| *Rhus coriaria* L. (A. p. 218) |
| *Ferula persica* Willd. (A. p. 223) |
| |
| |
| *Majorana hortensis* Moench (A. p. 225) |
| *Artemisia maritima* L. (LSJ) |
| *Castanea vulgaris* Lam. (A. p. 32) |
| *Astragalus fasciculifolius* Boiss. sp. (A. p. 227) |
| *Fritillaria graeca* L. (A. p. 228) |
| *Serapias cordigera* L. (A. p. 228) |
| *Ranunculus* L. sp. |
| *Ranunculus* L. sp. |
| *Apium graveolens* L. (A. p. 234) |
| *Orchis morio* L. sp. (A. p. 236) |
| *Cichorium endivia* L. (A. p.236) |
| *Cichorium endivia* L. (LSJ) |
| *Artemisia maritima* L. (A. p. 236) |
| *Tordylium officinale* L. (A. p. 237) |
| *Bupleurum fruticosum* L. (A. p. 237) |
| *Bupleurum fruticosum* L. (A. p. 237) |
| *Bupleurum fruticosum* L. (A. p. 237) |
| *Tordylium officinale* L. (A. p. 237) |
| *Ricinus communis* L. (A. p. 237) |
| *Seseli tortuosum* L. (A. p. 237) |
| *Malabaila aurea* Sibth. (A. p. 237) |
| *Malabaila aurea* Sibth. (A. p. 237) |
| *Beta maritima* L. (LSJ) |
| *Helleborus cyclophyllus* R. Br. |
| *Reseda alba* L. (A. p. 237) |
| *Aubrietia deltoides* L. (A. p. 237) |

| **Botanical name** |
|---|
| *Sesamum indicum* L. (A. p. 237) |
| *Ricinus communis* L. (A. p. 237) |
| *Mespilus germanica* L. (A. p. 237) |
| *Achillea millefolium* L. (A. p. 238) |
| *Ajuga hamaepitys* L. (A. p. 258) |
| *Sideritis romana* L. (A. p. 238) |
| *Parietaria officinalis* L. (A. p. 238) |
| *Sanguisorba minor* Scop. = *Poterium sanguisorba* L. (A. p. 238) |
| *Scrofularia lucida* L. (A. p. 238) |
| |
| *Citrullus colocynthis* Schrad. (A. p. 238) |
| *Cucumis sativus* L. (A. p. 80) |
| *Cucumis sativus* L. (A. p. 80) |
| *Ecballium elaterium* Rich. |
| *Cucumis sativus* L. (A. p. 80) |
| *Silybum marianum* Gaertn. (A. p. 240) |
| ~*Ferula tingitana* L. (A. p. 240) |
| *Sinapis alba* L. (A. p. 240) |
| *Sison amomum* L. (A. p. 241) |
| *Nasturtium officinale* R. Br. (A. p. 242) |
| *Sium angustifolium* L. (A. p. 242) |
| *Pastinaca sativa* L. (A. p. 241) |
| *Mentha silvestris* L., *M. viridis* L. (A. p. 241) |
| *Nasturtium officinale* R. Br. (A. p. 241) |
| *Convolvulus scammonia* L. (A. p. 228) |
| *Scandix pecten-Veneris* L. (A. p. 229) |
| *Urginea maritima Baker* = *Scilla maritima* L. (A. p. 229) |
| *Pancratium maritimum* L. (A. p. 230) |
| *Urginea maritima* Baker = *Scilla maritima* L. (A. p. 229) |
| *Ceterach officinarum* Willd. (A. p. 230) |
| *Scolymus maculatus* L. and *S. hispanicu* s L. (A. p. 231) |
| *Teucrium scordium* L. (A. p. 231) |
| *Allium sativum* L. (A. p. 232) |
| *Allium descendens* (LSJ) |
| *Coronilla scorpioides* Koch (A. p. 232) |
| *Ephedra distachya* L. (A. p. 232) |
| *Heliotropium europaeum* L., *H. villosum* L., *H. supinum* L. (A. p. 232) |
| *Glycyrrhiza glabra* L, G. echinata L. (A.. P. 233) |
| *Umbilicus pendulinu* s DC. |
| |

| **Botanical name** |
| --- |
| *Taxus baccata* L. (A. p. 161) |
| *Vigna sinensis* Endl. (A. p.161,) *Phaseolus vulgaris* L. (LSJ) |
| |
| *Taxus baccata* L. (A. p. 161) |
| *Commiphora myrrha* Engl. (A. p.167) |
| |
| *Smyrnium olusatrum* L. (A. p. 124) |
| *Smyrnium perfoliatum* Mill. (A. p. 242) |
| *Sonchus* L. sp. |
| *Sonchus asper* L. (A. p. 243) |
| *Sonchus oleraceus* L. (A. p. 243) |
| |
| |
| *Sparganium ramosum* Curtis, *S. simplex* Huds. (A. p. 244) |
| *Spartium junceum* L. (A. p. 244) |
| *Evernia* L. (A. p. 247) |
| *Lonicera etrusca* L. (A. p. 247) |
| *Ceterach officinarum* Willd. (A. p. 247) |
| *Scolopendrium hemionitis* Lag. (A. p. 247) |
| |
| |
| |
| *Delphinium staphisagria* L. (A. p. 248) |
| |
| *Daucus guttatus L.* (LSJ; see also A. pp. 57 and 248)) |
| *Daucus carota* L. (A. p. 248) |
| *Stachys* L. sp. (A. p. 247) |
| *Sempervivum arboreum* L. (A. p. 249) |
| *Ruscus hypoglossum* L. (LSJ) |
| *Poterium spinosum* L. (A. p. 250) |
| *Lavendula stoechas* L. (A. p. 250) |
| *Pistia stratiotes* L. (A. p. 250) |
| *Achillea millefolium* L. (A. p. 250) |
| *Achillea millefolium* L. (A. p. 250) |
| |
| *Pinus* sp. |
| *Pyrus Cydonia* (LSJ) |
| *Saponaria officinalis* L. (A. p. 251) |
| *Physalis alkekeng* i L. (A. p. 251) |
| *Physalis alkekengi* L. (A. p. 251) |

| **Botanical name** |
|---|
| *Solanum nigrum* L. (A. p. 251) |
| *Datura stramonium* L. ( See A. p. 251 regarding this identification ) |
| *Withania somnifera* Dun. (A. p. 251) |
| |
| |
| *Styrax officinalis* L. (A. p. 252) |
| |
| *Ficus carica* L. (A. p. 104) |
| *Morus nigra* L. (A. p. 253) |
| *Ficus sycomorus* L. (A. p. 253) |
| *Euphorbia chamaesyce* L. (A. p. 253) |
| *Euphorbia peplis* L. (A. 253) |
| *Ficus sycomorus* L. (A. p. 253) |
| *Inula helenium* L. (A. p. 253) |
| *Glycyrrhiza glabra* L. G. echinata (A. p. 253) |
| *Symphytum bulbosum* (LSJ) |
| *Symphytum tuberosum* L. (A. p. 253) |
| *Sorbus domestica* (LSJ) |
| *Sorbus domestica* (LSJ) |
| *Alhagi maurorum* L. (A. p. 244) |
| *Salvia* sp. |
| *Heracleum sphondylium* L. (A. p. 244) |
| *Pistacia lentiscus* L. (LSJ) |
| *Cymbopogon schoenanthus* Spreng. (A. p. 229) |
| *Cymbopogon schoenanthus* Spreng. sp. (A. p. 229) |
| *Cymbopogon schoenanthus* Spreng. sp. (A. p. 229) |
| *Scirpus* L. sp., *Juncus* L. sp. (A. p. 229) |
| *Taxus baccata* L. (A. p. 256) |
| *Ephedra distachya* L. |
| *Pistacia terebinthus* L. (A. p. 256) |
| *Polygonum aviculare* L. |
| *Teucrium creticum* L. (A. p. 303) |
| *Rubia tinctorum* L. (A. p. 257) |
| *Teucrium flavum* L. (A. p. 257) |
| *Teucrium chamaedrys* L., *T. lucidum* L. (A. p. 257) |
| *Cymbopogon schoenanthus* Spreng. (A. p. 257) |
| |
| |
| |
| |

| Greek name | English name | References |
|---|---|---|
| τηλέφιον | Houseleek, Third kind of | IV, 90 |
| τηλέφιον | Stonecrop | IV, 90 |
| τηλεφώνιον | *Telephonion* | II, 186 |
| τήλινον | Fenugreek unguent | I, 47 |
| τῆλις | Fenugreek | II, 102 |
| τιθυμαλλίς | Spurge | IV, 164 |
| τιθύμαλλος | Spurge | IV, 164 |
| τιθύμαλλος | Yew | IV, 79 |
| τιθύμαλλος θῆλυς | Myrtle spurge | IV, 164 |
| τόρδιλον | Cretan hartwort | III, 54 |
| τραγάκανθα | Tragacanth | III, 20 |
| τράγιον | Stinking tutsan | IV, 49 |
| τράγιον ἄλλο | Pimpinell | IV, 50 |
| τραγοπώγων | Salsify | II, 143 |
| τραγορίγανος | Goat's marjoram | III, 30 |
| τράγος | Spelt | II, 93 |
| τράγος | *Tragos* | IV, 51 |
| τρίβολος ἔνυδρος | Water chestnut | IV, 15 |
| τρίβολος χερσαῖος | Caltrops | IV, 15 |
| τριπόλιον | Sea starwort | IV, 132 |
| τρίφυλλον | Italian melilot | IV, 110 |
| τρίφυλλον | Man orchis | III, 128 |
| τρίφυλλον | Treacle clover | III, 109 |
| τριχομανές | Caper | II, 173 |
| τριχομανές | Waterwort | IV, 135 |
| Τρωγλοδυτική | Myrrh | I, 64 |
| τύφη | Reed mace | III, 118 |
| ὑάκινθος | Wild hyacinth | IV, 62 |
| ὑγιεινὴ ἀγρία | Pellitory | IV, 85 |
| ὕδνον | Truffle | II, 145 |
| ὑδρόμελι | Hydromel | V, 9 |
| ὑδρόμηλον | Water, honey, and quinces | V, 22 |
| ὑδροπέπερι | Smartweed | II, 161 |
| ὑοσκύαμος | Henbane | IV, 68 |
| ὑπερικόν | St. John's wort | III, 154 |
| ὑπερικόν | St. John's wort | III, 157 |
| ὑπήκοον | Horned cumin | IV, 67 |
| ὑπόγλωσσον | Horse tongue | IV, 129 |
| ὑπόγλωττον | Daphne Alexandreia | IV, 145 |
| ὑποκυστίς | Hypocist | I, 97 |

| **Botanical name** |
|---|
| *Sedum album* L., *S. stellatum* L. (A. p. 256) |
| *Sedum* L. sp. (A. p. 256) |
| *Andrachna telephioides* L. (A. p. 256) |
| |
| *Trigonella fenum graecum* L. (A. p. 256) |
| *Euphporbia parallias* L. (A. p. 262) |
| *Euphorbia* L. (A. p. 261) |
| *Taxus baccata* L. |
| *Euphorbia myrsinites* L. (A. p. 262) |
| *Tordylium officinale* L. (A. p. 262) |
| *Astragalus gummife* r Labill., *A. microcephalus* Willd. (A. p. 262) |
| *Pistacia palestina* Boiss. (A. pp. 262-263) |
| *Pimpinella tragium* Vill. (A. p. 263) |
| *Tragopogon porrifolius* L. (A. p. 263) |
| ~*Thymus graveolens* Sibth. sp, ~*Th. tragoriganum* L, sp. , ~*Origanum heraceoticum* R |
| *Triticum* L. sp. |
| *Ephedra distachya* L. sp. (A. p. 263) |
| *Trapa natans* L. (A. p. 263) |
| *Tribulus terrestris* L. (A. p. 263) |
| ~*Aster tripolium* L., ~*Limonium* L. sp. (A. p. 265) |
| *Melilotus* Adans. sp. (A. p. 264) |
| *Fritillaria graeca* L. (A. p. 265) |
| *Psorolea bituminosa* L. (A. p. 264) |
| *Capparis spinosa* L. |
| *Asplenium trichomanes* L. (A. p. 264) |
| |
| *Typha* L. sp. (A. p. 267) |
| *Scilla bifolia* L. (A. p. 126) |
| *Parietaria officinalis* L. |
| *Tuber cibarium* L. sp. (A. pp. 126 and 266) |
| |
| |
| *Polygonum hydropiper* L. (A. p. 127) |
| *Hyoscyamus* L. sp. ( A. p. 127) |
| *Hypericum crispum* L. (A. p. 128) |
| *Hypericum empetrifolium* Willd. , ~ *H. coris* L. (A. p. 128) |
| *Hypecoum procumbens* L. (A. p. 128) |
| *Ruscus hypoglossum* L. (A. p. 128) |
| *Ruscus hypophyllum* L. (LSJ) |
| *Cytinus hypocistis* L. (A. p. 128) |

| Greek name | English name | References |
|---|---|---|
| ὑσόβρυον | *Hysobryon* | III, 42 |
| ὕσσωπος | Hyssop | III, 25 |
| φακοειδές | Sea heath | IV, 179 |
| φακός | Lentil | II, 107 |
| φακός ὁ ἐπί τελμάτων | Duckweed | IV, 87 |
| φαλάγγιον | Spiderwort | III, 108 |
| φαλαγγῖτις | Spiderwort | III, 108 |
| φαληρίς | Canary grass | III, 142 |
| φασγάνιον | Corn flag | IV, 20 |
| φάσγανον | Broad-leaved burweed | IV, 136 |
| φασήλιον | Fumitory | IV, 120 |
| φέρομβρον | Squirting cucumber | IV, 150 |
| φηγός | Valonia oak | I, 106 |
| φιλάνθρωπον | Cleavers | III, 90 |
| Φιλεταίριον | Catchfly | IV, 28 |
| Φιλεταίριον | Jacob's ladder | IV, 8 |
| φιλοφαρές | Horehound | III, 105 |
| φιλύρα | Lime tree | I, 96 |
| φλομίς | Mullein | IV, 103 |
| φλομίς ἡ καλουμένη λυχνῖτις | Mullein | IV, 103 |
| φλόμος | Mullein | IV, 103 |
| φλὸμος ἀγρία | Sage of Jerusalem | IV, 103 |
| φλόμος Ἰδαῖος | Elecampane | I, 28 |
| φλονῖτις | Stone bugloss | III, 131 |
| φοῖνιξ | Date palm | I, 109 |
| φοῖνιξ | Rye grass | IV, 43 |
| φοῦ | Cretan spikenard | I, 11 |
| φρύνιον | Goat's thorn | III, 15 |
| φῦκος θαλάσσιον | Seaweed | IV, 99 |
| φῦκος θαλάσσιον ἐν Κρήτη | Seaweed, Cretan | IV, 99 |
| φῦκος θαλάσσιον πλατύ | Seaweed, Broad | IV, 99 |
| φῦκος θαλάσσιον ὑπόμηκες | Seaweed, Longish | IV, 99 |
| φυλλῖτις | Hart's tongue | III, 107 |
| φύλλον | Dog mercury | III, 125 |
| φύλλον | Tuberous thistle | III, 19 |
| φύτευμα | Montpellier rocket | IV, 128 |
| χαλβάνη | Galbanum | III, 83 |
| χαμαιάκτη | Deadwort | IV, 173 |
| χαμαιάκτη | Elder | IV, 173 |
| χαμαιβάλανος | Tuberous spurge | IV, 175 |

| Botanical name |
|---|
| *Amaracus sipyleus* Rafin. (A. p. 154) |
| *Satureia graeca* L. = *Micromeria graeca* Benth. (A. p. 129) |
| *Frankenia hirsuta* L. and *F. pulverulenta* L. (A. p. 195) |
| *Ervum lens* L. ( LSJ) |
| *Lemna minor* L. (A. p. 141) |
| *Lloydia graeca* L. (A. p. 195) |
| *Lloydia graeca* L. (A. p. 195) |
| *Phalaris canariensis* L. (A. p. 195) |
| *Gladiolus segetum* Gawler (A. p. 196) |
| *Xanthium strumarium* L. (A. p. 196) |
| *Corydalis claviculata* Pers. |
| *Ecballium elaterium* Rich. |
| *Quercus aegilops* L. (A. p. 196) |
| *Galium aparine* L. (A. p. 196) |
| *Silene gallica* L. |
| *Polemonium caeruleum* L. or *Hypericum olympicum* L. (A. p.196) |
| *Marrubium vulgare* L., *M. creticum* Miller |
| *Phillyrea* L. sp. (A. p. 197) |
| *Verbacum* L. sp. (A. p. 197) |
| *Verbascum* L. sp. (A. p. 197) |
| *Verbascum* L. sp. (A. p. 197) |
| V*erbascum* L. sp. (A. p. 197) |
| *Inula helenium* L. (A. p. 69) |
| *Onosma echinoides* L. (A. p. 197) |
| *Phoenix dactylifera* L. (LSJ) |
| *Lollium perenne* L. (A. p. 197) |
| *Valeriana phu* L. (A. p. 170) |
| *Astagalus poterium* Labıll. (A. p. 198) |
| |
| *Cystoseira foeniculosa* sp. (A. p. 198) |
| *Posidonia oceanica* Del. (A. p. 198) |
| *Nithrophyllum punctatum* L. (A. p. 198) |
| *Scolopendrium officinale* L. sp. (A. p. 105) |
| *Mercurialis perennis* L. (A. p. 198) |
| *Cnicus tuberosus* L. or *Cirstium tuberosum* All. (A. p. 199) |
| *Reseda phyteuma* L. (A. p. 199) |
| *Ferula galbaniflua* Boiss. and Buhse (A. p. 108) |
| *Sambucus ebulus* L. (A. p. 59) |
| *Sambucus nigra* L. (A. p. 4) |
| *Euphorbia apios* L. (A. p. 59) |

| **Botanical name** |
|---|
| *Cardopatium corymbosum* Pers. (A. pp. 59-60) |
| *Ruscus racemosus* L. (A. p. 59) |
| *Daphne laureola* L. (A. p. 59) |
| *Teucrium chamaedrys* L. and *T. lucidum* L. (A. p. 59) |
| *Glechoma hederacea* L. (A. p. 59) |
| *Atractylis gummifera* L. (A. p.59) |
| *Cardopatium corymbosum P* ers. (A. p. 60) |
| *Matricaria chamomilla* L. (A. p. 60) |
| *Ruscus aculeatus* L. (A. p. 60) |
| Unidentifiable (A. p. 60), *Chamaepeuce mutica* (LSJ) |
| *Ajuga chia* Schreb. (A. p. 60) |
| *Ajuga hamaepitys* Schreb. (A. p. 60) |
| *Ajuga iva* Schreb. (A. p. 60) |
| *Hypericum crispum* L. (A. p. 60) |
| *Ajuga chia* Schreb. (A. p. 60) |
| *Ajuga iva* Schreb. (A. p. 60) |
| *Teucrium chamaedrys* L. and ~*T. lucidum* L. (A. p. 59) |
| *Euphorbia chamaesyce* L. (A. p. 61) |
| *Daphne gnidium* L. (A. p. 61) |
| *Daphne oleides* L. and *D. oleafolia* L. (A. p. 61) |
| *Euphorbia Sibthorpii* Boiss. (A. p. 61) |
| *Xanthium strumarium* L. |
| *Bryonia dioica* Jacq. (A. p. 62) |
| *Chelidonium majus* L. (A. p. 62) |
| *Ficaria verna* Huds. (A. p. 62) |
| *Polemonium caeruleum* L. or *Hypericum olympicum* L. (A. p.203) |
| *Xanthium strumarium* L. |
| *Chondrilla juncea* L. (LSJ) |
| *Chondrlla ramosissima* L. (LSJ) |
| |
| *Anthemis tinctoria* L. (A. p. 63) |
| *Helichrysum orientale* L., *H. stoechas* L., *H. siculum* L. (A. p. 63) |
| *Aster linosyris* Bernh. (A. p. 64) |
| *Leontice chrysogonon* L. sp. (A. p. 64) |
| *Anthemis tinctoria* L. (A. p. 64) |
| *Aster linosyris* Bernh. (A. p. 64) |
| |
| |
| *Pimpinella cretica* L. (A. p. 209) |
| (see A. p. 52) |

| Greek name | English name | References |
|---|---|---|
| ψευδοκινάμωμον | *Pseudocinamomon* | I, 14 |
| ψευδοσέλινον | Cinquefoil | IV, 42 |
| ψίλωθρον | Bryony | IV, 182 |
| ψύλλιον | Fleawort | IV, 69 |
| ψυχροτρόφον | Betony | IV, 1 |
| ὠκίμινον | Basil unguent | I, 49 |
| ὠκιμοειδές | Catchfly | IV, 28 |
| ὠκιμοειδές | Chameleon thistle | III, 9 |
| ὠκιμοειδές | Horse thyme | III, 95 |
| ὤκιμον | Basil | II, 141 |

| **Botanical name** |
|---|
| *Cinnamomum tamala* Nees sp., *C. iners* Blume sp. (A. p.209) |
| *Potentilla reptans* L. (A. p. 209) |
| *Bryonia dioica* Jacq. (A. p. 209) |
| *Plantago psyllium* L. and *P. cynops* L. (A. p. 210) |
| *Stachys officinalis* L. (A. pp. 209-210) |
| |
| *Silene gallica* L. (A. p. 175) |
| *Cardopatium corymbosum* Pers. (A. p. 175) |
| *Calamintha clinopodium* Moris (A. p. 175) |
| *Ocimum basilicum* L. sp. (A. p. 175) |

| **Botanical name** |
|---|
| *Acacia arabica* (LSJ) |
| *Acacia catechu* Willd. (A. p. 149) |
| *Acacia* sp. (A. p. 209) |
| *Acanthus mollis* L. (A. p. 157) |
| *Acanthus mollis* L. (A. p. 185) |
| *Acanthus mollis* L. (A. p. 2) |
| *Acanthus spinosus* L. (A. p. 2) |
| *Acetabularia mediterranea* L. (A. p. 17) |
| *Achillea ageratum* L. (A. p. 7) |
| *Achillea millefolium* L. (A. p. 238) |
| *Achillea millefolium* L. (A. p. 250) |
| *Achillea millefolium* L. (A. p. 250) |
| *Achillea millefolium* L. (A. p. 3) |
| *Achillea ptarmica* L. (A. p. 210) |
| *Aconitum napellus* L. (A. p. 149) |
| *Aconitum napellus* L. (A. p. 4) |
| *Acorus calamus* L. (A. p. 45) |
| *Adiantum capillus Veneris* L. (A. p. 205) |
| *Adiantum capillus Veneris* L. (A. p. 5) |
| *Aegilops ovata* L. (A. p. 6) |
| *Agrimonia eupatoria* L. (A. p. 99) |
| *Agrostemma githago* L. (A. p. 149) |
| *Ajuga chia* Schreb. (A. p. 60) |
| *Ajuga chia* Schreb. (A. p. 60) |
| *Ajuga hamaepitys* L. (A. p. 258) |
| *Ajuga hamaepitys* Schreb. |
| *Ajuga hamaepitys* Schreb. (A. p. 125) |
| *Ajuga hamaepitys* Schreb. (A. p. 60) |
| *Ajuga iva* Schreb. (A. p. 18) |
| *Ajuga iva* Schreb. (A. p. 60) |
| *Ajuga iva* Schreb. (A. p. 60) |
| *Alhagi maurorum* L. (A. p. 244) |
| *Alhagi maurorum* L. (A. p. 28) |
| *Alhagi maurorum* L. (A. p. 88) |
| *Alhagi maurorum* L. (A. p. 98) |

| Greek name | English name | References |
| --- | --- | --- |
| ἀκακία ἡ ἐν Αἰγύπτῳ | Shittah tree | I, 101 |
| Ἰνδικὸν λύκιον | Indian *lycion* | I, 100 |
| ψευδοκασσία | *Pseudocassia* | I, 13 |
| μελάμφυλλον | Bear's-foot | III, 17 |
| παιδέρως | Bear's-foot | III, 17 |
| ἄκανθος | Bear's-foot | III, 17 |
| ἄκανθος ἀγρία | Bear's-foot, Wild | III, 17 |
| ἀνδρόσακες | Sea navel | III, 133 |
| ἀγήρατον | Pot marjoram | IV, 58 |
| σιδηρῖτις | Achilles woundwort | IV, 36 |
| στρατιώτης ὁ χιλιόφυλλος | Milfoil | IV, 102 |
| στρατιώτης ὁ χιλιόφυλλος | Yarrow | IV, 102 |
| Ἀχίλλειος | Achilles woundwort | IV, 36 |
| πταρμική | Sneezewort | II, 162 |
| λυκοκτόνον | Wolfsbane | IV, 77 |
| ἀκόνιτον ἕτερον | Wolfsbane | IV, 77 |
| κάλαμος ἀρωματικός | Sweet flag | I, 18 |
| πολύτριχον | Maidenhair | IV, 134 |
| ἀδίαντον | Maidenhair | IV, 134 |
| αἰγίλωψ | Haver grass | IV, 137 |
| Εὐπατόριος | Agrimony | IV, 41 |
| λυχνὶς ἀγρία | Corn cockle | III, 101 |
| χαμαίπιτυς | Ground pine | III, 158 |
| χαμαίπιτυς ἑτέρα | Mountain germander | III, 158 |
| σιδηρῖτις | Ground pine | III, 158 |
| ἰωνία | Ground pine | III, 158 |
| ὁλόκυρος | Ground pine | III, 158 |
| χαμαίπιτυς | Ground pine, Another | III, 158 |
| ἀνθυλλὶς ἑτέρα | Anthyllis, Another | III, 136 |
| χαμαίπιτυς | Ground pine, Third kind | III, 158 |
| χαμαιπὶτυς τρίτη | Herb ivy | III, 158 |
| σφάγνος | Camel's-thorn | I, 20 |
| ἀσπάλαθος | Camel's-thorn | I, 20 |
| διάξυλον | Camel's-thorn | I, 20 |
| ἐρυσίσκηπτρον | Camel's-thorn | I, 20 |

| **Botanical name** |
|---|
| *Alisma plantago* L. *A. arcuatum* Mich. |
| *Alisma plantago* L., *A. arcuatum* Mich. (A. p. 150) |
| *Alisma plantago* L., *A. arcuatum* Mich. (A. p. 86) |
| *Allium ambeloprasum* L. (A. p. 206) |
| *Allium cepa* (LSJ) |
| *Allium descendens* (LSJ) |
| *Allium nigrum L. (A. p. 163)~* |
| *Allium porrum* L. (A. pp. 206-207) |
| *Allium sativum* L. (A. p. 232) |
| *Aloe vera* L. (A. p. 11) |
| *Althaea cannabina* L. (A. p. 47) |
| *Althaea officinalis* L. |
| *Althaea officinalis* L. (A . p. 12) |
| *Amaracus sipyleus* Rafin (A. p. 154) |
| *Amaracus sipyleus* Rafin. (A. p. 154) |
| *Amaranthus blitum* L. (A. p. 36) |
| *Amomum subulatum* Roxb. (A. p. 14) |
| *Anacyclus pyrethrum* DC. = *Anthemis pyrhethrum* L. (A. p. 212) |
| *Anagallis arvensis* L. (A. p. 15) |
| *Anagallis arvensis* L. (A. p. 65) |
| *Anagallis caerulea* Schreb. (A. p. 15) |
| *Anagallis phoenicea* Scop. (A. p. 15) |
| *Anagyris foetida* L. (A. p. 4) |
| *Anagyris foetida* L. (A. p. 16) |
| *Anagyris foetida* L. (A. p. 16) |
| *Anchusa italica* Retz. (A. p. 40) |
| *Anchusa tinctoria* L. (A. p. 46) |
| *Anchusa tinctoria* L. (A. p.16) |
| *Anchusa tinctoria* L. (A. p. 178) |
| *Andrachna telephioides* L. (A. p. 16) |
| *Andrachna telephioides* L. (A. p. 16) |
| *Andrachna telephioides* L. (A. p. 256) |
| *Andrachna telephioides* L. (A. p. 8) |
| *Anemone coronaria* L. |
| *Anemone coronaria* L. |

| Greek name | English name | References |
|---|---|---|
| ἄλισμα | Water plantain | III, 152 |
| λύρον | Water plantain | III, 152 |
| δαμασώνιον | Water plantain | III, 152 |
| ἀμπελόπρασον | Wild leek | II, 150 |
| κρόμιον | Onion | II, 151 |
| σκορδόπρασον | Garlic leek | II, 153 |
| μῶλυ | Garlic | III, 47 |
| πράσον κεφαλωτόν | Leek | II, 149 |
| σκόρδον | Garlic | II, 152 |
| ἀλόη | Aloe | III, 22 |
| κάνναβις ἀγρία | Hemp mallow | III, 149 |
| ἐβίσκος | Marsh mallow | III, 146 |
| ἀλθαία | Marsh mallow | III, 146 |
| μᾶρον | *Maron* | III, 42 |
| ὑσόβρυον | *Hysobryon* | III, 42 |
| βλίτον | Blite | II, 117 |
| ἄμωμον | Nepal cardamom | I, 15 |
| πύρεθρος | Pellitory | III, 73 |
| ἀναγαλλίς | Pimpernel | II, 178 |
| κιχόριον | Pimpernel | II, 178 |
| ἀναγαλλὶς θήλεια | Pimpernel | II, 178 |
| ἀναγαλλὶς ἄρρην | Pimpernel | II, 178 |
| ἄκοπον | Stinking bean trefoil | III, 150 |
| ἀνάγυρις | Stinking bean trefoil | III, 150 |
| ἀνάγυρος | Stinking bean trefoil | III, 150 |
| βούγλωσσον | Bugloss | IV, 127 |
| κάλυξ | Alkanet | IV, 23 |
| ἄγχουσα | Alkanet | IV, 23 |
| ὀνόκλεια | Alkanet | IV, 23 |
| ἀνδράχνη ἀγρία | *Telephonion* | II, 186 |
| βρύον | *Telephonion* | II, 186 |
| τηλεφώνιον | *Telephonion* | II, 186 |
| ἀείζῳον ἄγριον | *Telephonion* | II, 186 |
| ἀργεμώνιον | Anemone poppy | II, 176 |
| ἀργεμώνιον | Scarlet windflower | II, 176 |

| **Botanical name** |
|---|
| *Anemone coronaria* L. |
| *Anemone coronaria* L. (A. p. 17) |
| *Anemone coronaria* L. (A. p. 17) |
| *Anemone coronaria* L. (A. p. 96) |
| *Anethum graveolens* L. (A. p. 17) |
| *Anthemis tinctoria* L. (A. p. 63) |
| *Anthemis tinctoria* L. (A. p. 64) |
| *Antirrhinum orontium* L. (A. p. 149) |
| *Antirrhinum orontium* L. (LSJ) |
| *Antirrhinum orontium* L. (LSJ) |
| *Apium graveolens* L. var. *silvestre* (A. p. 118) |
| *Apium graveolens* L. (A. p. 234) |
| *Aquilaria agallocha* Roxb. (A. p. 7) |
| *Aquilaria agallocha* Roxb. (A. p. 7) |
| *Arbutus unedo* L. (A. p. 72) |
| *Arctium lappa* L. (A. p. 208) |
| *Arctium lappa* L. (A. p. 208) |
| *Arctium lappa* L. (A. p. 23) |
| *Arisarum vulgare* Targ.-Tozz., *A. proboscideum* Savi (A. p. 24) |
| *Aristolochia clematitis* L. (A. p. 25) |
| *Aristolochia* L. (A. p. 25) |
| *Aristolochia longa* L. (A. p. 25) |
| *Aristolochia longa* L. (A. p. 25) |
| *Aristolochia longa* L. (A. p. 25) |
| *Aristolochia rotunda* L. (A. p. 25) |
| *Aristolochia rotunda* L. (A. p. 25) |
| *Artemisia abrotonon* L. |
| *Artemisia abrotonum L. (A. p. 115 s. v. (h)abrotonum)~* |
| *Artemisia abrotonum L.~* |
| *Artemisia abrotonum (A. p. 115 s.v (h)abrotonum)~* |
| *Artemisia arborescen* s L. (A. p. 26) |
| *Artemisia arborescens* L., *A. campestris* L., *A. genipi* Weber (A. p. 26) |
| *Artemisia campestris* L. (A. p. 26) |
| *Artemisia fragrans* (LSJ) |
| *Artemisia genipi* Weber (A. p. 26) |

| Greek name | English name | References |
|---|---|---|
| ἠρέμιον | Scarlet windflower | II, 176 |
| ἀνεμώνη | Anemone poppy | II, 176 |
| ἀνεμὼνη ἀγρία | Scarlet windflower | II, 176 |
| ἠρέμιον | Anemone poppy | II, 176 |
| ἄνηθον | Dill | III, 58 |
| χρυσάνθεμον | Camomile | III, 137 |
| χρυσοκαλλίας | Camomile | III, 137 |
| λυχνὶς ἀγρία | Calf's snout | IV, 130 |
| ἀνάρρινον | Calf's snout | IV, 130 |
| ἀντίρρινον | Calf's snout | IV, 130 |
| ἐλεοσέλινον | Celery, Marsh | III, 64, 2 |
| σέλινον κηπαῖον | Celery, Garden | III, 64 |
| ἀγάλοχον | Aloewood | I, 22 |
| ἀγάλοχον | Eaglewood | I, 22 |
| κόμαρος | Strawberry tree | I, 122 |
| προσώπιον | Burdock | IV, 106 |
| προσωπίς | Burdock | IV, 106 |
| ἄρκιον | Burdock | IV, 106 |
| ἀρίσαρον | Hooded arum | II, 168 |
| κληματῖτις | Birthwort | III, 4 |
| ἀριστολοχεία | Birthwort | III, 4 |
| ἀριστολοχεὶα ἄρρην | Birthwort | III, 4 |
| ἀριστολοχεὶα μακρά | Birthwort | III, 4 |
| δακτυλῖτις | Birthwort | III, 4 |
| ἁριστολοχεὶα θῦλεια | Birthwort | III, 4 |
| ἀριστολοχεὶα στρογγύλη | Birthwort | III, 4 |
| Ἡράκλειον | Southernwood | III, 24 |
| γλυκὺς ἀγκών | Wormwood | III, 24 |
| Ἡράκλειον | Wormwood | III, 24 |
| ἀβρότονον | Wormwood | III, 24 |
| ἀρτεμισὶα πλατυτέρα | Wormwood | III, 113 |
| ἀρτεμισία | Wormwood | III, 113 |
| ἀρτεμισὶα λεπτοτέρα | Wormwood | III, 113 |
| ἀβρότονον ἄρρεν | Southernwood | III, 24 |
| ἀρτεμισία τό ἐν μεσογείοις βοτάνιον | Wormwood | III, 113 |

| **Botanical name** |
|---|
| *Artemisia maritima* L. (A . p. 1) |
| *Artemisia maritima* L. (A . p. 1) |
| *Artemisia maritima* L. (A. p. 13) |
| *Artemisia maritima* L. (A. p. 236) |
| *Artemisia maritima* L. (A. p. 26) |
| *Artemisia maritima* L. (A. p. 37) |
| *Artemisia maritima* L. (LSJ) |
| *Arum dracunculus* L. (A. p. 90) |
| *Arum dracunculus* L. (A. p. 90) |
| *Arundines* (LSJ) |
| *Arundo dona* x L. |
| *Arundo donax* L. (A. p. 45) |
| *Arundo pliniana* Turra (A. pp. 45 and 170) |
| *Arundo* sp. |
| *Arundo* sp. |
| *Arundo* sp. (A. p. 45) |
| *Asarum europaeum* L. |
| *Asarum europaeum* L. (A. p. 27) |
| *Asparagus aspartilis* L. (A. p. 126) |
| *Asparagus officinalis* L. (A. pp. 28 and 166) |
| *Asperugo procumbens* L. (A. p. 166) |
| *Asperugo procumbens* L. (A. p. 166) |
| *Asphodelus* L. sp. (A. pp. 29-30) |
| *Aspidium lonchitis* L. (A. p. 147) |
| *Asplenium onopteris L. (LSJ,) Dryopteris L. sp. ~ (A. p. 91)~* |
| *Asplenium trichomanes* L. (A. p. 264) |
| *Astagalus poterium* Labill. |
| *Astagalus poterium* Labill. (A. p. 171) |
| *Astagalus poterium* Labill. (A. p. 198) |
| *Astagalus poterium* Labill. (A. p. 207) |
| *Aster amellus* L. (A. p. 29) |
| *Aster amellus* L. (A. p. 39) |
| *Aster linosyris* Bernh. (A. p. 64) |
| *Aster linosyris* Bernh. (A. p. 64) |
| *Aster tripolium L., Limonium L. sp. (A. p. 265)~* |

| **Greek name** | **English name** | **References** |
|---|---|---|
| ἀψίνθιον | Wormwood | III, 23 |
| ἀψίνθιον θαλάσσιον | Worm-seed | III, 23 |
| ἀμβροσία | Ambrose | III, 114 |
| σέριφον | Worm-seed | III, 23 |
| ἀρτεμισία | Ambrose | III, 114 |
| βότρυς | Ambrose | III, 114 |
| Σαντόνικον | Worm-seed | III, 23 |
| δρακόντιον | Dragon arum | II, 166 |
| δρακόντιον | Edderwort | II, 166 |
| κάλαμος(οι) | Reed(s) | I, 85 |
| κάλαμος, δονάξ | Reed, *donax* | I, 85 |
| κάλαμος, Κύπριος | Reed, Cyprian | I, 85 |
| κάλαμος, νάστος | Reed, *nastos* | I, 85 |
| κάλαμος, θῆλυς | Reed, *thelys* | I, 85 |
| κάλαμος, συριγγίας | Reed, *syringias* | I, 85 |
| κάλαμος, φραγμίτης | Reed, *phragmites* | I, 85 |
| νὰρδος ἀγρία | Hazelwort | I, 10 |
| ἄσαρον | Hazelwort | I, 10 |
| ὅρμινον | Asparagus | II, 125 |
| ἀσπάραγος πετραῖος ἤ μυάκανθος | Asparagus | II, 125 |
| μυὸς ὦτα | Madwort | II, 183 |
| μυὸς ὠτίς | Madwort | II, 183 |
| ἀσφόδελος | Asphodel | II, 169 |
| λογχῖτις ἑτέρα | Holy fern | III, 145 |
| δρυοπτερίς | Black oak fern | IV, 187 |
| τριχομανές | Waterwort | IV, 135 |
| ἀκιδωτὸν | Goat's thorn | III, 15 |
| νευράς | Goat's thorn | III, 15 |
| φρύνιον | Goat's thorn | III, 15 |
| ποτίρριον | Goat's thorn | III, 15 |
| ἀστὴρ Ἀττικός | Blue daisy | IV, 119 |
| βουβώνιον | Blue daisy | IV, 119 |
| χρυσῖτις | Immortelle | IV, 55 |
| χρυσοκόμη | Immortelle | IV, 55 |
| τριπόλιον | Sea starwort | IV, 132 |

| Botanical name |
|---|
| *Astragalus fasciculifolius* Boiss. sp. (A. p. 227) |
| *Astragalus gummife* r Labill., *A. microcephalus* Willd. (A. p. 262) |
| *Astragalu* s L. sp. (A. p. 29) |
| *Athamanta cretensis L. (A. p. 87)~* |
| *Athamanta cretensis* L. (LSJ) |
| *Athamanta macedonica L. (A. p. 181)~* |
| *Atractylis gummifera* L. (A. p. 134) |
| *Atractylis gummifera* L. (A. p. 59) |
| *Atriplex halimus* L. (A. p. 116) |
| *Atriplex hortensis* L. (A. p. 16) |
| *Aubrietia deltoides* L. (A. p. 237) |
| *Avena sativa* L. |
| *Ballota nigra* L. |
| *Ballota nigra* L. (A. p. 33) |
| *Beta maritima* L. (A. p. 146) |
| *Beta maritima* L. (A. p. 172) |
| *Beta maritima* L. (LSJ) |
| *Bifora testiculata Rich. (A. p. 124)~* |
| *Biscutella* L. sp. (A. p. 12) |
| *Boswellia* sp. (LSJ) |
| *Brassica oleracea* L. (A. p. 77) |
| *Brassica napus* L. (A. p. 41) |
| *Brassica oleracea, ~ var. silvestris, ~ B. cretica* (A. p. 38) ~ |
| *Brassica rapa* L. (A. p. 112) |
| *Bryonia dioica Jacq. (A. p. 14)* |
| *Bryonia dioica* Jacq. (A. p. 14) |
| *Bryonia dioica* Jacq. (A. p. 151) |
| *Bryonia dioica* Jacq. (A. p. 159) |
| *Bryonia dioica* Jacq. (A. p. 179) |
| *Bryonia dioica* Jacq. (A. p. 209) |
| *Bryonia dioica* Jacq. (A. p. 23) |
| *Bryonia dioica* Jacq. (A. p. 39) |
| *Bryonia dioica* Jacq. (A. p. 62) |
| *Bryonia dioica* Jacq., *B. cretica* Fr. (A. p. 54) |
| *Bunium ferulaceum* Sibth. and Sm. (A. p. 4) |

| Greek name | English name | References |
|---|---|---|
| σαρκοκόλλα | Sarcocolla | III, 85 |
| τραγάκανθα | Tragacanth | III, 20 |
| ἀστράγαλος | Milk vetch | IV, 61 |
| δαῦκος | *Daucos* | III, 72 |
| Κρητικὸς δαῦκος | Cretan *daucos* | III, 72 |
| ὀρεοσέλινον | Mountain parsley | III, 65 |
| ἰξία | Pine thistle | III, 8 |
| χαμαιλὲων λευκός | Pine thistle | III, 8 |
| ἅλιμον | Tree purslane | I, 91 |
| ἀνδράφαξυς | Orach | II, 119 |
| σησαμοειδὲς τὸ μικρόν | Purple rock cress | IV, 163 |
| βρόμος | Oats | II, 94 |
| μελαμπράσιον | Black horehound | III, 103 |
| βαλλλωτή | Black horehound | III, 103 |
| λειμώνιον | Sea lavender | IV, 16 |
| νευροειδές | Sea lavender | IV, 16 |
| σεῦτλον | Beet | II,123 |
| ἱππομάραθον ἕτερον | Horse fennel, Another | III, 71 |
| ἄλυσσον | Madwort | III, 91 |
| λίβανος | Frankincense | I, 68 |
| κράμβη ἥμερος | Cabbage, Cultivated | II, 120 |
| βουνιάς | French turnip | II, 111 |
| κράμβη ἀγρία | Cabbage, Wild | II, 121 |
| γογγύλη | Turnip | II, 110 |
| ἄγρωστις | Bryony | IV, 182 |
| ἄμπελος λευκή | Bryony | IV, 182 |
| μάδος | Bryony | IV, 182 |
| μήλωθρον | Bryony | IV, 182 |
| ὀφιοστάφυλον | Bryony | IV, 182 |
| ψίλωθρον | Bryony | IV, 182 |
| ἀρχεζῶστις | Bryony | IV, 182 |
| βρυωνία | Bryony | IV, 182 |
| χελιδόνιον | Bryony | IV, 182 |
| κέδρωστις | Bryony | IV, 182 |
| ἄκτιον | Earthnut | IV, 123 |

| **Botanical name** |
|---|
| *Bunium ferulaceum* Sibth. and Sm. (A. p. 41) |
| *Bupleurum fruticosum* L. (A. p. 237) |
| *Bupleurum fruticosum* L. (A. p. 237) |
| *Bupleurum fruticosum* L. (A. p. 237) |
| *Buxus sempervirens* L. (A. p. 42) |
| *Cachris libanotis Koch sp. (A. p. 46)~* |
| *Cachris libanotis Koch, Lecokia graeca* ~ (Andrews) *Prangos ferulea* L ~(A. p. 144) |
| *Cachrys libanotis Koch* sp. ~(A. p. 279) |
| *Cachrys libanotis Koch* sp.~ (A. p. 144) |
| *Calamagrostis epigeios Roth, ~Sorgum halepense L.,~* |
| *Calamintha* Lmk. sp. (A. p. 44) |
| *Calamintha clinopodium* L. (A. p. 69) |
| *Calamintha clinopodium* Moris (A. p. 175) |
| *Calamintha clinopodium* Moris. = *Clinopodium vulgare* L. (A. p. 69) |
| *Calamintha clinopodium* Moris. = *Clinopodium vulgare* L.(A. p. 280) |
| *Calamintha* Lmk. sp. (A. p. 44) |
| *Calamintha nepeta* Savi (A. p. 171) |
| *Campanula lingulata* L. ~ (A. p. 157) |
| *Cannabis sativa* L. (A. p. 47) |
| *Capparis spinosa* L. |
| *Capparis spinosa* L. |
| *Capparis spinosa* L. |
| *Capparis spinosa* L. |
| *Capparis spinosa* L. |
| *Capparis spinosa* L. |
| *Capparis spinosa* L. |
| *Capparis spinosa* L. (A. p. 179) |
| *Capparis spinosa* L. (A. p. 179) |
| *Capparis spinosa* L. (A. p. 258) |
| *Capparis spinosa* L. (A. p. 48) |
| *Capparis spinosa* L. (A. p. 84) |
| *Capparis spinosa* L. (A. pp. 123-124) |
| *Capsella bursa pastoris* L. (A. p. 259) |
| *Cardopatium corymbosum* Pers. (A. pp. 59-60) |
| *Cardopatium corymbosum* Pers. (A. p. 175) |

| **Greek name** | **English name** | **References** |
|---|---|---|
| βούνιον | Earthnut | IV, 123 |
| σέσελι Αἰθιοπικόν | Ethiopian hartwort | III, 53 |
| σέσελι Αἰθιοπικόν | Hare's ear | III, 53 |
| σέσελι Αἰθιοπικόν | Hartwort | III, 53 |
| πύξος | Boxthorn | I, Pref. |
| καμψάνεμα | Rosemary frankincense | III, 74 |
| λιβανωτίς | Rosemary frankincense | III, 74 |
| ζέα | Rosemary frankincense | III, 74 |
| λιβανωτὶς κάρπιμος | Rosemary frankincense | III, 74, 1 |
| καλαμάγρωστις | *Calamagrostis* | IV, 30 |
| γλήχων ἀγρία | Catmint | III, 35 |
| κλεόνικον | Horse thyme | III, 95 |
| ὠκιμοειδές | Horse thyme | III, 95 |
| κλινοπόδιον | Horse thyme | III, 95 |
| Ζωπύριον | Horse thyme | III, 95 |
| καλαμίνθη | Catmint | III, 35 |
| νεπέτα | Catmint | III, 35 |
| μήδιον | *Medion* | IV, 18 |
| κάνναβις | Hemp | III, 148 |
| ἀείχλωρος | Caper | II, 173 |
| ἰωνίτης | Caper | II, 173 |
| καπρία | Caper | II, 173 |
| μῆλον κόρακος | Caper | II, 173 |
| ὀλόφυτον | Caper | II, 173 |
| πετραία | Caper | II, 173 |
| τριχομανές | Caper | II, 173 |
| ὀφιόσκορδον | Caper | II, 173 |
| ὀφιοστάφυλον | Caper | II, 173 |
| θαλλία | Caper | II, 173 |
| κάππαρις | Caper | II, 173 |
| κυνόσβατος | Caper | II, 173 |
| ἱππομανές | Caper | II, 173 |
| θλάσπι | Sheparrd's purse | II, 156 |
| χαμαιδάφνη | Chameleon thistle | III, 9 |
| ὠκιμοειδές | Chameleon thistle | III, 9 |

| **Botanical name** |
|---|
| *Cardopatium corymbosum* Pers. (A. p. 275) |
| *Cardopatium corymbosum* Pers. (A. p. 60) |
| *Cardopatium corymbosum* Pers. (A. p. 60) |
| *Cardopatium corymbosum* Pers. (A. p. 84) |
| *Cardopatium corymbosum* Pers. (A. p. 84) |
| *Carduus pycnocephalus* L.~, *C. tenuiflorus* ~ Curtis (A. p. 67) |
| *Carthamus lanatus* L. (A. p. 30) |
| *Carthamus lanatus* L. (A. p. 69) |
| *Cartharmus tinctorius* L. (A. p. 69) |
| *Carum carvi* L. (A. p. 51) |
| *Carum copticum* B. and H. (A. p. 14) |
| *Carum copticum* B. and H. (A. p. 81) |
| *Carum copticum* B. and H. (A. p. 81) |
| *Castanea vulgaris* Lam. |
| *Castanea vulgaris* Lam. |
| *Castanea vulgaris* Lam. (A. p. 32) |
| *Castanea vulgaris* Lam. (A. p. 32) |
| *Castanea vulgaris* Lam. (A. p. 52) |
| *Castanea vulgaris* Lam. (A. p. 52) |
| *Caucalis grandiflora* L. (A. p. 87) |
| *Caucalis grandiflora* L. ~ (A. p. 53) |
| *Celtis australis* L. (A. p. 147) |
| *Centaurea centaurium* L. (A. p. 109) |
| *Centaurea centaurium* L. (A. p. 169) |
| *Centaurea centaurium* L. (A. p. 55) |
| *Centaurea spinosa* L. (A. p. 124) |
| *Ceratonia siliqua* L. (LSJ) |
| *Ceterach officinarum* Willd. (A. p. 119) |
| *Ceterach officinarum* Willd. (A. p. 210) |
| *Ceterach officinarum* Willd. (A. p. 230) |
| *Ceterach officinarum* Willd. (A. p. 247) |
| *Ceterach officinarum* Willd. (A. p. 29) |
| *Chamaelina sativa Crantz, var. microcarpa Andrz. (A. p. 166)~* |
| *Chamaelina sativa Crantz, var. microcarpa Andrz. (A. p. 157)~* |
| *Chamaepeuce mutica* (LSJ) |

| Greek name | English name | References |
|---|---|---|
| οὐλοφόνιον | Chameleon thistle | III, 9 |
| ἰξίας | Chameleon thistle | III, 9 |
| χαμαιλέων ὁ μέλας | Chameleon thistle | III, 9 |
| κυνόζολον | Chameleon thistle | III, 9 |
| κυνόμαζον | Chameleon thistle | III, 9 |
| κρίσσιον | Thistle | IV, 118 |
| ἀτρακτυλίς | Spindle thistle | III, 93 |
| κνῆκος ἄγριος | Spindle thistle | III, 93 |
| κνῆκος | Safflower | IV, 188 |
| καρώ | Caraway | III, 57 |
| ἄμι | Ajowan | III, 62 |
| Αἰθιοπικὸν κύμινον | Ajowan | III, 62 |
| βασιλικὸν κύμινον | Ajowan | III. 62 |
| Διὸς βάλανοι | Chestnuts, Sweet | I, 106 |
| λόπιμα | Chestnuts, Sweet | I, 106 |
| βάλανοι Διός | Chestnuts, Sweet | I, 106 |
| Σαρδιαναὶ βάλανοι | Chestnuts, Sweet | I, 106 |
| καστανίαι | Chestnuts, Sweet | I, 106 |
| μότα | Chestnuts, Sweet | I, 106 |
| δαῦκος ἄγριος | *Caucalis* | II, 139 |
| καυκαλίς | *Caucalis* | II, 139 |
| λωτὸς τὸ δένδρον | Nettle tree | I, 117 |
| γεντιανή | Centaury | III, 6 |
| νάρκη | Centaury | III, 6 |
| κενταύρειον τὸ μέγα | Centaury | III, 6 |
| ἱππόφαιστον | *Hippophaiston* | IV, 160 |
| κεράτια | Carob tree, Fruit of | I, 114 |
| ἡμιόνιον | Miltwaste | III, 134 |
| πτέρυξ | Miltwaste | III, 134 |
| σκολοπένδριον | Miltwaste | III, 134 |
| σπλήνιον | Miltwaste | III, 134 |
| ἄσπληνος | Miltwaste | III, 134 |
| μύαγρον | Ball mustard | IV, 116 |
| μελάμπυρον | Ball mustard | IV, 116 |
| χαμαιπεύκη | Fishbone thistle | IV, 126 |

| **Botanical name** |
|---|
| *Chamomilla* L. sp. |
| *Chamomilla* sp. |
| *Chelidonium majus* L. |
| *Chelidonium majus* L. (A. p. 62) |
| *Chenopodium botry* s L. (A. p. 3) |
| *Chondrilla juncea* L. (LSJ) |
| *Chondrlla ramosissima* L. (LSJ) |
| *Chrozophora tinctoria* Juss. (A. p. 119) |
| *Chrysanthemum coronarium* L. |
| *Chrysanthemum coronarium* L. (A. p. 41) |
| *Chrysanthemum parthenium* Bernh. |
| *Chrysanthemum parthenium* Bernh. (A. p. 189) |
| *Chrysanthemum parthenium* Bernh. (A. p. 189) |
| *Cicer arietinum* L. (A. p. 182) |
| *Cicer arietinum* L. (A. p. 78) |
| *Cicer arietinum* L. (A. p. 96) |
| *Cichorium endivia* L. (A. p. 236) |
| *Cichorium endivia* L. (LSJ) |
| *Cichorium intybus* L. (LSJ) |
| *Cinnamomum zeylanicum Blume, Pogostemon patchouli* ~ Pell. (A. p. 152) |
| *Cinnamomum cassia* Blume (A. p. 52) |
| *Cinnamomum cassia sp.* (LSJ) |
| *Cinnamomum* sp. (A. p. 278) |
| *Cinnamomum tamala* Nees ~, *C. iners~* Blume (A. p. 152) |
| *Cinnamomum tamala* Nees sp., *C. iners* Blume sp. (A. p. 209) |
| *Cinnamomum tamala Nees, ~C. iners Blume (A. p. 152)~* |
| *Cinnamomum tamala Nees , C. iners* Blume (A. p. 67) |
| *Cinnamomum tamala Nees, C. iners* Blume sp. |
| *Cinnamomun tamala* Nees, C. *iners* Blume sp. |
| *Cinnmomum cassia* sp. |
| *Cistus* L. sp. (A. p. 68) |
| *Cistus creticus* L. (A. p. 141) |
| *Cistus creticus* L., *C. cyprius* L. (A. p. 137) |
| *Cistus cyprius* (LSJ) |
| *Cistus* L. sp. (A. p. 68) |

| Greek name | English name | References |
|---|---|---|
| ἀνθεμίς | Camomile | III, 137 |
| καλλία | Camomile | III, 137 |
| κρίμνον | Celandine | II, 180 |
| χελιδόνιον τὸ μέγα | Celandine | II, 180 |
| ἀμβροσία | Oak of Jerusalem | III, 115 |
| χονδρίλη | Gum succory | II, 133 |
| χονδρίλη, ἕτερον εἶδος | Gum succory, another kind | II, 133 |
| ἡλιοτρόπιον τὸ μικρόν | Small heliotrope | IV, 191 |
| κάχλα | Oxeye | III, 139 |
| βούφθαλμον | Oxeye | III, 139 |
| λευκάνθεμον | Feverfew | III, 138 |
| παρθένιον | Feverfew | III, 138 |
| ἀμάρακον | Feverfew | III, 138 |
| ὀροβίας | Chickpea, Cultivated | II, 104 |
| κριός | Chickpea, Cultivated | II, 104 |
| ἐρέβινθος ὁ ἥμερος | Chickpea, Cultivated | II, 104 |
| σέρις | Chicory | II, 132 |
| σέρις | Endive | II, 132 |
| κιχόριον | Chicory | II, 132 |
| μαλάβαθρον | Malabar | I, 12 |
| κασσία | Cassia | I, 13 |
| βάτος Μοσυλῖτις | Mosilian bramble | I. 13, 2 |
| ξυλοκινάμωμον | *Xylocinamomon* | I, 14 |
| | Malabar | I, 12 |
| ψευδοκινάμωμον | *Pseudocinamomon* | I, 14 |
| μαλάβαθρον | Malabar | I, 12 |
| κινάμωμον | Cinnamon | I, 14 |
| ζιγγιβέρι | Cinnamon | I, 14 |
| Μόσυλον | Cinnamon | I, 14 |
| Μοσυλῖτις | Cassia | I, 13 |
| κίσθαρος | Rock rose | I, 97 |
| λῆδον | Rock rose | I, 97 |
| λάδανον | Gum ladanum | I, 97 |
| κὶσθου ἕτερον εἶδος | Rock rose | I, 97 |
| κίσθος | Rock rose | I, 97 |

| **Botanical name** |
|---|
| *Cistus* L. sp. (A. p. 68) |
| *Cistus salviaefolius* L. (A. p. 68) |
| *Cistus villosus* L. (A. p. 68) |
| *Citrullus colocynthis* Schrad. (A. p. 238) |
| *Citrullus colocynthis* Schrad. *(*A. p. 71*)* |
| *Citrullus colocynthis* Schrad. (A. p. 71) |
| *Citrullus sativus* Schrad. (A. p. 192) |
| *Citrus medica* Risso |
| *Citrus medica* Risso (A. p. 153) |
| *Citrus medica* Risso (A. pp. 68, 153) |
| *Clematis vitalba* L., *C. cirrosa* L., *C. flammula* L. (A. p. 69) |
| *Cnicus ferox* L. or C. acarna ~ (A. p. 2) |
| *Cnicus tuberosus* L. or *Cirstium tuberosum* All. |
| *Cnicus tuberosus* L. or *Cirstium tuberosum* All. (A. p. 199) |
| *Cnicus tuberosus* L. or *Cirstium tuberosum* All. (A. p. 133) |
| *Cnicus tuberosus* L. or *Cirstium tuberosum* All. (A. p. 142) |
| *Cnicus tuberosus* L. or *Cirstium tuberosum* All. (A. p. 204) |
| *Colchicum* L. (A. p. 95) |
| *Colchicum* L. sp. (A. p. 71) |
| *Colocasia antiquorum* Schott |
| *Colocasia antiquorum* Schott (A. p. 26) |
| *Commiphora kataf Forsk., ~Styrax benzoin Dryand. (A. p. 47)~* |
| *Commiphora mukul* Engl. (A. p. 34) |
| *Commiphora mukul* Engl. (A. p. 38) |
| *Commiphora mukul Engl. ~(A. p. 151-152)* |
| *Commiphora myrrha* Engl. (A. p. 167) |
| *Commiphora opobalsamum* Engl. (A. p. 33) |
| *Conium maculatum* L. (A. p. 73) |
| *Convolvulus arvensis* L. (A. p. 119) |
| *Convolvulus arvensis* L. (A. p. 67) |
| *Convolvulus arvensis* L. (LSJ) |
| *Convolvulus oleaefolius* Desr. (A. p. 116) |
| *Convolvulus oleaefolius* Desr. (A. p. 90) |
| *Convolvulus oleaefolius* Desr. (LSJ) |
| *Convolvulus scammonia* L. (A. p. 228) |

| **Greek name** | **English name** | **References** |
|---|---|---|
| κίσσαρος | Rock rose | I, 97 |
| κὶσθος θῆλυς | Rock rose, female | I, 97 |
| κὶσθος ἄρρην | Rock rose, male | I, 97 |
| σικὺα πικρά | Colocynth | IV, 176 |
| κολόκυνθα ἀγρία | Colocynth | IV, 176 |
| κολοκυνθίς | Colocynth | IV, 176 |
| πέπων | *Pepon* | II, 135 |
| Περσικά | Citrons | I, 115 |
| Μηδικά | Citrons | I, 115 |
| κίτρια | Citrons | I, 115 |
| κληματίς | Traveler's joy | IV, 180 |
| ἄκανθα λευκή | Fish thistle | III, 12 |
| λάδανον | Tuberous thistle | III, 19 |
| φύλλον | Tuberous thistle | III, 19 |
| ἰσχιάς | Tuberous thistle | III, 19 |
| λευκάκανθα | Tuberous thistle | III, 19 |
| πολυγόνατον | Tuberous thistle | III, 19 |
| ἐφήμερον | Meadow saffron | IV, 83 |
| Κόλχικον | Meadow saffron | I, 70 |
| λοῦφα | Cuckoopint | II, 167 |
| ἄρον | Cuckoopint | II, 167 |
| κάγκαμον | Bisabol | I, 24 |
| βδέλλιον | Bdellium | I, 67 |
| βλόχον | Bdellium | I, 67 |
| μάλδακον | Bdellium | I, 67 |
| σμύρνα | Myrrh | I, 64 |
| βάλσαμον | Mecca balsam | I, 19 |
| κώνειον | Hemlock | IV, 78 |
| ἑλξίνη | Bindweed | IV, 39 |
| κισσάμπελος | Bindweed | IV, 39 |
| ἀμερσίνη | Bindweed | IV, 39 |
| ἁλικάκκαβον | *Dorycnion* | IV, 74 |
| δορύκνιον | *Dorycnion* | IV, 74 |
| καλλέας | *Dorycnion* | IV, 74 |
| σκαμμωνία | Scammony | IV, 170 |

| **Botanical name** |
|---|
| *Convolvulus sepium* L. (A. p. 161) |
| *Convolvulus soldanella* L. (A. p. 38 s. v. brassica) |
| *Coriandrum sativum* L. (A. p. 75) |
| *Cornus mas* (LSJ) |
| *Coronilla scorpioides* Koch (A. p. 232) |
| *Coronopus procumbens Gilib. (A. p. 112)~* |
| *Corydalis claviculata* Pers. |
| *Corydalis claviculata* Pers. (A. p. 133) |
| *Corylus avellana* L. |
| *Corylus avellana* L. |
| *Cotoneaster pyracantha* Spach. (A. p. 183) |
| *Cotoneaster pyracantha* Spach. (A. p. 211) |
| *Cotoneaster pyracantha* Spach. (A. p. 212) |
| *Cressa cretic* a L. (A. p. 18) |
| *Crithmum maritimum* L. (A. p. 78) |
| *Crocus sativus* L. (A. p. 79) |
| *Cucumis sativus* L. (A. p. 80) |
| *Cucumis sativus* L. (A. p. 80) |
| *Cucumis sativus* L. (A. p. 80) |
| *Cucumis sativus* L. (A. p. 80) |
| *Cuminum cyminum* L. (A. p. 81) |
| *Cupressus sempervirens* L. (LSJ) |
| *Curcuma longa* L. (A. p. 85) |
| *Curcuma longa* L. (A. p. 85) |
| *Cuscuta epithymum* L. (A. p. 95) |
| *Cyclamen graecum* Link. (A. p. 82) |
| *Cymbopogon schoenanthus* Spreng. (A. p. 229) |
| *Cymbopogon schoenanthus* Spreng. (A. p. 229) |
| *Cymbopogon schoenanthus* Spreng. (A. p. 257) |
| *Cymbopogon schoenanthus* Spreng. sp. (A. p. 229) |
| *Cymbopogon schoenanthus* Spreng. sp. (A. p. 229) |
| *Cynanchum acutum* L., for Orient: *Marsdenia erect* a Br. |
| *Cynanchum acutum* L., for Orient: *Marsdenia erecta* Br. |
| *Cynanchum acutum* L., for Orient: *Marsdenia erecta* Br. (A. p. 83) |
| *Cynanchum acutum* L., for the Orient: *Marsdenia erecta* Br. (A. p. 189) |

| Greek name | English name | References |
|---|---|---|
| μῖλαξ λεία | Great bindweed | IV, 143 |
| κρὰμβη θαλασσία | Sea cole | II, 122 |
| κόριον | Coriander | III, 63 |
| κρανία | Cornelian cherry tree | I, 119 |
| σκορπιοειδές | Scorpionwort | IV, 192 |
| γλαύξ | Wart cress | IV, 138 |
| φασήλιον | Fumitory | IV, 120 |
| ἰσόπυρον | Fumitory | IV, 120 |
| κάρυον Ποντικόν | Filbert | I, 125 |
| λεπτοκάρυον | Filbert | I, 125 |
| ὀξυάκανθα | Fiery thorn | I, 93 |
| πυρακάνθη | Fiery thorn | I, 93 |
| πυρήν | Fiery thorn | I, 93 |
| ἀνθυλλίς | Anthyllis | III, 136 |
| κρῆθμον | Samphire | II, 129 |
| κρόκος | Saffron | I, 26 |
| πέπων | Cucumber, ripe | II, 135 |
| σικὺου ἡμὲρου ῥίζα | Cucumber, root | II, 135 |
| σικὺου ἡμὲρου ῥίζα | Cucumber, Cultıvated, Root | IV, 151 |
| σὶκυς ἥμερος | Cucumber | II, 135 |
| κύμινον ἥμερον | Cultivated cumin | III, 59 |
| κυπάρισσσος | Cypress | I, 74 |
| κυπὲρου ἕτερον | Turmeric | I, 5 |
| κυπὲρου ἕτερον | Galingale, Another | I, 5 |
| ἐπίθυμον | *Epithymon* | IV, 177 |
| κυκλάμινος | Cyclamen | II, 164 |
| βαβυλώνιον | Camel hay | I, 17 |
| σχοῖνος | Camel hay | I, 17 |
| τευχῖτις | Camel hay | I, 17 |
| σχοῖνος Ἀραβική | Camel hay | I, 17 |
| σχοῖνος ἐν Ναβαταίᾳ | Camel hay | I, 17 |
| κύναγχον | Dogbane | IV, 80 |
| κυνόμορον | Dogbane | IV, 80 |
| κυνοκράμβη | Dogbane | IV, 80 |
| παρδαλιαγχές | Dogbane | IV, 80 |

| **Botanical name** |
|---|
| *Cynanchum acutum* L., for the Orient: *Marsdenia erecta* Br. (A. p. 21) |
| *Cynodon dactylon* Pers. (A. p. 8) |
| *Cyperus papyrus* L. (A. p. 188) |
| *Cyperus rotundus* L. (A. p. 85) |
| *Cyperus rotundus* L. (A. p. 98) |
| *Cystoseira foeniculosa* sp. (A. p. 198) |
| *Cytinus hypocistis* L. (A. p. 128) |
| *Cytinus hypocistis* L. (A. p. 182) |
| *Cytinus hypocistis* L. (A. p. 85) |
| *Dactyloctenium aegyptiacum Willd. = Cynosurus aegyptius L. (A. p. 44)~* |
| *Daphne gnidium* L. |
| *Daphne gnidium* L. |
| *Daphne gnidium* L. (A. p. 212) |
| *Daphne gnidium* L. (A. p. 260) |
| *Daphne gnidium* L. (A. p. 61) |
| *Daphne gnidium* L. (A. p. 70) |
| *Daphne gnidium* L. (A. p. 70) |
| *Daphne laureola* L. |
| *Daphne laureola* L. (A. p. 59) |
| *Daphne laureola* L. (A. p. 87) |
| *Daphne laureola* L. (A. p. 99) |
| *Daphne oleides* L. (LSJ) |
| *Daphne oleide s* L. and *D. oleafolia* L. (A. p. 212) |
| *Daphne oleides* L. and *D. oleafolia* L. (A. p. 61) |
| *Daphne oleides* L. and *D. oleafolia* L. (A. p. 70) |
| *Datura stramonium* L. |
| *Datura stramonium* L. |
| *Datura stramonium* L. |
| *Datura stramonium* L. |
| *Datura stramonium* L. |
| *Datura stramonium* L. |
| *Datura stramonium* L. |
| *Datura stramonium* L. (A. p. 251) |
| *Daucus carota* L. (A. p. 248) |
| *Daucus guttatus L.* (LSJ), see also (A. pp. 57 and 248) |

| **Greek name** | **English name** | **References** |
|---|---|---|
| ἀπόκυνον | Dogbane | IV, 80 |
| ἄγρωστις | Dog's-tooth grass | IV, 29 |
| πάπυρος | Papyrus | I, 86 |
| κύπερος | Galingale | I, 4 |
| ἐρυσίσκηπτρον | Galingale | I, 4 |
| φῦκος θαλάσσιον ἐν Κρήτη | Seaweed, Cretan | IV, 99 |
| ὑποκυστίς | Hypocist | I, 97 |
| ὀρόβηθρον | Hypocist | I, 97 |
| κύτινος | Hypocist | I, 97 |
| καλαμάγρωστις | *Calamagrostis* | IV, 30 |
| ἀπόλινον | Spurge flax | IV, 172 |
| λίνον | Spurge flax | IV, 172 |
| πυρὸς ἄχνη | Spurge flax | IV, 172 |
| θυμελαία | Spurge flax | IV, 172 |
| χαμελαία | Spurge flax | IV, 172 |
| κνέωρον | Spurge flax | IV, 172 |
| κνῆστρον | Spurge flax | IV, 172 |
| εὔπεπλον | Spurge laurel | IV, 146 |
| χαμαιδάφνη | Spurge laurel | IV, 146 |
| δαφνοειδές | Spurge laurel | IV, 146 |
| εὐπέταλον | Spurge laurel | IV, 146 |
| ἄκνηστον | Spurge olive | IV, 171 |
| πυρὸς ἄχνη | Spurge olive | IV, 171 |
| χαμελαία | Spurge olive | IV, 171 |
| κὸκκος Κνίδιως | Spurge olive | IV, 171 |
| πέρσειον | Thorn apple | IV, 73 |
| ὀρθόγυιον | Thorn apple | IV, 73 |
| ἄνυδρον | Thorn apple | IV, 73 |
| ἔνορυ | Thorn apple | IV, 73 |
| θρύον | Thorn apple | IV, 73 |
| πεντόδρυον | Thorn apple | IV, 73 |
| περισσόν | Thorn apple | IV, 73 |
| στρὺχνον μανικόν | Thorn apple | IV, 73 |
| σταφυλῖνος κηπευτός | Carrot, Cultivated | III, 52 |
| κέρας | Wild carrot | III, 52 |

| **Botanical name** |
|---|
| *Daucus guttatus L.* (LSJ), see also (A. pp. 57 and 248) |
| *Delphinium staphisagria* L. (A. p. 248) |
| *Diospyrus ebenum* Koenig (A. p. 92) |
| *Diospyrus ebenum* Koenig, *D . melanoxylon* Roxb. (A. p. 92) |
| *Dipsacus fullorum* L., *D. silvestris* L. (A. p. 89) |
| *Doronicum pardalianches Jacq.* (~A. p. 46)~ |
| *Doronicum pardalianches Jacq.* ~ (A. p. 189) |
| *Doronicum pardalianches Jacq.* ~ (A. p. 4) |
| *Doronicum pardalianches Jacq. ~(A. p. 258)~* |
| *Doronicum pardalianches Jacq.~* |
| *Doronicum pardalianches Jacq.~* |
| *Ecballium elaterium* Rich. |
| *Ecballium elaterium* Rich. |
| *Echium diffusum* Sibth. (A. p. 16) |
| *Echium diffusum* Sibth. (A. p. 16) |
| *Echium diffusum* Sibth. (A. p. 178) |
| *Echium italicum* L sp. (A. p. 149) |
| *Echium plantagineum* L., *E. rubrum* L. (A. p. 9) |
| *Echium plantagineum* L., *E. rubrum* L. (A. p. 90) |
| *Echium plantagineum* L., *E. rubrum* L. (A. p. 92) |
| *Elettaria cardamomum* White and Maton and other spp. (A. p. 49) |
| *Ephedra distachya* L. |
| *Ephedra distachya* L. (A. p. 232) |
| *Ephedra distachya* L. sp. (A. p. 263) |
| *Epilobium angustifolium* L. (A. p. 178) |
| *Epilobium angustifolium* L. (A. p. 179) |
| *Epilobium angustifolium* L. (A. pp. 178-179) |
| *Equisetum maximum* Lmk = *E. telmateia* Ehr. (A. p. 124) |
| *Equisetum silvaticum* L. (A. p. 124) |
| *Equisetum silvaticum* L. (A. p. 124) |
| *Equisetum silvaticum* L. (A. p. 15) |
| *Erica arborea* L. (A. p. 96) |
| *Erodium malacoides* Willd. (A. p. 110) |
| *Eruca sativa Lam* . (A. p. 100) |
| *Erucaria aleppica* (LSJ) |

| Greek name | English name | References |
|---|---|---|
| σταφυλῖνος ἄγριος | Carrot, Wild | III, 52 |
| σταφὶς ἀγρία | Stavesacre | IV, 152 |
| Ἰνδικὴ ἔβενος | Indian ebony | I, 98 |
| ἔβενος | Ebony | I, 98 |
| δίψακος | Teasel | III, 11 |
| κάμμαρον | Leopard's bane | IV, 76 |
| παρδαλιαγχές | Leopard's bane | IV, 76 |
| ἀκόνιτον | Leopard's bane | IV, 76 |
| | Leopard's bane | IV, 76 |
| κυνοκτόνον | Leopard's bane | IV, 76 |
| μυοκτόνον | Leopard's bane | IV, 76 |
| σίκυς ἄγριος | Squirting cucumber | IV, 150 |
| φέρομβρον | Squirting cucumber | IV, 150 |
| ἄγχουσα ἑτέρα | Alkanet, Another | IV, 24 |
| Ἀλκιβιάδειον | Alkanet, Another | IV, 24 |
| ὀνοχειλές | Alkanet, Another | IV, 24 |
| λυκαψός | Viper's herb | IV, 26 |
| Ἀλκιβιάδειον | *Echion* | IV, 27 |
| Δωρίς | *Echion* | IV, 27 |
| ἔχιον | *Echion* | IV, 27 |
| καρδάμωμον | Cardamom | I, 6 |
| τάργανον | *Tragos* | IV, 51 |
| σκορπίον | *Tragos* | IV, 51 |
| τράγος | *Tragos* | IV, 51 |
| ὀνάγρα | Oleander | IV, 117 |
| ὀνό‹θο›υρις | Oleander | IV, 117 |
| ὀνοθήρας | Oleander | IV, 117 |
| ἵππουρις ἑτέρα | Horsetail, Another | IV, 47 |
| ἔφεδρον | Horsetail | IV, 46 |
| ἵππουρις | Horsetail | IV, 46 |
| ἀναβάσιον | Horsetail | IV, 46 |
| ἐρείκη | Tree heath | I, 88 |
| γεράνιον ἕτερον | Cranesbill, Another | III, 116 |
| εὔζωμον | Rocket | II, 140 |
| γογγύλη ἀγρία | Eastern cress | II, 110 |

| **Botanical name** |
|---|
| *Ervum lens* L. (LSJ) |
| *Eryngium campestre* L. |
| *Eryngium campestre* L. (A. p. 97-98) |
| *Eryngium campestre* L. (A. pp. 97-98) |
| *Eryngium maritinum* (LSJ) |
| *Erythraea centaurium* (A. p. 55) |
| *Erythraea centaurium* (A. p. 55) |
| *Erythraea centaurium* L. (A. p. 145) |
| *Euphorbia* L. (A. p. 261) |
| *Euphorbia peplis* L. (A. p. 156) |
| *Euphorbia peplis* L. (A. p. 192) |
| *Euphorbia acanthothamnos* Heldr. and Sart. (A. p. 124) |
| *Euphorbia acanthothamnos* Heldr. and Sart. (A. p. 124) |
| *Euphorbia apios* L. |
| *Euphorbia apios* L. (A. p. 133) |
| *Euphorbia apios* L. (A. p. 20) |
| *Euphorbia apios* L. (A. p. 216) |
| *Euphorbia apios* L. (A. p. 59) |
| *Euphorbia chamaesyce* L. (A. p. 253) |
| *Euphorbia chamaesyce* L. (A. p. 61) |
| *Euphorbia cyparissias* L. (A. p. 262) |
| *Euphorbia dendroides* L. (A. p. 262) |
| *Euphorbia helioscopia* L. (A. p. 118) |
| *Euphorbia helioscopia* L. (A. p. 262) |
| *Euphorbia lathyris* L. (A. p. 139) |
| *Euphorbia myrsinites* L. (A. p. 262) |
| *Euphorbia myrsinites* L. (A. 262) |
| *Euphorbia myrsinites* L. (A. p. 167) |
| *Euphorbia myrsinites* L. (A. p. 52) |
| *Euphorbia myrsinitis* L. (A. p. 52) |
| *Euphorbia paralias* L. (A. p. 261) |
| *Euphorbia peplis* L. (A. 253) |
| *Euphorbia peplis* L. (A. p. 16) |
| *Euphorbia peplis* L. (A. p. 192) |
| *Euphorbia peplis* L. (A. p. 192) |

| Greek name | English name | References |
|---|---|---|
| φακός | Lentil | II, 107 |
| κάρυον | Eryngo | III, 21 |
| ἠρύγγη | Eryngo | III, 21 |
| ἠρύγγιον | Eryngo | III, 21 |
| κροκοδείλεον | Sea holly | III, 10 |
| κενταύρειον λεπτόν | Feverfew | III, 7 |
| κενταύρειον μικρόν | Feverfew | III, 7 |
| λιμνήσιον | Feverfew | III, 7 |
| τιθύμαλλος | Spurge | IV, 164 |
| μὴκων ἀφρώδης | Wartweed | IV, 167 |
| πέπλος | Wartweed | IV, 167 |
| ἱπποφαές | Spurge | IV, 159 |
| ἱππόφαος | Spurge | IV, 159 |
| λινόζωστις | Tuberous spurge | IV, 175 |
| ἰσχάς | Tuberous spurge | IV, 175 |
| ἄπιος | Tuberous spurge | IV, 175 |
| ῥάφανος ἀγρία | Tuberous spurge | IV, 175 |
| χαμαιβάλανος | Tuberous spurge | IV, 175 |
| συκῆ | Thyme spurge | IV, 169 |
| χαμαισύκη | Thyme spurge | IV, 169 |
| κυπαρισσίας | Spurge | IV, 164 |
| δενδροειδής | Spurge | IV, 164 |
| ἡλιοσκόπιος | Sun spurge | IV, 164 |
| ἡλιοσκόπιος | Spurge | IV, 164 |
| λαθυρίς | Caper spurge | IV, 166 |
| τιθύμαλλος θῆλυς | Myrtle spurge | IV, 164 |
| μυρσινίτης | Spurge | IV, 164 |
| μυρσινίτης | Myrtle spurge | IV, 164 |
| καρυίτις | Myrtle spurge | IV, 164 |
| καρυίτης | Spurge | IV, 164 |
| παράλιος | Spurge | IV, 164 |
| συκῆ | Wartweed | IV, 167 |
| ἀνδράχνη ἀγρία | Wild purslane | IV, 168 |
| πέπλιον | Wild purslane | IV, 168 |
| πεπλίς | Wild purslane | IV, 168 |

| **Botanical name** |
|---|
| *Euphorbia pityusa* L. |
| *Euphorbia pityusa* L. (A. p. 69) |
| *Euphorbia pityusa* L. (A. p. 188) |
| *Euphorbia pityusa* L. (A. p. 262) |
| *Euphorbia pityusa* L. (A. p. 77) |
| *Euphorbia platyphyllos* L. (A. p. 262) |
| *Euphorbia resinifera* Berg. (A. p. 99) |
| *Euphorbia Sibthorpii* Boiss. |
| *Euphorbia Sibthorpii* Boiss. (A. p. 61) |
| *Euphorbia Sibthorpii* Boiss. (A. p. 70) |
| *Euphorbia Sibthorpii* Boiss. (A. p. 73) |
| *Euphporbia parallias* L. (A. p. 262) |
| Evax pygmaea Pers. ,~E. asterifolia Pers., (A. p. 55) ~Plantago cretica L.,~ |
| *Evernia* L. (A. p. 247) |
| *Evernia* L. (A. p. 39) |
| *Ferula galbaniflua* Boiss. And Buhse (A. p. 58) |
| *Ferula communis* L. (A. p. 170) |
| *Ferula ferulago* L . = *Ferulago galbanifera* Koch (A. p. 144) |
| *Ferula galbaniflua* Boiss. & Buhse (A. p. 160) |
| *Ferula galbaniflua* Boiss. and Buhse (A. p. 108) |
| *Ferula marmarica* L. (A. p. 116) |
| *Ferula marmarica* L. (A. p. 7) |
| Ferula nodosa L. or ~Echinophora tenuifolia L. (A. p. 186)~ |
| *Ferula persica* Willd. (A. p. 223) |
| *Ferula tingitana* L. ~ (A. p. 240) |
| *Ficaria verna* Huds. (A. p. 212) |
| *Ficaria verna* Huds. (A. p. 62) |
| *Ficus carica* L. (A. p. 104) |
| *Ficus carica* L. (A. pp. 48 and 96) |
| *Ficus sycomorus* L. (A. p. 253) |
| *Ficus sycomorus* L. (A. p. 253) |
| *Foeniculum vulgare* Gaertn. (A. p. 155) |
| *Frankenia hirsuta* L. and *F. pulverulenta* L. (A. p. 195) |
| *Frankenia hirsuta* L. and *F. pulverulenta* L. (A. p. 94) |
| *Fraxinus ornus* L. (LSJ) |

| Greek name | English name | References |
|---|---|---|
| Κανωπικόν | Quacksalver's spurge | IV, 165 |
| κλῆμα | Quacksalver's spurge | IV, 165 |
| παράλιος | Quacksalver's spurge | IV, 165 |
| πιτυούσα | Quacksalver's spurge | IV, 165 |
| κράμβιον | Quacksalver's spurge | IV, 165 |
| πλατύφυλλος | Spurge | IV, 164 |
| εὐφόρβιον | Spurge | III, 82 |
| ἀμυγδαλίτης | Spurge | IV, 164 |
| χαρακίας | Spurge | IV, 164 |
| κωβιός | Spurge | IV, 164 |
| κομήτης | Spurge | IV, 164 |
| τιθυμαλλίς | Spurge | IV, 164 |
| κῆμος | *Cemos* | IV, 133 |
| σπλάχνον | Tree moss | I, 21 |
| βρύον | Tree moss | I, 21 |
| πάνακες | Allheal | III, 83 |
| νάρθηξ | Giant fennel | III, 77 |
| λιβανωτὶς ἑτέρα | Rosemary, The other | III, 74, 2, l. 6 |
| μέτωπον | Galbanum | III, 83 |
| χαλβάνη | Galbanum | III, 83 |
| ἀμμωνιακόν | Gum ammoniac | III, 84 |
| ἀγασυλλίς | Gum ammoniac | III, 84 |
| πάνακες Ἀσκληπί‹ει›ον | Asculapius' allheal | III, 49 |
| σαγάπηνον | *Sagapenon* | III, 81 |
| σίλφιον | Laserwort | III, 80 |
| πυρὸς ἄγριος | Pilewort | II, 181 |
| χελιδόνιον τὸ μικρόν | Pilewort | II, 181 |
| σῦκα | Figs | I, 128 |
| ἐρινεός | Wild fig | I, 128 |
| συκάμινον | Sycamore fig | I, 127 |
| συκόμορον | Sycamore fig | I, 127 |
| μάραθον | Fennel | III, 70 |
| φακοειδές | Sea heath | IV, 179 |
| ἔμπετρον | Sea heath | IV, 179 |
| μελία | Manna ash | I, 80 |

| **Botanical name** |
|---|
| *Fritillaria graeca* L. (A. p. 228) |
| *Fritillaria graeca* L. (A. p. 265) |
| *Fumaria officinalis* L. (A. p. 48) |
| *Fungi* |
| *Galium aparine* L. |
| *Galium aparine* L. (A. p. 177) |
| *Galium aparine* L. (A. p. 19) |
| *Galium aparine* L. (A. p. 196) |
| *Galium verum* L. |
| *Galium verum* L. |
| *Galium verum* L. (A. p. 108) |
| *Genista acanthoclada* (LSJ) |
| *Genista acanthoclada* (LSJ) |
| *Gentiana lutea* L., *G. purpurea* L. (A. p. 109) |
| *Geranium tuberosum* L. (A. p. 110) |
| *Gladiolus segetum* Gawler (A. p. 151) |
| *Gladiolus segetum* Gawler (A. p. 196) |
| *Gladiolus segetum* Gawler (A. p. 278) |
| *Glaucium corniculatum* Curtis (A. p. 112) |
| *Glaucium flavum* Crantz |
| *Glaucium flavum* Crantz (A. p. 188) |
| *Glaucium flavum* Crantz (A. p. 57) |
| *Glechoma hederacea* L. (A. p. 59) |
| *Globularia alypum* L. (A. p. 12) |
| *Glycyrrhiza glabra* L, G. echinata L. (A. p. 233) |
| *Glycyrrhiza glabra* L. (LSJ) |
| *Glycyrrhiza glabra* L. G. echinata (A. p. 253) |
| *Glycyrrhiza glabra* L., G. echinata L. (A. p. 112) |
| *Glycyrrhiza glabra* L., G. echinata L. (A. p. 109) |
| *Glycyrrhiza glabra* L., G. echinata L. (A. p. 5) |
| *Gnaphalium* L. sp., *Filago* L. sp. (A. p. 112) |
| *Gnaphalium leontopodium ~ (A. p. 55)* |
| *Hedera helix* L. (A. p. 67) |
| *Helichrysum orientale* L., *H. stoechas* L., *H. siculum* L. (A. p. 118) |
| *Helichrysum orientale* L., *H. stoecha* s L., *H. siculum* L. (A. p. 13) |

| Greek name | English name | References |
|---|---|---|
| σατύριον | Man orchis | III, 128 |
| τρίφυλλον | Man orchis | III, 128 |
| καπνός | Fumitory | IV, 109 |
| μύκητες | Mushrooms | IV, 82 |
| ἀμπελόκαρπον | Cleavers | III, 90 |
| ὀμφαλόκαρπον | Cleavers | III, 90 |
| ἀπαρίνη | Cleavers | III, 90 |
| φιλάνθρωπον | Cleavers | III, 90 |
| γαλαίριον | Bedstraw | IV, 95 |
| γαλάτιον | Bedstraw | IV, 95 |
| γάλιον | Bedstraw | IV, 95 |
| ἀκακία ἡ ἐν Καππαδοκίᾳ | Shittah tree, another | I, 101 |
| ἀκακία ἡ ἐν Πόντῳ | Shittah tree, another | I, 101 |
| γεντιανή | Gentian | III, 3 |
| γεράνιον | Cranesbill | III, 116 |
| μαχαιρίων | Corn flag | IV, 20 |
| φασγάνιον | Corn flag | IV, 20 |
| ξίφιον | Corn flag | IV, 20 |
| γλαύκιον | *Glaucion* | III, 86 |
| μὴκων ἀγρία | Horned poppy | IV, 65 |
| μὴκων παράλιος | Horned poppy | IV, 65 |
| μὴκων κερατῖτις | Horned poppy | IV, 65 |
| χαμαίκισσος | Ground ivy | IV, 125 |
| ἄλυπον | Herb terrible | IV, 178 |
| Σκύθιον | Licorice | III, 5 |
| Ποντικὴ ῥίζα | Licorice | III, 5 |
| σύμφυτον | Licorice | III, 5 |
| γλυκύρριζα | Licorice | III, 5 |
| γεντιανή | Licorice | III, 5 |
| ἄδιψον | Licorice | III, 5 |
| γναφάλλιον | Cottonweed | III, 117 |
| κῆμος | *Cemos* | IV, 133 |
| κισσός | Ivy | II, 179 |
| ἑλίχρυσον | Gold flower | IV, 57 |
| ἀμάραντον | Gold flower | IV, 57 |

| Greek name | English name | References |
|---|---|---|
| χρυσάνθεμον | Gold flower | IV, 57 |
| βάκχαρις | Sowbread | III, 44 |
| σκορπίουρον | Large heliotrope | IV, 190 |
| ἡλιοτρόπιον τὸ μέγα | Large heliotrope | IV, 190 |
| ἐλλέβορος μέλας | Black hellebore | IV, 162 |
| σησαμοειδές | Black hellebore, Fruit of | IV, 162 |
| πολύρριζον | Black hellebore | IV, 162 |
| Μελαμπόδιον | Black hellebore | IV, 162 |
| ἔκτομον | Black hellebore | IV, 162 |
| σφονδύλιον | Cow parsnip | III, 76 |
| πολύγονον θῆλυ | Mare's tail | IV, 5 |
| μάκιρ | Mace | I, 82 |
| κριθή | Barley | II, 86 |
| κίννα | Wall barley | IV, 32 |
| ἄγρωστις ἡ ἐν Κιλικίᾳ | Wall barley | IV, 32 |
| ἰξός | Oak mistletoe | III, 89 |
| ὑοσκύαμος | Henbane | IV, 68 |
| ἀδάμας | Henbane | IV, 68 |
| ὑπήκοον | Horned cumin | IV, 67 |
| χαμαίπιτυς | St. John's wort | III, 154 |
| ὑπερικόν | St. John's wort | III, 154 |
| ἀνδρόσαιμον | St. John's wort | III, 154 |
| κόριον | St. John's wort | III, 154 |
| ὑπερικόν | St. John's wort | III, 157 |
| κόρις | St. John's wort | III, 157 |
| πάνακες Χειρώνιον | Chiron's allheal | III, 50 |
| ἀνδρόσαιμον | St. John's wort | III, 156 |
| ἄσκυρον | St. John's wort | III, 156 |
| Διονυσιάς | St. John's wort | III, 156 |
| ἀνδρόσαιμον | St. John's wort | III, 155 |
| ἀσκυροειδές | St. John's wort | III, 155 |
| ἄσκυρον | St. John's wort | III, 155 |
| κόνυζα, τρίτον εἶδος | Fleabane | III, 121 |
| ἄρκτιον | Bearwort | IV, 105 |
| ἀρκτοῦρος | Bearwort | IV, 105 |

| **Botanical name** |
| --- |
| *Inula graveolens* Desf. (A. p. 74) |
| *Inula helenium* L. (A. p. 157) |
| *Inula helenium* L. (A. p. 171) |
| *Inula helenium* L. (A. p. 181) |
| *Inula helenium* L. (A. p. 181) |
| *Inula helenium* L. (A. p. 253) |
| *Inula helenium* L. (A. p. 253) |
| *Inula helenium* L. (A. p. 69) |
| *Inula helenium* L. (LSJ) |
| *Inula helenium* L.(A. p. 118) |
| *Inula* sp. |
| *Inula viscosa* Aiton (A. p. 74) |
| *Iris florentina* L., *I. germanica* L., *I. pallida* Lamk. (A. p. 133) |
| *Iris* L. sp. (A. p. 278) |
| *Iris* L. sp. (A. p. 278) |
| *Iris* L. sp. (A. p. 278) |
| *Iri* s L. sp. (A. p. 278) |
| *Iris pseudacorus* L. (A. p. 4) |
| *Iris pseudacorus* L. (A. p. 4) |
| *Isatis agrestis* L. (A. p. 133) |
| *Isatis tinctoria* L. (A. p. 133) |
| *Juglans regia* L. (A. p. 52) |
| *Juglans regia* L. (A. p. 52) |
| *Juncus acutus* L. (A. p. 184) |
| *Juniperus* L. (LSJ) |
| *Juniperus* L. (LSJ) |
| *Juniperus sabina* L. (A. p. 38) |
| *Juniperus sabina* L. (A. p. 38) |
| *Lactuca sativa* L. (A. p. 260) |
| *Lactuca scariola* L. (A. p. 260) |
| *Lagenaria vulgaris* Ser. (A. p. 71) |
| *Lagoecia cuminoides* L. (A. p. 81) |
| *Lamium album* L. (A. p. 143) |
| *Laurus nobilis* L. (LSJ) |
| *Lavendula stoechas* L. (A. p. 250) |

| **Greek name** | **English name** | **References** |
|---|---|---|
| κόνυζα μικρά | Fleabane | III, 121 |
| νεκτάριον | Elecampane | I, 28 |
| βάτος Ἰδαία | Elecampane | I, 28 |
| κλεώνιον | Elecampane | I, 28 |
| Ὀρέστιον | Elecampane | I, 28 |
| Μηδική | Elecampane | I, 28 |
| σύμφυτον | Elecampane | I, 28 |
| φλόμος Ἰδαῖος | Elecampane | I, 28 |
| Περσική | Elecampane | I, 28 |
| Ἑλένιον | Elecampane | I, 28 |
| κόνυζα | Fleabane | III, 121 |
| κόνυζα μείζων | Fish thistle | III, 121 |
| ἶρις | Iris | I, 1 |
| γλαδίολος | Gladwyn | IV, 22 |
| ἶρις ἀγρία | Gladwyn | IV, 22 |
| ξιρίς | Gladwyn | IV, 22 |
| ξυρίς | Gladwyn | II, 22 |
| ἄκορον | Yellow flag | I, 2 |
| ἄσπληνον | Yellow flag | I, 2 |
| ἰσὰτις ἀγρία | Wild woad | II, 185 |
| ἰσάτις | Woad | II, 184 |
| κάρυον βασιλικόν | Walnut | I, 125 |
| κάρυον Περσικόν | Walnut | I, 125 |
| ὀξύσχοινος | Rush | IV, 52 |
| ἄρκευθος | Juniper | I, 75 |
| κέδρος | Cedar | I, 77 |
| βόρατον | Savin | I, 76 |
| βράθυ | Savin | I, 76 |
| θριδάξ ἥμερος | Lettuce, Cultivated | II, 136 |
| θριδάξ ἀγρία | Lettuce, Wild | II, 136 |
| κολόκυνθα ἐδώδιμος | Bottle gourd, Edible | II, 134 |
| κύμινον ἄγριον | Wild cumin | III, 60 |
| λευκάς | Dead nettle | III, 99 |
| δάφνη | Sweet bay | I, 78 |
| στοιχάς | French lavender | III, 26 |

| **Botanical name** |
|---|
| *Lawsonia inermis* L. (A. p. 85) |
| *Lemna minor* L. (A. p. 141) |
| *Leontice chrysogonon* L. sp. (A. p. 64) |
| *Leontice chrysogonon* L. sp. (LSJ) |
| *Leontice chrysogonon* L. sp. (LSJ) |
| *Leontice leontopetalum* (LSJ) |
| *Leontice leontopetalum* L. (A. p. 142) |
| *Leontice leontopetalum* L. (A. p. 143) |
| *Leontice leontopetalum* L. (A. p. 189) |
| *Leontice leontopetalum* L. (A. p. 259) |
| *Leonurus cardiaca L., ~ L. marrubiastrum L. (A. p. 211)~* |
| *Lepidium draba* L. (A. p. 90) |
| *Lepidium latifolium* L. (A. p. 110) |
| *Lepidium latifolium* L. (A. p. 142) |
| *Lepidium sativum* L. (A. p. 49) |
| *Levisticum officinale* Koch (A. p. 145) |
| *Levisticum officinale* Koch (A. p. 187 ) |
| *Lilium candidum* L. (A. p. 145) |
| *Lilium candidum* (LSJ) |
| *Lilium martagon* L. (A. p. 119) |
| *Lilium martagon* L. (A. p. 119) |
| *Linaria spuria* Miller (A. p. 93) |
| *Linum usitatissimum* (LSJ) |
| *Lithospermum fruticosum* L. (A. p. 16) |
| *Lithospermum officinale* (A. p. 100) |
| *Lithospermum officinale* L. |
| *Lithospermum officinale* L. (A. p. 89) |
| *Lithospermum officinale* L. (A. p. 120) |
| *Lithospermum officinale* L. (A. p. 147) |
| *Lloydia graeca* L. |
| *Lloydia graeca* L. (A. p. 195) |
| *Lloydia graeca* L. (A. p. 195) |
| *Lolium temulentum* L. (A. p. 6) |
| *Lollium perenne* L. (A. p. 16) |
| *Lollium perenne* L. (A. p. 197) |

| Greek name | English name | References |
|---|---|---|
| κύπρος | Henna | I, 95 |
| φακός ὁ ἐπί τελμάτων | Duckweed | IV, 87 |
| χρυσόγονον | Black turnip | IV, 56 |
| ἴασπις | Black turnip | IV, 56 |
| λίνον | Black turnip | IV, 56 |
| λεοντοπέταλον | *Leontopetalon* | III, 96 |
| λεοντοπέταλον | *Leontopodion* | III, 96 |
| λεύκηθρον | *Leontopetalon* | III, 96 |
| παρδάλιον | *Leontopetalon* | III, 96 |
| θορύβηθρον | *Leontopetalon* | III, 96 |
| πυκνόκομον | Motherwort | IV, 174 |
| δράβη | Arabian mustard | II, 157 |
| γιγγίδιον | Pepperwort | II, 174 |
| λεπίδιον | Pepperwort | II, 174 |
| κάρδαμον | Garden cress | II, 155 |
| λιγυστικόν | Lovage | III, 51 |
| πάνακες | Lovage | III, 51 |
| λείριον | Lily | III, 102 |
| κρίνον | Lily | III, 102 |
| ἡμεροκαλλές | Martagon lily | III, 122 |
| ἡμεροκατάλλακτον | Martagon lily | III, 122 |
| ἐλατίνη | Cankerwort | IV, 40 |
| λινόσπερμον | Linseed | II, 103 |
| ἄγχουσα ἄλλη | Alkanet, Another | IV, 25 |
| ἐξώνυχον | Groomwell | III, 141 |
| ἀετώνυχον | Groomwell | III, 141 |
| Διὸς πυρός | Groomwell | III, 141 |
| Ἡρακλεία | Groomwell | III, 141 |
| λιθόσπερμον | Groomwell | III, 141 |
| λευκάκανθον | Spiderwort | III, 108 |
| φαλάγγιον | Spiderwort | III, 108 |
| φαλαγγῖτις | Spiderwort | III, 108 |
| αἶρα | Darnel | II, 100 |
| ἀγχύνωψ | Rye grass | IV, 43 |
| φοῖνιξ | Rye grass | IV, 43 |

| **Botanical name** |
|---|
| *Lollium perenne* L. (A. p. 218) |
| *Lonicera etrusca* L. (A. p. 192) |
| *Lonicera etrusca* L. (A. p. 247) |
| *Lonicera etrusca* L. (A. p. 69) |
| *Lonicera periclimenum* (A. p. 67) |
| *Lonicera periclymenum* L. (A. p. 82) |
| Lunaria alba L., ~ Sinapis alba L., ~ Brassica nigra Koch (A. p. 259) |
| *Lupinus* L. (LSJ) |
| *Lychnis coronaria* Desr. (A. p. 149) |
| *Lycopus europaeus* L. (A. p. 193) |
| *Lysimachia vulgaris* L. (A. p. 150) |
| *Madragora* L. sp. (A. pp. 153-154) |
| *Madragora* L. sp. (LSJ) |
| *Madragora* L. sp. (LSJ) |
| *Majorana hortensis* Moench (A. p. 13) |
| *Majorana hortensis* Moench (A. p. 225) |
| *Malabaila aurea* Sibth. (A. p. 237) |
| *Malabaila aurea* Sibth. (A. p. 237) |
| *Malabaila sekakul* Russ. (A. p. 110) |
| *Malope malacoides* L. (A. p. 9) |
| *Malum* sp. (LSJ) |
| *Malum medica* Risso (A. pp. 68, 153) |
| *Malva silvestris* (LSJ) |
| *Mandragora autumnalis* Sprengel (A. p. 259) |
| *Mandragora autumnalis* Sprengel (A. p. 154) |
| *Mandragora* L. sp. (LSJ) |
| *Mandragora vernalis* Bert. (A. p. 154) |
| *Mandragora vernalis* Bert. (A. p. 164) |
| *Marrubium vulgare* L. (LSJ) |
| *Marrubium vulgare* L., *M. creticum* Miller |
| *Matricaria chamomilla* |
| *Matricaria chamomilla* L. |
| *Matricaria chamomilla* L. (A. p. 157) |
| *Matricaria chamomilla* L. (A. p. 60) |
| *Matthiola incana* L. (A. p. 142) |

| Greek name | English name | References |
|---|---|---|
| ῥοῦς | Rye grass | IV, 43 |
| περικλύμενον | Honeysuckle | IV, 14 |
| σπλήνιον | Honeysuckle | IV, 14 |
| κλύμενον | Honeysuckle | IV, 14 |
| κισσάνθεμον | Cyclamen, Another | II, 165 |
| κυκλάμινος ἑτέρα | Cyclamen, Another | II, 165 |
| Περσικὸν σίνηπι | Sheparrd's purse | II, 156 |
| θέρμος | Lupine | II, 109 |
| λυχνὶς στεφανωματική | Rose campion | III, 100 |
| περιστέριον | Vervain | IV, 59 |
| λυσιμάχειος | Loosestrife | IV, 3 |
| μανδραγόρας | Mandrake | IV, 75 |
| Κιρκαία | Mandrake | IV, 75 |
| ἀντίμιμον | Mandrake | IV, 75 |
| ἀμάρακον | Marjoram | III, 39 |
| σάμψουχον | Marjoram | III, 39 |
| σέσελι τό ἐν Πελοποννήσῳ | Peloponnesian hartwort | III, 53 |
| σέσελι τό ἐν Πελοποννήσῳ | Golden cow-parsnip | III, 53 |
| γιγγίδιον | *Gingidion* | II, 137 |
| ἀλκαία | Vervain mallow | III, 147 |
| ὀρβικλᾶτα | Rose apple | I, 115 |
| κεδρόμηλα | Citrons | I, 115 |
| μολόχη | Mallow | II, 118 |
| θριδακίας | Mandrake, female | IV, 75 |
| μανδραγὸρας θῆλυς | Mandrake, female | IV, 75 |
| βομβόχυλον | Mandrake | IV, 75 |
| μανδραγὸρας ἄρρην | Mandrake, male | IV, 75 |
| μώριος | Mandrake, male | IV, 75 |
| πράσιον | Horehound | III, 105 |
| φιλοφαρές | Horehound | III, 105 |
| ἐράνθεμον | Camomile | III, 137 |
| λευκάνθεμον | Camomile | III, 137 |
| μηλάνθεμον | Camomile | III, 137 |
| χαμαίμηλον | Camomile | III, 137 |
| λευκόιον | Gillyflower | III, 123 |

| **Botanical name** |
|---|
| *Medicago arborea* L. (A. p. 85) |
| *Medicago sativa* L. (A. p. 157) |
| *Medicago sativa* L. (A. p. 157) |
| *Melilotus* Adans. sp. (A. p. 158) |
| *Melilotus* Adans. sp. (A. p. 264) |
| *Melilotus Adans*. sp. (A. pp. 147-148) |
| *Melissa officinalis* L., *M. altissima* Sibth. and Sm. (A. p. 158) |
| *Melissa officinalis* L., *M. altissima* Sibth. and Sm. (A. p. 158) |
| *Mentha* L. |
| *Mentha* L. |
| *Mentha pulegium* L. (A. p. 112) |
| *Mentha pulegium* L. (A. p. 36) |
| *Mentha silvestris* L., *M. viridis* L. (A. p. 122) |
| *Mentha silvestris* L., *M. viridis* L. (A. p. 241) |
| *Mercurialis annua* L. (A. p. 122) |
| *Mercurialis annua* L. (A. p. 146) |
| *Mercurialis annua* L. (A. p. 189) |
| *Mercurialis perennis* L. (A. p. 198) |
| *Mespilus germanica* L. |
| *Mespilus germanica* L. (A. p. 160) |
| *Mespilus germanica* L. (A. p. 237) |
| *Mespilus germanica* L. (A. p. 95) |
| *Metricaria camomilla* L. (A. p. 96) |
| *Meum athamanticum* Jacq. (A. pp. 160-161) |
| *Meum athamanticum* Jacq. (A. pp. 160-161) |
| *Mimusops Schimperi* L. (A. p. 193) |
| *Moringa* sp. |
| *Morus nigra* L. (A. p. 164) |
| *Morus nigra* L. (A. p. 253) |
| *Muscari comosum* Miller (A. p. 40) |
| *Myriophyllum spicatum* L. (A. p. 167) |
| *Myrrhis odorata* Scop. (A. p. 167) |
| *Myrrhis odorata* Scop. (A. p. 167) |
| *Myrtus communis* L. (LSJ) |
| *Narcissus poeticus* L. (A. p. 169) |

| Greek name | English name | References |
|---|---|---|
| κύτισος | Tree medick | IV, 112 |
| Μηδική | Alfalfa | II, 147 |
| Μηδική | Lucerne | II, 147 |
| μελίλωτος | King's clover | III, 40 |
| τρίφυλλον | Italian melilot | IV, 110 |
| λωτός ἐν παραδείσοις | Italian melilot | IV, 110 |
| μελιτταίνα | Balm | III, 104 |
| μελισσόφυλλον | Balm | III, 104 |
| ἡδύοσμον | Green mint | III, 34 |
| μίνθη | Green mint | III, 34 |
| βλήχων | Pennyroyal | III, 31 |
| γλήχων | Pennyroyal | III, 31 |
| ἕρπυλος ἄγριος μέγας | Bergamot mint | III, 41 |
| σισύβριον | Bergamot mint | III, 41 |
| Ἑρμοῦ βοτάνιον | Mercury | IV, 189 |
| λινόζωστις | Mercury | IV, 189 |
| παρθένιον | Mercury | IV, 189 |
| φύλλον | Dog mercury | III, 125 |
| ἀρωνία | Medlar | I, 118 |
| μέσπιλον | Medlar tree | I, 118 |
| σητάνιον | Medlar | I, 118 |
| ἐπιμηλίς | Medlar | I, 118 |
| ἠράνθεμον | Camomile | III, 137 |
| μῆον | Bald money | I, 3 |
| μῆον | Spignel | I, 3 |
| περσαία | Persea | I, 129 |
| βάλανος μυρεψική | Ben | IV, 157 |
| μορέα | Mulberry tree | I, 126 |
| συκάμινον | Mulberry tree | I, 126 |
| βολβὸς ἐδώδιμος | Purse tassels | II, 170 |
| μυριόφυλλον | Water milfoil | IV, 114 |
| μύρρα | Sweet cicely | IV, 115 |
| μυρρίς | Sweet cicely | IV, 115 |
| μυρσὶνη ἥμερος | Cultivated myrtle | I, 112 |
| νάρκισσος | Narcissus | IV, 158 |

| **Botanical name** |
|---|
| Narcissus tazetta (LSJ) see also (A. p. 41) |
| *Nardostachys jatamansi* DC (A. p. 109) |
| *Nardostachys jatamansi* DC (A. p. 170) |
| *Nardostachys jatamansi* DC (A. p. 170), *Patrinia scabiosifolia* Fisch. (A. p. 170) |
| *Nardostachys jatamansi* DC. (A. p. 170) |
| *Nasturtium officinale* R. Br. (A. p. 241) |
| *Nasturtium officinale* R. Br. (A. p. 242) |
| *Nasturtium officinale* R. Br. (A. p. 49) |
| *Nelumbo nucifera* Gaert. (A. p. 148) |
| *Nelumbo nucifera* Gaert. (A. p. 82) |
| *Nelumbo nucifera* Gaert. (A. p. 82) |
| *Nerium oleander* L. |
| *Nerium oleander* L. (A. p. 171) |
| *Nerium oleander* L. (A. p. 217) |
| *Nigella arvensis* (LSJ) |
| *Nigella sativa* L. (A. p. 157) |
| *Nithrophyllum punctatum* L. (A. p. 198) |
| *Notobasis syriaca* Cass. = *Cirsium syriacum* Gaertn. (A. p. 2) |
| *Nuphar luteum* Sm. (A. p. 174) |
| *Nymphaea alba* L. (A. p. 174) |
| *Ocimum basilicum* L. sp. (A. p. 175) |
| *Ocinum pilosum Willd, ~ Thymus acinos L. ~* (A. p. 4) |
| *Ocinum pilosum Willd, ~ Thymus acinos L. ~(* A. p. 4) |
| *Olea europaea* L. var. *sativa* Hoffm. and Lk. (A. p. 176) |
| *Olea europaea* L. var. *silvestris* Miller (A. p. 176) |
| *Olea europaea* L. var. *silvestris* Miller (A. p. 176) |
| *Olea europaea* L. var. *silvestris* Miller (A. p. 76) |
| *Onobrychis caput galli* Link. and *O. viciaefolia* Scop. (A. p. 178) |
| *Ononis antiquorum* L. (A. p. 17) |
| *Ononis antiquorum* L. (A. p. 178) |
| *Onopordum acanthium* L., *O. illyricum* (A. p. 2) |
| *Onosma echinoides* L. |
| *Onosma echinoides* L. (A. p. 178) |
| *Onosma echinoides* L. (A. p. 178) |
| *Onosma echinoides* L. (A. p. 197) |

| Greek name | English name | References |
|---|---|---|
| βολβὸς ἐμετικός | Narcissus tazetta | IV, 156 |
| Γαγγῖτις | Gangitis | I, 7 |
| Ἰνδικὴ νάρδος | Indian spikenard | I, 7 |
| νάρδος | Spikenard | I, 7 |
| νὰρδος Ἰνδική | Indian spikenard | I, 7 |
| σισύμβριον | Water cress | II, 128 |
| σίον | Water cress | II, 128 |
| καρδαμίνη | Water cress | II, 128 |
| λωτός ὁ ἐν Αἰγύπτῳ | Egyptian lotus | IV, 113 |
| κύαμος Αἰγύπτιος | Bean, Egyptian | II, 106 |
| κύαμος Ποντικός | Bean, Egyptian | II, 106 |
| ῥοδοδάφνη | Oleander | IV, 81 |
| νήριον | Oleander | IV, 81 |
| ῥοδόδενδρον | Oleander | IV, 81 |
| κύμινον ἕτερον γένος | Wild cumin, Another | III, 61 |
| μελάνθιον | Black cumin | III, 79 |
| φῦκος θαλάσσιον ὑπόμηκες | Seaweed, Longish | IV, 99 |
| ἄκανθα Ἀραβική | Milk thistle, smaller | III, 13 |
| νυμφαὶα ἄλλη | White water lily, Another | III, 132 |
| νυμφαία | White water lily | III, 132 |
| ὤκιμον | Basil | II, 141 |
| ἄκινος | Wild basil | III, 43 |
| ἄκονος | Wild basil | III, 43 |
| ἐλαὶα ἥμερος | Olive tree, Cultivated | I, 105 |
| ἀγριελαία | Wild olive tree | I, 105 |
| ἐλαὶα Αἰθιοπική | Olive tree, Wild | I, 105 |
| κότινος | Wild olive tree | I, 105 |
| ὀνοβρυχίς | Cock's head | III, 153 |
| ἀνωνίς | Rest harrow | III, 18 |
| ὀνωνίς | Rest harrow | III, 18 |
| ἀκάνθιον | Cotton thistle | III, 16 |
| ὀσμάς | Stone bugloss | III, 131 |
| ὄνοσμα | Stone bugloss | III, 131 |
| ὄνωνις | Stone bugloss | III, 131 |
| φλονῖτις | Stone bugloss | III, 131 |

| **Botanical name** |
|---|
| *Opopanax hispidus* Grisb. (A. p. 179 and p.186 s.v *panaces*) |
| *Opoponax hispidus* Grisb. (A. p. 186) |
| *Orchis morio* L. sp. (A. p. 236) |
| *Orchis morio* . L. sp. (.A. p. 180) |
| *Orchis papilionacea L., ~ O. longicruris ~ L.* (A. p. 180) |
| *Orchis papilionacea* L., ~ O. longicruris L. (A. p. 84)~ |
| *Origanum dictamnus* L. |
| *Origanum dictamnus* L. |
| *Origanum dictamnus* L. (A. p. 88) |
| *Origanum heracleoticum* Rchb. and *O. vulgare* L. |
| *Origanum heracleoticum* Rchb. and *O. vulgare* L. (A. p. 181) |
| *Origanum heracleoticum* sp. Rchb. |
| *Origanum viride Boiss.* ~ (A. p. 120) |
| *Origanum viride Boiss.* ~ (A. p. 187) |
| *Origanum viride Boiss.* ~ (A. p. 73) |
| Origanum viride Boiss. sp. ~ |
| *Ornithogalum umbellatum* L. (A. p. 181) |
| *Ornithopus compressu* s L. (A. p. 53) |
| *Orobanche crenata* Forsk. (A. p. 141) |
| *Orobanche crenata* Forsk. (A. p. 260) |
| *Orobanche crenata* Forsk. (A. p. 84) |
| *Orobanche crenata* Forsk. (A. pp. 181-182) |
| *Oryza sativa* (LSJ) |
| *Osiris alba* L. (A. p. 183) |
| *Ottelia alismoide* s Pers. (A. p. 206) |
| *Paeonia* L. sp (A. p. 112) |
| *Paeonia* L. |
| *Paeonia* L. (A. p. 191) |
| *Paeonia* L. sp. (A. p. 185) |
| *Paeonia* L. sp. (A. p. 7) |
| *Paliurus australis* Gaertn. = *P. spina Christi* Mill. (A. 185) |
| *Pancratium maritimum* L. (A. p. 187) |
| *Pancratium maritimum* L. (A. p. 230) |
| *Panicum miliaceum* L. (LSJ) |
| *Papaver argemone* L. (A. p. 23) |

| **Botanical name** |
|---|
| *Papaver rhoeas* L. (A. p. 156) |
| *Papaver somniferum* L. |
| *Papaver somniferum* L. |
| *Papaver somniferum* L. |
| *Papaver somniferum* L. (A. p. 156) |
| *Parietaria officinalis* L. |
| *Parietaria officinalis* L. (A. p. 119) |
| *Parietaria officinalis* L. (A. p. 119) |
| *Parietaria officinalis* L. (A. p. 120) |
| *Parietaria officinalis* L. (A. p. 189) |
| *Parietaria officinalis* L. (A. p. 192) |
| *Parietaria officinalis* L. (A. p. 204) |
| *Parietaria officinalis* L. (A. p. 238) |
| *Parietaria officinalis* L. (A. p. 69) |
| *Parnassia palustris* L. (A. p. 8) |
| *Paronychia* Mill. sp. (A. p. 189) |
| *Pastinaca sativa* L. (A. p. 241) |
| *Pastinaca sativa* L. (A. p. 93) |
| *Pastinaca sativa* L. (A. p. 93) |
| *Patrinia scabiosifolia* Fisch. (A. p. 170) |
| *Peganum harmala* L. |
| *Peganum harmala* L. |
| *Peganum harmala* L. (A. p. 163) |
| *Peganum harmala* L. (A. p. 163) |
| *Petasites officinalis* Moench (A. p. 194) |
| *Petroselinum hortense* Hoffm. (A. p. 195) |
| *Peucedanum officinale* L. (A. p. 195) |
| *Phalaris canariensis* L. (A. p. 195) |
| *Phillyrea* L. sp. (A. p. 197) |
| *Phoenix dactylifera* L. (LSJ) |
| *Physalis alkekengi* L. (A. p. 115) |
| *Physalis alkekeng* i L. (A. p. 251) |
| *Physalis alkekengi* L. (A. p. 251) |
| *Pimpinella anisum* L. (A. p. 17) |
| *Pimpinella cretica* L. (A. p. 209) |

| Greek name | English name | References |
|---|---|---|
| μὴκων ῥοιάς | Corn poppy | IV, 63 |
| μὴκων θυλακῖτις | Opium poppy | IV, 64 |
| μὴκων πιθῖτις | Opium poppy | IV, 64 |
| μὴκων ῥοιάς | Opium poppy | IV, 64 |
| μήκων | Opium poppy | IV, 64 |
| ὑγιεινὴ ἀγρία | Pellitory | IV, 85 |
| ἑλξίνη | Pellitory | IV, 85 |
| ἔλυμος | Italian millet | II, 98 |
| Ἡράκλεια | Pellitory | IV, 85 |
| παρθένιον | Pellitory | IV, 85 |
| περδίκιον | Pellitory | IV, 85 |
| πολυώνυμον | Pellitory | IV, 85 |
| σιδηρῖτις | Pellitory | IV, 85 |
| κλύβατις | Pellitory | IV, 85 |
| ἄγρωστις ἡ ἐν τῶ Παρνασσῷ | Grass of Parnassus | IV, 31 |
| παρωνυχία | *Paronychia* | IV, 54 |
| σίσαρον | Parsnip | II, 113 |
| ἐλαφοβόσκον | Parsnip | III, 69 |
| ἐλαφόβοσκον | Parsnip | III, 69 |
| νὰρδος Συριακή | Syrian spikenard | I, 7 |
| ἁρμαλά | Wild rue | III, 46 |
| βήσσασα | Wild rue | III, 46 |
| μῶλυ | Wild rue | III, 46 |
| πήγανον ἄγριον | Wild rue | III, 46 |
| πετασῖτις | Butterbur | IV, 107 |
| πετροσέλινον | Parsley | III, 66 |
| πευκέδανον | Sulphurwort | III, 78 |
| φαληρίς | Canary grass | III, 142 |
| φιλύρα | Lime tree | I, 96 |
| φοῖνιξ | Date palm | I, 109 |
| ἁλικάκκαβον | Winter cherry | IV, 71 |
| στρὺχνον ἕτερον | Hound's berry, another | IV, 71 |
| στρὺχνον ἕτερον | Winter cherry | IV, 71 |
| ἄνησσον | Anise | III, 56 |
| ψευδοβούνιον | Cretan pimpinnell | IV, 124 |

| **Botanical name** |
|---|
| *Pimpinella tragium* Vill. (A. p. 263) |
| *Pinus* sp. |
| *Pinus* sp. |
| *Pinus* sp. |
| *Pinus* sp. |
| *Piper album* L. (A. p. 200) |
| *Piper nigrum* L. (A. p. 200) |
| *Piper officinarum* DC. (A. p. 200) |
| *Pirus malus* L. (A. p. 115) |
| *Pistacia lentiscus* L. (LSJ) |
| *Pistacia palestina* Boiss. (A. pp. 262-263) |
| *Pistacia terebinthus* L. (A. p. 256) |
| *Pistacia vera* L. (LSJ) |
| *Pistia stratiotes* L. (A. p. 250) |
| *Plantago* L. sp. (A. p. 120) |
| *Plantago Bellardii All., ~ P. albicans L. ~* (A. p. 125) |
| *Plantago coronopus* (LSJ) |
| *Plantago* L. sp. (A. p. 26) |
| *Plantago major* L. sp. (A. p. 204) |
| *Plantago psyllium* L. and *P. cynops* L. |
| *Plantago psyllium* L. and *P. cynops* L. (A. p. 210) |
| *Plantago psyllium* L. and *P. cynops* L. (A. p. 79) |
| *Plantago psyllium* L. and *P. cynop* s L. (A. p. 84) |
| *Platanus orientalis* L. (LSJ) |
| *Polemonium caeruleum L. ~ Hypericum olympicum ~* L. (A. p. 203) |
| *Polemonium caeruleum* L. or *Hypericum olympicum* L. (A. p. 196) |
| *Polemonium caeruleum* L. or *Hypericum olympicum* L. (A. p. 203) |
| *Polygala venulosa* Sibth. (A. p. 203) |
| *Polygonatum multiflorum* All. and *P. verticillatum* All. (A. p. 133) |
| *Polygonatum multiflorum* All., P. *verticillatum* All. (A. p. 95) |
| *Polygonatum verticillatum* All., *P. officinale* All., *P. multiflorum* L. (A. p. 204) |
| *Polygonum aviculare* L. |
| *Polygonum aviculare* L. (A. 203) |
| *Polygonum aviculare* L. (A. 69) |
| *Polygonum aviculare* L. (A. p. 168) |

| Greek name | English name | References |
|---|---|---|
| τράγιον ἄλλο | Pimpinell | IV, 50 |
| πεύκη | *Peuce* pine | I, 69 |
| πίτυς | *Pitys* pine | I, 69 |
| πίτυς | Stone pine *cembra* | I, 69 |
| στρόβιλος | *Stobilos* pine | I, 69 |
| πέπερι λευκόν | Pepper, White | II, 159 |
| πέπερι | Pepper | II, 159 |
| πέπερι μακρόν | Pepper, Long | II, 159 |
| μηλέα | Apple | I, 115 |
| σχῖνος | Mastic | I, 70 |
| τράγιον | Stinking tutsan | IV, 49 |
| τέρμινθος | Terebinth | I, 71 |
| πιστάκια | Pistachio nut | I, 124 |
| στρατιώτης ὁ ἐπὶ τῶν ὑδάτων | Water lettuce | IV, 101 |
| ἑπτάπλευρον | Plantain | II, 126 |
| ὁλόστεον | Allbone | IV, 11 |
| κορωνόπους | Hartshorn | II, 130 |
| ἀρνόγλωσσον | Plantain | II, 126 |
| πολύπλευρον | Plantain | II, 126 |
| κυνοκέφαλον | Fleawort | IV, 69 |
| ψύλλιον | Fleawort | IV, 69 |
| κρυστάλλιον | Fleawort | IV, 69 |
| κυνόμυια | Fleawort | IV, 69 |
| πλάτανος | Plane tree | I, 79 |
| πολεμώνιον | Jacob's ladder | IV, 8 |
| Φιλεταίριον | Jacob's ladder | IV, 8 |
| χιλιοδύναμον | Jacob's ladder | IV, 8 |
| πολύγαλον | Milkwort | IV, 139 |
| ἶρις ἀγρία | *Ephemeron* | IV, 84 |
| ἐφήμερον | *Ephemeron* | IV, 84 |
| πολυγόνατον | Solomon's seal | IV, 6 |
| τευθαλίς | Knotgrass | IV, 4 |
| πολύκαρπον | Knotgrass | IV, 4 |
| κλῆμα | Knotgrass | IV, 4 |
| μυρτοπέταλον | Knotgrass | IV, 4 |

| **Botanical name** |
|---|
| *Polygonum aviculare* L. (A. p. 204) |
| *Polygonum aviculare* L. (A. p. 49) |
| *Polygonum hydropiper* L. (A. p. 127) |
| *Polygonum persicaria* L. (A. p. 77) |
| *Polypodium vulgare* L. (A. p. 204) |
| *Polyporus* sp. (A. p. 7) |
| *Polystichum filix mas* Roth. (A. p. 205) |
| *Polystichum filix mas* Roth. (A. p. 210) |
| *Polystichum filix mas* Roth. (A. p. 36) |
| *Populus alba* L. (A. p. 143) |
| *Populus nigra* L. (A. p. 6) |
| *Portulaca oleracea* L. (A. p. 16) |
| *Posidonia oceanica* Del. (A. p. 198) |
| *Potentilla reptans* L. |
| *Potentilla reptans L.* (A. p. 191) |
| *Potentilla reptans* L. (A. p. 191) |
| *Potentilla reptans* L. (A. p. 191) |
| *Potentilla reptans* L. (A. p. 191) |
| *Potentilla reptans* L. (A. p. 209) |
| *Potentilla reptans* L. (A. p. 278) |
| *Potentilla reptans* L. (A. p. 278) |
| *Poterium spinosum* L. (A. p. 250) |
| *Prangos ferulacea* L. sp. ~ (A. p. 124) |
| *Prunus amygdalus* Stokes esp. var. *sativa* Asch. (A. p. 15) |
| *Prunus amygdalus* Stokes, var. *amara* Schn. (A. p. 15) |
| *Prunus armeniaca* L. |
| *Prunus armeniaca* L. (A. p. 157) |
| *Prunus avium (* LSJ) |
| *Prunus domestica* L. (A. p. 71) |
| *Prunus persica* Sieb. and Z. (A. p. 153) |
| *Psorolea bituminosa* L. (A. p. 162) |
| *Psorolea bituminosa* L. (A. p. 183) |
| *Psorolea bituminosa* L. (A. p. 264) |
| *Psorolea bituminosa* L. (A. p. 28) |
| *Psorolea bituminosa* L. (A. p. 319) |

| **Greek name** | **English name** | **References** |
|---|---|---|
| πολύγονον ἄρρεν | Knotgrass | IV, 4 |
| καρκίνωθρον | Knotgrass | IV, 4 |
| ὑδροπέπερι | Smartweed | II, 161 |
| κραταιόγονον | Willow weed | III, 124 |
| πολυπόδιον | Polypody | IV, 186 |
| ἀγαρικόν | Agaric | III, 1 |
| πολύρριζον | Male fern | IV, 184 |
| πτερίς | Male fern | IV, 184 |
| βλῆχρον | Male fern | IV, 184 |
| λεύκη | White poplar | I, 81 |
| αἴγειρος | Black poplar | I, 83 |
| ἀνδράχνη | Purslane | II, 124 |
| φῦκος θαλάσσιον πλατύ | Seaweed, Broad | IV, 99 |
| ξυλοπέταλον | Cinquefoil | IV, 42 |
| πενταδάκτυλον | Cinquefoil | IV, 42 |
| πενταπετές | Cinquefoil | IV, 42 |
| πεντάτομον | Cinquefoil | IV, 42 |
| πεντέφυλλον | Cinquefoil | IV, 42 |
| ψευδοσέλινον | Cinquefoil | IV, 42 |
| καλλιπέταλον | Cinquefoil | IV, 42 |
| ξυλόλωτον | Cinquefoil | IV, 42 |
| στοιβή | Thorny burnet | IV, 12 |
| ἱππομάραθον | Horse fennel | III, 71 |
| ἀμυγδάλη | Almond | I, 123 |
| ἀμύγδαλων πικρόν | Almond, bitter | I, 123 |
| μῆλα ἀρμενιακά | Apricots | I, 115 |
| βρεκόκκια | Apricots | I, 115 |
| κεράσια | Cherries, Fruit of cherry tree | I, 113 |
| κοκκυμηλέα | Plum tree | I, 121 |
| Περσικὰ μῆλα | Peaches | I, 115 |
| μινυανθές | Treacle clover | III, 109 |
| ὀξύφυλλον | Treacle clover | III, 109 |
| τρίφυλλον | Treacle clover | III, 109 |
| ἀσφάλτιον | Treacle clover | III, 109 |
| κνήκιον | Treacle clover | III, 109 |

| **Botanical name** |
|---|
| *Pteris aquilina* L. (A. p. 258) |
| *Pteris aquilina* L.(A. p. 174) |
| *Punica granatum* (LSJ) |
| *Pyrus acerba* (LSJ) |
| *Pyrus amygdaliformis* Vill. (A. p. 3) |
| *Pyrus communis* (LSJ) |
| *Pyrus Cydonia* (LSJ) |
| *Pyrus praecox* (LSJ) |
| *Quercus aegilops* L. (A. p. 196) |
| *Quercus coccifera* L. (A. p. 70) |
| *Quercus ilex* L. (A. p. 207) |
| *Quercu* s L sp. (A. p. 91) |
| *Quercus* L. sp. (A. p. 32) |
| *Ranunculus* L. sp. |
| *Ranunculus* L. sp. |
| *Ranunculus* L. sp. |
| *Ranunculus* L. sp. |
| *Ranunculus* L. sp. |
| *Ranunculus* L. sp. (A. p. 34) |
| *Raphanus raphanistrum* (LSJ) |
| *Raphanus raphanistrum* L. (A. p. 138) |
| *Raphanus sativus* (LSJ) |
| *Reseda alba* L. (A. p. 237) |
| *Reseda alba* L. (A. p. 94) |
| *Reseda phyteuma* L. (A. p. 199) |
| *Rhamnus cathartica* L. (A. p. 217) |
| *Rhamnus petiolaris* , *Rh. lycoides* , *Rh. punctata* Boiss. (A. p. 212) |
| *Rhamnus petiolaris, Rh. lycoides, Rh. punctata* Boiss. (A. p. 149) |
| *Rheum officinale* (LSJ) |
| *Rheum ribes* L. (A. p. 217) |
| *Rhus coriaria* L. (A. p. 218) |
| *Rhus coriaria* L. (LSJ) |
| *Ricinus communis* L. (A. p. 237) |
| *Ricinus communis* L. (A. p. 237) |
| *Ricinus communi* s L. (A. p. 66) |

| Greek name | English name | References |
|---|---|---|
| θηλυπτερίς | Bracken | IV, 185 |
| νυμφαία πτερίς | Bracken | IV, 185 |
| ῥοά | Pomegranate | I, 110 |
| μῆλον ἄγριον | Crab apple | I, 115 |
| ἀχράς | Wild pear | I, 116 |
| ἄπιος | Pear | I, 116` |
| στρούθια | Quinces | I, 115 |
| μελίμηλον | Summer apple | I, 115 |
| φηγός | Valonia oak | I, 106 |
| κὸκκος βαφική | Kermes oak | IV, 48 |
| πρῖνος | Holm oak | I, 106 |
| δρῦς | Oak | I, 106 |
| βάλανος | Acorn | I, 106 |
| βατράχιον ἕτερον | Ranunculus | II, 175 |
| βατράχιον τέταρτον | Ranunculus | II, 175 |
| βατράχιον τρίτον | Ranunculus | II, 175 |
| σέλινον ἄγριον | Ranunculus | II, 175 |
| σέλινον ἄγριον ἕτερον | Ranunculus | II, 175 |
| βατράχιον | Ranunculus | II, 175 |
| ἀγρὶα ῥαφανίς | Wild radish | II, 112 |
| λαμψάνη | Charlock | II, 116 |
| ῥαφανίς | Radish | II, 112 |
| σησαμοειδὲς τὸ μέγα | Bastard rocket | IV, 149 |
| ἐλλέβορος | Bastard rocket | IV, 149 |
| φύτευμα | Montpellier rocket | IV, 128 |
| ῥάμνος | Boxthorn | I, 90 |
| πυξάκανθα | Dyer's buckthorn | I, 100 |
| λύκιον | Dyer's buckthorn | I, 100 |
| ῥῆον | Rhubarb | III, 2 |
| ῥά | Rhubarb | III, 2 |
| ῥοῦς ὁ ἐπὶ τὰ ὄψα | Sumac | I, 108 |
| ἐρυθρόν | Sumac | I, 108 |
| σέσελι Κύπριον | Castor oil tree | IV, 161 |
| σήσαμον ἄγριον | Castor oil tree | IV, 161 |
| κίκι | Castor oil tree | IV, 161 |

| **Botanical name** |
|---|
| *Ricinus communis* L. (A. p. 79) |
| *Rosa* (LSJ) |
| *Rosa sempervirens* L. (A. p. 183) |
| *Rosa sempervirens* L. (A. p. 84) |
| *Rosmarinum sterile* (LSJ) |
| *Rosmarinus officinalis* L. (A. p. 144) |
| *Rubia tinctorum* L. (A. p. 257) |
| *Rubia tinctorum* L., *R. per'a* L. (A. p. 96) |
| *Rubia tinctorum* L., *R. per'a* L. (A. p. 98) |
| *Rubus idaeus* L. (A. p. 34) |
| *Rubus ulmifolius* Schott (LSJ) |
| *Rumex* L. sp. (A. p. 137) |
| *Rumex* L. sp. (LSJ) |
| *Rumex aquaticus* L. (A. p. 123) |
| *Rumex aquaticus* L. (A. p. 39) |
| *Rumex conglomeratus* L. (LSJ) |
| *Rumex crispus* L. (A. p. 183) |
| *Rumex* sp. |
| *Ruscus aculeatus* L. |
| *Ruscus aculeatus* L. |
| *Ruscus aculeatus* L. |
| *Ruscus aculeatus* L. |
| *Ruscus aculeatus* L. |
| *Ruscus aculeatus* L. (A. p. 167) |
| *Ruscus aculeatus* L. (A. p. 183) |
| *Ruscus aculeatus* L. (A. p. 60) |
| *Ruscus hypoglossum* L. (A. 130) |
| *Ruscus hypoglossum* L. (A. p. 128) |
| *Ruscus hypoglossum* L. (LSJ) |
| *Ruscus hypoglossum* L. (LSJ) |
| *Ruscus hypophyllum* L. (LSJ) |
| *Ruscus hypophyllum* L. (LSJ) |
| *Ruscus hypophyllum* L. (LSJ) |
| *Ruscus hypophyllum* L. (LSJ) |
| *Ruscus racemosus* L. (A. p. 59) |

| **Greek name** | **English name** | **References** |
|---|---|---|
| κροτών | Castor oil tree | IV, 161 |
| ῥόδον | Rose | I, 99 |
| ὀξυάκανθα | White rose | I, 94 |
| κυνόσβατος | White rose | I, 94 |
| λιβανωτὶς ἄκαρπος | Rosemary frank'se, fruitless | III, 74, 2, 1.9 |
| λιβανωτίς | Rosemary | III, 75 |
| τεύθριον | Madder | III, 143 |
| ἐρευθέδανον | Madder | III, 143 |
| ἐρυθρόδανον | Madder | III, 143 |
| βάτος Ἰδαία | Raspberry | IV, 38 |
| βάτος | Bramble | IV, 37 |
| λάπαθον | Monk's rhubarb | II, 114 |
| ἀναξυρίς | Monk's rhubarb | II, 114 |
| ἱππολάπαθον | Dock sorrel | II, 115 |
| βρεττανική | Water dock | IV, 2 |
| λάπαθον ἄγριον | Dock | II, 114 |
| ὀξυλάπαθον | Curled dock | II, 114 |
| ὀξαλίς | Monk's rhubarb | II, 114 |
| ἄκαιρον | Butcher's broom | IV, 144 |
| γοργυνθία | Butcher's broom | IV, 144 |
| κίνη | Butcher's broom | IV, 144 |
| λειχήνη | Butcher's broom | IV, 144 |
| μυρσὶνη ἀγρία | Butcher's broom | IV, 144 |
| μυρτάκανθος | Butcher's broom | IV, 144 |
| ὀξυμυρσίνη | Butcher's broom | IV, 144 |
| χαμαιμυρσίνη | Butcher's broom | IV, 144 |
| Ἰδαία | Daphne Alexandreia | IV, 145 |
| ὑπόγλωσσον | Horse tongue | IV, 129 |
| Ἰδαὶα ῥίζα | *Idaia rhiza* | IV, 44 |
| στέφανος | Daphne Alexandreia | IV, 145 |
| Δανάη | Daphne Alexandreia | IV, 145 |
| δάφνη Αλεξάνδρεια | Daphne Alexandreia | IV, 145 |
| ζαλεία | Daphne Alexandreia | IV, 145 |
| ὑπόγλωττον | Daphne Alexandreia | IV, 145 |
| χαμαιδάφνη | Chamaidaphne | IV, 147 |

| **Botanical name** |
|---|
| *Ruscus racemosus* L. (A. p. 9) |
| *Ruta chalepensis L. (A. p. 191)* |
| *Ruta graveolens* L. (A. p. 191) |
| *Salix* L. sp. (A. p. 134) |
| *Salvia aethiopis* L., *S. argentea* L. (A. p. 7) |
| *Salvia horminum* L. (A. p. 126) |
| *Salvia* L. sp. (A. p. 93) |
| *Salvia* sp. |
| *Sambucus ebukus* L. |
| *Sambucus ebulus* L. (A. p. 59) |
| *Sambucus nigra* L. (A. p. 4) |
| *Sambucus nigra* L. (A. p. 4) |
| *Sambucus nigra* L. (A. p. 4) |
| *Sanguisorba minor* Scop. = *Poterium sanguisorba* L. (A. p. 238) |
| *Santolina chamaecyparissus* (A. p. 115) |
| *Saponaria officinalis* L. (A. p. 251) |
| *Satureia graeca* L. = *Micromeria graeca* Benth. (A. p. 129) |
| *Satureia thymbra* L. sp. (A. p. 260) |
| *Satureia thymbra* L. (A. p. 260) |
| *Saussurea lappa* Clarke (A. p. 76) |
| *Saxifrage* L. sp. (A. p. 77) |
| *Scandix pecten-Veneris* L. (A. p. 229) |
| *Scilla bifolia* L. (A. p. 126) |
| *Scirpus holoschoenus* L. (A. p. 125) |
| *Scirpus* L. sp., *Juncus* L. sp. (A. p. 229) |
| *Scirpus* L. sp., *Juncus* L. sp. (A. p. 229) |
| *Scolopendrium hemionitis* Lag. (A. p. 120) |
| *Scolopendrium hemionitis* Lag. (A. p. 247) |
| *Scolopendrium officinale* L. sp. (A. p. 105) |
| *Scolymus maculatus* L. and *S. hispanicu* s L. (A. p. 231) |
| *Scorpiurus vermiculatus* L. (A. p. 69) |
| *Scrofularia lucida* L. (A. p. 238) |
| *Scrofularia lucida* L. (LSJ) |
| *Scrofularia peregrina* L. |
| *Scrofularia peregrina* L. (A. p. 108) |

| Greek name | English name | References |
|---|---|---|
| Ἀλεξάνδρεια | Chamaidaphne | IV, 147 |
| πήγανον ὀρεινόν | Rue | III, 45 |
| πήγανον | Rue | III, 45 |
| ἰτέα | Willow | I, 104 |
| Αἰθιοπίς | Silver sage | IV, 104 |
| ὅρμινον | Clary | III, 129 |
| ἐλελίσφακον | Sage | III, 33 |
| σφάγνος | Sage | III, 33 |
| ἕλειος ἀκτῆ | Deadwort | IV, 173 |
| χαμαιάκτη | Deadwort | IV, 173 |
| ἀκτῆ | Elder | IV, 173 |
| ἀκτῆ ἕλειος | Elder | IV, 173 |
| χαμαιάκτη | Elder | IV, 173 |
| σιδηρῖτις ἄλλη | Burnet | IV, 34 |
| ἀβρότονον θῆλυ | Lavender cotton | III, 24 |
| στρούθιον | Soapwort | II, 163 |
| ὕσσωπος | Hyssop | III, 25 |
| θύμβρα | Savory | III, 37 |
| θύμος | Cretan thyme | III, 36 |
| κόστος | Costusroot | I, 16 |
| κοτυληδών, ἕτερον εἶδος | Navelwort, Another | IV, 92 |
| σκάνδιξ | Wild chervil | II, 138 |
| ὑάκινθος | Wild hyacinth | IV, 62 |
| ὁλόσχοινος | Club-rush | IV, 52 |
| Εὐριπικὴ σχοῖνος | Euripic rush | IV, 52 |
| σχοῖνος Εὐριπική | Rush | IV, 52 |
| ἡμιονῖτις | Mule fern | III, 135 |
| σπλήνιον | Mule fern | III, 135 |
| φυλλῖτις | Hart's tongue | III, 107 |
| σκόλυμος | Golden thistle | III, 14 |
| κλύμενον | Bearbind | IV, 13 |
| σιδηρῖτις ἑτέρα | Figwort | IV, 35 |
| Ἡρακλεία | Figwort | IV, 35 |
| γάληψις | Brownwort | IV, 94 |
| γαλεόβδολον | Brownwort | IV, 94 |

| Botanical name |
|---|
| *Scrofularia peregrina* L. (A. p. 108) |
| *Securigera securidaca* (A. p. 117) |
| *Securigera securidaca* L. (A. p. 191) |
| *Sedum* L. sp. (A. p. 8) |
| *Sedum* L. sp. (A. p. 8) |
| *Sedum album* L., *S. stellatum* L. (A. p. 16) |
| *Sedum album* L., *S. stellatum* L. (A. p. 256) |
| *Sedum cepaia* L. (A. p. 56) |
| *Sedum* L. sp. (A. p. 16) |
| *Sedum* L. sp. (A. p. 256) |
| *Sedum* L. sp. (A. p. 8) |
| *Sedum roseum* Scop., *S. rhodiola* DC. (A. p. 217) |
| *Sempervivum arboreum* L. (A. p. 249) |
| *Sempervivum arboreum* L. (A. p. 41) |
| *Sempervivum arboreum* L. (A. p. 13) |
| *Sempervivum arboreum* L. (A. p. 280) |
| *Sempervivum arboreum* L. (A. p. 8) |
| *Sempervivum tectorum* L. (A. p. 8) |
| *Senecio thapsoides DC.* ~ *Mercurialis tomentosa* L. (A. pp. 140-141) |
| *Senecio thapsoides DC.* ~, *Mercurialis tomentos* a L. ~ (A. p. 43) |
| *Senecio vulgaris* L. (A. p. 96) |
| *Serapias cordiga* L. (A. p. 228) |
| *Serapias cordigera* L. (A. p. 228) |
| *Serapias lingua* L. (A. p. 147) |
| *Sesamum indicum* L. (A. p. 237) |
| *Seseli tortuosum* L. (A. p. 237) |
| *Setaria italica* P. B. (A. p. 158) |
| *Sideritis romana* L. (A. p. 120) |
| *Sideritis romana* L. (A. p. 238) |
| *Silene gallica* L. |
| *Silene gallica* L. (A. 92) |
| *Silene gallica* L. (A. p. 175) |
| *Silene inflata* Sm., *S. muscipula* L. (A. p. 120) |
| *Silene inflata* Sm., *S. muscipula* L. (A. p. 156) |
| *Silybum marianum* Gaertn. (A. p. 240) |

| Greek name | English name | References |
|---|---|---|
| γαλήοψις | Brownwort | IV, 94 |
| ἡδύσαρον | Axweed | III, 130 |
| πελεκῖνος | Axweed | III, 130 |
| ἀείζῳον, τρίτον εἶδος | Stonecrop | IV, 90 |
| ἀείζῳον, τρίτον εἶδος | Houseleek | IV, 90 |
| ἀνδράχνη ἀγρία | Houseleek, Third kind of | IV, 90 |
| τηλέφιον | Houseleek, Third kind of | IV, 90 |
| κηπαία | *Cepaia* | III, 151 |
| ἀνδράχνη ἀγρία | Stonecrop | IV, 90 |
| τηλέφιον | Stonecrop | IV, 90 |
| ἰλλεκέβρα | Houseleek, Third kind of | IV, 90 |
| ῥοδία ῥίζα | *Rhodia rhiza* | IV, 45 |
| στέργηθρον | Houseleek | IV, 88 |
| βούφθαλμον | Houseleek | IV, 88 |
| ἀμβροσία | Houseleek | IV, 88 |
| ζῳόφθαλμον | Houseleek | IV, 88 |
| ἀείζῳον μέγα | Houseleek | IV, 88 |
| ἀείζῳον τὸ μικρόν | Houseleek | IV, 89 |
| λεαντική | *Caccalia* | IV, 122 |
| κακκαλία | *Caccalia* | IV, 122 |
| ἠριγέρων | Groundsel | IV, 96 |
| Ἐρυθραικὸν σατύριον | Man orchis | III, 128 |
| σατύριον ἐρυθραϊκόν | Man orchis | III, 128 |
| λογχῖτις | *Lonchitis* | III, 144 |
| σήσαμον | Sesame | II, 99 |
| σέσελι Μασσαλιώτικον | Massilian hartwort | III, 53 |
| μελίνη | Italian millet | II, 98 |
| Ἡρακλεία | Ironwort | IV, 33 |
| σιδηρῖτις | Ironwort | IV, 33 |
| Φιλεταίριον | Catchfly | IV, 28 |
| ἔχιον | Catchfly | IV, 28 |
| ὠκιμοειδές | Catchfly | IV, 28 |
| Ἡρακλεία | Frothy poppy | IV, 66 |
| μήκων ἀφρώδης | Frothy poppy | IV, 66 |
| σίλλυβον | Milk thistle | IV, 155 |

| **Botanical name** |
|---|
| *Sinapis alba* L. (A. 169) |
| *Sinapis alba* L. (A. p. 240) |
| *Sison amomum* L. (A. p. 241) |
| *Sisymbrium officinale* Scop., *S. iri* o L. (A. p. 98) |
| *Sium angustifolium* L. (A. p. 242) |
| *Smilax aspera* L. (A. p. 161) |
| *Smyrnium olusatrum* L. |
| *Smyrnium olusatrum* L. (A. p. 124) |
| *Smyrnium olusatrum* L. (A. p. 124) |
| *Smyrnium olusatrum* L. (LSJ) |
| *Smyrnium olusatrum* L. (LSJ) |
| *Smyrnium olusatrum* sp. ~ |
| *Smyrnium olusatrum* sp. ~ |
| *Smyrnium perfoliatum* Mill. (A. p. 195) |
| *Smyrnium perfoliatum* Mill. (A. p. 242) |
| *Solanum nigrum* L. (A. p. 251) |
| *Sonchus asper* L. (A. p. 243) |
| *Sonchus* L. sp. |
| *Sonchus oleraceus* L. (A. p. 243) |
| *Sorbus domestica* (LSJ) |
| *Sorbus domestica* (LSJ) |
| *Sorbus domestica,* L. (LSJ) |
| *Sparganium ramosum* Curtis, *S. simplex* Huds. (A. p. 244) |
| *Spartium junceum* L. (A. p. 244) |
| *Spiraea filipendula* L. (A. p. 177) |
| *Stachys* L. sp. (A. p. 247) |
| *Stachys officinalis* L. (A. pp. 209-210) |
| *Stachys officinalis* L. (A. pp. 209-210) |
| *Styrax officinalis* L. (A. p. 252) |
| *Symphytum bulbosum* (LSJ) |
| *Symphytum bulbosum* (LSJ) |
| *Symphytum tuberosum* L. (A. p. 253) |
| *Tamarix articulata* (LSJ) |
| *Tamarix tetrandra* Pall. (A. p. 167) |
| *Tamus communis* L. (A. p. 14) |

| Greek name | English name | References |
|---|---|---|
| νᾶπυ | Mustard | II, 154 |
| σίνηπι | Mustard | II, 154 |
| σίνων | Stone parsley | III, 55 |
| ἐρύσιμον | Hedge mustard | II, 158 |
| σίον | Water parsnip | II, 127 |
| μῖλαξ τραχεῖα | Rough bindweed | IV, 142 |
| ὀλέσαθρον | Alexanders | III, 67 |
| ἱπποσέλινον | Alexanders | III, 67 |
| σμύρνιον | Alexanders | III, 67 |
| ἀγρίολον | Alexanders | III, 67 |
| ἀγριοσέλινον | Alexanders | III, 67 |
| Βοιωτιακὴ σμύρνα | Boeotian myrrh | I, 65 |
| ἱπποσέλινον | Alexanders ~ | III, 67 |
| πετροσέλινον | Cretan alexanders | III, 68 |
| σμύρνιον | Cretan alexanders | III, 68 |
| στρὺχνον κηπαῖον | Hound's berry | IV, 70 |
| σὸγχος ἀκανθωδέστερος | Sow thistle, more wild | II, 131 |
| σόγχος | Sow thistle | II, 131 |
| σὸγχος τρυφερώτερος | Sow thistle, more tender | II, 131 |
| σῦον | Serviceberry | I, 120 |
| σῦον | Service tree | I, 120 |
| οὖον | Sorb apple | I,120 |
| σπαργάνιον | Bur reed | IV, 21 |
| σπάρτιον | Spanish broom | IV, 154 |
| οἰνάνθη | Dropwort | III, 120 |
| στάχυς | Base horehound | III, 106 |
| κέστρον | Betony | IV, 1 |
| ψυχροτρόφον | Betony | IV, 1 |
| στύραξ | Storax | I, 66 |
| πηκτή | Comfrey | IV, 10 |
| σύμφυτον ἄλλο | Comfrey | IV, 10 |
| σύμφυτον πετραῖον | Low pine | IV, 9 |
| μυρίκη ἡ ἐν Αἰγύπτῳ | Oriental tamarisk | I, 87 |
| μυρίκη | Tamarisk | I, 87 |
| ἄμπελος μέλαινα | Black bryony | IV, 183 |

| **Botanical name** |
|---|
| *Tamus communis* L. (A. p. 14) |
| *Tamus communis* L. (A. p. 39) |
| *Taxus baccata* L. |
| *Taxus baccata* L. (A. p. 161) |
| *Taxus baccata* L. (A. p. 161) |
| *Taxus baccata* L. (A. p. 256) |
| *Teucrium chamaedrys* L. *and ~T. lucidum L. (A. p. 59)* |
| *Teucrium chamaedrys* L. *and T. lucidum* L. *(A. p. 146)* |
| *Teucrium chamaedrys* L. and *T. lucidum* L. (A. p. 59) |
| *Teucrium chamaedrys* L., *T. lucidum* L. (A. p. 257) |
| *Teucrium creticum* L. (A. p. 303) |
| *Teucrium flavum* L. (A. p. 257) |
| *Teucrium polium* L. (A. p. 203) |
| *Teucrium scordium* L. (A. p. 231) |
| *Thalictrum flavum* L., *Th. minus* L. (A. p. 258) |
| *Thapsia garganica* L. (A. p. 258) |
| *Thelygonum cynocrambe* L. = *Cynocrambe prostrata* Gaertn. (A. p. 11) |
| *Thelygonum cynocrambe* L. = *Cynocrambe prostrata* Gaertn. (A. p. 166) |
| *Thymus graveolens* Sibth. ~ |
| *Thymus graveol. Sibth* sp.,*~Th. tragoriganum* L. sp.,*~Origanum heraceoticum Richb* sp.(A. 263) |
| *Thymus incanus* L. (A. p. 118) |
| *Thymus Sibthorpii* (LSJ) |
| *Thymus Sibthorpii* (LSJ) |
| *Thymus tragoriganum* L. ~ |
| *Tordylium officinale* L. (A. p. 237) |
| *Tordylium officinale* L. (A. p. 237) |
| *Tordylium officinale* L. (A. p. 262) |
| *Tragopogon porrifolius* L. (A. p. 263) |
| *Tragopogon porrifolius* L. (A. p. 73) |
| *Trapa natans* L. (A. p. 263) |
| *Tribulus terrestris* L. (A. p. 263) |
| *Trifolium arvense* L. (A . p. 137) |
| *Trigonella elatior* Sibth. sp., *T. gladiata* L. sp. (A. p. 148) |
| *Trigonella fenum graecum* L. |
| *Trigonella fenum graecum* L. (A. p. 256) |

| Greek name | English name | References |
|---|---|---|
| ἄμπελος Χειρώνιος | Black bryony | IV, 183 |
| βρυωνία | Black bryony | IV, 183 |
| τιθύμαλλος | Yew | IV, 79 |
| σμῖλαξ | Yew | IV, 79 |
| σμῖλος | Yew | IV, 79 |
| τάξος | Yew | IV, 79 |
| χαμαίρωψ | Wall germander | III, 98 |
| λινόδρυς | Wall germander | III, 98 |
| χαμαίδρυς | Wall germander | III, 98 |
| Τεύκριον | Wall germander | III, 98 |
| τεύθριον | Hulwort | III, 110 |
| Τεύκριον | Tree germander | III, 97 |
| πόλιον | Hulwort | III, 110 |
| σκόρδιον | Garlic germander | III, 111 |
| θαλίητρον | Meadow rue | IV, 97 |
| θαψία | Deadly carrot | IV, 153 |
| ἀλσίνη | Lichwort | IV, 86 |
| μυὸς ὦτα | Lichwort | IV, 86 |
| πράσιον | Goat's marjoram | III, 30 |
| τραγορίγανος | Goat's marjoram | III, 30 |
| Ἑλένιον ἄλλο | Elecampane, Another | I, 29 |
| ἕρπυλος | Tufted thyme | III, 38 |
| ζυγίς | Tufted thyme | III, 38 |
| πράσιον | Goat's marjoram | III, 30 |
| σέσελι | Hartwort | III, 53 |
| σέσελι Κρητικόν | Cretan hartwort | III, 54 |
| τορδιλον | Cretan hartwort | III, 54 |
| τραγοπώγων | Salsify | II, 143 |
| κόμη | Salsify | II, 143 |
| τρίβολος ἔνυδρος | Water chestnut | IV, 15 |
| τρίβολος χερσαῖος | Caltrops | IV, 15 |
| λαγώπουν | Hare's foot trefoil | IV, 17 |
| λωτὸς ἄγριος | Wild fenugreek | IV, 111 |
| κὲρας αἴγειον | Fenugreek | II, 102 |
| τῆλις | Fenugreek | II, 102 |

| **Botanical name** |
|---|
| *Trigonella fenum graecum* L. (A. p. 39) |
| *Trigonella fenum graecum* L. (A. p. 51) |
| *Trigonella fenum graecum* L. (A. p. 148) |
| *Trigonella fenum graecum* L. (A. p. 6) |
| *Triticcum* L. sp. |
| *Triticum dicoccum* (LSJ) |
| *Triticum dicoccum* Schrek. (A. p. 279) |
| *Triticum* L. |
| *Triticum* L. sp. |
| *Triticum monoccocum* Schrek. (A. p. 279) |
| *Tuber cibarium* L. sp. (A. pp. 126 and 266) |
| *Tussilago farfara* L. |
| *Tussilago farfara* L. |
| *Tussilago farfara* L. |
| *Tussilago farfara* L. (A. p. 35) |
| *Typha* L. sp. (A. p. 267) |
| *Ulmus glabra* (LSJ) |
| *Ulva lactuca* L., and *U. latissima* L. (A. p. 39) |
| *Umbilicus pendulinus* DC. |
| *Umbilicus pendulinu s* DC. |
| *Umbilicus pendulinus* DC. (A. p. 77) |
| *Urginea maritima Baker* = *Scilla maritima* L. (A. p. 229) |
| *Urginea maritima* Baker = *Scilla maritima* L. (A. p. 229) |
| *Urtica* L. sp. (A. p. 2) |
| *Urtica* L. (A. p. 70) |
| *Valeriana celtica* L. (A. p. 170) |
| *Valeriana phu* L. (A. p. 170) |
| *Valeriana phu* L. (A. p. 170) |
| *Valeriana tuberosa* L. (A. p. 170) |
| *Valeriana tuberosa* L. (A. p. 170) |
| *Valeriana tuberosa* L. (A. p. 260) |
| *Veratrum album* L. (A. p. 94) |
| *Verbacum* L. sp. (A. p. 197) |
| *Verbascum* L. sp. (A. p. 197) |
| *Verbascum* L. sp. (A. p. 149) |

| Greek name | English name | References |
|---|---|---|
| βούκερως | Fenugreek | II, 102 |
| κάρφος | Fenugreek | II, 102 |
| λωτός | Fenugreek | II, 102 |
| αἰγόκερας | Fenugreek | II, 102 |
| ζέα | Wheat *zea* | II, 89 |
| ὄλυρα | Rice-wheat | II, 91 |
| ζὲα δίκοκκος | Wheat *zea* , two-seeded | II, 89 |
| πυρός | Wheat | II, 85 |
| τράγος | Spelt | II, 93 |
| ζὲα μονόκκοκος | Wheat *zea* , one-seeded | II, 89 |
| ὕδνον | Truffle | II, 145 |
| πετρώνιον | Coltsfoot | III, 112 |
| πίθιον | Coltsfoot | III, 112 |
| πήχιον | Coltsfoot | III, 112 |
| βήχιον | Coltsfoot | III, 112 |
| τύφη | Reed mace | III, 118 |
| πτελέα | Elm | I, 84 |
| βρύον θαλάσσιον | Sea lettuce | IV, 98 |
| κυμβάλιον | Navelwort | IV, 91 |
| σκυτάλιον | Navelwort | IV, 91 |
| κοτυληδών | Navelwort | IV, 91 |
| σκίλλα | Scilla | II, 171 |
| σκίλλα | Squill | II, 171 |
| ἀκαλήφη | Stinging nettle | IV, 93 |
| κνίδη | Stinging nettle | IV, 93 |
| νὰρδος Κελτική | Celtic spikenard | I, 8 |
| νὰρδος ἀγρία | Cretan spikenard | I, 11 |
| φοῦ | Cretan spikenard | I, 11 |
| νάρδος ὀρεινή | Mountain sipkenard | I, 9 |
| πυρῖτις | Mountain spikenard | I, 9 |
| θυλακῖτις | Mountain spikenard | I, 9 |
| ἐλλέβορος λευκός | White hellebore | IV, 148 |
| φλομίς | Mullein | IV, 103 |
| φλόμος | Mullein | IV, 103 |
| λυχνῖτις | Phlome | IV, 103 |

| **Botanical name** |
|---|
| *Verbascum* L. sp. (A. p. 197) |
| Verbascum L. sp. (A. p. 197) |
| *Verbascum* L. sp. (A. p. 260) |
| *Verbascum* L. sp. (A. p. 260) |
| *Verbascum* L. sp. (A. p. 260) |
| *Verbascum* L. sp.(A. p. 149) |
| *Verbena officinalis* L. (A. p. 123) |
| *Verbena officinalis* L. (A. p. 193) |
| *Verbascum* L. sp. (A. p. 149) |
| *Vicia ervilia* Willd. (A. p. 182) |
| *Vicia faba* L. (LSJ) |
| *Vicia sativa* var. *angustifolia* L., *V. articulata* Hornem. (A. p. 19) |
| *Vigna sinensis* Endl. (A. p.161,) *Phaseolus vulgaris* L. (LSJ) |
| *Vinca minor* L. (A. p. 204) |
| *Vinca minor* L. (A. p. 69) |
| *Vinca minor* L. (A. p. 87) |
| *Vinca minor* L. (A. p.167) |
| *Vincetoxicum nigrum* Moench (LSJ) |
| *Vincetoxicum nigrum* Moench (LSJ) |
| *Vincetoxicum officinale* Moench (A. p. 27) |
| *Viola odorata* L. (A. p. 132) |
| *Vitex agnus-castus* L. (A. p. 150) |
| *Vitex agnus-castus* L. (A. p. 8) |
| Vitis silvestris Gmel. (A. p. 176) |
| *Vitis silvestris* L. (LSJ) |
| *Vitis silvestris* Gmel. (A. p. 14) |
| *Vitis vinifera* L. (LSJ) |
| *Withania somnifera* Dun. (A. p. 251) |
| *Withania somnifera* Dun. |
| *Withania somnifera* Dun. (A. p. 115) |
| *Withania somnifera* Dun. (LSJ) |
| *Xanthium strumarium* L. |
| *Xanthium strumarium* L. |
| *Xanthium strumarium* L. |
| *Xanthium strumarium* L. (A. p. 19) |

| Greek name | English name | References |
|---|---|---|
| φλομίς ἡ καλουμένη λυχνῖτις | Mullein | IV, 103 |
| φλὸμος ἀγρία | Sage of Jerusalem | IV, 103 |
| θρυαλλίς | Mullein | IV, 103 |
| θρυαλλίς | Mullein | IV, 103 |
| θρυαλλίς | Sage of Jerusalem | IV, 103 |
| λυχνῖτις | Mullein | IV, 103 |
| ἱερὰ βοτάνη | Holy vervain | IV, 60 |
| περιστερεών | Holy vervain | IV, 60 |
| λυχνῖτις | Sage of Jerusalem | IV, 103 |
| ὄροβος | Bitter vetch | II, 108 |
| κύαμος Ἑλληνικός | Bean, Greek | II, 105 |
| ἀφάκη | Tare | II, 148 |
| σμῖλαξ κηπαία | Kidney bean | II, 146 |
| πολυγονοειδές | Periwinkle | IV, 7 |
| κληματίς | Periwinkle | IV, 7 |
| δαφνοειδές | Periwinkle | IV, 7 |
| μυρσινοειδές | Periwinkle | IV, 7 |
| διρκαία | Black swallowwort | III, 119 |
| κιρκαία | Black swallowwort | III, 119 |
| ἀσκληπιάς | Swallowwort | III, 92 |
| ἴον | Violet | IV, 121 |
| λύγος | Chaste tree | I, 103 |
| ἄγνος | Chaste tree | I, 103 |
| οἰνάνθη | Grape, Inflo'ce of wild | V, 2; V, 4 |
| ἄμπελος ἀγρία | Wild grapevine | V, 2 |
| ἄμπελος ἀγρία | Wild grapevine | IV, 181 |
| ἄμπελος οἰνοφόρος | Grapevine | V, 1 |
| στρὺχνον ὑπνωτικόν | Sleepy nightshade | IV, 72 |
| κακκαλία | Sleepy nightshade | IV, 72 |
| ἁλικάκκαβον | Sleepy nightshade | IV, 72 |
| μώριος ἑτέρα | Sleepy nightshade, Another | IV, 75 |
| ἀντιθέσιον | Broad-leaved burweed | IV, 136 |
| χάσκανον | Broad-leaved burweed | IV, 136 |
| χοιραδόλεθρον | Broad-leaved burweed | IV, 136 |
| ἀπαρίνη | Broad-leaved burweed | IV, 136 |

| Greek name | English name | References |
|---|---|---|
| φάσγανον | Broad-leaved burweed | IV, 136 |
| ξάνθιον | Broad-leaved burweed | IV, 136 |
| ζιγγίβερι | Ginger | II, 160 |
| πολύκνημον | Field basil | III, 94 |

| English name | Greek name | References |
|---|---|---|
| Leather | δέρμα | II, 48 |
| Lizard | σαύρα | II, 64; 65 |
| Locust | ἀκρίς | II, 52 |
| Locust | τρωξαλλίς | II, 52 |
| Locust | ὄνος | II, 52 |
| Lung | πνεύμων | II, 38 |
| *Lyngourion* | λυγγούριον | II, 81 |
| Lynx | λύγξ | II, 81 |
| *Mainis* | μαινίς | II, 29 |
| Marine snail | κοχλίας θαλάσσιος | II, 9 |
| Marrow | μυελός | II, 77 |
| Mice | μύες | II, 69 |
| Milk | γάλα | II, 70 |
| *Oisypos* | οἴσυπος | II, 74 |
| *Omotarichos* | ὠμοτάριχος | II, 31 |
| Perch | περκίς | II, 33 |
| *Phene* | φήνη | II, 53 |
| *Phycis* | φυκίς | II, 33 |
| Pig | χοῖρος | II, 38 |
| Pontic sea mussel | μύακες ποντικοί | II, 5 |
| Propolis | πρόπολις | II, 84 |
| Purple murex | πορφύρα | II, 4 |
| Red mullet | τρίγλα | II, 22 |
| Rennet | πιτύα | II, 19; 75 |
| Reptile | ὄφις | II, 17 |
| Riverine snail | κοχλίας ποτάμιος | II, 9 |
| Salamander | σαλαμάνδρα | II, 62 |
| Sea hare | λαγοὼς θαλάσσιος | II, 18 |
| Sea horse | ἱππόκαμπος | II, 3 |
| Sea mussel | μύαξ | II, 5 |
| Sea scolopendra | σκολοπένδρα θαλασσία | II, 14 |
| Sea scorpion | σκορπίος θαλάσσιος | II, 12 |
| Sea urchin | ἐχῖνος θαλάσσιος | II, 1 |
| *Seps* | σήψ | II, 65 |
| Serpent | ὄφις | II, 17 |
| Shearwater | αἴθυια | II, 55 |
| Sheatfish | σίλουρος | II, 27 |

| English name | Greek name | References |
|---|---|---|
| Shrewmouse | μυογαλῆ | II, 68 |
| Skink | σκίγκος | II, 66 |
| *Smaris* | σμαρίς | II, 28 |
| Snail | κοχλίας | II, 9 |
| Soot | λίγνυς | II, 72; 74 |
| Spider | ἀράχνη | II, 63 |
| Spider | ὁλκός | II, 63 |
| Spider | λύκος | II, 63 |
| Sponges | σπόγγοι | V, 120 |
| Stag | ἔλαφος ἄρρην | II, 41 |
| Stingray | τρυγὼν θαλασσία | II, 20 |
| Swallow | χελιδών | II, 56 |
| Swine | χοῖρος | II, 38 |
| *Tellinai* | τελλῖναι | II, 6 |
| Trumpet shell | κήρυξ | II, 4 |
| Tuna | θύννος | II, 31 |
| Urine | οὖρον | II, 81 |
| Viper | ἐχίδνα | II, 16 |
| Viper | ἔχις | II, 17 |
| Vulture | φήνη | II, 53 |
| Wax | κηρός | II, 83 |
| Wood lice | ὄνοι οἱ ὑπὸ τὰς ὑδρίας | II, 35 |
| Wool | ἔρια | II, 73 |
| Wrasse | ἰουλίς | II, 33 |

| English name | Greek name | References |
|---|---|---|
| *Adarces* | ἀδάρκης | V, 119 |
| Aerugo vermicularis | ἰὸς σκώλυκος | V, 79 |
| Alabaster | ὄνυξ | V, 135 |
| Alabaster | ἀλαβαστρίτης λίθος | V, 135 |
| Alum | στυπτηρία | V, 106 |
| *Ambelitis* earth | ἀμπελῖτις γῆ | V, 160 |
| Antimony | στίβι | V, 84 |
| Antimony | πλατυόφθαλμον | V, 84 |
| Antimony | λάρβασον | V, 84 |
| *Antispoda* | ἀντίσποδα | V, 75 |
| *Apochyma* | ἀπόχυμα | I, 72 |
| Arabian stone | Ἀραβικὸς λίθος | V, 131 |
| Arsenic sulfide | σανδαράκη | V, 105 |
| Asbestos | ἀμίαντος λίθος | V, 138 |
| Asphalt | ἄσφαλτος | I, 73 |
| Assian stone | Ἄσσιος λίθος | V, 124 |
| Azurite | Ἀρμένιον | V, 90 |
| Brine | ἅλμη | V, 111 |
| Brine vinegar | ὀξάλμη | V, 15 |
| Brine vinegar w/ Cretan thyme | θυμοξάλμη | V, 16 |
| Builders' red earth | τεκτονικὴ μίλτος | V, 96 |
| Calamine | καδμεία | V, 74 |
| Calamine | βοτρυῖτις | V, 74 |
| Calamine | πλακωτή | V, 74 |
| Calamine | ζωνῖτις | V, 74 |
| Calamine | ὀστρακῖτις | V, 74 |
| Calamine | ὀνυχῖτις | V, 74 |
| Chian earth | Χία γῆ | V, 155 |
| Basic copper carbonate | χρυσοκόλλα | V, 89 |
| Cimolian earth | Κιμωλία | V, 156 |
| Cinnabar | κιννάβαρι | V, 94 |
| Clay stone | ὀστρακίτης λίθος | V, 146 |
| Copper ore | μίσυ | V, 100 |
| Copper ore, Flake of | λεπὶς Κυπρίων μετάλλων | V, 78 |
| Copper ore, Flake of | ἠλῖτις | V, 78 |
| Copper pyrites | πυρίτης λίθος | V, 125 |
| Copper pyrites | διφρυγές | V, 125 |

| English name | Greek name | References |
|---|---|---|
| Copper pyrites | διφρυγές | V, 125 |
| Copper sulfate | χαλκανθές | V, 98 |
| Copper, Burned | χαλκὸς κεκαυμένος | V, 76 |
| Copper, Flower of | χαλκοῦ ἄνθος | V, 77 |
| Copper, Slug of | χαλκοῦ σκωρία | V, 76 |
| Earth | γῆ | V, 151 |
| Earth-like stone | γεὼδης λίθος | V, 150 |
| Emery | σμύρις | V, 147 |
| Eretrian earth | Ἐρετριάδος γῆ | V, 152 |
| Galena | μολύβδαινα | V, 85 |
| Gypsum | γύψος | V, 116 |
| Haematite | αἱματὶτης λίθος | V, 126 |
| Honeystone | μελιτὶτης λίθος | V, 133 |
| Indigo | Ἰνδικόν | V, 92 |
| Ink, Black | μέλαν | V, 162 |
| Iron rust | σιδὴρου ἰός | V, 80 |
| Iron slag | σιδὴρου σκωρία | V, 80 |
| Iron, Flake of | λεπὶς στομὼματος | V, 78 |
| Iron, Red-hot | σίδηρος πεπυρωμένος | V, 80 |
| Itch salve | ψωρικόν | V, 99 |
| Jasper | λὶθος ἴασπις | V, 142 |
| Jasper | ἄστριος | V, 142 |
| Jasper | τερεβινθίζων | V, 142 |
| Judaic stone | Ἰουδαικὸς λίθος | V, 137 |
| Lapis lazuli | κύανος | V, 91 |
| Lapis lazuli | λίθος σάπφειρος | V, 139 |
| Lead dross | μολύβδου σκωρία | V, 82 |
| Lead stone | μολυβδοειδὴς λίθος | V, 83 |
| Lead, Washed | μολυβδος πεπλυμένος | V, 81 |
| Lemnian earth | Λημνία γῆ | V, 97 |
| Lignite | Γαγάτης | V, 128 |
| Lime, Unslaked | ἄσβεστος | V, 115 |
| Litharge | λιθάργυρος | V, 87 |
| Litharge | χρυσῖτις | V, 87 |
| Litharge | ἀργυρῖτις | V, 87 |
| Litharge | σκαλαυθρῖτις | V, 87 |
| Magnate | Μαγνῆτις λίθος | V, 130 |

| **English name** | **Greek name** | **References** |
|---|---|---|
| Melanterite | σῶρι | V, 102 |
| Melian earth | Μηλία γῆ | V, 159 |
| Memphitic stone | Μεμφίτης λίθος | V, 140 |
| Mercury | ὑδράργυρος | V, 95 |
| Milkstone | γαλακτίτης | V, 132 |
| *Minion* | μίνιον | V, 95 |
| Naxian whetsone powder | Ναξίας ἀκόνης ἀπότριμμα | V, 149 |
| *Pharmacitis* earth | ἀμπελῖτις γῆ | V, 160 |
| Phrygian stone | Φρύγιος λίθος | V, 123 |
| Pipe clay | μόροχθος λίθος | V, 134 |
| Pipe clay | γαλαξίας | V, 134 |
| Pipe clay | λευκογραφίς | V, 134 |
| *Pnigitis earth* | πνιγῖτις γῆ | V, 157 |
| Pompholyx | πομφόλυξ | V, 75 |
| Potsherds | ὄστρακα τὰ ἐξ ἰπνῶν | V, 158 |
| Pumice stone | κίσηρις | V, 108 |
| Pyrite from copper mines | διφρυγές | V, 103 |
| Red earth from furnaces | γῆ πυρρὰ καμίνων | V, 158 |
| Rock alum | χαλκῖτις | V, 99 |
| Salt | ἅλς | V, 109 |
| Salt froth | ἁλὸς ἄχνη | V, 110 |
| Salt, efflorescence | ἁλὸς ἄνθος | V, 112 |
| Salt scum | ἁλὸς ἄνθος | V, 112 |
| Samian earth | κολλούριον | V, 153 |
| Samian earth | ἀστήρ | V, 153 |
| Samian earth | Σαμία γῆ | V, 153 |
| Samian earth, Stone in | λίθος ἐν τῇ Σαμίᾳ γῇ | V, 154 |
| Sand | ἄμμος | V, 148 |
| Seawater | θαλάττιον ὕδωρ | V, 11 |
| Seawater with honey | θαλασσόμελι | V, 12 |
| Selenite | σεληνίτης | V, 141 |
| Selenite | ἀφροσέληνον | V, 141 |
| Selinus earth | Σελινουσία γῆ | V, 155 |
| Serpentine | ὀφίτης λίθος | V, 143 |
| Shoemaker's black | μελαντηρία | V, 101 |
| Silver dross | ἀργύρου σκωρία | V, 86 |
| Silver dross | ἕλκυσμα | V, 86 |

| Greek name | English name | References |
|---|---|---|
| Ἐρετριάδος γῆ | Eretrian earth | V, 152 |
| ζωνῖτις | Calamine | V, 74 |
| ἠλῖτις | Copper ore, Flake of | V, 78 |
| θαλασσόμελι | Seawater with honey | V, 12 |
| θαλάττιον ὕδωρ | Seawater | V, 11 |
| Θρακὶας | Thracian stone | V, 129 |
| θυΐτης | *Thyites* | V, 136 |
| θυΐτης | Turquoise | V, 136 |
| θυμοξάλμη | Brine vinegar w/ Cretan thyme | V, 16 |
| Ἰνδικόν | Indigo | V, 92 |
| ἰὸς ξυστός | Verdigris | V, 79 |
| ἰὸς σκώλυκος | Aerugo vermicularis | V, 79 |
| Ἰουδαικὸς λίθος | Judaic stone | V, 137 |
| καδμεία | Calamine | V, 74 |
| Κιμωλία | Cimolian earth | V, 156 |
| κιννάβαρι | Cinnabar | V, 94 |
| κίσηρις | Pumice stone | V, 108 |
| κολλούριον | Samian earth | V, 153 |
| κονία | Soap powder | I, 128 |
| κύανος | Lapis lazuli | V, 91 |
| λάρβασον | Antimony | V, 84 |
| λεπὶς Κυπρὶων μετάλλων | Copper ore, Flake of | V, 78 |
| λεπὶς στομώματος | Iron, Flake of | V, 78 |
| λευκογραφίς | Pipe clay | V, 134 |
| Λημνία γῆ | Lemnian earth | V, 97 |
| λιθάργυρος | Litharge | V, 87 |
| λίθοι οἱ ἐν τοῖς σπόγγοις | Stone in sponges | V, 144 |
| λιθοκόλλα | Stone glue | V, 145 |
| λίθος ἐν τῇ Σαμίᾳ γῃ | Stone in Samian earth | V, 154 |
| λίθος ἴασπις | Jasper | V, 142 |
| λίθος σάπφειρος | Lapis lazuli | V, 139 |
| Μαγνῆτις λίθος | Magnate | V, 130 |
| μέλαν | Ink, Black | V, 162 |
| μελαντηρία | Shoemaker's black | V, 101 |
| μελιτίτης λίθος | Honeystone | V, 133 |
| Μεμφίτης λίθος | Memphitic stone | V, 140 |
| Μηλία γῆ | Melian earth | V, 159 |

| Greek name | English name | References |
|---|---|---|
| μίλτος Σινωπική | Sinopic red earth | V, 96 |
| μίνιον | *Minion* | V, 95 |
| μίσυ | Copper ore | V, 100 |
| μολύβδαινα | Galena | V, 85 |
| μολυβδοειδὴς λίθος | Lead stone | V, 83 |
| μόλυβδος πεπλυμένος | Lead, Washed | V, 81 |
| μολύβδου σκωρία | Lead dross | V, 82 |
| μόροχθος λίθος | Pipe clay | V, 134 |
| Ναξίας ἀκόνης ἀπότριμμα | Naxian whetsone powder | V, 149 |
| νίτρον | Soda | V, 113 |
| νίτρου ἀφρός | Soda, Foam of | V, 113 |
| ὄνυξ | Alabaster | V, 135 |
| ὀνυχίτης | Calamine | V, 74 |
| ὀξάλμη | Brine vinegar | V, 15 |
| ὄστρακα τὰ ἐξ ἰπνῶν | Potsherds | V, 158 |
| ὀστρακίτης λίθος | Clay stone | V, 146 |
| ὀστρακῖτις | Calamine | V, 74 |
| ὀφίτης λίθος | Serpentine | V, 143 |
| πλακωτή | Calamine | V, 74 |
| πλατυόφθαλμον | Antimony | V, 84 |
| πνιγῖτις γῆ | *Pnigitis earth* | V, 157 |
| πομφόλυξ | *Pompholyx* | V, 75 |
| πομφόλυξ | Zinc oxide | V, 75 |
| πυρίτης λίθος | Copper pyrites | V, 125 |
| Σαμία γῆ | Samian earth | V, 153 |
| σανδαράκη | Arsenic sulfide | V, 105 |
| σεληνίτης | Selenite | V, 141 |
| Σελινουσία γῆ | Selinus earth | V, 155 |
| σίδηρος πεπυρωμένος | Iron, Red-hot | V, 80 |
| σιδήρου ἰός | Iron rust | V, 80 |
| σιδήρου σκωρία | Iron slag | V, 80 |
| σκαλαυθρῖτις | Litharge | V, 87 |
| σμύρις | Emery stone | V, 147 |
| σποδός | *Spodos* | V, 75 |
| σποδός/σπόδιον | Zinc oxide | V, 75 |
| στίβι | Antimony | V, 84 |
| στυπτηρία | Alum | V, 106 |

| Greek name | English name | References |
|---|---|---|
| σχιστὸς λίθος | Talc | V, 127 |
| σῶρι | Melanterite | V, 102 |
| τεκτονικὴ μίλτος | Builders' red earth | V, 96 |
| τερεβινθίζων | Jasper | I, 142 |
| ὑδράργυρος | Mercury | V, 95 |
| ὕδωρ | Water | V, 10 |
| φαρμακῖτις γῆ | Ampelitis earth | V, 160 |
| Φρύγιος λίθος | Phrygian stone | V, 123 |
| χαλκανθές | Copper sulfate | V, 98 |
| χαλκανθές | Vitriol | V, 98 |
| χαλκῖτις | Rock alum | V, 99 |
| χαλκὸς κεκαυμένος | Copper, Burned | V, 76 |
| χαλκοῦ ἄνθος | Copper, Flower of | V, 77 |
| χαλκοῦ σκωρία | Copper, Slag of | V, 76 |
| Χία γῆ | Chian earth | V, 155 |
| χρυσῖτις | Litharge | V, 87 |
| χρυσοκόλλα | Basic copper carbonate | V, 89 |
| ψιμύθιον | White lead | V, 88 |
| ψωρικόν | Itch salve | V, 99 |
| ὤχρα | Yellow ocher | V, 93 |

## Medical Index

# Medical Index

# Medical Index

| Conditions | References |
| --- | --- |
| | 153,2; 155. |
| Anus | I, 26,3; 47,2; 68,2; 70,1; 72,2; 99,1; 100,3; 103,3; 112,2; 115,2. II, 10; 15; 29; 50; 74,4; 78,3; 107,3; 118,2; 131; 164,2; 178,2. |
| Anus (cont'd) | III, 11,2; 40,1; 74,2; 80,1; 123; 146,1. IV, 10,2; 96,2; 119; 121. V, 1,2; 13,1; 15; 30; 77,2; 81,3. |
| Aphrodisiac | I, 16,2; 26,3; 71,1. II, 66; 103; 110,1; 124,1; 140; 149,2; 155,1; 166,3; 167; 170,1. III, 34,1; 52,2; 56; 126,2; 128,1; 128,2; 129. IV, 20,2; 93,2; 95. |
| Appetite | I, 113. II, 109,2; 110,1; 113; 151,1; 159,3. III, 23,1. V, 3,1; 6,10; 8,1; 9,2; 13,1; 32,2; 25, 39, 3; 49; 52; 64; 65. |
| Armpit odor, see Deodorant | |
| Arthritis | I, 73,3; 102. II, 49,2; 120,2. III, 104,2. IV, 162,3. V, 7,1; 14; 16. |
| Asthma | I, 24; 25,1; 33,2; 72,1; 73,3; 128,1. II, 39; 49,2; 126,2; 171,3. III, 1,3; 2,2; 4,5; 25,1; 36,2; 83,1; 84,2; 105,1; 138; 150,2. IV, 134,1; 153,3. V, 38,2; 40,2; 105,2; 107,1. |
| Atrabilious, see Melancholia | |
| Bald spots | I, 72,3; 85; 125, 2; 125,3. II, 2; 3; 19; 26; 44; 76,18; 80,3; 80,5; 112,1; 123; 151,2; 152,3; 154,2; 164,3; 169,3; 175,2. III, 80,3; 132,2. IV, 134,2; 135; 153,4. V, 80,1; 105,1; 118,3; 149. |
| Barrenness | I, 77,2; 81;104. II, 19; 75,1; 75,2; 79,2; 120,3; 159,3; 179,3. III, 34,2;130; 134,2. IV 19; 185. V, 80,1; 106,6; 146. |
| Bile | I, 1,2; 52, 5; 115,1; 125,1. II, 141,2; 156,2. III, 138. IV, 75,3; 109; 149; 150,2; 150,6; 161,2; 162,2; 163; 164,2; 166,2; 167; |

## Medical Index

# Medical Index

## Medical Index

| Conditions | References |
|---|---|
| | IV, 169. |
| Catarrh, see also Rheum | I, 40,2; 56,3; 64,5; 66,2; 73,3; 125,3. II, 50; 166,2. III, 25,1; 79,2. IV, 57; 68,4. V, 34,2; 107,3. |
| Cathartic, see Purgative | |
| Cervix, dilation | I, 13,3; 19,4; 23; 66,3; 67,2. III, 78,3. |
| Cervix, induration | I, 66,3. |
| Chafing, see Abrasion | |
| Chalkstone | I, 30,5. III, 84,3; 149. V, 93. |
| Chap, see Fissure | |
| Chest | I, 2,2; 3; 16,2; 64,3; 69,3; 71,2; 72,1; 75; 78,2, 128,1. II, 50; 75,1; 103; 112,1; 149,1; 149,2; 155,2; 158; 159,3; 166,2. III, 2,2; 5,2; 23,4; 26; 36,2; 45,2; 54; 74,3; 81,1; 84,2. IV, 93,2; 120. V, 13,3; 37; 38,2; 40,2; 48; 54,2; 56; 60; 63. |
| Chilblain | I, 45,2; 47,2; 68,3; 101,2; 108, 128,3. II, 10; 37; 42; 76,18; 107,3; 108,2; 110,1;114,2; 123; 164,3; 166,3; 169,3; 171,4; 175,2. IV, 91; 105. V, 11,1; 106,5. |
| Childbirth | II, 165. III, 4,1; 44,2; 122; 146,2. IV, 115; 134,1. V, 47; 69; 72,3; 154,2; 155; 156,2. IV, 23,2; 88,2; 95; 103,3; 105; 158,2; 173,3. |
| Chills | I, 4,2; 19,4. III, 35,2; 53,1; 73; 81,1. V, 11,2; 13,2; 18,3; 42; 43; 49. |
| Choking | I, 116. III, 23,2; 104,2. IV, 83,2; 148,1; 148,2; 148,3; 182,3. |
| Cholera | I, 115,1. III, 34,1; 35,2. IV, 4,1; 5. V, 80,2. |
| Cicatrize | I, 68,2; 69,1; 77,3; 84,2 109,3. II, 4,1; 72,3; 73,1; 78,3; 118,1; |

# Medical Index

| Conditions | References |
|---|---|
| | 69,4; 70,1; 70,3; 71,2; 71,3; 72,1; 73,3; 74,1; 75; 77,4; 82; 92; 97,4; 100,3; 113; 123,1; 123,2; 125,1; 125,3; 128,1. II, 82,3; 84; 85,2; 94; 103; 105,1; 112,1; 152,2; 158; 163; 166,2; 169,1; 171,3. III, 6,2; 20,2; 25,1; 27,1; 30,2; 44,1; 45,2; 48,4; 53,1; 64,2; 68,2; 72,2; 78,3; 80,5; 81,1; 83,1; 98,1; 105,1; 111,2; 112,2. IV, 46,2; 64,2; 64,3; 68,4; 85,2; 103,3; 120; 122; 182,3. V, 3,3; 9,1; 13,3; 34,2; 37; 38,2; 40,2; 55; 60; 61; 105,2; 107,1. |
| Craving for strange food | I, 115,5. V, 1,1; 2; 6,14. |
| Cyst, see Impetigo contagiosa | |
| Dandruff | I, 30,3; 33,2; 39,2; 45,2; 47,2; 52,5; 68,3; 104; 105,4; 112,2; |
| Dandruff (cont'd) | I, 128,5. II, 21; 78,3; 81,1; 102,2; 118,1; 123; 152,3; 170,2. III, 102,2. IV, 134,2. V, 15; 29; 106,6. |
| Deafness | I, 85. |
| Delirium | IV, 68,5. |
| Delivery, see Childbirth | |
| Delusions | V, 17,3. |
| Dentifrice, see Teeth cleaner | |
| Deodorant | I, 64,4; 99,3. V, 106,6. |
| Depilatory, see Hair remover | |
| Diarrhea | I, 64,3; 69,1; 70,1; 74,1; 82; 83; 92; 93; 94; 99,2; 101,2; 109,1; 109,5; 110,2; 115 passim; 116; 128,1. II, 19; 50; 70,5; 79,1; 81,3; 85,3; 86,2; 105,1; 107,2; 126,4; 148. III, 17,2; 43; 45,1; 56; 58; 64,1; 68,2; 71; 95; 107; 127; 140,2; 146,3; 152,2. IV, 4,1; |

| Conditions | References |
|---|---|
| | 17; 22,2; 23,2; 31; 37; 42,2; 43; 44; 52,2; 61; 62; 64,3; 79; 88,2; 103,3; 134,1. V, 3,1; 4,1; 6,5; 6,10; 6,17; 13,1; 27; 28; 96,2. |
| Digestion | I, 17,2; 27; 47,2; 66; 71,2. II, 112,1; 159,3; 170,1; 171,4. III, 31,1; 53,1; 57. V, 6 passim; 17,3; 27; 34,2; 38,2. |
| Discharges | II, 59; 75,1. IV, 9,2; 36; 51. V, 3,3; 5,2; 34,2; 134; 153,2. |
| Diuretic | I, 2,2; 4,2; 7,3; 8,3; 10,2; 12,2; 13,3; 14,4; 16,1; 17, 2; 19,4; 19,5; 26,2; 26,3; 27; 52,5; 56,4; 58,2; 69,4; 70,2; 71,1; 71,2; 75; 97,4; 106,1; 110,1; 112,1; 114; 115,1; 115,2; 123,1; 123,2. II, 1; 86,1; 87; 104; 108,2; 110,1; 112,1; 112,2; 113; 120,1; 128; 135,1;137; 138; 139; 140; 141; 146; 149,1; 150; 151,2; 152,2; 163; 166,3; 173,2. III, 23,1; 30,2; 35,2; 36,2; 45,1; 52,2; 57;64,1; 64,2; 65; |
| Diuretic (cont'd) | III, 66; 70,1; 111,1; 137,2; 143,2; 144; 154,2. IV, 1,3; 22,2; 31; 46,2; 62; 71; 72,2; 93,2; 123; 144,2; 182,3; 183,2. V, 4,1; 6 passim; 7,1; 8,1; 26; 32,2; 34,2; 36,2; 39,3; 40,2; 52; 56; 58; 60; 70. |
| Dizziness | I, 19,5. II, 70,6. III, 78,1; 78,2; 83,2. IV, 182,3; 183,3. V, 17,3; 18,3; 34,2. |
| Dropsy, see Edema | |
| Drunkenness | I, 123,2. II, 164,1. V, 6 passim. |
| Duct, see Fistule | |
| Dysentery | I, 22; 42,1; 64,3; 70,1; 73,3; 74,1; 82; 97,1; 97,2; 100,3; 106,1; 107,2; 108,2; 108,3; 109,2; 110,2; 115,1; 117; 119; 128,6; 128,7. II, 27; 32; 59; 72,2; 75,1; 76,17; 79,1; 83,3; 96; 102,2; 105,1; 106,2; 114,2; 126,2; 126,3; 127; 179,1. III, 2,2; 104,2; 107; 111,1; |

| Conditions | References |
| --- | --- |
| | 117; 132,2; 146,2;146,3; 147; 152,2. IV, 3; 7; 8,2; 9,2; 12; 16; 36; 40; 41,2; 42,2; 46,2; 50; 88,2. V, 1,1; 3,2; 3,3; 5,2; 15; 20; 25; 27; 34,2; 80; 111. |
| Dyspnea | I, 19,4; 73,3. III, 6,2; 44,1; 45,2; 78,3; 79,2; 83,1. IV, 150,6; 182,3. |
| Dysuria | III, 62,2. |
| Ear, broken | I, 68,3. |
| Ear, bruised | I, 64,4. II, 99; 170,2. V, 107,3. |
| Ear, discharges | I, 72,1; 105,2; 112,2. II, 81,1; 151,2; 169,2; 179,2. III, 23,2; 56; 76,2. IV, 4,2; 12. V, 5,2; 29; 113,3. |
| Ear, fissure | II, 78,3. |
| Ear, hissing, see Ear, singing in | |
| Ear, inflammation | I, 26,3; 64,4. III, 25,2. |
| Ear, itching | I, 128,3. |
| Ear, lacerated | III, 76,2. |
| Ear, purulent, see Ear, discharges | |
| Ear, rheum | V, 106,5. |
| Ear, ringing, see Ear, singing | |
| Ear, singing in | I, 33,2; 34; 56,3; 66,2; 77,2; 78,2; 128,3. II, 78,3; 82,2; 149,3; 151,2; 154,3. V, 13,2; 113,3. |
| Ear, sores | II, 78,4. |
| Ear, water in | II, 151,2. |
| Ear worm | II, 81. III, 35,3. |
| Earache | I, 32,2; 33,2; 34; 35; 40,2; 78,2; 81; 97,4; 99,1; 104; 110,2. II, 17; |

# Medical Index

| Conditions | References |
|---|---|
| Eyes, affliction | I, 87,1; 101,2. V, 126,2. |
| Eyes, cataract, see Eyes, shadow | |
| Eyes, cloud-like opacities | II, 151,1; 166,4; 167, 177. IV, 65,2; 110; 169. |
| Eyes, corneal defect | 1, 68,5; 105,2; 109,3. II, 105,2. V, 127,2; 139. |
| Eyes, dim-sightedness | I, 24; 33,2; 81; 105,6. II, 9,2; 12; 22; 76,19; 120,1; 136,1;141,1; 149,1; 151,1; 154,3; 164,2; 178,2. III, 23,3; 36,2; 45,4; 46,2; 81,2. IV, 72,2; 169. V, 112,2. |
| Eyes, discharges from | I, 68,8; 79; 100,3. |
| Eyes, eroded corners | I, 69,3. II, 74,4. |
| Eyes, inflammations | I, 12,2; 15,2; 68,8; 74,2; 79; 112,1; 115,3. II, 50; 71; 99; 107,3; 124,1; 132,2; 134; 135,1;176,2. III ,3,2; 24,3; 39,2; 40,1; 44,2; 64,1; 122. IV, 38; 40; 64,4; 68,3; 75,4; 86; 88,2; 103,3; 119; 121; 161,2. |
| Eyes, itching corners | III, 22,5. |
| Eyes, leucoma | I, 64,5; 73,2; 77,2; 105,6. II, 5; 9,2; 12; 21; 166,4. III, 84,3; 129. |
| Eyes, leucoma (cont'd) | IV, 110. V, 112,2. |
| Eyes, medications | I, 7,4; 77,2; 89; 98,2; 99,1; 100,2; 101,4; 102; 105,2; 105,3. II, 17; 21; 72,3; 73,2; 74,4; 126,3; 159,1; 163; 169,2; 182,2. III, 3,2; 22,5; 70,2; 82,3. IV, 31; 64,6; 75,4; 76; 88,2; 148,2. V, 4,2; 6,8; 74,2; 78,2; 78,4; 87,13; 88,2; 94,3; 100; 114,3; 120,2; 126,1; 126,2; 134. |
| Eyes, membraneous growths | I, 101,2; 108,2; 112,3; 128,2. II, 21. III, 5,2; 22,4. IV, 42,3; 164,4. V, 13,1; 80,1; 109,2. |
| Eyes, missing | II, 78,2; 81,2; 136,2; 141,1; 166,4. III, 98,2. IV, 169. V, 114,3. |

# Medical Index

## Medical Index

# Medical Index

| Conditions | References |
| --- | --- |
| | 17; 22,2; 33; 36; 38; 40; 53; 55; 60,1; 63,2; 64,2; 64,4; 68,3; 75,4; 85,1; 85,2; 86; 87; 88,2; 93,2; 96,2; 98; 99; 101; 103,3; 114; 119; 121; 161,2; 173,3; 182,2. V, 1,1; 1,2; 3,2; 3,3; 4,2; 5,2; 6,11; 9,1; 9,2; 13,1; 79,9; 92; 93; 99,2; 106,6; 109.3; 146; 150; 153,2; 156,2. |
| Inflation | III, 1,4; 25,2; 31,2; 45,2; 48,4; 56; 58; 59,1; 68,2; 80,3; 116; 137,2; 146,1. V, 38,2; 41; 42; 113,3. |
| Injury, see Wound | |
| Insanity, see Madness | |
| Insomnia, see Soporific | |
| Intestinal worm | I, 30,2; 32,2; 64,4; 77,3. II, 109,1; 120,3; 155,1. III, 23,5; 26,1; 36,2; 45,3; 63. V, 37. |
| Intestine | I, 6; 16,2; 30,2; 32,2; 43,4; 56,4; 64,4; 67,2; 74,2; 77,3; 104; 110,2; 110,3; 115,3; 119. II, 70 passim; 71; 85,1; 86,2; 103; 107,1; 109,1; 118,1; 118,2; 120,3; 124,1; 124,2; 155,1; 171,1. III, 23,5; 25,1; 36,2; 45,2; 45,3; 63; 137,2. IV, 9,2; 20,2; 42,3; 46,2; 178. V, 6,5; 6,7; 6,14; 30; 37; 45. |
| Itching | I, 71,2; 100,3; 128,3. II, 14; 72,1; 81,2; 108,2; 114,2; 154,3. III, 5,2; 22,5; 27,2; 28; 31,2; 33,2; 45,5; 48,4; 151. IV, 10,2; 100; 152,2; 157,2. V, 11,1; 13,2; 74,6; 106,5; 107,2; 109,2; 108,3; 158. |
| Jaundice | I, 7,4; 8,3; 87,1; 100,4. II, 35; 59; 80,1; 104; 114,3; 119; 125; 129; 158; 163; 164,2; 171,3; 180,2. III, 1,3; 22,3; 23,1; 27,2; 35,2; 71; 74,3; 75; 76,2; 80,5; 105,2; 110; 121,2; 134,2; 137,2; |

# Medical Index

## Medical Index

| Conditions | References |
|---|---|
| Membrane | I, 68,2. II, 49,1; 72,2; 79,1; 87. V, 84,2; 139. |
| Meninx, see Membrane | |
| Menses | I, 1,2; 3; 4,2; 10,2; 11,2; 13,3; 14,4; 18; 24; 28,2; 48,2; 50; 58,2; 64,3; 66,3; 73,3; 77,4; 81; 96; 103,2; 105,6; 115,3; 123,1; 125,2; 128,3. II, 9,2; 19; 24,1; 61,2; 74,4; 75,1; 75,2; 79,2; 104; 109,1; 112,1; 114,3; 120,2; 120,3;127; 129; 133,1; 136,3; 149,1; 150; 151,1; 152,3; 155,1; 156,2; 163;164,1; 169,1; 173,2; 176,2; 179,3. III, 1,4; 4,4; 6,3; 7,2; 21,2; 23,2; 24,2;27,1; 30,2; 31,1; 33,2; 35,2; 36,2; 38,2; 39,2; 43; 44,1; 48,4; 48,5; 51,3; 52,2; 53,1; 54; 55; 59,2; 62,2;65; 66; 67,2; 68,2; 70,1; 71; 72,2; 74,3; 79,2; 81,2; 83,1; 80,6; 95; 98,2;102,2; 104,2; 105,2; 106; 110; 111,2; 113,2; 121.2; 123; 124; 137,2; 140,2; 143,2; 150,2; 152,2; 157. IV, 1,4; 18; 19; 20,2; 49; 57; 68,4; 75,4; 93,1; 93,2; 115; 134,1; 135; 144,2; 146; 147; 148,2; 150,7; 162,3; 183,2; 189,2; 190,2.V, 32,2; 39,3; 40,2; 47; 54,2; 60; 61; 62; 106,6; 146. |
| Menstruation, see Menses | |
| Micturition | I, 3; 6; 11,2; 14,4; 18; 19,5; 20; 28,2; 33,2; 58,2; 69,1; 74,1; 105,6; 115,4; 123,1. II, 34; 35; 52; 61,2; 67; 82,3; 97; 108,2; 109,2; 125; 127; 129; 141,2; 169,1; 171,3. III, 1,3; 8,2; 12,2; 24,2; 38,2; 39,1; 44,1; 51,3; 52,2; 54; 55; 56; 58; 62,1; 68,2; 83,2; 98,1; 109,2; 111,1;136,2; 146,2; 151; 153; 157; 158,1. IV, 8,2; 29; 52,2; 57; 105; 112;124; 134,1; 135, 144,2; 182,1. V, 18,3; 20; 21; 22; 54,2; 57; 59; 63; 64; 118,3; 121,3; 122,2; |

| Conditions | References |
|---|---|
| | 126,2; 137. |
| Milk | I, 19,2; 19,4; 26,2; 68,2; 91; 103,2; 106,1; 124,1; 128,3; 128,5. |
| Milk (cont'd) | II, 10; 19; 70 passim; 27,1; 7 passim; 78,3; 83,3; 85,2; 86,1; 101,2; 104; 105,1; 107,3; 118,2; 131; 135,1; 140; 149,3; 174; 176,2. III, 27,2; 34,2; 56; 58; 64,1; 70,1; 79,2; 80,5; 90; 119; 126,2; 136,2. IV, 7; 27; 64,4; 78,2; 83,2; 95; 138; 139; 150,7; 182,4; 188,2. V, 6,4; 11,1; 13,3; 15; 32,2; 84,3; 95,3; 114,3; 126,1; 127,2; 154. |
| Mind | II, 179,2. III, 63. IV, 72,2; 182,3. |
| Miscarriage, see also Abortif't | I, 93. II, 164,1; 164,2; 166,2. III, 68,2; 131. V, 72,2; 72,3. |
| Mole, see Birthmark | |
| Mood enhancer, see Psychoactive plants | |
| Mortification | II, 100. III, 4,5. |
| Mouth | I, 4,2; 12,2; 86; 87,1; 96; 101,2; 105,1; 107,1; 110,2. II, 29; 69; 70,5; 78,4; 126,3; 152,2; 173,3. III, 5,2; 22,5; 127. IV,2; 15,2; 37; 42,2; 60,2. V, 4,2; 105,2; 106,6. |
| Mouthwash | I, 12,2; 20; 22; 43,4; 64,4; 69,2; 70,2; 77,2; 79; 87,2; 105,4, 105,5; 110,2; 126,2. II, 17; 26; 29; 70,5; 114,3; 126,3; 126,4; 173,2. III, 12,2; 18; 25,2; 73; 79,2; 80,4; 104,2. IV, 68,5; 103,3; 162,3; 176,2. V, 13,3. |
| Muscle | I, 58,2; 59,2. |
| Nails | I, 72,2; 74,2; 105,4. II, 96; 103; 114,2; 170,2; 175,2; 181. |

## Medical Index

## Medical Index

# Medical Index

## Medical Index

## Medical Index

# Medical Index

## Medical Index

# Medical Index

## Medical Index